Neurological Rehabilitation:
Optimizing Motor Performance

Neurological Rehabilitation:
Optimizing Motor Performance

Janet H. Carr EdD, FACP

Associate Professor

School of Physiotherapy
Faculty of Health Sciences
The University of Sydney
Australia

and

Roberta B. Shepherd EdD, FACP

Professor

School of Physiotherapy
Faculty of Health Sciences
The University of Sydney
Australia

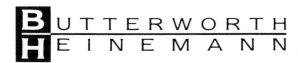

EDINBURGH LONDON NEW YORK OXFORD PHILADELPHIA ST LOUIS
SYDNEY TORONTO

BUTTERWORTH-HEINEMANN
An imprint of Elsevier Limited

First published 1998
 Reprinted 1999 (twice), 2000, 2001, 2002, 2003, 2004, 2005

ISBN 0 7506 0971 0

British Library Cataloguing in Publication Data
A catalogue record for this book is available from the British Library

Library of Congress Cataloging in Publication Data
A catalog record for this book is available from the Library of Congress

Notice
Medical knowledge is constantly changing. Standard safety precautions
must be followed, but as new research and clinical experience broaden our
knowledge, changes in treatment and drug therapy may become necessary
or appropriate. Readers are advised to check the most current product
information provided by the manufacturer of each drug to be administered
to verify the recommended dose, the method and duration of
administration, and contraindications. It is the responsibility of the
practitioner, relying on experience and knowledge of the patient, to
determine dosages and the best treatment for each individual patient.
Neither the Publisher nor the editors/contributor assumes any liability for
any injury and/or damage to persons or property arising from this
publication.

The Publisher

ELSEVIER your source for books,
journals and multimedia
in the health sciences

www.elsevierhealth.com

Working together to grow
libraries in developing countries

www.elsevier.com | www.bookaid.org | www.sabre.org

ELSEVIER   BOOK AID International   Sabre Foundation

Composition by Genesis Typesetting, Rochester, Kent
Printed and bound in Great Britain by
The Bath Press plc, Bath

The Publisher's
policy is to use
**paper manufactured
from sustainable forests**

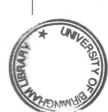

Contents

Preface

This book represents an attempt to set down a philosophy and model of rehabilitation for individuals with movement dysfunction which is an alternative to models most commonly in use throughout the world, the eponymous facilitation-inhibition models. The view taken here is that research in the areas of neuromuscular control, biomechanical aspects of performance, the link between cognition and action, together with recent developments related to pathology and adaptation can inform rehabilitation methods.

In this book, we argue that consideration of movement science research implies that movement rehabilitation should focus on motor performance, on exercises and training to ensure appropriate muscle strength, on endurance and physical fitness to enable the desired physical activities to be carried out and on increased cognitive engagement with the environment. The clinician is then coach to the individual with the disability, one who is skilled in methods of training action, and of organizing independent practice. Too often therapists underestimate the capacity of individuals, including small children and the elderly, to work hard, pay attention and actively engage with a training regime over which they have some control. One-to-one therapy remains the preferred style in many rehabilitation settings, yet the available evidence points to the need for disabled individuals to be actively involved in their rehabilitation for several hours a day. This requires that there be a plan for group practice, and work stations for independent practice; that therapists

work with engineers, computer scientists, orthotists and the makers of gymnasium equipment to design training devices which will enable independent practice and promote the wanted actions. The clinician as problem-solving scientist is both a user of research and an adaptor of technology.

The chapters are clustered into three groups. Chapters 1 to 3 focus on three major issues critical to neurorehabilitation: the nature of the adaptive system, the optimization of functional motor performance, and methods of measurement. It is increasingly being shown that the brain, neural system, muscles and other soft tissues reorganize and adapt according to patterns of use and experience. We argue that what happens to an individual and what that person does, will affect positively or negatively the reorganization and adaptation which are naturally occurring phenomena. Focus in the second chapter is therefore on skill learning, physical training and exercise in neurorehabilitation, stressing the importance of cognitive engagement and practice. The third chapter sets out a selection of, for the most part, reliable and valid measures which are appropriate for use in neurorehabilitation. Tests are grouped according to the level of measurement – whether global tests of function or specific biomechanical measures of motor performance, tests of muscle strength or perception; whether tests of impairment or of anxiety or self-efficacy. Emphasis throughout the book is on the need to measure the effects of the interventions that make up rehabilitation.

Chapters 4 to 7 focus on actions critical to an independent and effective lifestyle: standing up and sitting down, walking, reaching and manipulation, and balancing, in which biomechanical models of the action are presented as a framework upon which training and exercise to improve performance are based.

Chapters 8 to 10 focus on pathological and adaptive aspects of lesions of the motor system (upper motor neuron, cerebellum) and of the sensory-perceptual system. Chapters 11 to 14 contain descriptions of the particular pathological impairments, adaptations and disabilities associated with stroke, traumatic brain injury, Parkinson's disease and multiple sclerosis, with specific points about rehabilitation which are of significance for these conditions.

Throughout the book, we have provided references in order to illustrate the process of utilizing theoretical and data-based information in clinical practice. Where these are available, we have included reference to outcome studies because it is such evidence-based material which is a powerful determinator of theory and direction, enabling the development and testing of protocols (or strictly observed guidelines) as a means of establishing best practice. Our aim in writing this book was to assist clinicians to become more informed and effective practitioners and to raise questions intended to stimulate clinical and laboratory research which will in turn lead to dynamic and effective methodologies. Finally, we hope the book will give the reader an appreciation for what are currently unexplored possibilities of movement rehabilitation.

J.H.C.
R.B.S.

Acknowledgements

We particularly wish to thank the teaching team in neurological physiotherapy at The University of Sydney for their comments on various chapters and for many stimulating discussions over the years: Dr Louise Ada, Colleen Canning, Dr Cath Dean, Virginia Fowler, Dr Sharon Kilbreath. Other members of the staff of the School of Physiotherapy have also made helpful comments on sections of the manuscript: Dr Roger Adams, Associate Professor Jack Crosbie, Dr Elizabeth Ellis and Associate Professor Nicholas O'Dwyer. We would also like to express our thanks to those individuals whose photographs appear throughout the book and to David Robinson, who took the photographs.

Much of this book was written by the shores of Lake Como, in the splendid environment of the Villa Serbelloni. We express our grateful thanks to the Rockefeller Foundation who made this possible and to the staff of the Villa.

J.H.C.
R.B.S

Part One
Introduction: Adaptation, Training and Measurement

1

The adaptive system: plasticity and recovery

All living organisms have an inherent capacity/ability to self-organize throughout life, and organizational processes affecting all systems are reflective of the organism's history (including experience and use). Specific molecular, biochemical, electrophysical and structural changes take place throughout life in CNS neurons and neuronal networks in response to activity and behaviour (Cotman and Nieto-Sampedro 1982). The aetiology and mechanisms of organizational processes in humans are increasingly being understood and such knowledge provides insights into how these processes can be manipulated to drive optimal recovery.

A brain lesion affects both the anatomy and the physiology of the nervous system. That is, the lesion directly interferes with (or destroys) nerve cell bodies, dendrites and axons and indirectly affects the 'programming' of nerve impulses throughout intact brain tissue. It is reasonable to hypothesize, as we have in several texts (Carr and Shepherd 1987a,b; Shepherd 1995), that training following the lesion, given that it involves the person learning again how to perform actions and mental processes which were performed with ease pre-lesion, is a critical stimulus to the making of new or more effective functional connections within remaining brain tissue. Of course, if recovery/reorganization is successful, patients may have different connections mediating action than before the lesion.

This chapter addresses briefly issues related to neural reorganization after a brain lesion as a means of stressing the potential for rehabilitation to affect such processes. Concurrent with brain changes, muscles and other soft tissues also reorganize and adapt according to patterns of use, and this issue is also discussed. It is our view that too little consideration is given to the details of movement rehabilitation with little critical examination of the scientific validity and functional effectiveness of techniques in common use. What seems certain from the material presented here is that for rehabilitation (including physiotherapy) to be effective in aiding an individual to regain optimal functional recovery, there needs to be more emphasis on methods of 'forcing' use of affected limbs and providing task-related experience and training. There is mounting evidence that neural reorganization reflects patterns of use. Even at the peripheral level, specific goal-directed exercise has been shown to enhance recovery in animals and humans in acute and chronic neuropathies (Bailliet *et al.* 1982; van Meeteren *et al.* 1996).

Following an acute brain lesion, those individuals who do not die begin to demonstrate behavioural recovery, and the underlying biological manifestations of recovery reflect the inherent reorganizational ability of the system. Gradually the notion of the brain (indeed the entire human system) as adaptable is filtering through to the clinical community. However, although there is increasing acceptance of a link between brain plasticity (i.e., anatomical, physiological and functional reorganization) and recovery potential, it is still not generally accepted that there might be a link between recovery potential and events occurring post-lesion, in particular, events related to rehabilitation. There are many clinicians who argue that rehabilitation appears critical to recovery (e.g., Bach-y-Rita 1990, 1996), but there are still only a few who would take the next step and argue that the nature, the process, the methods used in rehabilitation would also affect recovery; that some methods may facilitate and others actually inhibit recovery. Bach-y-Rita (1990) has proposed that a relative lack of interest in functional recovery has resulted in little research into recovery itself and therefore a poorly developed theoretical foundation in rehabilitation. It has, therefore, been difficult for clinicians to argue that particular aspects of rehabilitation might have specific effects upon brain recovery. Major clinical research emphasis should now be placed, in our view, on studying the effects of different rehabilitation methods upon brain morphology and function as well as on behaviour.

Plasticity of the intact brain

The term 'plasticity' refers, in general, to the capacity of the central nervous system to adapt to functional demands and therefore to the system's capacity to reorganize. Following from experimental studies of both animals and humans, brain processes are now acknowledged to be continuously remodelled by our experiences throughout life, particularly by the use to which we put the system. In its broadest sense, therefore, plasticity includes the process of learning. This view is in contrast to an earlier view of the brain as functionally static (for discussion, see Merzenich *et al.* 1991).

Mechanisms of brain plasticity include the capacity for neurochemical, neuroreceptive and neuronal structural changes. Furthermore, the parallel and distributed nature of brain organization appears to play an important role in the brain's capacity for flexibility and adaptation. Extensive intracortical axonal collaterals provide input to many different movement representations of a given body part and their pattern of recruitment may determine the execution of complex movements. There is a wide overlap in cortical neuronal networks targeting different body parts and these networks, in part, share common neuronal elements (Schieber 1992). In monkey, the motor cortex projection area to a single motor neuron in the spinal cord is relatively large (it can be up to 13 mm square) and colonies of cortical neurons overlap (Phillips and Porter 1977). Cellular populations within the brain are dynamically organized, with the possibility for variability in structure and function according to behavioural needs (Edelman 1987). That is, individual cells and neuronal systems have the ability to subserve more than one function. Regulation of both transient and long-term effectiveness of synapses occurs daily throughout life and is also determined by experience. Receptors themselves demonstrate plasticity, synaptic transmission becoming stronger or weaker according to use. (Specific mechanisms underlying brain reorganization are described in detail elsewhere, e.g., Finger and Stein 1982; Held 1987; Goldstein 1993; Kolb 1995).

Remodelling of cortical neuron responses occurs between columnarly arrayed and cooperative groups of neurons of which there are hundreds of millions. Merzenich and colleagues (1991) describe a continual competition between neural groups for the domination of neurons on their mutual borders. This competition for cortical territory appears to be use-dependent. Cortical maps differ in ways that reflect their use (Merzenich *et al.* 1983), appearing to be subject to modification on the basis of activity of peripheral sensory pathways. For example, in an animal experiment, use of the middle three fingers to obtain food was followed by an expansion of the area of cortex that serves the middle fingers (Jenkins *et al.* 1990) (Fig. 1.1). (Note that this occurred with several thousand repetitions.) In this example, practice may have acted on pre-existing patterns of connections to strengthen their effectiveness (Kandel 1991). Such organizational changes in the nervous system are considered to be a general property of the somatosensory system.

Studies of humans following surgery to transpose muscle or with congenital blindness have also shown the capacity of the brain to reorganize. For example, reorganization of cortical outputs has been reported in individuals with an amputation of a limb (Hall *et al.* 1990; Cohen et al. 1991; Fuhr *et al.* 1992). In congenital upper limb amputees and early following amputation of part of one upper limb, the remaining muscles in the limb received more descending connections than those muscles

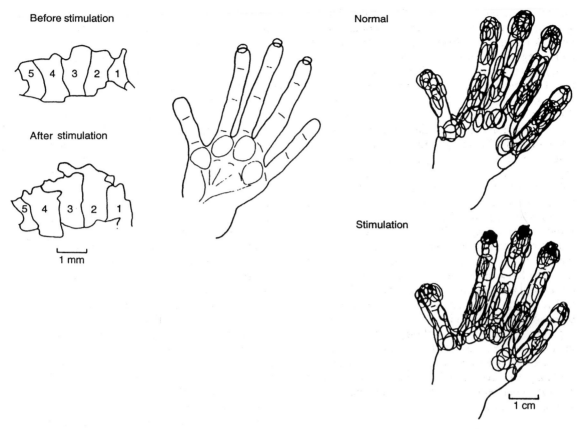

Fig. 1.1 Repetitive use of fingers 2, 3, 4 caused expansion of the cortical representation of these fingers. Outlines of regions in cortical area 3b represent surfaces of fingers before and after training. Maps of glabrous fields are identified for recording sites within area 3b before and after training. (Reprinted from Jenkins, W. M., Merzenich, M. M., Ochs, M. T. *et al.* (1990) Functional reorganization of primary somatosensory cortex in adult owl monkeys after behaviorally controlled tactile stimulation. *Journal of Physiology*, **63**, 82–104, with permission)

of the uninvolved limb (Hall *et al.* 1990). Changes reported include increased size of cortical motor representation area and recruitment of a larger percentage of the alpha motor neuron pool of muscles ipsilateral and immediately proximal to the side of the amputation. It seems clear, therefore, that neuronal elements are inherently flexible, responding according to usage patterns and the capacity for functional gain for that individual.

Motor learning, training and plasticity

Flexibility and adaptability of the nervous system, including the brain, are illustrated in studies involving training. Evidence for the effectiveness of training on brain reorganization, including functional changes in cortical motor and sensory neurons, comes from many studies on animals (e.g., Merzenich *et al.* 1990; Aou *et al.* 1992; Recanzone *et al.* 1992; Sanes *et al.* 1992). Experience has been shown in animals to lead to changes in the strength of existing neuronal connections and the emergence of new connections (Greenough *et al.* 1993). Findings from studies of rats taught complex skills suggest that increased demands of repeated physical activity stimulate angiogenesis and synaptogenesis (Black and Greenough 1989; Isaacs *et al.* 1992).

Training animals (rats) on specific tasks such as reaching, for example, has been shown to increase selectively the dendritic arborisation in the fore-limb representation of the motor and sensory cortex (Greenough *et al.* 1985). Such changes have been found for both unimanual and bimanual reaching (Kolb 1995), either on one side of the motor cortex or on both sides. Intensity of training has been shown with animals to enhance recovery (e.g., Goldberger and Murray 1980; Bach-y-Rita 1981). Behavioural recovery and concomitant neural changes (in geniculate nucleus and visual cortex) have been reported in cats who received vigorous training with positive and negative rewards (Chow and Stewart 1972). It was the forced usage of vision in this study which was considered to aid in the recovery of function.

Of particular interest to physiotherapists working with neurologically impaired individuals (who need to 'relearn' previously learned skills) is the evidence that skill learning in humans has been shown to be associated with similar nervous system changes as seen in animals (e.g., Asanuma and Keller 1991; Jacobs and Donoghue 1991; see Merzenich 1986 for review). That is, humans with an intact brain have shown functional changes in the brain associated with training and use, specifically, with increased use of a body part or enhanced sensory feedback from it. This is particularly so where the increase in use is accompanied by functional gain for the subject. Learning a complicated sequence of voluntary finger movements has been shown to be associated with modifications of cortical activity (Niemann *et al.* 1991) and with increases in regional blood flow in the cerebellum (Seitz *et al.* 1990). Learning a pursuit rotor task is associated with an increase in regional blood flow in primary and supplementary motor areas and thalamus (Grafton *et al.* 1992).

Increased use of a body part or enhanced sensory feedback from it may lead to a shift in the balance of intracortical networks towards that body part (Gracies 1996). For example, skilled Braille reading is associated with a relative enlargement of the cortical sensorimotor representation of the reading finger (Pascual-Leone and Torres 1993), brain changes being mapped using focal transcranial magnetic stimulation (TMS). Learning is reflected in changes in the pattern of interconnections in those sensory and motor systems involved in learning a specific task (Kandel 1991), in particular, changes in the effectiveness of neural connections.

Modulation of cortical motor output by which the motor cortex increases its influence on a motor neuron pool may be due to increased synaptic efficiency in existing intracortical circuits, for example, by long-term potentiation (Iriki *et al.* 1989); unmasking of existing intracortical connec-

tions (Asanuma and Keller 1991); by learning-dependent changes in pre-motor cortex or cerebellum (Gilbert and Thach 1977; Mitz and Wise 1987); and by a shift in segmental excitability at relevant spinal levels. Flexible modulation may represent a first stage in learning with further practice of a task eventually leading to structural changes in intracortical and subcortical networks (Pascual-Leone *et al.* 1995).

There is now substantial evidence from biomechanical studies that neural as well as musculoskeletal adaptations occur in response to physical activity, strength training and immobilization (Enoka 1995). The gain in strength occurring in the first few weeks of a strength-training programme is accompanied by a comparable increase in electrical activity in muscle which precedes a significant change in muscle size (Moritani and deVries 1979; Narici *et al.* 1989). This time course implicates a role for neural adaptation. Qualitative and quantitative changes in neural drive occurring in association with exercise appear to be task-specific. Evidence for this comes from studies showing the velocity-dependent effects of isokinetic training (Behm and Sale 1993), differences in amplitude of EMG signal for (intended) concentric and eccentric contractions (Grabiner *et al.* 1995), and reduction in coactivation and improved coordination amongst synergists (Rutherford and Jones 1986; Carolan and Cafarelli 1992).

There is increasing evidence that altered physical activity is likely to involve functional and structural changes in the motor pathway (e.g., Cracraft and Petajan 1977; Sale et al. 1982; Hakkinen and Komi 1983). It has been shown that strength training results in a greater improvement in performance than in either muscle bulk or muscle strength (Rutherford and Jones 1986). Descending drive on to spinal motor neurons appears to increase following strength training and decrease after a period of inactivity (McComas 1993). The person following stroke for example, may have degeneration in a proportion of nerve fibres descending from the brain and inactivity is likely to be extreme (McComas 1993). The number of functional motor units has been shown to decrease by approximately half between the second and sixth months after a stroke (McComas *et al.* 1973), suggesting transsynaptic changes in α-motoneurons after degeneration of corticospinal fibres. Increasing periods of inactivity may also be implicated together with the direct effects of the lesion.

Mental practice (Chapter 2) has been shown to be sufficient to promote modulation of neural circuits in the early stage of learning a complicated finger exercise (Pascual-Leone *et al*. 1995). In mental simulation of motor actions, cerebral blood flow studies suggest that prefrontal and supplementary motor areas, basal ganglia and cerebellum (the same central structures required for performance of the actual movements) are part of the network involved (Roland *et al*. 1987). Furthermore, changes to cortical motor output maps show that mental practice alone can lead to the same plastic changes in the motor system as those occurring with repetitive physical practice (Pascual-Leone *et al*. 1995). Results of studies of muscle force production, although not demonstrating direct effects of mental practice on neural adaptation, infer that such changes take place. For example, a study in which subjects imagined muscle contractions over a four-week period (Yue and Cole 1992), showed that the resultant increase in the maximum voluntary contraction they produced, although less than in those who trained physically, was greater than in those who did no training.

Do comparable brain changes occur in ageing brains? Histologically there is a loss of neurons as we age. However, there is evidence that one mechanism that enables the adaptation associated with learning a new skill at any age is an increase in the number of synapses per neuron (Buell and Coleman 1981). That is, it appears that the effectiveness of existing connections is increased by practice and learning at any age.

Plasticity following brain lesion

The logical question arising from studies of brain plasticity is whether an enriched environment, use, training and experience have similar effects on the damaged brain and whether these effects would enhance functional recovery (Kolb 1995, p. 149). Conversely, would impoverishment and non-use inhibit recovery? Technological advances are enabling brain processes to be more closely examined and it is becoming increasingly apparent that recovery of function following a brain lesion is in large part due to similar reorganization processes as occur in response to learning and experience in the intact brain; i.e., reorganization after a brain lesion takes place as a result of structural and functional changes. Anatomical changes include dendritic and axonal sprouting; physiological changes include changes in the sensitivity of certain sites to certain neurotransmitters. Much of the investigation of these mechanisms has been carried out on experi-

mentally lesioned animals using microelectric mapping techniques. However, studies have also been performed recently on humans who have had stroke using functional imaging techniques or transcranial magnetic stimulation.

As might be expected, recovery mechanisms are widespread throughout the brain. It is well known that the cerebellum for example, has the capacity to compensate for changed processing resulting from a cortical lesion (Evarts 1980). There is evidence that one cerebral hemisphere can take over functions normally subserved by the lesioned hemisphere (Glees 1980). More recently, several studies of humans using positron emission tomography (PET) have demonstrated that ipsilateral motor pathways may play a role in recovery of motor function (Chollet *et al*. 1991; Fisher 1992; Weiller *et al*. 1992; Silvestri *et al*. 1993). Extensions of cortical motor fields into undamaged areas have also been demonstrated (Asanuma 1991; Weiller *et al*. 1993). Differences in levels of motor unit synchronization have been found during recovery following stroke, paralleling improvements in fine motor control (Farmer *et al*. 1993).

A recent study (using PET) of 10 patients (DiPiero *et al*. 1992) has shown that post-stroke metabolic changes differed between patients. (Metabolism is considered an index of transynaptic activity.) Motor recovery was associated in some patients with an increase in oxygen metabolism in structures normally involved in motor function in the affected hemisphere; in others without such changes, there were relative increases in metabolism in the contralateral non-lesioned cortical hemisphere. Although motor recovery was better in this group than in those who had no cortical metabolism increase in either hemisphere, it was not as pronounced as in those with increased metabolism in the appropriate but lesioned hemisphere.

Recovery has been shown, therefore, to be associated with bilateral activation of the motor system, with use of ipsilateral pathways and recruitment of additional motor areas. Activation of attentional and intentional states also appears to be important to the process (Weiller *et al*. 1992). Task-related neurons in putamen, for example, have been shown to be more active in relation to intention to move and to the attentiveness of the performer (Boussaoud and Wise 1992).

Environmental factors and learning bring out specific capabilities by altering the effectiveness (and anatomical connections) of pre-existing pathways (Kandel 1991) and these two factors probably play key roles in determining the extent of functional recovery. Partly due to a perceived dichotomy between body and mind, learning has been considered an abstract function related to the mind and not the brain. New experimental evidence of neural processes associated with learning are enabling it to be considered in a biological sense rather than as abstract. In learning a motor skill, the learner must combine the appropriate movements into a pattern or synergy, in both spatial and temporal domains, that ensures successful performance. Practice enables the movements to become smoother, coordinated and usually more rapid. Such biomechanical changes are reflective of changes at the neural level. For example, Grafton and colleagues (1992) found an increase in neuronal activation in the left motor cortex, left supplementary motor area and thalamus during motor skill assimilation (or learning) and in a more widely distributed network involving cortex, basal ganglia and cerebellum during motor execution. It appears from recent evidence that different aspects of motor learning are processed at different parts of the sensorimotor system (Glickstein 1992; Halsband and Freund 1993).

The physiological basis of learning includes modification of synapses (Bear *et al.* 1987). Although the plastic changes which represent learning appear to be localized to specific neurons, these neurons are probably widely distributed in the nervous system, given the complex nature of learning (Kupferman 1991). This neuronal distribution probably accounts for the apparent ability of individuals after an extensive brain lesion to relearn tasks. Wyke (1971), for example, reported that learning a motor task after a stroke was illustrated by improved performance of the task, with a decrease in errors and in time to complete the task.

It is known that everyday events, including sensory stimulation, deprivation and learning, can cause an effective disruption of synaptic connections under some circumstances and reactivation of connections under others (Kandel 1991). Recent work on the effects of activity-dependent enrichment of neural connections and use-dependent modification of cellular structure and function makes it clear that, just as a brain lesion affects brain function, so also do the person's experiences following the lesion. As a consequence, the patient who has had an acute lesion has to contend not only with impairments resulting from the lesion itself but also with the emotional effects, such as depression and lack of motivation which may be associated with their own sense of loss, and the debilitating effects of a non-stimulating environment in which they may feel they can have no active participation. It is quite possible, therefore, that what happens to an individual after, for example, a stroke, can have a negative effect, not only by inhibiting the recovery of the brain from the effects of the lesion, but also by inhibiting synaptic connections which were not directly affected by the lesion and which, potentially, could adapt and mediate some improvement in functional effectiveness.

It is of interest that consideration is now being given to the possible effects of drugs on recovery processes, both the enhancing or potentially harmful effects (Goldstein 1993). For example, in one study, patients who received amphetamine and physiotherapy showed greater increments in motor scores than those with physiotherapy alone (Crisosomo *et al.* 1988).

In summary, it is apparent that learning new motor skills with an intact CNS and regaining skill after a lesion of the CNS are similar in many respects. At the motor performance level, the changes that take place in biomechanical parameters are similar in the regaining of skill after stroke as when non-lesioned individuals are learning a new skill. Hence, the physiological reorganization underlying the behavioural changes may be the same for motor learning and for recovery of motor skills after brain lesion (Lee and van Donkelaar 1995).

Nature of spontaneous recovery

Recovery can be categorized as

1. *spontaneous recovery* due to reparative processes occurring immediately following the lesion, and
2. *reorganization of neural mechanisms* which is influenced by use and experience.

However, this distinction is not typically made, physicians often assuming that all recovery, even as long as two years post-lesion, is 'spontaneous' and that no relationship exists between what the person does (including physiotherapy) and recovery (Wade et al. 1985). The implicit assumption appears to be that rehabilitation enables the person to take advantage of a 'natural' recovery process unaffected in itself by what the person does and experiences. Such a view may underlie the reluctance to test different forms of rehabilitation in order to find the most effective and to adopt newer methods of intervention. Another consequence of this view is that it is said to be difficult to test the effects of rehabilitation since these effects are additional to the 'spontaneous recovery' and cannot, therefore, be separated.

Early spontaneous recovery after an acute lesion probably represents the return to function of undamaged parts of the brain, the capacity of which is diminished by reparative processes, for example, *resolution of local factors such as oedema and the absorption of necrotic tissue debris, and opening of collateral channels for circulation to the lesioned area*. This takes place over a relatively short period, 3 to 4 weeks (Lee and van Donkelaar 1995). An accumulation of intracellular fluid (oedema) can produce local functional depression in areas immediately surrounding the primary area of injury and remote functional depression of distant structures. Early clinical worsening and spontaneous improvement may therefore be due to development and resolution of oedema (Goldstein 1993).

The term *diaschisis* is used to describe a sudden functional depression of brain distant to the lesion site, with reduced blood flow and metabolism. The mechanism underlying this phenomenon is not understood, but it has been proposed that persistence of diaschisis in supplementary motor area (which could play a role in reorganization of motor cortex after lesion; Aizawa *et al.* 1991), could be responsible for both prolonged muscle flaccidity and poor motor recovery. A recent finding that disruption of regional blood supply to the brain may result in death of nerve cells that were not injured as a direct result of the lesion suggests that to enhance recovery and reorganization potential may require methods of preventing cell death and controlling subsequent growth of nerve cells that survive (Almli and Finger 1992).

Lee and van Donkelaar (1995, p. 257) point out that later recovery, that occurring after 3 to 4 weeks, must be due to other mechanisms, those which underlie what is called plasticity. These mechanisms include *unmasking* of pathways previously functionally inactive, *sprouting* of fibres from surviving nerve cells with formation of new synapses and *redundancy* in neural circuitry, i.e., multiple parallel pathways subserving similar functions.

Too broad an interpretation of spontaneous recovery reflects a lack of understanding of how all recovery beyond the immediate reparative stage must be affected by what the person experiences, by what the person actually does and learns. It is certain that the brain will reorganize (adapt) after a lesion whatever happens to the individual.

However, given the evidence from investigations of the differential and context-dependent effects on reorganization, it is possible to hypothesize that the nature of that reorganization must depend on the inputs received and the outputs demanded post-lesion, and particularly during the rehabilitation process.

Physiotherapy intervention is typically regarded as enabling the individual to make the most of what is left after the lesion, inferring a static system, rather than actually affecting or driving the recovery (reorganization) process itself. There is, however, increasing support in the neurosciences for the argument that what the person does and experiences in rehabilitation, and the rehabilitation environment itself, affects the recovery process. Methods used in intervention should logically, therefore, have the potential either for a negative effect or a positive one.

Accordingly, we would propose that it is now possible to monitor a person's recovery after the immediate reparative period in terms of that person's experiences, their immobility or activity, opportunities for training and practice (i.e., the specific intervention available) and the physical features of the environment and its demands. Such data could be matched against changes occurring within the nervous system itself, via such techniques as PET, magnetic resonance imaging (MRI) and transcranial magnetic stimulation (TMS). The results may enable us to determine the critical components of best practice in rehabilitation and to identify those factors that have the potential for a negative effect.

In the absence of appropriate experience, new connections may be maladaptive. This mechanism may underlie the development over time of stiff 'spastic' muscles and the use of inappropriate force by intact muscles (see Chapter 8). In addition, maladaptive changes will also occur in the musculoskeletal system, with a negative impact on the capacity of the effectors to carry out the intended action. The opportunity for interaction with and exploration of the environment may therefore be critical to an optimally effective recovery process. It was suggested long ago that lesions of the motor cortex or upper part of the pyramidal tract in humans do not necessarily eliminate function, but put it in abeyance until such time as the appropriate conditions are present for production of movement (Franz *et al.* 1915). Setting up conditions which 'force' the required movements and enable intensive practice must surely become a major part of rehabilitation. The opportunity to do this may only be available if an enriched and challenging environment is built within the rehabilitation setting for humans as has been done for animal experimentation, and if staff attitudes can shift to a more stimulating 'coaching' role.

The effect of the environment on behaviour and recovery

Active interaction with the environment is known to be necessary for an animal or human to extract the appropriate information from that environment. It is apparent from studies of animals that the nature of the environment (physical structure; possibilities for social interaction, physical activity and exercise) affect brain organization and reorganization after a lesion. In humans, behavioural and ecological studies are illustrating the close relationship between the environment and behaviour, including the extent and type of physical activity the individual engages in. Motor control research and clinical observations also make it clear that the environment (i.e., objects, their position and orientations) drives the motor pattern in an action. For example, reaching to grasp objects is dependent upon the features of the object and where it is in the environment. The environment is increasingly being seen as a potent facilitator or inhibitor of behaviour.

Anatomical, physiological, biochemical and behavioural differences are known to occur in lesioned and non-lesioned animals kept in an enriched environment compared to those in an impoverished environment (e.g., Rosenzweig *et al.* 1973; Finger 1978; Rosenzweig 1980; Walsh 1981; Held *et al.* 1985; Camel *et al.* 1986; Isseroff and Isseroff 1987). Furthermore, the beneficial effects of enrichment are decreased if the animal is subsequently moved to an impoverished milieu. Housing animals in an enriched environment can result in such brain changes as greater cortical depth and weight, increased glial proliferation, an increase in number of synapses in the cortex, and in the number of dendritic spines, and increased capillary density. (See Kolb 1995 for review.)

In animals, the aspects of the enriched environment which appear to be critical as enhancers are social stimulation, the opportunity for interaction with objects (Bennett 1976) and an increased level of arousal (Walsh and Cummins 1975). It is important, therefore, to consider what effects the typical post-lesion or rehabilitation environment has on human brain reorganization. There are few experiments on brain reorganization in humans and none that we know of which have investigated the effect of environmental modification on reorganization. However, there have been several ecological studies which give us information about the behaviour of people under these conditions. From these findings it is possible to infer that human brain reorganization may occur as it does in animals according to the richness or poverty of the environment in which the person finds themselves post-lesion. A person's environment of course includes the physical structure and the people within it.

The field of human ecology offers many insights into the effects of the environment on human behaviour since investigations are made by observing people in their natural settings. Such observations, when made in rehabilitation units in particular (see Canter and Canter 1979), have the potential to offer explanations about a patient's behaviour after a lesion. For example, we have argued for some time that, after a stroke, a person's poor recovery may be explained by the impoverished non-challenging environment the person is in rather than solely by the lesion (Carr and Shepherd 1987a,b). Even casual observation of rehabilitation units around the world shows a remarkable similarity in physical structure, which typically has limited physical signs of activity, but plentiful evidence of disability and handicap.

Studies of environments in several rehabilitation settings have been reported. For example, a group of individuals with spinal cord injury were found to be more 'independent' in corridors and the cafeteria than in the therapy rooms (Willems 1972). Another study of spinal cord injured patients, this time in a rehabilitation centre designed for this population (Kennedy *et al.* 1988), showed that only 16% of time (75 minutes) was spent in face-to-face contact with therapists, while 40% was spent in the ward in 'isolated disengagement' or being inactive. Interestingly, only 6% of time was spent in interactions with other patients. Although plans to implement change were drawn up and staff agreed to increase patient time in therapy departments, follow-up investigation 8 months later showed virtually no change in how patients spent their time.

It is generally suggested that intensive rehabilitation after stroke promotes recovery. However, the evidence from environmental studies so far is that rehabilitation tends not to be intensive for many groups of patients even when it is planned to be so, and it appears that more time is spent in passive pursuits than in meaningful and task-related activity and exercise. One study (Lincoln *et al.* 1989) observed patients in a specialized stroke unit designed to provide intensive rehabilitation. As in Kennedy and colleagues' study, approximately 40% of the day was spent in passive pursuits. Keith (1980) also addressed the issue of how stroke patients spent their time during a waking day and followed up with another study several years later (Keith and Cowell 1987). In the follow-up, they found little had changed over the 20 years. One-third of the day was spent in treatment, with only 93 minutes spent in physiotherapy and occupational therapy. They used a useful clinical research tool, a behaviour map (see p. 59), to provide a distribution of certain behaviours within relevant settings. Another study of 15 stroke patients (Tinson 1989) showed that only 11% (53 minutes) of a working day was spent in physiotherapy and occupational therapy. The 40% of the day which could have been spent in exercising was spent 'watching others or looking out of the window', most of it on the ward. There was little evidence of

self-directed exercise (Fig. 1.1). Other studies have shown similar results (e.g., Lincoln *et al.* 1989; Mackey *et al.* 1996).

What is the nature of a therapeutic environment? It has been suggested that even small increments in environmental quality can result in a disproportionate increase in the quality of life (Lawton 1979) and this may well be the case in terms of the rehabilitation environment. Does the typical rehabilitation environment actually facilitate or inhibit recovery or functional optimization in individuals with acute or chronic brain lesion. The evidence is that the typical environment may cause depression or disorientation, may give messages to the patient which are not congruent with the goals of the rehabilitation staff, may encourage inappropriate behaviour and may not offer any opportunity for the person to practise the functional actions required for independence in the outside world.

Decline in intellectual activity seen in some individuals after stroke may be explained by the

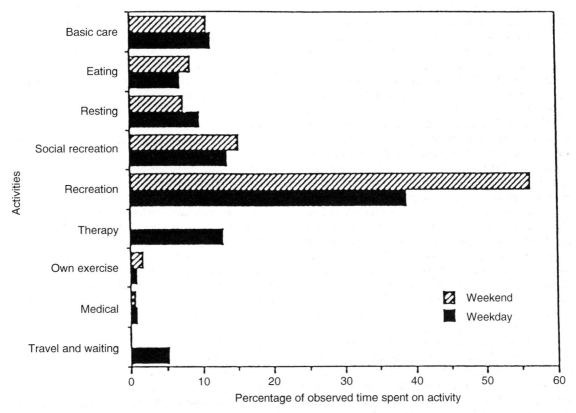

Fig. 1.2 Pattern of patients' activities during structured observations on weekdays and weekend. (From Tinson, D. J. (1989) How stroke patients spend their days. *International Disabilities Study*, **11**, 45–49, by permission)

lesion and/or by the person's age. However, such decline can also be explained by other factors (Baltes and LaBouvie 1973). The rehabilitation environment is complex, unfamiliar and unpredictable to those who suddenly find themselves in it and such situations have been suggested to evoke less adaptive responses in the older person, particularly when there are also high stress levels and limited processing or response time is available (Lawton 1979). Difficulty coping with an unfamiliar environment can cause an erosion of the feeling of competence. It has been suggested that 'learned helplessness' generated by an overly assistive and protective environment may cause symptoms of passivity and poor performance in individuals where they have little control over their role in an institutional environment (Seligman 1975; Peterson *et al.* 1993).

It has been clearly shown that the physical setting, for example, the structure of a room and the furniture in it, can also affect behaviour (Sommer 1969), even motor performance itself. Biomechanical studies for example, make it clear that inability to stand up from a seat may be due to an obstacle to the necessary foot placement backward or to the therapist or nurse standing too close in front of the patient. Standing up from a higher chair, by decreasing the extensor muscle force required through the lower limbs, is therefore easier than from a low seat, but height-adjustable chairs are not a common sight in hospitals or rehabilitation centres (although they are available).

Not only are rehabilitation units similar the world over, they also tend to be furnished in a remarkably similar fashion – with parallel bars, walking aids and substitutes such as canes, quadripod sticks and wheelchairs, mats on the floor, so-called 'high mats' or wide, low beds. There is typically little sign that arm and hand activities are practised, little exercise equipment of the type found in a gymnasium, few electronic devices to give feedback or enable challenging interactions (although stationary bicycles with electronic feedback are becoming more evident).

There are, however, some promising new developments. Treadmills are becoming more evident (although they may not be used) and video may be available to enable patients to see themselves in action. Entertaining games and interactive machines are being reported to lead to improved performance (Smedley *et al.* 1986).

There may sometimes be a mismatch between rehabilitation equipment and goals of therapy. Compare, for example, what might be a patient's impression on sighting a treadmill or a wheelchair. A wheelchair signifies an alternative mode of getting about, to be used when walking is difficult or impossible. Once a person is an occupant of a wheelchair, subtle (and not so subtle) changes occur in the behaviours and attitudes of others. Social interactions can be severely affected. Kerr (1970) provides a valuable description of her personal experiences as a professional person moving about a hospital in a wheelchair. She describes how, apparently because she was in a wheelchair, she was thought to be a patient and many staff interacted with her quite differently from the way in which they would have done had they known she was there as a clinical psychologist. On one occasion, she was wheeled to a dining room without any conversation with the staff member, i.e., without being asked if that was where she wanted to go. It is very likely that being relegated to spend all day in a wheelchair can affect in a negative way the behaviour of both patient and staff in the facility.

In conclusion, it is very likely that the provision of a challenging environment structured in a way that is relevant to the everyday tasks that patients need to learn and stimulating to mental and physical functioning may be found to have direct effects upon the reorganization of the brain after a lesion. However, to bring this about would take massive changes in the ways in which health professionals typically function. In physiotherapy, for example, the dominance of therapy which discourages practice by patients without their therapist lest they should practise in error, the preference of many physiotherapists for hands-on therapy rather than a more coaching or training role, and the relative paucity of any technological aids to enable interesting and stimulating interactions, are all environmental factors which may mitigate against optimal recovery.

Adaptation of motor performance

Compensatory or adaptive behaviour illustrates the individual's attempt to respond, immediately after the lesion, on the basis of the best neural systems available (LeVere 1980). It is illustrated by the person's attempts to achieve a goal using movement patterns or strategies which differ from those that would normally be used. A different movement pattern may be illustrated by different angular displacements or a different hand path in reaching. A different strategy may involve using the upper limb(s) for support or balance.

There is clinical evidence that adaptive behaviour occurs early after an acute lesion, as soon as the person attempts to fulfil some motor goal, and gradually over time when a lesion is progressive. It has typically been considered by clinicians that post-lesion movement patterns are a direct result of the brain lesion. These so-called 'abnormal movement patterns' have been considered, for example, to be a manifestation of spasticity (e.g., Bobath 1981, 1990; Levin 1996) rather than adaptive. As a consequence, therapeutic efforts are typically directed at 'normalizing' movement patterns since this is believed to be required for 'normal' function.

However, we have argued that these patterns represent in large part secondary adaptations which emerge as the individual with impairments in motor control attempts a purposeful action in order to achieve a goal (Carr and Shepherd 1987a,b; Shepherd and Carr 1991; Ada *et al.* 1994; Shepherd 1995). They represent the anatomical and functional constraints on the system (see Kugler *et al.* 1980; Kugler and Turvey 1987), and possibly, as Latash and Anson (1996) have recently suggested, an altering by the CNS of its priorities. That is, there are multiple (but finite) ways in which muscle activations and segmental rotations can be coordinated in order to achieve a single desired movement outcome. (See Bernstein 1967 for discussion of 'degrees of freedom'.) Nevertheless, as we acquire skill in a relatively simple task like standing up, performance becomes remarkably consistent and the system has apparently made a choice regarding the optimal movement pattern for effective performance. Of course, small changes may occur in a movement pattern as a result of changes in environmental features or goal. The choices, however, may become very limited for a person after an acute lesion and one of the problems presented by adaptive motor patterns is that they often represent the *only* action available for many similar tasks. For example, the man in Fig. 6.8 can get his hand to the page but this is *all* he could do with this adaptation. He could not touch the book if it was held even a few centimetres to his left. If he cannot be trained to use a more functional pattern which allows flexibility according to environmental features and goal of the action, then he will gradually stop using this limb. Training may, therefore, make a difference, and there is some evidence that this is so (see Chapter 6).

The way in which a person attempts to achieve a goal at this stage illustrates, in a sense, the 'best' that can be done given the state of the musculoskeletal as well as the neural system (Shepherd and Carr 1991). It seems that the action is performed in the most biomechanically advantageous manner given the effects of the lesion, the dynamic possibilities inherent in the musculoskeletal linkage and the environment in which the action is performed (Carr and Shepherd 1996); what, in other words, appears to be functionally preferred. After an acute lesion such as stroke, the person will use whatever muscles can generate sufficient force to move the necessary body segments in an attempt to achieve the goal of the action. The biomechanical flexibility inherent in the musculoskeletal system will often enable a rough approximation of the action to be accomplished, even in individuals with considerable weakness. Therefore, the movement patterns are reflective of the imbalance caused by greater activity of some muscles of a synergy compared to others. The imbalance is the direct result of the lesion which causes reduced cortico-motor neuronal connectivity and absent or reduced and slowed intensity of muscle activation. The movement pattern reflects this imbalance.

Another factor that dictates what motor patterns will emerge post-lesion is the state of the musculoskeletal system, the effector apparatus which is put into motion by the neural system. Enforced immobility, even for relatively short periods, results in length-associated changes in muscle and other soft tissues. Loss of muscle extensibility affects not only the joint over which a muscle passes but also affects segments at a distance from the contracted muscle. For example, contracture of the soleus muscle not only prevents ankle dorsiflexion but also prevents hip extension and, as a result, translation of the body mass forward over the foot in standing and walking. There is some evidence that adaptive muscle changes may affect the neural system itself. Dietz and Berger (1983), for example, have shown in patients following stroke that muscles held short not only develop structural changes but also generate tension at shorter lengths. Muscles are also affected by the process of thixotropy, and unused muscles may become stiff, which in turn can impact on the nervous system (see Chapter 8).

The third factor that influences motor patterns is the external environment and the person's experiences, that is, what they do, what they practise and learn. When most of the day is spent in a wheelchair, muscle length adapts accordingly and lower limb flexor muscles shorten. When the individual propels the wheelchair with one arm, it is this unaffected arm which is exercised. Kolb points out the probable effects of using one limb to substitute for a limb with an impairment (1995, p. 153). Part of learning to depend on one hand involves reducing the use of the affected hand, therefore a patient may actually lose any residual capacity they had in this limb. Taub and Berman (1963) called this phenomenon 'learned non-use'.

What is particularly complex about this issue for rehabilitation is that there appears to be a strong drive in patients for reorganization of motor patterns in order to adapt to lesion effects and enable some functional independence. This is aided by the fact that such adaptations may be effective in a limited way, enabling the individual to 'get by' given that assistance is provided by others, the patient's responsibilities are few, and the rehabilitation environment is less demanding than real life. It is, therefore, interesting that several studies of 'forced use' of the affected upper limb in humans have shown a positive result in terms of functional use (e.g., Ostendorf and Wolf 1981; Wolf *et al.* 1989; Taub *et al.* 1993).

In study of monkeys, 4 months following a lesion (Nudo and Grenda 1992), the loss of cortical representation of movement on electrical stimulation of the hand area was found to be greater than would be predicted by the lesion alone. However, when another group of monkeys were similarly lesioned then forced to use the affected limb, remapping of the cortex showed the animals still had an extensive region from which movement of fingers and hands could be elicited. That is, training had prevented a loss of function which was probably due to disuse.

The effect of early adaptive motor behaviour upon the initial reorganization processes in the CNS and the relationship between repetitive practice of maladaptive muscle activations and reorganization are not known. However, it seems likely from the evidence presented briefly in this chapter that both these issues pose significant questions relevant to the potential for functional recovery. Adaptive motor patterns, although they may be relatively ineffective, represent the individual's experience and use, two factors which appear to drive reorganization. These adaptive patterns are repeated and in the absence of any rehabilitation intervention appear to become learned or habitual which must reflect patterns of neural reorganization. Is it possible that training,

including 'forcing' more effective task-related muscle activations and movement patterns, would promote a more efficient and effective reorganization and hence a more optimal functional recovery?

These are complex issues. They have, we believe, been misunderstood in clinical circles with the result that therapists may prevent a person from practising an action, preferring to wait until movement patterns are more 'normal'. In reaction to this, some writers have recently proposed that patients should do what they can without therapeutic intervention but with unskilled assistance. Both approaches probably encourage maladaptation. Following acute brain lesion, there are, therefore, two broad, and quite opposed, options for the therapist in terms of how he or she addresses a patient's impairments. On the one hand, emphasis could be placed on helping the person learn to use the unaffected limbs, usually referred to as substitution or compensation; on the other, emphasis could be placed on enabling the person to learn to activate muscles and use the affected limbs. The former method prevailed early in the history of neurological rehabilitation and physiotherapy, and was based on the belief that lesions caused irretrievable loss of function with no possibility for recovery in the static circuitry of the CNS. Interestingly, although most physiotherapists, occupational therapists and rehabilitation physicians would now hold the view that improving function in the affected limbs is an important goal, much of what takes place in rehabilitation in reality still emphasizes the use of the unaffected limbs. For example, the use of one-arm drive wheelchairs, whilst enabling the individual to be independent in the undemanding environment of the hospital, ensures that more time is engaged in practising use of the unaffected limbs to locomote during the day than is spent in walking practice. The assumptions that the patient 'waits for' recovery before practising walking or that walking should not be practised until the movement pattern is 'correct' and 'tone is normal', which is common in Bobath therapy (see e.g. Hesse *et al.* 1993) remain dominant despite evidence that such assumptions are in error. Similarly, the term 'transfers', (which originated in reference to the need of individuals with spinal cord injury to adapt to moving about using the arms and upper body), continues to be used to refer to standing up and sitting down. Teaching 'transfers' infers that a new skill has to be learned, and indeed standing up from one seat and 'transferring' to another without achieving the erect position is not common in the everyday life of a healthy person. Unfortunately, in clinical practice, teaching transfers may take the place of training standing up, an action which would better enable the person to develop independence. At the very least, transfers, standing up and sitting down should be seen as three different actions.

We, and others, have argued that task-related training strategies such as modifying the task and structuring the environment (using a treadmill with supportive harness; raising the seat height) provide the opportunity to drive neural reorganization and optimize functional effectiveness. It is evident that motor tasks comprise some critical biomechanical features without which the task would not be possible (see Chapters 4–7). Task-related training probably needs to take account of these and emphasize them as part of the training process. Together with exercise and feedback, we assume that training will strengthen existing and potential neural connections and prevent adaptive muscle weakness and soft tissue change. The notion of training is rather different from that of much current therapy since it implies active participation by a motivated individual. Of course, a great deal is expected of the patient and active participation may not be the easiest option. Explanations by staff, provision of motivating tasks to practise, together with patience, diligence and great motivation on the part of the patient are therefore required for this natural and spontaneous drive toward substitution to be replaced by a drive to activate muscles and use the affected limbs.

Muscle adaptation

Following an acute brain lesion, the potential exists for muscle adaptation (and adaptation of other soft tissues) directly as a result of the muscle inactivity imposed by the brain lesion and secondarily as a result of subsequent disuse. Adaptations appear to occur rather quickly, atrophy of quadriceps, for example, occurring after only 3 days of immobilization (Lindboe and Platou 1984). Muscle structure, like any physical structure, is dependent upon and reflects patterns of use. Repetitive and strong force production through exercise is known to increase muscle mass; conversely, decreased force production reduces muscle mass.

Disuse of muscle results in wasting due to decrease in protein synthesis, apparently occurring earliest in slow contracting muscles and depending on the amount of stretch applied to the muscle. Disuse is also associated with length-associated changes in muscle (Herbert 1988). It has been shown in muscles immobilized in plaster casts that when muscles are immobilized in the shortened position sarcomeres are lost and the remaining sarcomeres adapt their length to enable the muscle to develop its maximum tension in the immobilized position (Williams and Goldspink 1978). As a result, length/tension curves of the shortened muscles shift to the left. Conversely, muscles immobilized at a lengthened position, add on sarcomeres.

Disused muscle also shows changes in connective tissue. It has been noted that muscles which are held immobile at a shortened length show an increased resistance to passive stretch (Williams and Goldspink 1973). Biochemical studies show that, in muscles immobilized in a shortened position, there is an increase in the proportion of collagen to muscle fibre tissue. The proportional increase in endomysium and perimysium could explain why the muscle is stiffer (Williams and Goldspink 1984). Connective tissue changes appear in particular to be related to the lack of activity. It should be noted that adaptive changes occur also in joints in association with immobilization (Akeson *et al.* 1987).

Of relevance to the rehabilitation of older individuals, changes also occur in muscle and connective tissue in association with ageing. Muscle mass decreases as does muscular performance. However, the relative contributions of an ageing process and a lack of activity are not known. There is some evidence that regular exercise in older individuals might reduce age-related fibrosis and increase muscle performance.

The type of activity affects muscle differentially. Fast and slow contracting fibres are recruited according to the type of activity. For example, if exercise is of low intensity, fast fibres may rarely be recruited and may, as a consequence atrophy while the slow fibres hypertrophy. Muscles also respond to repetitive training by producing more mitochondria, more oxidative enzymes and a greater number of capillaries per fibre (Hoppeler and Lindstedt 1985). Adaptation as a result of exercise can, therefore, increase fatigue resistance.

Following stroke in particular, adaptation of muscle probably plays a large part in determining the degree of subsequent recovery of the patient. Not only is the person immobilized by the poor recruitment of motor units and subsequent disuse, but there may also be pre-existing adaptive changes associated with getting older and becoming less active. It has been shown that disuse affects in particular the normally highly active antigravity muscles such as soleus (Fischback and Robbins 1969). These muscles show rapid and extensive atrophy in the absence of normal activity patterns (Goldspink and Williams 1990). Muscle changes which are particularly evident in antigravity lower limb muscles following disuse have been reported in both animals and humans. It should be noted that such changes take place in *both* lower limbs in the absence of weight-bearing (Gossman *et al.* 1986), a point that needs consideration in those with a hemiplegia.

The degree of activity is also affected by the amount of stretch a muscle undergoes, hence the importance in rehabilitation of the patient practising exercises and activities which both train force production by the muscle and also stretch the muscle. Exercises such as those shown in Figs. 5.22, 5.23 accomplish both and are directed at strengthening the lower limb extensors as well as training coordination of the necessary muscle synergies. This type of exercise, as well as practice of the actions to be regained, also provides the intermittent stretch and shortening under conditions typical of daily life. Such exercises and task-related training instituted early in rehabilitation may be sufficient to gain and maintain optimal muscle length. Although prolonged passive stretch (in a cast) may sometimes be necessary when a muscle is extremely shortened, it has the disadvantage of placing an antagonist muscle in a shortened position which would induce muscle wasting (Williams and Goldspink 1973). (For further discussion of adaptive changes to soft tissues, including muscle, see Chapter 8.)

It needs also to be noted that for our daily lives we need to be able to produce the necessary muscle force to accomplish our different goals and we need to be able to do this with the muscles at the lengths at which such force must be generated for successful function. As we know from our own experience, when we are about to undertake an activity which differs from usual, such as cross country skiing, it is advisable to do preparatory exercises which gain the greater muscle length necessary (e.g., in hip flexors). A patient may therefore require to stretch particular muscles in order to return to a favourite recreation.

It should be clear to neurological physiotherapists that activity (including intensive exercise) is critical following a brain lesion to ensure that the muscle and connective tissue adaptations that take place have a positive effect rather than a negative effect upon recovery of function. Emphasis in physiotherapy on preventing unwanted adaptive changes in the musculoskeletal system as a result of disuse may be critical to effective motor training. Length-associated changes in soft tissues, in particular those changes associated with shortening, can make it impossible for a person to generate muscle force, particularly when the ability to do so is fragile. That is, an impaired musculoskeletal system will compromise recovery, as has been shown in animal studies (Travis and Woolsey 1956).

The current rehabilitation methodologies in common use do not appear to prevent negative adaptations. It is common for individuals following acute lesions such as stroke, for example, to develop soft tissue contracture, particularly in the upper limb, and to fail to recover activity in muscles of the affected side. This has recently been reported in a large group of patients treated by the Bobath approach (Nakayama *et al.* 1994). Therapists using this approach do not consider the muscle itself to be of consequence following a brain lesion. Strengthening exercises are, therefore, not a common part of the commonly used forms of neurological physiotherapy.

In conclusion, over a number of years, the authors have been developing a systematic approach to training of motor actions for individuals with brain lesions, using post-stroke as a major example. Emphasis is on training control of muscles and preserving integrity of the musculoskeletal system, as well as on promoting the learning of relevant actions (motor learning). The assumption has been that, if training is effective, it will be associated with cellular changes such as those referred to in this chapter. Emphasis is, therefore, on driving the reorganization of the brain and ensuring flexibility of the musculoskeletal system by enabling active participation by the patient, by exercise and training and by 'forced' use. Therapist-induced responses as in the commonly used approach of Bobath (Bobath 1990; Davies 1990; Johnstone 1987) are replaced in this new model by patient-initiated interactions with objects in the environment and by exercises to elicit muscle activity when it is paralysed and to strengthen muscle force production when it is weak. All practice, including most exercise, is task- and context-related, meaning that the actions to be learned are practised in an appropriate environment, with exercises directed specifically at the muscles (and muscle synergies) required for the performance of that action, working through the range at which they must generate force. Patients practise the tasks which are difficult, for example walking, with the therapist as coach, encouraging the performance of most critical biomechanical features and discouraging behavioural adaptations which have limited effectiveness through their interference with cadence or balance. Patients also practise on their own and under supervision, with a checklist of those components to which they need to direct their attention. Repetition and extensive practice are probably critical to the motor learning process, and thus to brain reorganization.

In testing the effects of neurological rehabilitation, including physiotherapy, consideration needs to be given to the various levels at which efficacy can be tested. Although we consider outcome needs to be tested in terms of the individual's performance on the actions necessary for independence, personal well-being and social integration also provide essential information about efficacy of intervention. However, it is also necessary for physiotherapists to collaborate with neuroscientists in determining the effects of various interventions, such as task-related training, on the brain's processes of reorganization. That is, although measurement of motor performance is critical for the gaining of information about the behavioural effects of brain processes or of rehabilitation, it is also crucial to understand what is happening at the biological level. Recovery at biochemical, neural and muscle levels forms the basis of behavioural (including motor) recovery (see Rose and Johnson 1992). Studies using TMS and MRI, for example, have the capacity to demonstrate reorganization after brain injury (Dominkus et al. 1990; Cohen *et al.* 1991; Escudero *et al.* 1992; Heald *et al.* 1993) and enable the relationship between specific training and reorganization to be tested. We would hypothesize that task-related practice of a meaningful action may provide the best input conditions for achieving the most effective reorganization (see Jenkins and Merzenich 1987). Task-related training may alter the access to remaining motor neural circuitry and excitability of an alternate motor pathway may reflect the development of a new neural strategy for that movement.

Developments in cell and molecular biology are expanding our understanding of the relationship between biological and psychological phenomena and usage patterns. Future developments in brain imaging techniques may enable the effects of use, experience, environmental stimulation and training on brain reorganization to be more easily evaluated. As yet we do not know what the lesioned brain can achieve under optimal conditions. We do not even know how to categorize patients according to the likelihood of intensive training resulting in true independence or the probable need for more assistance. However, we are currently gaining increasing insights into how dynamic physiological processes associated with reorganization and learning might be best manipulated to accelerate and optimize recovery of function.

References

Ada, L., Canning, C.G., Kilbreath, S.L. and Shepherd, R.B. (1994) Task-specific training of reaching and manipulation. In *Insights into the Reach to Grasp Movement* (eds K.M.B. Bennett and U. Castiello) Elsevier, Amsterdam, pp. 239–268.

Aizawa, H., Inase, M., Mushiake, H. *et al.* (1991) Reorganisation of activity in the supplementary motor area associated with motor learning and functional recovery. *Experimental Brain Research,* **84**, 668–671.

Akeson, W.H., Amiel, D., Abel, M.F. et al. (1987) Effects of immobilization on joints. *Clinical Orthopaedics and Related Research,* **219**, 28–37.

Almli, C.R. and Finger, S. (1992) Brain injury and recovery of function: theories and mechanisms of functional reorganisation. *Journal of Head Trauma Rehabilitation,* **7**, 70–77.

Aou, S.A., Woody, C.D. and Birt, D. (1992) Increases in excitability of neurons of the motor cortex of cats after rapid acquisition of eye blink conditioning. *Journal of Neurophysiology,* **12**, 560–569.

Asanuma, C. (1991) Mapping movements within a moving motor map. *Trends in Neuroscience,* **14**, 217–218.

Asanuma, H. and Keller, A. (1991) Neuronal mechanisms of motor learning in mammals. *Neuroreport,* **2**, 217–224.

Bach-y-Rita, P. (1981) Central nervous system lesions: sprouting and unmasking in rehabilitation. *Archives of Physical Medicine and Rehabilitation,* **62**, 413–417.

Bach-y-Rita, P. (1990) Receptor plasticity and volume transmission in the brain: Emerging concepts with relevance to neurologic rehabilitation. *Journal of Neurological Rehabilitation,* **4**, 121–128.

Bach-y-Rita, P. (1996) Conservation of space and energy in the brain. *Restorative Neurology and Neuroscience,* **10**, 1–3.

Bailliet, R., Shin, J.B. and Bach-y-Rita, P. (1982) Facial paralysis rehabilitation: retraining selective muscle control. *International Rehabilitation Medicine, 4,* 67–74.

Baltes, P.B. and LaBouvie, G.V. (1973) Adult development of intellectual performance: description, explanation and modification. In *The Psychology of Adult Development and Aging* (eds C. Eisdorfer and M.P. Lawton), American Psychological Association, Washington, DC.

Bear, M.F., Cooper, L.N. and Ebner, F.F. (1987) A physiological basis for a theory of synapse modification. *Science,* **237,** 42–48.

Behm, D.G. and Sale, D.G. (1993) Intended rather than actual movement velocity determines velocity-specific training exercise. *Journal of Applied Physiology,* **74,** 359–368.

Bennett, E.L. (1976) Cerebral effects of differential experience and training. In *Neural Mechanisms of Learning and Memory* (eds M.R. Rosenzweig and E.L. Bennett), MIT Press, Cambridge, MA, 279–287.

Bernstein, N. (1967) *The Coordination and Regulation of Movements,* Pergamon Press, New York.

Black, J.E. and Greenough, W.T. (1989) Metabolic support of neural plasticity: implications for the treatment of Alzheimer's disease. In *Novel Approaches to the Treatment of Alzheimer's Disease* (eds E. Meyer, J. Simpkins and J. Yamamoto), Plenum Press, New York.

Bobath, B. (1981) *Abnormal Postural Reflex Activity Caused by Brain Lesions,* Heinemann, London.

Bobath, B. (1990) *Adult Hemiplegia: Evaluation and Treatment,* 3rd edn, Butterworth Heinemann, Oxford.

Boussaoud, D. and Wise, S. P. (1993) Primate frontal cortex neuronal activity following atteutional versus inteutional cues. *Experimental Brain Research,* **92,** 15–27.

Buell, S.J. and Coleman, D.P. (1981) Dendritic growth in aged human brain and failure of growth in senile dementia. *Science,* **206,** 854–856.

Camel, J.E., Withers, G.S. and Greenough, W.T. (1986) Persistence of visual cortex dendritic alterations induced by post-weaning exposure to a 'super-enriched' environment in rats. *Behavioral Neuroscience,* **100,** 810–813.

Canter, S. and Canter, D. (eds) (1979) *Designing for Therapeutic Environments. A Review of Research,* John Wiley, New York.

Carolan, B. and Cafarelli, E. (1992) Adaptations in coactivation after isometric resistance training. *Journal of Applied Physiology,* **73,** 911–917.

Carr J.H. and Shepherd R.B. (1987a) *A Motor Relearning Programme for Stroke,* Butterworth Heinemann, Oxford.

Carr J.H. and Shepherd R.B. (1987b) A motor learning model for rehabilitation. In *Movement Science. Foundations for Physical Therapy in Rehabilitation* (eds J.H. Carr and R.B. Shepherd), Aspen Publishers, Rockville, MD, pp. 31–92.

Carr, J.H. and Shepherd, R.B. (1996) 'Normal' is not the issue: it is 'effective' goal attainment that counts. *Behavioral and Brain Science,* **19,** 72–73.

Chollet, F., DiPiero, V., Wise, R.J.S. *et al.* (1991) The functional anatomy of motor recovery after stroke in humans: a study with positron emission tomography. *Annals of Neurology,* **29,** 63–71.

Chow, K.L. and Stewart, D.L. (1972) Reversal of structural and functional effects of long-term visual deprivation in cats. *Experimental Neurology,* **34,** 409–433.

Cohen, L.G., Roth, B.J., Wasserman, E.M. *et al.* (1991) Magnetic stimulation of the human cerebral cortex, an indicator of reorganisation in motor pathways in certain pathological conditions. *Journal of Clinical Neurophysiology,* **8,** 56–65.

Cotman, C.W. and Nieto-Sampedro, M. (1982) Brain function, synapse renewal and plasticity. *Annual Review of Psychology,* **33,** 371–401.

Cracraft, J.D. and Petajan, J.H. (1961) Effect of muscle training on the pattern of firing of single motor units. *American Journal of Physical Medicine,* **56,**183–194.

Crisosomo, E.A., Duncan, P.W., Propst, M. *et al.* (1988) Evidence that amphetamine with physical therapy promotes recovery of motor function in stroke patients. *Annals of Neurology,* **23,** 94–97.

Davies, P.M. (1990) *Right in the Middle,* Springer-Verlag, London.

Dietz, J. and Berger, W. (1983) Normal and impaired regulation of muscle stiffness in gait. A new hypothesis about muscle hypertonia. *Experimental Neurology,* **79,** 680.

DiPiero, V., Collet, F.M., MacCarthy, P. *et al.* (1992) Motor recovery after acute ischaemic stroke: a metabolic study. *Journal of Neurology, Neurosurgery, and Psychiatry,* **55,** 990–996.

Dominkus, M., Grisold, W. and Jelinek, V. (1990) Transcranial electrical motor potentials as a prognostic indicator for motor recovery in stroke patients. *Journal of Neurology, Neurosurgery, and Psychiatry,* **53,** 745–748.

Edelman, G.M. (1987) *Neuronal Darwinism: The Theory of Neuronal Group Selection,* Basic Books, New York.

Enoka, R.M. (1995) Neural adaptations with chronic physical activity. *Proceedings of XVth Congress of ISB.,* Jyvaskyla, Finland, pp. 20–21.

Escudero, J., Sancho, J., Escudero, M. *et al.* (1992) Clinical applications of magnetic transcranial stimulation in patients with ischaemic stroke. In *Clinical Applications of Magnetic Transcranial Stimulation* (ed. M. Lissens), Peeters Press, Leuven, pp. 146–165.

Evarts, E. (1980) Brain control of movement: possible mechanisms of function. In *Recovery of Function: Theoretical Considerations for Brain Injury Rehabilitation* (ed. P. Bach-y-Rita), Hans Huber, Bern, pp. 173–186.

Farmer, S.F., Swash, M., Ingram, D.A. and Stephens, J.A. (1993) Changes in motor unit synchronisation following central nervous lesions in man. *Journal of Physiology, 463*, 83–105.

Finger, S. (1978) Environmental attenuation of brain-lesion symptoms. In *Recovery from Brain Damage* (ed. S. Finger), Plenum Press, London, pp. 297–329.

Finger, S. and Stein, D.G. (1982) *Brain Damage and Recovery: Research and Clinical Perspectives,* Academic Press, New York.

Fischback, G.D. and Robbins, N. (1969) Changes in contractile properties of disused soleus muscles. *Journal of Physiology (London), 201*, 305.

Fisher, C.M. (1992) Concerning the mechanism of recovery in stroke hemiplegia. *Canadian Journal of Neurology Science, 19*, 57–63.

Franz, S.I., Scheetz, M. and Wilson, A. (1915) The possibility of recovery of motor function in long-standing hemiplegia. *Journal of American Medical Association, 65*, 2150–2154.

Fuhr, P., Cohen, L.G., Dang, N. *et al.* (1992) Physiological analysis of motor reorganisation following lower limb amputation. *Electroencephalography and Clinical Neurophysiology, 85*, 53–60.

Gilbert, P.F.C. and Thach, W.T. (1977) Purkinje cell activity during motor learning. *Brain Research, 128*, 309–328.

Glees, P. (1980) Functional reorganisation following hemispherectomy in man and after small experimental lesions in primates. In *Recovery of Function: Theoretical Considerations for Brain Injury Rehabilitation* (ed. P. Bach-y-Rita), Hans Huber, Berne, pp. 106–126.

Glickstein, M. (1992) The cerebellum and motor learning. *Current Opinion in Neurobiology, 2*, 802–806.

Goldberger, M. and Murray, M. (1980) Locomotor recovery after deafferentation of one side of the cat's trunk. *Experimental Neurology, 67*, 103–117.

Goldspink, G. and Williams, P. (1990) Muscle fibre and connective tissue changes associated with use and disuse. In *Key Issues in Neurological Physiotherapy.* (eds. L. Ada and C. Canning), Butterworth-Heinemann, Oxford, pp. 197–218.

Goldstein, L.B. (1993) Basic and clinical studies of pharmacologic effects on recovery from brain injury. *Journal of Neural Transplantation and Plasticity, 4*, 175–192.

Gossman, M.R., Sahrmann, S.A. and Rose, S.J. (1986) Review of length-associated changes in muscle. *Physical Therapy, 62*, 1799–1808.

Grabiner, M.D., Owings, T.A., George, M.R. *et al.* (1995) Eccentric contractions are specified *a priori* by the CNS. *Proceedings of XVth Congress of ISB*, Jyvaskyla, Finland, pp. 338–339

Gracies, J.M. (1996) Personal communication.

Grafton, S.T., Mazziotta, J.C., Presty, S. *et al.* (1992) Functional anatomy of human procedural learning determined with regional blood flow and PET. *Journal of Neuroscience, 12*, 2542–2548.

Greenough, W.T., Larson, J.R. and Withers, G.S. (1985) Effects of unilateral and bilateral training in a reaching task on dendritic branching of neurons in the rat motor-sensory forelimb cortex. *Behavioral and Neural Biology, 44*, 301–314.

Greenough, W.T., Black, J.E. and Wallace, C.S. (1993) Experience and brain development. In *Brain Development and Cognition* (ed. M.H. Johnson), Blackwell, Oxford, pp. 290–322.

Hakkinen, K. and Komi, P.V. (1983) Electromyographic changes during strength training and detraining. *Medicine and Science in Sport and Exercise, 15*, 455–460.

Hall, E.J., Flament, D., Fraser, C. and Lemon, R.N. (1990) Non-invasive brain stimulation reveals reorganised cortical outputs in amputees. *Neuroscience Letters, 116*, 379–386.

Halsband, U. and Freund, H-J. (1993) Motor learning. *Current Opinion in Neurobiology, 3*, 940–949.

Heald, A., Bates, D., Cartlidge, N.E.F. *et al.* (1993) Longitudinal study of central motor conduction time following stroke. 2: Central motor conduction measured 12–72 h after stroke as a predictor of functional outcome at 12 months. *Brain, 116*, 1371–1385.

Held, J.M. (1987) Recovery of function after brain damage. In *Movement Science. Foundations for Physical Therapy and Rehabilitation* (eds J.H. Carr and R.B. Shepherd), Aspen Publishers, Rockville, MD, pp. 155–177.

Held, J.M., Gordon, J. and Gentile, A.M. (1985) Environmental influences on locomotor recovery following cortical lesions in rats. *Behavioral Neuroscience, 99*, 678–690.

Herbert, R. (1988) The passive mechanical properties of muscle and their adaptations to altered patterns of use. *Australian Journal of Physiotherapy, 34*, 141–149.

Hesse, S.A., Jahnke, M.T., Schreiner, C. and Mauritz, K-H. (1993) Gait symmetry and functional walking performance in hemiparetic patients prior to and after a 4-week rehabilitation programme. *Gait and Posture, 1*, 166–171.

Hoppeler, H. and Lindstedt, S.L. (1985) Malleability of skeletal muscle in overcoming limitations: structural elements. *Journal of Experimental Biology, 115*, 355.

Iriki, A., Pavlides, C., Keller, A. *et al.* (1989) Long-term potentiation of motor cortex. *Science, 245*, 1385–1387.

Isaacs, K.R., Anderson, B.J., Alcantara, A.A. *et al.* (1992) Exercise and the brain: angiogenesis in the adult rat cerebellum after vigorous physical activity and motor skill learning. *Journal of Cerebral Blood Flow and Metabolism, 12*, 110–119.

Isseroff, A. and Isseroff, R. (1987) Experience aids recovery of spontaneous alternation following hippocampal damage. *Physiology and Behavior, 21*, 469–472.

Jacobs, K.M. and Donoghue, J.P. (1991) Reshaping the cortical motor map by unmasking latent intracortical connections. *Science, 251*, 944–947.

Jenkins, W.M. and Merzenich, M.M. (1987) Reorganization of neocortical representations after brain injury: a neurophysiological model of the bases of recovery from stroke. In *Progress in Brain Research, No. 71* (eds F.J. Seil, E. Herbert and B.M. Carlson), Elsevier Science, New York, pp. 249–266.

Jenkins W.M., Merzenich M.M., Ochs M.T. *et al.* (1990) Functional reorganisation of primary somatosensory cortex in adult owl monkeys after behaviorally controlled tactile stimulation. *Journal of Neurophysiology*, **63**, 82–104.

Johnstone M. (1987) *Restoration of Motor Function in the Stroke Patient*, 3rd edn, Churchill Livingstone, Edinburgh.

Kandel E. (1991) Cellular mechanisms of learning and the biological basis of individuality. In *Principles of Neural Science* (eds E.R. Kandel, J.H. Schwartz and T.M. Jessell), 3rd edn, Appleton and Lange, Norwalk, CT, pp.1009–1031.

Keith, R.A. (1980) Activity patterns in a stroke rehabilitation unit. *Social Science and Medicine*, **14A**, 575–580.

Keith, R.A. and Cowell, K.S. (1987) Time use of stroke patients in three rehabilitation hospitals. *Social Science and Medicine*, **24**, 529–533.

Kennedy, P., Fisher, K. and Pearson, E. (1988) Ecological evaluation of a rehabilitative environment for spinal cord injured people: behavioural mapping and feedback. *British Journal of Clinical Psychology*, **27**, 239–246.

Kerr, N. (1970) Staff expectations for disabled persons: helpful or harmful. *Rehabilitation Counseling Bulletin*, **14**, 85–94.

Kolb, B. (1995) *Brain, Plasticity and Behavior*, Lawrence Erlbaum Associates, Mahwah, NJ.

Kugler, P.N., Kelso, J.A.S. and Turvey, M.T. (1980) On the concept of coordinative structure as dissipative structures: 1. Theoretical lines of convergence. In *Tutorials in Motor Behavior* (eds G.E. Stelmark and J. Requin), North-Holland, Amsterdam.

Kugler, P.N. and Turvey, M.T. (1987) *Information, Natural Law, and the Self-Assembly of Rhythmic Movement*, Erlbaum, New York.

Kupferman I. (1991) Learning and memory. In *Principles of Neural Science* (eds E.R. Kandel, J.H. Schwartz and T.M. Jessell), 3rd edn, Appleton and Lange, Norwalk, CT, pp. 997–1008.

Latash, M.L. and Anson, J.G. (1996) What are 'normal movements' in atypical populations? *Behavioral and Brain Science*, **19**, 55–106.

Lawton, P. (1979) Therapeutic environments for the aged. In *Designing for Therapeutic Environments. A Review of Research* (eds S. Canter and D. Canter), John Wiley, New York, pp. 233–276.

Lee, R.G. and van Donkelaar, P. (1995) Mechanisms underlying functional recovery following stroke. *Canadian Journal of Neurological Sciences*, **22**, 257–263.

LeVere, T.E. (1980) Recovery of function after brain damage: a theory of the behavioral deficit. *Physiological Psychology*, **8**, 297–308.

Levin, M.F. (1996) Should stereotyped movement synergies in hemiplegic patients be considered adaptive? *Behavioral and Brain Science*, **19**, 79–81.

Lincoln, N.B., Gamlen, R. and Thomason, H. (1989) Behavioural mapping of patients on a stroke unit. *International Disability Studies*, **11**, 149–154.

Lindboe, C.F. and Platou, C.S. (1984) Effect of immobilization of short duration on the muscle fibre size. *Clinical Physiology*, **4**, 183–188.

McComas, A.J. (1993) Human neuromuscular adaptations that accompany changes in activity. *Medicine and Science in Sports and Exercise*, **26**, 1498–1509.

McComas, A.J., Sica, R.E.P., Upton, A.R.M. *et al.* (1973) Functional changes in motor neurones of hemiparetic patients. *Journal of Neurology, Neurosurgery, and Psychiatry*, **36**, 183–193.

Mackey, F., Ada, L., Heard, R. and Adams, R. (1996) Stroke rehabilitation: are highly structured units more conducive to physical activity than less structured units? *Archives of Physical Medicine and Rehabilitation*, **77**, 1066–1070.

Merzenich, M.M. (1986) Sources of intraspecies and interspecies cortical map variability in mammals: conclusions and hypotheses. In *Comparative Neurobiology: Modes of Communication in the Nervous System*, M.J. Cohen and F. Strumwasser (eds), John Wiley and Sons, New York.

Merzenich, M.M., Allard, T.T. and Jenkins, W.M. (1991) Neural ontogeny of higher brain function: implications of some recent neurophysiological findings. In *Information Processing in the Somatosensory System* (eds O. Franzen and J. Westman), Macmillan, London.

Merzenich, M.M., Kaas, J.H., Wall, J.T. *et al.* (1983) Topographic reorganization of somatosensory cortical areas 3b and 2 in adult monkeys following restricted deafferentation. *Neuroscience*, **10**, 33–55.

Merzenich, M.M., Recanzone, G.H., Jenkins, W.M. *et al.* (1990) Adaptive mechanisms in cortical networks underlying cortical contributions to learning and nondeclarative memory. *Cold Spring Harbor Symposium of Quantitative Biology*, **55**, 873–887.

Mitz, A.R. and Wise, S.P. (1987) The somatotopic organization of the supplementary motor area: intracortical microstimulation mapping. *Journal of Neuroscience*, **7**, 1010–1021.

Moritani, T. and deVries, H.A. (1979) Neural factors versus hypertrophy in the time course of muscle strength gain. *American Journal of Physical Medicine*, **58**, 115–130.

Nakayama, H., Jorgensen, H.S., Raaschou, H.O. *et al.* (1994) Compensation in recovery of upper extremity function after stroke: The Copenhagen Stroke Study. *Archives of Physical Medicine and Rehabilitation*, **75**, 852–857.

Narici, M.V., Roi, G.S., Landoni, L. *et al.* (1989) Changes in force, cross-sectional area and neural activation during strength training and detraining of the human quadriceps. *European Journal of Applied Physiology*, **59**, 310–319.

Niemann, J., Winker, T., Gerling, J. *et al.* (1991) Changes in slow cortical negative DC-potentials during the acquisition of a complex finger motor task. *Experimental Brain Research,* **85**, 417–422.

Nudo, R. and Grenda, R. (1992) Reorganization of distal forelimb representations in primary motor cortex of adult squirrel monkeys following focal ischemic infarct. *Society for Neuroscience Abstracts,* **18**, 216.

Ostendorf, C.G. and Wolf, S.L. (1981) Effect of forced use of the upper extremity of a hemiplegic patient on changes in function. *Journal of the American Physical Therapy Association,* **61**, 1022–1028.

Pascual-Leone, A. and Torres, F. (1993) Plasticity of the sensorimotor cortex representation of the reading finger in Braille readers. *Brain,* **116**, 39–52.

Pascual-Leone, A., Dang, N., Chen, L.G. *et al.* (1995) Modulation of muscle responses evoked by transcranial magnetic stimulation during the acquisition of new fine motor skills. *Journal of Neurophysiology,* **74**, 1037–1045.

Peterson, C., Maier, S.F. and Seligman, M.E.P. (1993) *Learned Helplessness. A Theory for the Age of Personal Control,* Oxford University Press, Oxford.

Phillips, C.G. and Porter, R. (1977) *Corticospinal Neurones: Their Role in Movement,* Academic Press, London.

Recanzone, G.H., Jenkins, W.M., Hradek, G.T. *et al.* (1992) Progressive improvement in discriminative abilities in adult owl monkeys performing a tactile frequency discrimination task. *Journal of Neurophysiology,* **67**, 1015–1030.

Roland, P.E., Ericksson, L., Stone-Elander, S. *et al.* (1987) Does mental activity change the oxidative metabolism of the brain? *Journal of Neurosience,* **7**, 2373–2389.

Rose F.D. and Johnson D.A. (1992) Research on recovery. In *Recovery from Brain Damage* (eds F.D. Rose and D.A. Johnson), Plenum Press, New York, pp. 187–198.

Rosenzweig, M.R., Bennet, E.L. and Diamond, M. (1973) Effects of differential experience on dendritic spine counts in rat cerebral cortex. *Journal of Comparative Physiology and Psychology,* **82**, 175–181.

Rosenzweig, M. (1980) Animal models for effects of brain lesions and for rehabilitation. In *Recovery of Function: Theoretical Considerations for Brain Injury Rehabilitation* (ed. P. Bach-y-Rita) University Park Press, Baltimore, MD, pp. 172.

Rutherford, O.M. and Jones, D.A. (1986) The role of learning and coordination in strength training. *European Journal of Applied Physiology,* **55**, 100–105.

Sale, D.G., McComas, A.J., MacDougall, J.D. *et al.* (1982) Neuromuscular adaptations in human thenar muscles following strength training and immobilization. *Journal of Applied Physiology,* **53**, 419–424.

Sanes, J.N., Wang, J. and Donoghue, J.P. (1992) Immediate and delayed changes of rat motor cortical output representation with new forelimb configurations. *Cerebral Cortex,* **2**, 141–152.

Schieber, M.H. (1992) Widely distributed neuron activity in primary motor cortex area during individuated finger movements. *Society of Neuroscience Abstracts,* **18**, 504.

Seitz, R.J., Roland, E., Bohm, C. *et al.* (1990) Motor learning in man: a positron emission tomographic study. *Neuroreport,* **1**, 57–60.

Seligman, M. (1975) *Helplessness. On Depression, Development and Death,* W.H. Freeman, San Francisco.

Shepherd, R.B. (1995) *Physiotherapy in Paediatrics,* 3rd edn, Butterworth Heinemann, Oxford.

Shepherd, R.B. and Carr, J.H. (1991) An emergent or dynamical systems view of movement dysfunction. *Australian Journal of Physiotherapy,* **37**, 4, 5–17.

Silvestri, M., Caltagirone, C., Cupini, L.M. *et al.* (1993) Activation of healthy hemisphere in post-stroke recovery. *Stroke,* **24**, 1673–1677.

Smedley, R.R., Fiorino, A.J., Soucar, E. and Reynolds, D. (1986) Slot machines: their use in rehabilitation after stroke. *Archives of Physical Medicine and Rehabilitation,* **67**, 546–549.

Sommer, R. (1969). *Personal Space: The Behavioural Basis of Design,* Saxon House, Englewood Cliffs, NJ.

Taub, E. and Berman, A.J. (1963) Avoidance conditioning in the absence of relevant proprioceptive and exteroceptive feedback. *Journal of Comparative Physiology and Psychology,* **56**, 6, 1012–1016.

Taub, E., Miller, N.E., Novack, T.A. *et al.* (1993) A technique for improving chronic motor deficit after stroke. *Archives of Physical Medicine and Rehabilitation,* **74**, 347–354.

Tinson, D.J. (1989) How stroke patients spend their days. *International Disability Studies,* **11**, 45–49.

Travis, A.M. and Woolsey, C.N. (1956) Motor performance of monkeys after bilateral partial and total cerebral decortication. *American Journal of Physical Medicine,* **35**, 273–310.

Van Meeteren, N.L.U., Brakkee, J.H., Biessels, G-J. *et al.* (1996) Effect of exercise training on acute (crush lesion) and chronic (diabetes mellitus) peripheral neuropathy in the rat. *Restorative Neurology and Neuroscience,* **10**, 85–93.

Wade, D.T., Hewer, R.L., Skilbeck, C.E. and David, R.M. (1985) *Stroke. A Critical Approach to Diagnosis, Treatment and Management,* Chapman & Hall Medical, London.

Walsh, R. (1981) Sensory environments, brain damage, and drugs: a review of interactions and mediating mechanisms. *International Journal of Neuroscience,* **14**, 129–137.

Walsh, R.N. and Cummins, R.A. (1975) Mechanisms mediating the production of environmentally induced brain changes. *Psychology Bulletin,* **82**, 986–1000.

Weiller, C., Chollet, F., Friston, K.J. *et al.* (1992) Functional reorganisation of the brain in recovery from striatocapsular infarction in man. *Annals of Neurology,* **31**, 463–472.

Weiller, C., Ramsay, S.C., Wise, R.J.S. *et al.* (1993) Individual patterns of functional reorganisation in the human cerebral cortex after capsular infarction. *Annals of Neurology,* **33**, 181–189.

Willems, E.P. (1972) The interface of the hospital environment and patient behaviour. *Archives of Physical Medicine and Rehabilitation,* March, 115–122.

Williams, P.E. and Goldspink, G. (1973) The effect of immobilisation on the longitudinal growth of striated muscle fibres. *Journal of Anatomy,* **116**, 445–454.

Williams, P.E. and Goldspink, G. (1978) Changes in sarcomere length and physiological properties in immobilised muscle. *Journal of Anatomy,* **127**, 459–468.

Williams, P.E. and Goldspink, G. (1984) Connective tissue changes in immobilised muscle. *Journal of Anatomy,* **138**, 2, 343–350.

Wolf, S.L., LeCraw, D.E., Barton, L.A. and Jann, B.B. (1989) Forced use of hemiplegic upper extremities to reverse the effect of learned nonuse among chronic stroke and head-injured patients. *Experimental Neurology,* **104**, 125–132.

Wyke, M. (1971) The effects of brain lesions on the performance of bilateral arm movements. *Neuropsychologia,* **9**, 33–42.

Yue, G. and Cole, K.J.J. (1992) Strength increases from the motor program: comparison of training with maximum voluntary and imagined muscle contractions. *Journal of Neurophysiology,* **67**, 1114–1123.

Further reading

Bortz, W.M. (1982) Disuse and aging. *Journal of the American Medical Association,* **248**, 1203–1208.

Fries, W., Danek, A., Scheidtmann, K. *et al.* (1993) Motor recovery following capsular stroke. *Brain,* **116**, 369–382.

Fuglsang-Frederiksen, A. and Scheel, U. (1978) Transient decrease in number of motor units after immobilisation in man. *Journal of Neurology, Neurosurgery, and Psychiatry,* **41**, 924–929.

Kolb, B. (1995) *Brain Plasticity and Behavior,* Lawrence Elbaum Associates, Mahwah, NJ.

Singer W. (1982) The role of attention in developmental plasticity. *Human Neurobiology,* **1**, 41–43.

Thompson, R.F. (1986) The neurobiology of learning and memory. *Science,* **233**, 941–947.

2

Training motor control, increasing strength and fitness and promoting skill acquisition

Introduction: training motor control

The aim of physiotherapy in neurorehabilitation is to enable individuals with acute or chronic brain lesions to function as effectively as possible in everyday life. The individual with a motor impairment must attempt, therefore, to regain optimal (effective) motor performance in everyday actions critical to independence and to a desirable lifestyle. Essential to the regaining of effective motor performance is the provision of an expert coach or trainer (the therapist) and the opportunity for intensive practice and exercise.

A major purpose of this chapter (in conjunction with Chapters 4–7), is to show how everyday actions can be trained in adults whose motor disabilities are the result of a brain lesion. Effective performance of standing up and sitting down, walking, reaching out for a variety of objects and manipulating them to achieve desired goals is critical to independent living. Given the importance of the erect posture to most of our goal-directed motor behaviour, the individual needs the opportunity to concentrate on gaining control over body segments in the two erect postures (sitting and standing) most critical for independence. Early emphasis on being upright is particularly important following acute brain lesions, enabling individuals to learn the necessary orienting behaviours that enable them to explore and attend to their environment and develop the ability to formulate and carry out their goals.

An understanding of the biomechanics of everyday actions, of biological characteristics of muscle and nerve and how these change according to patterns of use, and of how skill is acquired is essential in physiotherapy practice. The training of motor control in individuals with impairments in control involves (1) ensuring adequate soft tissue flexibility, muscle strength and physical fitness for the activities required and (2) ensuring through exercise and practice that training methods are directed at the acquisition of skill (i.e., motor learning) in those activities.

The first section of this chapter contains a discussion on specificity in training. The role of muscle strengthening in training is emphasized since it is not possible for an individual to regain the ability to perform effective functional actions in the absence of appropriate muscle strength (the capacity of a group of muscles to generate and time the necessary forces). Techniques proposed for strengthening muscles in neurorehabilitation are those used by able-bodied subjects to improve motor performance and consist of intensive task-related exercises and practice of necessary actions.

The second section contains a brief review of some of the factors that underlie motor learning or the acquisition of skill. Learning a motor skill for the able-bodied requires monitored practice, motivation, awareness of the goal and a knowledge of results (Singer 1980). To some extent, the success of a person in rehabilitation depends on the capacity of the lesioned system to reorganize. It is likely, therefore, that the rehabilitation process may be able to drive that reorganization so that the best possible outcome is achieved by the individual.

We have proposed, therefore, that the methods used in training in individuals with lesions of the CNS could be similar to those already shown to be effective in increasing motor skill in non-disabled subjects (Carr and Shepherd 1980, 1987a,b). The rehabilitative teaching techniques used include demonstration and instruction, auditory and visual feedback and guidance.

Methods of intervention take into account motor control processes, movement biomechanics, muscle characteristics and environmental context as well as the underlying primary pathological impairments, secondary adaptations and recovery processes. Intervention is designed to ensure the optimal length and flexibility of muscles, activate muscles, strengthen muscle groups and promote synergic activity between muscles. Training is task-related, that is to say the individual practises a particular desired action in a variety of relevant environmental contexts. If it is not possible to practise the whole action, exercise may need to be given to enable muscles to be activated and strengthened, and to increase their compliance.

Muscle strengthening to optimize functional motor performance

It is intuitive that what people practise is what they learn, that, if an individual wants to learn to ski, or to learn again with a lesioned CNS how to walk or to stand up from a seat, then that action will itself need to be practised.

The area of research related to the specificity of exercise training is producing information of particular relevance to the rehabilitation of patients with central lesions resulting in weakness of muscle force production and lack of muscle coordination. It is becoming increasingly evident at different levels of analysis (behavioural, biological, biomechanical) that training aimed at improving motor performance needs to be specific to what is to be achieved. Even at the muscle level, muscle activation patterns, amplitude and timing of muscle forces, type of muscle contraction (eccentric–concentric, isometric–isokinetic), the length of muscle when peak force is produced, all appear to be specific to the action and the context in which it is being performed. This is not surprising given the potential for complex interactions both within the multisegmental linkage that makes up the human body and between this linkage and the opportunities offered by the external environment.

What is required for the coordination of the multijoint movements which make up most human actions is the control of many muscles performing together (i.e., synergistically) in combinations that vary, to a small or large degree, from action to action. A muscle may act as a prime mover or a fixator; it may contract to accelerate movement of a segment or to brake (decelerate) movement of a segment. Biarticular muscles may accelerate one segment and stabilize another. Muscles can affect distant segments by their contraction through reactive forces. Overall, the relative timing of contraction of all muscles involved in an action is critical and may be a major factor in fine-tuning an action.

Strength training: the specificity issue

A common finding from laboratory studies is that the major change accompanying strength training occurs in the training context itself (e.g., Sale and MacDougall 1981; Rutherford 1988); i.e., the exercise is shown to be action-specific, velocity-specific or angle-specific, and the transfer effect is typically not great. One early experiment by Rasch and Morehouse (1957) showed that men who exercised in standing to increase strength in elbow flexor muscles showed an increase in strength in standing but less so when in supine. That is, there was little transfer of training effect from one position to another. The authors suggested the result reflected the learning component of strength training. It is evident that the muscles which would need to be coordinated in order to stabilize the body while producing a forceful contraction of elbow flexors in standing would be different from those which would be active in supine. In particular, postural muscle activation patterns in standing would have involved lower limb muscles, timed to contract prior to as well as during the weight lifting exercise in order to control the anticipated perturbation caused by the exercise.

Rutherford and colleagues (Rutherford *et al.* 1986) reported a study illustrating the *action-specificity of exercise*. Able-bodied subjects, trained to lift through a range a maximum load with the knee extensors, were found to increase the load lifted by 200% over 12 weeks. However, maximum isometric force increased only 11%. In addition, when the maximum power output generated during isokinetic cycling was measured after the strength training, no change was found either at slow or fast speeds. That is, weight training for a muscle group that plays a critical part in generating leg extension force in cycling (quadriceps) was not effective in either increasing power output during cycling or in increasing muscle force under isometric conditions. A major reason for lack of transfer from muscle strengthening exercises performed with foot free to exercises with the foot as base of support (closed chain exercises) is the different muscle coordination patterns involved in these two quite different types of action. When knee extensor muscles contract to lift the shank and foot by angular movement at the knee, the muscles involved as synergists and the timing of muscle activations are different compared to when the knee extensors function to generate force through a fixed foot. For example, in cycling hip and ankle extensors, as well as knee extensors, function to produce force through the pedal.

Everyday actions typically involve both concentric (shortening) and eccentric (lengthening) modes of muscle contraction. That the two modes of contraction involve different physiological processes seems to be indicated by studies so far. The eccentric mode of isokinetic exercise has been found to have a more highly specific strength training effect than the concentric mode (e.g., Duncan *et al.* 1989). Furthermore, there is evidence from studies of able-bodied subjects that muscle strengthening exercises have specific effects that differ according to which mode is used in the exercise (Komi and Buskirk 1972; Friden *et al.* 1983). Komi and Buskirk (1972) reported that eccentric exercise was followed by a greater increase in strength than concentric exercise. Eccentric muscle action has been found to produce greater loading of elastic components of muscle (Stanish et al. 1986). Lesser levels of muscle activation for greater levels of force are produced in eccentric work compared to concentric (Westing *et al.* 1990). Eccentric contractions appear to involve lower motor unit discharge rates than concentric contractions (Tax *et al.* 1990). Eccentric exercise has been found to produce changes in the myofibrillar architecture (Friden 1984). Friden and colleagues (1983) had proposed that the tension placed on a muscle during lengthening contractions caused a preferential recruitment of type IIB muscle fibres.

A characteristic of muscle action in functional activities is its use in stretch–shortening cycles (e.g., Asmussen and Bonde-Petersen 1974; Bosco *et al.* 1982; Komi 1986). It has been shown, principally in the vertical jump, that eccentric muscle contraction immediately before the major concentric force generation can augment the amount of force delivered by the prime mover muscles. The stretch–shortening cycle has also been suggested to be one of the mechanisms enabling upper body flexion at the hips to potentiate lower limb extensor force in sit-to-stand (Shepherd and Gentile 1994).

In summary, eccentric contractions produce more muscle force, have greater mechanical efficiency, involve less metabolic cost, than concentric contractions (Asmussen 1953; Knuttgen *et al.* 1971; Komi and Buskirk 1972; Komi 1973; Komi *et al.* 1987; Chandler and Duncan 1988).

The *velocity-specificity of exercise* has been demonstrated in several studies (Moffried and Whipple 1970; Thorstensson *et al.* 1976; MacDougall *et al.* 1980; Caizzo *et al.* 1981; Kanehisa and Miyashita 1983; Narici *et al.* 1989), with little carryover of effect from one speed to another. The mechanisms responsible for the velocity-specific response are unknown. As Rutherford (1988) points out, it is possible that exercise affects the force-velocity characteristics of the muscle itself, and/or the motor neuron recruitment pattern within the nervous system. One study (Ellenbecker *et al.* 1988) has reported that, despite significant strength improvements in shoulder rotator muscles through both concentric and isokinetic (fixed-speed variable resistance) training, tennis serving speed increased only in the group of subjects who received concentric training. However, findings from another more recent study (Behm and Sale 1994) suggest that the intention to produce a high rate of force for a fast action appears more important than whether or not the ensuing contraction is concentric or eccentric.

Angle-specific training effects have also been reported, showing little transfer from one angle to another in isometric and isokinetic training (Lindh 1979; Knapik *et al.* 1983; Pavone and Moffatt 1985; Kitai and Sale 1989). When muscles are trained isometrically or isokinetically, the greatest increase in strength appears to occur at the angle of training (Lindh 1979; Sale and MacDougall 1981). There is some evidence from EMG findings of a greater increase in muscle activity at joint angles trained (Thepaut-Mathieu *et al.* 1985, 1988). These results suggest that neural adaptation allows more force to be generated at a particular muscle length (Rutherford 1988; Sale 1988).

It appears, therefore, that strength training is primarily the acquisition of an effective pattern of coordination (i.e., skill), specific to the contexts in which the action is performed. During training, major changes in strength (load lifted) have been consistently noted to occur early in the training period (Rutherford and Jones 1986) and improvement in strength (force output) is accompanied by increases in neural activation (IEMG) of strengthened muscles (Moritani and DeVries 1979; Hakkinen and Komi 1983). It is concluded, therefore, that the early changes in strength may be accounted for principally by neural factors, with hypertrophy of the muscles themselves becoming a gradually increasing contribution as training proceeds (Hakkinen and Komi 1983).

The context in which muscles must generate force varies from action to action. As Rutherford (1988) points out, particular neural adaptations that become established as a result of, say, lower limb extensor muscle training, may not be the adaptations necessary for other actions. In addition, just as training has neural and muscle effects, these effects are reversed by detraining, i.e., by relative immobility and disuse. The clinical implications from this work are that patients should practise specific actions under as near to natural conditions as possible and at close to natural speed. Therefore, for individuals with weak lower limb muscles who are attempting to regain the ability to perform actions with the feet on the ground (for example, sit-to-stand, walking, stair climbing), exercises are practised which involve lower limb extension over a fixed foot (see Figs 5.22, 5.23).

The muscle activations and segmental movements which stabilize and balance the body as we move about (reach for a cup of tea in sitting or standing, walk up a hill, stand up from a chair) are also specific to both action being carried out and environmental context. This has been shown in many biomechanical investigations of *postural adjustments* carried out on able-bodied subjects, particularly in standing, but more recently in sitting also (see Chapter 7). The muscles that act to balance and stabilize the body mass vary according to such factors as size of base of support, which segments make up the base of support, speed of

movement, direction of movement, whether support surface is stationary or moving (moving walkway or escalator).

Research findings illustrate the ability of the system to utilize whatever muscles are optimally situated to provide support or stability. In standing, when the floor (support) surface is stable, leg muscles ensure a balanced standing position as we pull a lever. By being active prior to the self-initiated voluntary arm movement, they set up the conditions in which the potentially destabilizing pulling movement can be performed effectively. When the floor surface is unstable, we may use a hand for support to ensure that the predicted perturbations will not cause us to lose our balance and fall. Even resting a finger on a stable support surface like a table decreases the work done by lower limbs in balancing.

Sensory training

Methods of treatment developed several decades ago in neurorehabilitation were based on the belief that certain sensory inputs were likely to initiate muscle activity and improve movement control; for example, fast brushing to specific dermatomes (Stockmeyer 1967); approximation to a joint (Semans 1967; Knott and Voss 1968; Bobath 1990). Others have proposed sensory stimulation or retraining programmes, involving bombardment with multiple sensory inputs including ice and vibration (e.g., de Jersey 1979). There is no evidence to suggest that such sensory stimulation techniques accomplish what was intended; i.e., improve functional performance. Pressure and cutaneous stimulation of forearm, hand and fingers, for example, have been found to have no significant effect on stereognosis or graphaesthesia (Van Deusen Fox 1964). Notably, although sensory stimulation techniques may have an immediate effect on muscle activity or on a simple joint movement, the effect does not appear to last beyond the administration of the technique (Matyas *et al.* 1986; Bohannon 1987a), and carryover into improved function has not been shown.

It is unlikely that sensory stimulation unrelated to any particular voluntary action (cognitive or motor) would affect motor function. Following a central lesion such as stroke, although normal sensory input may be received and transmitted by an intact peripheral nervous system, inputs are received in a reduced and distorted form (Yekutiel and Guttman 1993). It is, therefore, the ability of the patient to interpret the meaning and relevance of sensory input which may need to be trained.

Research from both neuroscience and cognitive science provides evidence that relatively arbitrary or non-specific sensory stimulation of a passive recipient is unlikely to affect either the awareness of specific sensations in people with discriminative sensory dysfunction or motor performance. Neuroscience findings suggest that sensory information is specific to the current state of the system and therefore to the action to be or being performed. Forssberg and colleagues (1975), for example, showed that if a cat's paw is touched with a rod during the swing phase of walking, there is an increase in flexion; if it is touched during stance phase, extension of the limb is enhanced. That is, the same stimulus had opposite effects depending on the timing of its application and the requirements of the action. Similar observations have been made in humans (Nashner *et al.* 1979).

In the normal waking state, we are bombarded with sensory inputs from our internal state and from the environment. At any particular point in time, the system selects for attention only those inputs which are relevant. Although the system receives many different sensory inputs from labyrinths, skin, muscle, joint, eyes, ears, it appears to 'take note of' and act only upon those inputs which provide information relevant to the action we are about to or are performing, extinguishing all others. That is, we select what it is we must pay attention to (Wise and Desimone 1988).

There have been several studies with the finding that specific sensory training can be effective in terms of the sensory attributes trained. Wynn Parry and Salter (1975) showed that sensory re-education could have a positive effect on recovery after median nerve lesions. Recognition of double simultaneous inputs (Goldman 1966) and identification of the midline of the back in response to touch (Weinberg *et al.* 1979) have been shown to improve with specific training of these perceptual-cognitive tasks. Whether there would have been any generalization to other sensory attributes is not known but may be unlikely. Findings from studies of animals with brain lesions suggest that training on a specific sensory task may not generalize to other tasks which are not trained (Schwartzman 1972; Weese *et al.* 1973).

Two recent reports of specific sensory retraining give strong support to the view that patients with CNS lesions may benefit from specific training programmes. Yekatiel and Guttman (1993) compared 20 men and women at least 2 years after a stroke with a similar control group. The retraining group received 45 minute lessons three times a week for 6 weeks. Training consisted of exploring with the patient the nature and extent of sensory loss and the practice of interesting tasks. Vision and the unaffected hand were used to teach 'tactics of perception'. Each lesson started and ended with a sensory task which the person was able to perform successfully. The tasks included identification of the number of touches or lines, numbers and letters drawn on the arm and hand; discrimination of shape, weight and texture of objects placed in the hand and passive drawing in which the therapist held the patient's hand, holding a pencil, and draws with it. The blindfolded patient had to identify the figure by choosing from four figures on a card. The unaffected and affected hands were used alternately. At the conclusion of the 6 weeks, subjects were tested on touch location, sense of elbow position, two-point discrimination and stereognosis. The training group overall showed a large and significant improvement in the sensory function of the hand. Although individual gains varied widely, no subject in the training group showed a decrease in score and some subjects made a marked improvement. No subjects in the control group showed any improvement.

There are several points of interest in this study. Subjects were two or more years post-stroke, a period when impairment is generally considered to be irreparable. In addition, as the authors point out, emphasis in training was on 'multi-modality problem-solving', with patients being 'encouraged to seek and use input from the paretic hand'. There is no evidence that motor performance improved since it was not tested. However, it is likely, if such a programme was carried out in addition to task-related motor training and exercise, that there might be a carryover effect. A similar study was carried out by Carey and colleagues (1993), who report the results of a programme of specific sensory stimulation on certain aspects of sensory discrimination in a group of people following a recent stroke (see Chapter 9).

In clinical practice, training of an action such as sit-to-stand, manipulating objects or walking, will provide the sensory inputs which normally are utilized in the control of those movements. It may be necessary to have the individual pay conscious attention to certain critical inputs, for example, the sense of pressure through the soles of the feet in sit-to-stand, the shape or texture of an object. However, it is very likely that any extraneous and irrelevant inputs provided by the therapist would have either a confusing effect or are merely seen as redundant and are therefore ignored by the system. It is possible, as a result of practice with relevant inputs and feedback, that individuals may be better able to use the information available (Proteau 1992; Abrams and Pratt 1993).

Muscle strengthening and physical conditioning in neurorehabilitation

A muscle or muscle group has to be strong enough for what it has to do, i.e., capable of generating sufficient force to bring about an intended action. The force generated has to be timed appropriately and synergistic muscle activity coordinated. In addition, muscles have to be capable of generating force over relatively long periods of time. We need endurance, for example, to walk up a long flight of stairs. We need to be able to build up the necessary force fast enough for the demands of the environment (crossing the street at traffic lights) and the task (using a keyboard or pushing buttons).

We also need to be conditioned for the type of activities in which we are involved. Hence, walking up stairs requires the lower limb muscles to generate more force than walking on a level surface; walking up stairs carrying a load of books requires more strength and endurance than walking up without an additional load. Normally our muscles are strong enough and our cardiovascular system sufficiently conditioned to enable us to carry out the actions of our daily lives. If, however, we want to do something that requires more muscle power, we need to undergo strengthening, endurance and fitness training to enable us to perform as well as possible. The link between muscle strength and function is therefore intuitively obvious.

An acute lesion affecting the central motor system commonly results in a disruption to the motor neurons normally activating muscles, with the result that the individual experiences paralysis or weakness of muscles (Chapter 8). Following a traumatic brain injury, there may be a long period of immobility imposed by skeletal fractures or by a comatose state. Following a stroke, immobility may result from an initial period of unconsciousness and also from spending a large part of the day, even in rehabilitation, sitting in a wheelchair and inactive. The older person who has a stroke may also have previously led a sedentary lifestyle, and have become deconditioned even before the stroke.

It is known that imposed immobility is associated with a secondary atrophy and weakness of muscles (MacDougall et al. 1977; Grimby *et al.* 1980; Imms 1980; White and Davies 1984; Rutherford *et al.* 1990) and investigations of muscle following disuse have shown decreased muscle volume and cross-sectional area (Sargeant *et al.* 1977; Ingemann-Hansen and Halkjaer-Kristensen 1980; Young *et al.* 1982). It has been suggested that muscles which are atrophied may respond more quickly to training, and to a greater extent than muscles which are not. For example, increases in muscle strength and size with training following musculoskeletal injury have been reported as greater than those reported in able-bodied subjects (Imms *et al.* 1977; Ingemann-Hansen and Halkjaer-Kristensen 1980; Jones and Rutherford 1987).

Despite the fact that both the neural lesion and imposed immobility are known to be associated with muscle weakness, for four decades there has been an insistence by many therapists that strength training plays only a minor part in neurorehabilitation (e.g., Bobath 1970; O'Sullivan 1998; 1990; Cornall 1991). In part, this idea arose as a reaction to the traditional strengthening paradigm in which single joint movements were performed against resistance, a paradigm which did not fit easily with the idea that patients needed to improve functional movement. However, the idea persists, apparently due to the continued belief that resisted exercise would increase spasticity. There is no evidence that this is so, and increasing evidence that exercise can be associated with a decrease in hyperreflexia and muscle stiffness (see Chapter 8).

Rather than increasing spasticity, it is more likely that repetitive strengthening exercises (utilizing appropriate force-generation) might decrease spastic stiffness both by improving the neural control of muscle and by maintaining the extensibility of muscle. Stiffening of a limb (co-contraction) is typically associated with a lack of skill in motor performance. The gradual acquisition of skill is accompanied by a decrease in muscle force, a decrease in co-contraction of agonist and antagonist and more efficient motor unit recruitment (Milner-Brown *et al.* 1975; Sale *et al.* 1983). Exercise has been shown to affect motor unit activation (Sale 1987). Exercise, including strength training, should therefore be beneficial where there are decreases in spinal motor neuron activation due to central lesion and secondary disuse. Increases in strength considered to be due to neural adaptation have been reported in patients with neuromuscular disease (McCartney *et al.* 1987). It is quite clear that exercise (activity) affects both structure and function of muscle.

According to Nativ (1993), dynamic or isokinetic resistance training invokes both autogenic and reciprocal inhibition and it should, therefore, lengthen stiff, shortened (spastic) muscles. He points out that the process of repeatedly contracting a muscle against resistance then stretching it should help increase rather than decrease the range of motion around the targeted joint. He suggests this occurs by way of reciprocal inhibition to the antagonist muscle, followed by autogenic inhibition to the eccentrically working agonist. Isometric resistance training in able-bodied subjects has been shown to decrease coactivation of antagonists, due, according to the authors, to an adaptation of the neuromuscular system (Carolan and Cafarelli 1992).

If resisted exercise is carried out as task-related practice (with at least body weight or weight of a limb as resistance), as in repeated standing up and sitting down or reaching to pick up an object (of light or heavy weight), then such exercise is likely to result in:

- Increased muscle strength (increased force-generating capacity).
- Increased skill (increased coordination of muscle activations).
- Increased extensibility and decreased stiffness of muscle.

The first two involve improved firing and synchronization of motor units, and improved agonist–antagonist and synergic coordination; the third, an increase in muscle length and improved muscle mechanics. Task-related exercises have, therefore, the potential to increase the control of movement and functional performance of the everyday actions which are the focus of the exercise.

The profound effect of the negative features of the upper motor neuron syndrome as a result of a decrease in descending fibres from cortex to final motor neuron population is well known and the weakness and loss of coordination is well documented.

There have recently been a few interesting reports showing the effects of muscle strengthening in neurorehabilitation. As one would expect, significant relationships have been found between measures of muscle strength and measures of motor performance and functional activity in patients following stroke and in elderly subjects. For example:

- Grip strength with Motor Club assessment scores (Sunderland *et al.* 1989).
- Wrist extension strength with upper limb function (Wilson *et al.* 1984).
- Lower limb muscle strength with:
    Fugl-Meyer motor scores (Sjostrom *et al.* 1980).
    Alternating movements of the lower limb (Bohannon and Dubuc 1984).
    Gait (Bohannon 1986, 1987b, 1991a,b; Wade and Hewer 1987; Olesen et al. 1988).
    Stair climbing (Bohannon and Walsh 1991).
    Balance in standing (Bohannon 1987c, 1988; Tinetti 1987; Lord *et al.* 1991).

Muscle weakness has also been found to be a predictor of poor outcome after stroke (e.g., Logigian *et al.* 1983; Fullerton *et al.* 1988; Olsen 1990).

Several studies have shown positive effects of physical conditioning programmes (involving strength, endurance, flexibility and coordination) in older individuals and in individuals following brain lesion (Cohadon 1981; Cardenas and Clawson 1990; Posner *et al.* 1990; Sullivan *et al.* 1990; Lord and Castell 1994). Significant increases in muscle strength have been reported in elderly subjects following strength training (Larsson 1982; Frontera *et al.* 1988), including high-intensity training (Fiatarone *et al.* 1990). Even in patients with progressive neurological disease, increases in muscle strength and endurance and a decrease in fatiguability have been found initially after strength training (Milner-Brown *et al.* 1986; Milner-Brown and Miller 1988a,b).

The issue of fatiguability is of interest when rehabilitation includes exercise and training protocols. The findings of a study of able-bodied adults, in which subjects trained to increase strength of elbow flexors with or without rests, have shown a greater short-term increase in strength when subjects exercised without rests (Rooney *et al.* 1994). Subjects performed 6 (progressing to 10) lifts of a 6RM load (the largest load which could be lifted 6 times) at each session. Those in the rest group rested for 30 seconds between lifts. These results are interesting since following acute brain lesion patients are typically given too few repetitions to enable an increase in muscle strength (or to optimize learning). The reason given is often that the patient may experience fatigue. The dilemma is, of course, that the less people do the more fatigued they feel. We suggest that, provided the person's medical condition is satisfactory, repetition is critical to a successful training programme and that patients need to understand that a degree of fatigue (principally muscle fatigue) is normal after exercise.

Increased strength (i.e. skill) may be due to an increase in the 'efficiency' of motor neuron recruitment as noted for able-bodied subjects (Sale *et al.* 1983), comprising such factors as improved neural coordination between agonists and antagonists and synchronization of motor unit activity (Milner-Brown *et al.* 1975). In a disabled population, with primary impairments affecting muscle activation and secondary disuse changes, it is likely that a large part of any initial strength increases associated with exercise and training will be from an increase in neural activation and neural adaptation (see McCartney *et al.* 1987). It is also likely that there is improved coordination of the muscles within the specific synergy trained, as well as an increase in the mechanical efficiency of the muscle.

Supraspinal influence from motor cortex on spinal motor neurons appears to be enhanced by strength training leading to an elevated level of motor unit synchronization. This was suggested by Milner-Brown and colleagues (1975) in discussing the findings of their study of able-bodied weightlifters undergoing strength training. It is likely, therefore, as we and others (e.g., Nativ 1993) have suggested, that strength training in individuals with brain lesions, particularly if it is related to the performance of everyday tasks, may have a neural retraining effect.

In summary, it is likely that muscle strengthening exercise in this population can consist of three types of exercise according to the individual's needs at a particular time:

- Repetitive graded exercise in which a weakened muscle group is exercised with the aim of it regaining the capacity to generate force both to move and brake a segment.
- Repetitive graded exercise in which a weakened muscle group is exercised at length and in modes of contraction related to a particular action/task.
- Repetitive practice of those functional actions which have been made ineffective by muscle weakness.

The first type of exercise is aimed at increasing the ability of a muscle to contract. The second is more specific to particular actions and is followed by practice of that action. For example, strengthening of lower limb extensor muscles on a isokinetic machine can be followed by the more task-related stepping exercises and by practice of stair walking.

The first types of exercise can be effective in helping a person elicit activity in a muscle group which appears paralysed. At this time, feedback about torque generated, for example, provides incentive. Attempts to control the muscles eccentrically may be more successful initially than concentric action. Also, a patient who cannot activate a muscle in a shortened position may be able to do so when that muscle is lengthened (Carr and Shepherd 1987a), where more torque can typically be generated (Bohannon 1986). We have found that a short period using an isokinetic exercise machine to train quadriceps eccentrically and concentrically, with feedback on torque produced, can enable a person after acute brain lesion, with no apparent ability to activate the muscles prior to exercise, to sustain sufficient contraction to prevent knee collapse in standing. It is also possible that modified gymnasium equipment would provide a means by which disabled individuals could practise generating, grading and timing muscle force. To achieve the necessary strength improvements, progressive application of resistance is required, at 80% of maximum voluntary strength (see Fiatarone *et al.* 1990). Some part of exercise and training of actions should also involve having the patient move as fast as possible (or at least to increase speed). Difficulty generating the high forces needed to move at higher speeds is known to be a problem following acute brain lesion (Bohannon 1987b).

Everyday actions that require substantial muscle force may need to be modified early in training in order to provide graded practice. For example, sit-to-stand requires a strong burst of muscle activity in knee extensor muscles in particular, but also in coordination with hip and ankle extensor muscles, around the time the thighs lift off the seat. Practice of sit-to-stand without sufficient strength in the muscles of one leg results in adaptive performance in which the other leg is favoured and the hands are used to aid vertical propulsion and balance. If the action is modified by increasing the height of the seat, less muscle force has to be produced at thighs-off as the body mass does not have to move so far and the amplitude of segmental movement is not so great. As the muscles become stronger, the seat can be incrementally lowered, in this way providing progressive resistance exercise (body mass providing resistance) in a task-related manner. It is likely that exercise such as this for the lower limb extensor muscles might transfer to improved performance of similar actions in which the body mass pivots over the feet as base of support, such as stair climbing, hill climbing and bending to pick up an object from the floor.

Finally, there has yet to be a substantial body of experimental evidence collected regarding the effect of task-related strengthening exercise on both muscle strength and motor performance in neurological rehabilitation and no studies of the effects of exercise on brain function or reorganization. Resisted exercise of various types, electrical stimulation and EMG feedback have been shown to improve both strength and performance (Bohannon 1993). Furthermore, the results of studies such as those of treadmill walking, finger exercises, stepping exercise and sit-to-stand as exercise, although reporting only measures of function and not of strength, also suggest that the improvements seen in performance are very likely to be due to increases in muscle strength and synergic control.

It is well known that inactivity leads to significant changes to muscle (MacDougall *et al.* 1980; Rutherford *et al.* 1990). Given the older age group of many individuals with acute brain lesion, it is very likely that muscle weakness arises in part from pre-lesion inactivity and particularly from inactivity in the post-lesion period, in addition to the direct effects of the lesion on muscle activation. Many older individuals are probably in need of intensive exercise to improve their general strength and fitness, in addition to exercise and training specific to their neural impairments.

It is important to further developments of intervention that future studies test whether strengthening exercises not only lead to a measurable improvement in functional performance but also an increase in dynamic or static strength.

Skill acquisition in the restoration of optimal functional motor performance

Skill has been defined in many ways. However, one definition which has explanatory value for the clinic is from Annett (1971, pp. 266–271):

> a skill is any human activity which becomes better organized and more effective as the result of practice.

When an adult has a brain lesion affecting the motor control system, as a result of muscle weakness and inability to control the pattern of muscle activations, skill in action is either lost or severely impaired. The person can no longer perform actions which were previously easily performed as the individual interacted with the world around. After the period in which the immediate effects of the lesion wear off, any change in motor performance probably occurs through a process of learning (adapting). However, what is it that is learned and what does this involve at the neural level? Is there a difference between this process and that which occurs in non brain-lesioned individuals when they learn a novel action?

We take the view, and there is theoretical support from animal experiments and increasingly in investigations of humans, that the process is likely to be similar, with, however, some important differences. Some of the neural 'equipment' previously used in initiating and controlling action is impaired as a result of the lesion. In a system that utilizes multiple connections in order to translate a goal into action, damage to one part of it will require reorganization. As a result, the re-learning process must resemble in some ways the process that occurs when someone learns a completely new action that they have never performed before. Since the physical structure of the brain has been altered and function disrupted, the neural mechanisms underlying the performance of a new version of an 'old' action (say, sit-to-stand) may be different both anatomically and functionally from those processes which brought about the action prior to the brain lesion. Neural mechanisms underlying learning and processes affecting learning are discussed elsewhere. (See Chapter 1 for discussion.)

Fluency of movement is an important criterion of skilled motor behaviour. Movement becomes more efficient with learning and this is probably due to improvements in timing, tuning and coordination of muscle activations (Rosenbaum 1991). The learning (relearning) process of disabled individuals with muscle paralysis or weakness is closely related to the greater efficiency arising out of increased muscle strength, i.e., increased force-generating capacity, endurance and physical fitness.

When patients attempt to move after an acute lesion, their first attempts reflect the distribution of muscle weakness and the resultant adaptive motor pattern. At the initial attempt, the adaptive movement emerges spontaneously. If it is reasonably effective it is repeated and may become learned or habitual. In the able-bodied, as skill increases, counterproductive or unnecessary movements tend to decrease (Sparrow 1983; Sparrow and Irizarry-Lopez 1987). Vincken (1984) showed that when subjects were confronted with a novel skill, they moved slowly with tense muscles. After practice, Vincken found performance took less time and the movement was smoother. He linked the increased ease of movement with decreased muscle 'stiffness', i.e., tension. There have been many reports describing the changes in muscle activation patterns associated with lack of skill together with the need to generate large forces. For example, additional muscles were recruited when there was an increased need for force generation (Gellhorn 1947; Gregg *et al.* 1957; Devine *et al.* 1981). Precision tasks may also be associated with a spread of muscle activity beyond the task muscles (Carey *et al.* 1983) when performed by the relatively unskilled.

Much of the training of actions for some individuals with a brain lesion may need to be directed toward ineffective motor adaptations. In attempting to generate muscle force, the force output is typically relatively uncontrolled. This may be manifested by muscle co-contraction with the appearance of stiffness, or by difficulty reducing agonist muscle force to the level required for the action. Training may, therefore, consist of teaching the person to control muscle activity, in other words, to match force generation to the needs of the task. It is generally considered that there should be a minimum expenditure of energy consistent with the goal to be achieved (MacConaill and Basmajian 1969) and that increased skill equates with greater efficiency of force production. Decreased EMG output has been noted in several investigations as able-bodied subjects increased their skill (e.g., Mulder and Hulstijn 1985; Sale 1987). This is considered to be due to increased muscular efficiency; i.e., as a result of training, muscles become more effective in producing tension, recruiting fewer motor units or lowering the firing rate of motor units.

It has been observed that unskilled learners demonstrate different patterns of interlimb coordination as they attempt to deal with the complexity of controlling several body segments during movement. Bernstein (1967) suggested that novices control the segmental linkages by cutting down on the joints that are free to move, i.e., by locking some joints, only freeing them up as they gain more experience. This proposal was confirmed in a study of pistol shooting (Arutyunyan *et al.* 1968). Novices initially held wrists and elbows rigid, then released them as they developed skill. A similar result has been reported for dart throwing (McDonald *et al.* 1989).

Movements made with tense muscles are more energy-consuming and lead to fatigue more quickly than relaxed movements (Whiting *et al.* 1987). The fact that a skilled performer demonstrates less energy expenditure than one who is unskilled is probably due to a number of factors associated with the elimination of unnecessary muscular activity. These include the minimizing of postural work by the development of more efficient balance and coordination and the modification of necessary movements to ensure they are of appropriate speed and direction (Shephard 1972).

Since the environment plays a significant role in modulating motor performance, specific aspects of the environment in training can be utilized to channel and direct the motor output. Similarly, if an action is too difficult for an individual with movement dysfunction, some feature of the environment can be modified to make the task possible without too much physical struggle.

The environment can be altered to set up conditions that force muscles to contract. Examples include object placement that forces the person to increase external rotation of the glenohumeral joint; applying pressure down along the shank forces quadriceps to rotate the thigh over the fixed shank (see Fig. 5.17b); walking on a treadmill forces an increased amplitude of hip extension and stretches the soleus muscle prior to ankle plantarflexion (push-off) (see Fig. 5.23).

The environment may be modified to provide constraint of unwanted actions. For example, a seat may be modified to prevent an undesirable body alignment.

Perceptual-cognitive factors

Action comprises not only motor factors but also cognitive/perceptual factors. The obvious conceptual links between knowing and doing (Newell 1981), i.e. cognition and action, are increasingly being recognized in the neurosciences. However, the traditional emphasis in neurorehabilitation remains largely on the motor system and perceptual-cognitive aspects of function tend to be ignored (Mulder 1991). There is, however, an increasing body of theoretical clinical literature in which the need to recognize and incorporate the action–cognition link in rehabilitation is advocated (Carr and Shepherd 1987a,b; Mulder 1991).

In everyday life, virtually every movement we make is linked to an intention. As we move we are selecting, from all the information that is available (both internally derived sensations and those coming from the environment), the most essential to the task at hand. It is unlikely, therefore, that skill in action will be (re)gained unless that action is practised under the appropriate environmental conditions. We are learning not only the appropriate motor pattern but also to select the most appropriate information in order to match the intention or the goal to the action and the environment (Higgins 1972). One of the important functions of the therapist (as coach) is setting up the conditions of practice to facilitate this process.

In rehabilitation, attentiveness is a necessary part of practice and improved performance has been found to be associated with improved attention (Diller 1970). In primate research, it has been shown that attention can have a powerful effect on the responses of individual neurons. In some cases it leads to enhancement of neuronal responses to items attended to; in others to suppression of those which are unattended (Wise and Desimone 1988). Eye contact between patient and therapist encourages attentiveness and increases motivation (Mehrabian 1969). A reminder to watch the object may be necessary when an individual is easily distracted or when attention is inappropriately focused.

Motivation

We have to want to do what we are learning to do. Success appears a motivating force, and in the early stages of learning probably increases the person's level of aspiration. Motivation can be provided by reward, by positive reinforcement, by an understanding of the goals and their relevance. Belmont and colleagues (1969) suggested that the possibility of brain-damaged patients requiring 'unique motivating conditions for performance has received little consideration' and this is probably true 30 years later.

It is evident that some individuals following acute brain lesions tend to be unmotivated and relatively passive if left to practise on their own during rehabilitation. There may be a number of reasons for this, including poor memory, distractibility, perceptual-cognitive dysfunction, depression and even boredom in non-stimulating surroundings. Stress, tension and anxiety, although they may not adversely affect motor performance, may depress it under certain conditions (Singer 1980), particularly in terms of complex tasks.

There is said to be a tendency for individuals in an institutional environment to develop what has been termed 'learned helplessness' (Seligman 1975). Perception of lost effectiveness in events that a person tries repeatedly to control is said to result first in anxiety. This is followed by depression which is characterized by apathy and a giving up of

trying that generalizes to other facets of life (Abrahamson *et al.* 1978).

Apparent lack of motivation, however, may also indicate that the tasks to be practised have little meaning or relevance for the patient. Physiotherapy may lack motivating impact by not being immediately and obviously relevant to the person's needs, or not sufficiently difficult or challenging to require concentration. The rehabilitation environment may also be non-motivating by being too undemanding and insufficiently geared to the patient as active learner.

The following sections describe some methods to promote motor learning/skill acquisition and thereby improve motor performance.

Information: instruction, demonstration and feedback

Information about performance that is available to the learner, either before, during or after the performance, is an important factor in optimizing skill acquisition (Newell 1981) and is, therefore, of practical importance for both therapist and patient in rehabilitation.

The most commonly used methods for conveying information about the goal and appropriate action sequences are verbal instructions and demonstrations (e.g., Newell 1981; Johnson 1984; Gentile 1987). Information may focus on kinematic description, for example, angular displacements, paths of body parts, which requires an understanding by the therapist of linked segment dynamics and the biomechanical necessities of the action to be learned.

Instructions

Instructions are given in such a way as to present a clear goal and to reduce uncertainty. In addition, it seems that the goal, in order for it to be pursued with enthusiasm, needs to be perceived as worthwhile and meaningful to that individual. As an example, tasks that have goals which are directed toward controlling one's physical interaction with objects or persons in the immediate environment seem to have more meaning than goals which are directed at movement for its own sake, and there is evidence that individuals perform better when an action is presented as a concrete task as opposed to an abstract task. These two types of task differ in the degree to which the required action is directed toward controlling physical interaction with the environment as opposed to merely moving a limb.

Van der Weel and colleagues (1991) have recently described an experiment in which the difference between performance on a concrete task compared to an abstract task which required the same action, pronation and supination of the forearm, was examined. The subjects were 9 children with cerebral palsy (CP) of hemiplegic distribution aged between 3 and 7 years and a group of non-disabled children. The authors found that the children with CP significantly increased movement range into both pronation and supination during performance of the concrete task (beating two drums by alternately supinating and pronating) compared to the abstract task in which they were asked to supinate and pronate the forearm as far as they could. Given that supination is often a particularly difficult movement to perform in individuals with brain dysfunction, it is interesting that supination range increased by more than 20% in the children with CP.

In explanation, the authors point out that movement is not an independent process but an integral part of an act. The extent and quality of movement depend on how much practice the individual has in performing the action, how interested the person is and the quality of the information available. Concrete tasks are associated with more information from the environment than abstract tasks. The drum in this experiment would have provided visual, auditory and tactile information about the individual's relationship with it and feedback information about the attainment of the goal. The abstract task would have depended primarily upon proprioceptive inputs about sense of muscle effort and limb configuration, together with visual inputs.

As another example, Leont'ev and Zaporzhets (1960) had patients with restricted range of motion of the elbow or shoulder as a result of injury raise their forearm or whole arm (depending on the site of injury) in four actions that varied from abstract to concrete. The actions were to raise the arm: (1) as far as possible with eyes shut; (2) as far as possible with eyes open; (3) to a specific point on a ruled screen; and (4) to grasp an object. The results indicated that the amplitude of movement increased progressively from task 1 to task 4, i.e., as the task became more concrete.

Demonstration

The goal of the action and the movements to be executed can be demonstrated either live or on videotape. The empirical work on the effectiveness

of demonstration, however, has been sporadic and the results equivocal. One of the reasons for equivocal results is that the videotaped demonstration is sometimes distant from actual practice in both time and place. Gonella and colleagues (1981), however, demonstrated that self-instruction using an audiovisual medium was effective in enabling able-bodied subjects to learn the new skill of crutch walking. The hypothesis that subjects could learn the cognitive aspects of the motor task in one viewing of the film was supported and transfer of learning to the physical performance of the task was found to occur.

Modelling of an action, either by videotape or by the 'teacher' performing the action, can help the learner develop an understanding, a conceptual representation (Carroll and Bandura 1982), or template (Keele and Summers 1976) of the action. Demonstration can be given by the therapist (see Fig. 4.17), and by a videotape of the desirable performance (the model). As a general rule, instruction is kept to a minimum in order to avoid overloading the individual with information.

Cognition plays a significant role in this observational learning since the patient must attend selectively to the model and to the critical features ('essential components': Carr and Shepherd 1987a) of the model. Observation seems to assist an individual to learn the temporal and spatial aspects of an action. The spatial relationship of therapist to patient may therefore be critical to the success of modelling, certainly in the initial stages when the patient is striving to understand the action. For example, observational learning has been found to be better if both model and subject maintain the same spatial orientation, i.e. reaching with the same hand side by side (Greenwald and Albert 1968), providing an 'image of the act' (Whiting and den Brinker 1982). Observation allows the patient to see the amplitude of the movement, appreciate the timing and fluency of the action, and the relationship between body parts. Whiting *et al.* (1987) showed that able-bodied subjects learning a new action who had access to a dynamic model of an expert performer produced more coordinated action than subjects who did not.

Feedback

Feedback refers to the use of sensory information for the control of action and the process of skill acquisition (Winstein and Schmidt 1989). It can be positive or negative, subjective or objective, and it may motivate the learner as well as provide information. Knowledge of results (KR) is information related to achievement of the goal of the action and is known to be one of the most potent variables in learning (Annett and Kay 1957; Newell 1976). KR provides guidance so that the individual knows what to do on the next attempt. After all, error identification is probably not useful in itself, the individual needs to know what to do about it. KR may provide an energizing function (Adams 1987), the individual striving to do better on the next attempt. KR that involves the kinematics and/or the kinetics of the action (Wallace and Hagler 1979; Newell and Walter 1981; Wood *et al.* 1992) may be particularly useful where individuals are learning a complex movement sequence as in sit-to-stand or walking.

A second type of feedback, commonly referred to as knowledge of performance (KP), provides information about how the movement was performed. Both KP and KR can be provided by the therapist verbally, through demonstration and through the use of electronic devices (e.g., videotape, EMG, forceplate system, computer games).

The physiotherapist uses *verbal (auditory) feedback* as a training technique in the clinic to provide reinforcement in the attainment of a goal, 'Yes, you did it', and to give information related to performance, 'Try again – this time push down more through your left foot'. With individuals who have an auditory perception impairment (as in receptive dysphasia), such feedback needs to be modified according to the person's capacity to understand the spoken word and a smile or a nod can also indicate whether an action should be repeated as before. Since accurate feedback is essential to learning, the therapist should avoid using positive feedback, 'Good', when it is inaccurate, and instead confine its use to situations in which it will encourage the individual to repeat a successful or nearly successful performance. That is, there should not be a mismatch between the consequence of an action and the feedback. For example, when a person can see that a goal, 'Pick up the glass', has not been achieved, it is meaningless if the therapist (as coach) says 'Good'.

As long ago as 1927, Thorndike showed that practice with right/wrong feedback was more effective in bringing about learning than practice alone. His subjects, with vision obstructed, drew 3-, 4-, 5- and 6-inch (5-, 7-, 13-, 15-cm) lines and the experimenter said 'right' if the line was within a tolerance band around the correct length, or 'wrong' if it was not. The subjects who had practised with feedback improved their percentage of right scores from 13% at pre-test to 55% in the final session (after 4200 lines were drawn). When subjects had no feedback, the percentage of correct lines remained similar after 5400 lines were drawn. The findings of Trowbridge and Cason (1932) supported Thorndike's work but added another dimension to it. They showed that quantitative feedback about the extent of error produced faster learning than qualitative feedback such as 'right' or 'wrong'.

Augmented feedback utilizes visual or auditory feedback to give objective information related to some aspect of performance or a physiological process of which a person is not normally aware. For example, feedback about critical kinematic or kinetic features of an action provides information which is directly relevant to the action the individual is striving to learn. A major advantage is that the person can practise relatively independently, with some supervision from the therapist, and gain pleasure and a sense of achievement from their own intended actions.

One potential value of biofeedback devices is their use in training or work 'stations', set up by the therapist, where patients can spend a period of time practising different functional actions with monitoring but without the one-to-one presence of the therapist. Feedback devices described in the literature include *pressure-sensitive devices* (forceplate, foot pad) to detect force through a lower limb in walking (Wolf and Binder-McLeod 1982) or sit-to-stand (Enghardt *et al.* 1993; Fowler and Carr 1996), and to give feedback about postural sway in standing (Shumway-Cook *et al.* 1988); *electrogoniometers* to monitor joint angle (Colbourne *et al.* 1993); and *various electronic devices* which provide auditory or visual feedback (e.g., Sachs *et al.* 1976; Smith *et al.* 1985); and *EMG monitors* to provide information about the presence of muscle activity and its amplitude (Wolf *et al.* 1979, 1980).

Biofeedback is not a substitute for motor training but an adjunct. The rationale for such augmented feedback is that an increase in the amount of information available to the individual will lead to an increase in learning and to improved performance (Mulder and Hulstijn 1988). Although there have been a number of investigations of efficacy, the results are ambiguous.

It is likely that failure to demonstrate efficacy in terms of a long-term transfer effect could result either from an inappropriate application of feedback (i.e., not directed at an appropriate goal) or from a failure to incorporate the use of the feedback device into the practice of real-life actions (i.e., lack of specificity). It is also possible that feedback given concurrently, i.e., during practice, may not be retained because the individual learns to rely on it. Once the feedback is withdrawn, however, the individual must rely on other feedback mechanisms. Winstein and colleagues (1996) have recently shown that concurrent feedback appears to have a positive effect during performance but does not aid learning.

Emphasis in several studies has been on using EMG feedback to improve contraction of a muscle or muscles. Although the aim may have been ultimately to improve an action such as walking, the feedback may not have been given during the practice of walking but in such a way that patients focused on the individual muscle rather than on the action required. (See Mulder and Hulstijn 1988, for discussion.) Compare, for example, Enghardt's successful use of a feedback device incorporated into standing up practice and designed to give meaningful feedback about a critical aspect of the action.

The withdrawal of the device is not necessarily followed by a continuation of the desired behaviour. The individual may lack the ability to generalize a newly learned skill to different environments. Augmented feedback would probably be optimally effective when combined with training of specific actions and withdrawn gradually so that the individual learns to perform the action using naturally occurring feedback mechanisms and with the realization by the individual that there are important benefits to be gained from the improved performance gained during the feedback training.

Future developments of electronic devices (including interactive computer games) to provide feedback and motivation should enable patients to enjoy performing exercise programmes designed to increase strength and control of specific muscle groups, accuracy of movement and to improve physical fitness in the context of specific goal-directed and meaningful actions. A major use should be made, in our view, of EMG feedback from paralysed muscles, for both patient and therapist, as a guide to whether or not muscles are activated in the early stage after an acute lesion. Feedback from deltoid muscle, for example, as the patient attempts to move the arm (see Fig. 6.17), could help determine optimum position(s) and action(s) for the patient to practise without the therapist.

The potential of electronic devices in motor training has not yet been realized, perhaps partly because of continued emphasis on the 'handling' techniques of the therapist rather than on the patient as an active participant in an intensive training process. The most neglected issue in the debate on augmented feedback may be in relation to the timing of muscle activity, i.e., force production. Devices which force the patient to focus on timing during the performance of an action may well prove to be more effective than devices commonly described in which the focus is more on the amplitude of the signal.

Manual guidance

In the skill acquisition literature, there are said to be two types of manual guidance used in training, *passive movement* and *spatio-temporal constraint* or *physical restriction* (Holding 1965, 1970, 1989; Newell 1981). During training in the clinic, passive movement may involve placing a limb in a position that enables a movement to take place (see Fig. 11.11) or moving a limb passively to give an idea of the action required, i.e., the goal and the spatial characteristics of the action. Spatial constraint may involve holding part of a limb stable, constraining the action spatially while the individual has only to control part of the limb (see Fig. 4.15a). As more control is gained, the physical restraint is reduced, increasing the number of degrees of freedom to be controlled. Manual guidance is replaced by verbal feedback or environmentally driven guidance.

Newell (1981) considered the second type of manual guidance decreases the likelihood of the learner making serious errors and developing bad habits. However, he also pointed out that, provided fundamentally inappropriate actions (which would include what we refer to as ineffective adaptive movements) that would hinder learning are prevented, errors of execution in spatio-temporal details of the action may actually be beneficial to learning. It is only by attempting to carry out a movement to achieve a goal that a person knows whether or not the action attempted is actually successful. Learning requires an element of trial and error. It is possible for the therapist to impede the patient's active attempts at carrying out an action, either by giving so much manual guidance that the person has to do little, or by physically blocking the path of a body part.

Practice

Practice of an action, both with and without supervision, is a necessary condition for acquiring skill in that action. One of the advantages of task-related training is that it enables the individual to see the future benefits of training to improve performance. Ability to stand up independently, for example, means that walking becomes a real possibility.

Practice can be considered as a continuum of procedures from overt practice at one extreme to covert or mental practice at the other (Johnson 1984). As a general rule, skill in performance increases as a direct result of the amount of practice. Repetition is an important part of that practice. It has been shown, for example, that repetition of a task or an exercise can improve performance in disabled as well as in able-bodied individuals (Asanuma and Keller 1991; Butefisch *et al.* 1995). Thousands of repetitions may be necessary (Crossman 1959; Beggs and Howarth 1972; Canning 1987) in order to improve performance to the necessary level of skill.

Repetitive practice is known to be important for learning to occur, as the repetitions enable the system to coordinate the muscular synergies which move the segmental linkage in the desired manner to accomplish the goal of action. Repetition can be described at the cognitive level as repeated attempts to solve a goal-related movement problem by building on the previous attempts; i.e., repetition without repetition (see Bernstein 1967). Repetition with feedback and with the knowledge of what is required (e.g., path of hand in reaching) develops the patient's problem-solving abilities, a cognitive skill which can be transferred to the practice of another action. However, in rehabilitation, repetitive practice of an action is also necessary to increase the strength of the muscle contractions to a level which is necessary to accomplish the goal.

One issue in the motor learning literature which has some interest for rehabilitation is the whole-vs-part method of practice. As a general rule, it seems that the action should be practised in its entirety, particularly when one part of the action is to a large part dependent upon the performance of a preceding part. For example, several studies of sit-to-stand (Schenkman *et al.* 1990; Pai and Rogers 1991; Shepherd and Gentile 1994) have pointed to the importance of flexion of the upper body at the hip in setting up the conditions for ascent into standing. The implication from these studies is that the vertical movement of the body mass is potentiated by the initial upper body flexion, and that the two movements overlap.

Performing the whole action seems important for giving the individual the idea of the action to be achieved (Johnson 1984). However, in rehabilitation, when the individual is having difficulty in activating muscles and generating and timing force, it may be necessary to practise eliciting activity in a particular group of muscles, or to practise one part of the action in order to strengthen a muscle group critical to the performance of the action.

Selecting components which are critical across similar actions may increase the generalizability of exercise. It is becoming evident that the actions possible in using our multisegmental linkage to interact with the environment can be classified into functional groups (see Chapter 6 for discussion of functional groupings of fingers). A major functional grouping of the lower limbs involves the hips, knees and ankles flexing and extending over the feet as fixed base of support (Fig. 2.1). One could consider, therefore, as one class of action, all

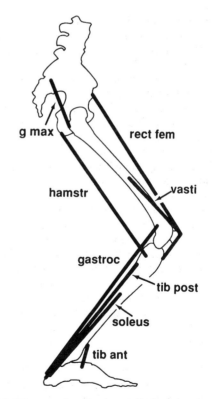

Fig. 2.1 Diagram showing lower limb segments and eight functional muscle groups affecting segmental rotation (reprinted from Kuo and Zajac (1993) by kind permission of Elsevier Science, Amsterdam, The Netherlands)

actions in which the lower limb extensor muscles (monoarticular and biarticular) contract concentrically and eccentrically to raise and lower the body mass, for example, sit-to-stand, squat-to-stand, bending to pick up an object, stance phase of walking including stair walking. The patient has to learn the 'rules' of this class of action, rules which can be applied to similar actions with some minor modification. This may be why practice of exercises such as the stepping exercise appears to generalize into improvement of other similar actions, such as walking (Nugent *et al.* 1994). There is some evidence in the motor learning literature of a positive transfer to similar tasks (Oxendine 1984; Gottlieb *et al.* 1988).

As another example, to reach for an object in sitting requires the ability to balance and move the body mass over the base of support (the thighs and feet). Practice of moving about by reaching for objects on the floor and reaching in a horizontal plane in different directions enables the individual to test the limits of stability and to expand these limits to increase the reaching distance. By varying the tasks or the placement of objects, the individual can be 'pushed' to the limits of stability. Reaching to one side requires that the lower limb on that side be used actively as the base of support, the extent of active use varying according to conditions such as direction, speed and distance to be moved (Dean 1997). Such exercise not only improves balance and reaching ability in sitting but also gives practice of generating force (weight-bearing) through the foot of the affected leg (Dean and Shepherd 1997). Since reaching forward beyond arm's length is similar biomechanically to the pre-extension phase of sit-to-stand, it is not surprising that there is some evidence of generalizability of such practice into improved sit-to-stand performance (Dean and Shepherd 1997). Variable practice, i.e., practice on a range of related tasks, has been found to lead to better performance than consistent practice of the one task (e.g., Newell 1981; Johnson 1984; Gentile 1987).

Mental practice

Also called mental rehearsal or visualization, mental practice involves thinking through the action to be performed. The relationship between motor and mental activity has been described by many authors over the years (Jacobson 1932; Jones 1965; Cardinall 1977; Yue and Cole 1992). Mapping of brain activity (using PET) during passive observation of someone else's hand, and while imagining grasping objects with their own hand, has shown different patterns of brain activity for each mental activity, despite no movement having occurred (Decety *et al.* 1994). When subjects were observing hand movements, activation was principally in visual cortical areas, but also in areas involved in motor behaviour (e.g., basal ganglia and cerebellum). When they imagined moving their own hand, cortical and subcortical areas involved in motor preparation and programming were active. Roland and colleagues (1980a,b), using regional cerebral blood flow (rCBF), have previously found the supplementary motor area exclusively involved. Decety and co-workers' findings suggest that their two mental tasks involve neural mechanisms which are involved in planning and programming. This provides considerable impetus to the increasing move for maximizing a patient's participation in active rehabilitation.

Cardinall (1977) suggested that 2–3 minutes' mental practice at a time, done between therapy sessions, may be sufficient, but suggests that mental practice may only be suitable for patients who do not have communication or perceptual problems and who are able to understand the idea. Care should be taken that the patient understands the details of the task to be practised in this way.

Unsupervised practice

Just as a person who wants to become skilled at a sporting activity, or in music or chess playing, will spend many hours a day in practice, so also a person who wants to regain skill in everyday actions needs to practise intensively in rehabilitation, not only during formal training sessions with the therapist giving individual advice and assistance. This situation, however, is not common in rehabilitation units, where only a very small proportion of the day may be spent in therapy sessions (see Chapter 1), with little if any time spent by the patient in unsupervised practice.

It is apparent that patients do not always carry out the instructions for independent practice expected of them by their therapists. Belmont and colleagues (1969) observed individuals with hemiplegia and non brain-injured individuals in sessions with the therapist present and without the therapist, who had been given instructions to keep working on their exercises. The proportion of time spent in practice fell from 82% to 52% when the therapist left the disabled group and from 91% to 87% for the able-bodied group. This result may reflect as much on the organization of unsupervised practice by the therapist as on the patients themselves. Nevertheless, unsupervised practice needs to take this factor into account.

For meaningful and intensive practice to take place outside formal training sessions requires that:

- The environment is organized to enable safe, independent, relatively unsupervised practice to take place.
- Therapists change their attitudes to rehabilitation so that some time is allocated to instructing the patient during intensive training periods, in providing workbooks, and in organizing a suitable physical environment that is challenging and which provides interesting and motivating feedback.
- An attitude is instilled into patients and nursing staff through which it is clear that the patient will need to work hard if the process of rehabilitation is to be optimally successful.

Part of planning for independent practice involves organizing methods of prompting the patient's attention to the actions to be practised. Canning and Adams (1985) report the results of planned covert monitoring of the independent practice of walking in a woman with hemiplegia following stroke. Although she could walk relatively normally in the physiotherapy area, elsewhere she reverted to a short-stepped and wide-based walking pattern. She agreed to being covertly monitored by a group of unknown observers, who would score her on stride width and step length. Observations were tallied daily. After 11 days an improved gait pattern was evident. The use of verbal cueing to help focus attention on particular tasks to be practised has also been reported (Loomis and Boersma 1982).

The issue of time spent in practice is a critical one for motor training in rehabilitation. It is generally considered in the able-bodied population that shorter practice sessions with shorter rest periods extending over a longer period of time are more effective than long practice sessions with longer rest periods (Singer 1980). If patients spent periods of the day positioned at work stations set up to encourage practice of particular actions (similar to circuit training), with therapists within the area but only indirectly supervising (with the help of aides), as well as an intensive period of one-to-one training, the time spent on training and practice could probably be more than doubled without increasing the therapist's load. The work space can be set up to

enable not only task-related exercise and practice (with treadmill for walking, harness for balancing tasks in standing) but also electrical stimulation for, say, paretic shoulder muscles, and practice with electronic feedback and computer-aided devices and exercise machines such as isokinetic dynamometers. Cooperation between physiotherapists and occupational therapists of course also ensures a greater proportion of the patient's day is spent in meaningful practice (see Poole 1991; Sabari 1991). Group work with patients helping each other is another way of increasing the time spent in practice, exercise and activity.

It is not clear with disabled learners how many repetitions of an action are necessary to promote improved performance. Although investigation into the relative effectiveness of consistent versus variable practice supports the prediction that variable practice, in the able-bodied population at least, leads to better performance than consistent practice, there have also been opposite findings (for reviews, see Johnson 1984; Newell 1981; Schmidt 1988; van Rossum 1990). It appears, therefore, that individuals with movement dysfunction may be more likely to regain effective performance of an action if they have the opportunity to practise the action under a variety of relevant conditions. However, where muscle weakness or paralysis interferes with the performance of an action, making it either impossible or ineffective, repetitive exercise in a stable environment may be critical in the initial stage of rehabilitation just to get the muscles contracting and generating force.

In general, it can be said that intensive practice is required:

- To enable a movement pattern to be learned (i.e., to refine the neural commands to the muscles (Gottlieb *et al.*, 1988).
- To strengthen muscles specifically for similar actions.
- To enable a stable pattern to be modified as necessary according to environmental and other demands (i.e., to develop flexibility of performance; to learn the 'rules' of movement in specific contexts).

In summary, the primary purpose of this chapter is to stress the importance of skill learning and physical training in neurorehabilitation. What seems certain at the present time is that the process of rehabilitation must become more active and more intensive for individuals with impairments resulting from brain lesions than it currently seems to be. Evaluation and an understanding of the impairments clarifies the particular emphasis for individuals. However, it is probable that all could benefit from being stronger and more physically conditioned.

References

Abrahamson, L.Y., Seligman, M.E.P. and Teasdale, J.D. (1978) Learned helplessness in humans: critique and reformulation. *Journal of Abnormal Psychology*, **87**, 49–74.

Abrams, R.A. and Pratt, J. (1993) Rapid aimed limb movements: differential effects of practice on component submovements. *Journal of Motor Behaviour*, **25**, 4, 288–298.

Adams, J.A. (1987) Historical review and appraisal of research on the learning, retention, and transfer of human motor skills. *Psychological Bulletin*, **101**, 41–74.

Annett, J. (1971) Acquisition of skill. *British Medical Bulletin*, **27**, 3, 266–271.

Annett, J. and Kay, H. (1957) Knowledge of results and skilled performance. *Occupational Psychology*, **31**, 69–79.

Arutyunyan, G.H., Gurfinkel, V.S. and Mirskii, M.L. (1968) Investigation of aiming at a target. *Biophysics*, **13**, 536–538.

Asanuma, H. and Keller, A. (1991) Neuronal mechanisms of motor learning in mammals. *Neuroreport*, **2**, 217–224.

Asmussen, E. (1953) Positive and negative muscular work. *Acta Physiologica Scandinavia*, **28**, 364–382.

Asmussen, E. and Bonde-Petersen, F. (1974) Storage of elastic energy in skeletal muscles in man. *Acta Physiologica Scandinavia*, **91**, 385–392.

Beggs, W.D.A. and Howarth, C.I. (1972) The movement of the hand towards a target. *Quarterly Journal of Experimental Psychology*, **24**, 448–453.

Behm, D.G. and Sale, D.G. (1994) Intended rather than actual movement velocity determines velocity-specific training response. *Journal of Applied Physiology*, **74**, 359–368.

Belmont, I., Benjamin, H., Ambrose, J. *et al.* (1969) Effect of cerebral damage on motivation in rehabilitation. *Archives of Physical Medicine and Rehabilitation*, **50**, 507.

Bernstein, N. (1967) *The Coordination and Regulation of Movements*, Pergamon Press, London.

Bobath, B. (1970) *Adult Hemiplegia: Evaluation and Treatment*, 3rd edn, Butterworth Heinemann, Oxford.

Bobath, B. (1990) *Adult Hemiplegia: Evaluation and Treatment*, 3rd edn, Butterworth Heinemann, Oxford.

Bohannon, R.W. and Dubuc, W.E. (1984) Documentation of the resolution of weakness in a patient with Guillain-Barré syndrome. *Physical Therapy*, **64**, 1388–1389.

Bohannon, R.W. (1986) Strength of lower limb muscle related to gait velocity and cadence in stroke patients. *Physiotherapy Canada*, **38**, 204–206.

Bohannon, R.W. (1987a) Relative decreases in knee extension torque with increased knee extension velocities in stroke patients with hemiparesis. *Physical Therapy*, **67**, 1218–1220.

Bohannon, R.W. (1987b) Relationship between strength and movement in the paretic lower limb following cerebrovascular accidents. *International Journal of Rehabilitation Research*, **10**, 420–422.

Bohannon, R.W. (1987c) The relationship between static standing capacity and lower limb static strength in hemiparetic stroke patients. *Clinical Rehabilitation*, **1**, 287–291.

Bohannon, R.W. (1988) Determinants of transfer capacity in patients with hemiparesis. *Physiotherapy Canada*, **40**, 236–239.

Bohannon, R.W. (1991a) Interrelationships of trunk and extremity muscle strengths and body awareness following unilateral brain lesions. *Perception and Motor Skills*, **73**, 1016–1018.

Bohannon, R.W. (1991b) Relationship among paretic knee extension strength, maximum weight-bearing, and gait speed in patients with stroke. *Journal of Stroke and Cerebrovascular Disease*, **1**, 65–69.

Bohannon, R.W. (1993) Muscle strength in patients with brain lesions: measurement and implications. In *Muscle Strength* (ed. K. Harms-Ringdahl), Churchill Livingstone, Edinburgh, pp. 187–225.

Bohannon, R.W. and Walsh, S. (1991) Association of paretic lower extremity strength and balance with stair climbing ability in patients with stroke. *Journal of Stroke and Cerebrovascular Disease*, **1**, 129–133.

Bosco, C., Viitasalo, J.T., Komi, P.V. *et al.* (1982) Combined effect of elastic energy and myoelectrical potentiation during stretch–shortening cycle exercise. *Acta Physiologica Scandinavia.*, **114**, 557–565.

Butefisch, C., Hummelsheim, H. and Denzler, P. *et al.* (1995) Repetitive training of isolated movements improves the outcome of motor rehabilitation of the centrally paretic hand. *Journal of the Neurological Sciences*, **130**, 59–68.

Caizzo, V.J., Perrine, J.J. and Edgerton, V.R.(1981) Training-induced alterations of the *in vivo* force-velocity relationship of human muscle. *Journal of Applied Physiology*, **51**, 3, 750–754.

Canning, C. (1987) Training standing up following stroke – a clinical trial. In *Proceedings of the Tenth International Congress of the World Confederation for Physical Therapy*, Sydney, pp. 915–919.

Canning, C. and Adams, R. (1985) Covert monitoring to promote consistency of walking performance: a case study. *Australian Journal of Physiotherapy*, **31**, 152.

Cardenas, D.D. and Clawson, D.R. (1990) Management of lower extremity strength and function in traumatically brain-injured patients. *Journal of Head Trauma Rehabilitation*, **5**, 43.

Cardinall, N. (1977) Mental practice. Paper presented at 53rd Congress of American Physical Therapy Association, St. Louis, MS.

Carey, J.R., Allison, J.D., Mundale, M.O. (1983) Electromyographic study of muscular overflow during precision handgrip. *Physical Therapy*, **63**, 4, 505–511.

Carey, L.M., Matyas, T.A. and Oke, L.E. (1993) Sensory loss in stroke patients: effective training of tactile and proprioceptive discrimination. *Archives of Physical Medicine and Rehabilitation*, **74**, 602–611.

Carolan, B. and Cafarelli, E. (1992) Adaptations in coactivation after isometric resistance training. *Journal of Applied Physiology*, **73**, 911–917.

Carr, J.H. and Shepherd, R.B. (1980) *Physiotherapy in Disorders of the Brain*, Heinemann, London.

Carr, J.H. and Shepherd, R.S. (1987a) *A Motor Relearning Programme for Stroke*, 2nd edn, Butterworth Heinemann, Oxford.

Carr, J.H. and Shepherd, R.B. (1987b) A motor relearning model for rehabilitation. In *Movement Science. Foundations for Physical Therapy in Rehabilitation* (eds. J.H. Carr and R.B. Shepherd) Aspen Publishers, Rockville, MD, p. 31–92.

Carroll, W.R. and Bandura, A. (1982) The role of visual monitoring in observational learning of action patterns: making the unobservable observable. *Journal of Motor Behaviour*, **14**, 2, 153–167.

Chandler J.M. and Duncan, P.W. (1988) Eccentric vs concentric force velocity relationships of the quadriceps femoris muscle. *Physical Therapy*, **68**, 5, 800.

Cohadon, F. (1981) The importance of rehabilitation programmes in the prevention and alleviation of head injury sequelae. *Progress in Neurological Surgery*, **10**, 344.

Colborne, G.R., Olney, S.J. and Griffin, M.P. (1993) Feedback of ankle joint angle and soleus electromyography in the rehabilitation of hemiplegic gait. *Archives of Physical Medicine and Rehabilitation*, **74**, 1100–1106.

Cornall, C. (1991) Self-propelling wheelchairs: the effects on spasticity in hemiplegic patients. *Physiotherapy Theory and Practice*, **7**, 13.

Crossman, E.R.F.W. (1959) A theory of the acquisition of speed-skill. *Ergonomics*, **2**, 153–166.

Dean, C. (1997) Stroke rehabilitation: factors affecting the performance and training of seated reaching tasks. Unpublished doctoral thesis.

Dean, C.M. and Shepherd, R.B. (1997) Task-related training improves performance of seated reaching tasks following stroke: a randomised controlled trial. *Stroke*, **28**, 722–728.

Decety, J., Perani, D., Jeannerod, M. *et al.* (1994) Mapping motor representations with positron emission tomography. *Nature*, **371**, 600–602.

de Jersey, M. (1979) Report on a sensory programme for patients with sensory deficits. *Australian Journal of Physiotherapy*, **25**, 165.

Devine, K.L., LeVeau, B.F. and Yack, H.J. (1981) Electromyographic activity recorded from an unexercised muscle during maximal isometric exercises of the contralateral agonists and antagonists. *Physical Therapy*, **61**, 898–903.

Diller, L. (1970) Psychomotor and vocational rehabilitation. In *Behavioural Change in Cerebrovascular Disease* (ed. A.L. Benton), Harper and Row, New York, pp. 81–116.

Duncan, P.W., Chandler, J.M., Cavanaugh, D.K. *et al.* (1989) Mode and speed specificity of eccentric and concentric exercise training. *Journal of Sports Physical Therapy*, **11**, 70–75.

Ellenbecker, T.S., Davies, G.J. and Rowinski, M.J. (1988) Concentric and eccentric isokinetic strengthening of the rotator cuff. *American Journal of Sports Medicine*, **16**, 65–69.

Enghardt, M., Ribbe, T. and Olsson, E. (1993) Vertical ground reaction force feedback to enhance stroke patients' symmetrical body-weight distribution while rising/sitting down. *Scandinavian Journal of Rehabilitation Medicine*, **25**, 41–48.

Fiatarone, M.A., Marks, E.C., Ryan, N.D. *et al.* (1990) High-intensity strength training in nonagenarians. *Journal of the American Medical Association*, **263**, 3029–3034.

Fowler, V. and Carr, J. (1996) Auditory feedback: effects on vertical force production during standing up following stroke. *International Journal of Rehabilitation Research*, **19**, 265–269.

Forssberg, H., Grillner, S. and Rossignol, S. (1975) Phase dependent reflex reversal during walking in chronic spinal cats. *Brain Research*, **55**, 247–304.

Friden, J. (1984) Changes in human skeletal muscle induced by long-term eccentric exercise. *Cell Tissue Research*, **236**, 365–372.

Friden, J., Seger, J., Sjostrom, M. *et al.* (1983) Adaptive responses in human skeletal muscle subjected to prolonged eccentric training. *International Journal of Sports Medicine*, **4**, 177–183.

Frontera, W.R., Meredith, C.N., O'Reilly, K.P. *et al.* (1988) Strength conditioning in older men: skeletal muscle hypertrophy and improved function. *Journal of Applied Physiology*, **64**, 1038–1044.

Fullerton, K.J., Mackenzie, G. and Stout, R.W. (1988) Prognostic indices of stroke. *Quarterly Journal of Medicine*, **66**, 147–162.

Gellhorn, E. (1947) Patterns of muscular activity in man. *Archives of Physical Medicine and Rehabilitation*, **28**, 568–574.

Gentile, A.M. (1987) Skill acquisition: action, movement, and neuromotor processes. In *Movement Science. Foundations for Rehabilitation* (eds J.H. Carr and R.B. Shepherd) Aspen Publishers, Rockville, MD, pp. 93–154.

Goldman, H. (1966) Improvement of double simultaneous stimulation perception in hemiplegic patients. *Archives of Physical Medicine and Rehabilitation*, **47**, 681–687.

Gonella, C., Hale, G., Ionta, M. *et al.* (1981) Self-instruction in a perceptual motor skill. *Physical Therapy*, **61**, 177–184.

Gottlieb, G.L., Corcos, D.M., Jaric, S. *et al.* (1988) Practice improves even the simplest movements. *Experimental Brain Research*, **73**, 436–440.

Greenwald, A.G. and Albert, S.M. (1968) Observational learning: a technique for elucidating S-R mediation processes. *Journal of Experimental Psychology*, **76**, 267–272.

Gregg, R.A., Mastellone, A.F. and Gersten, J.W. (1957) Cross exercise: A review of the literature and study utilizing electromyographic techniques. *American Journal of Physical Medicine*, **36**, 269–280.

Grimby, G., Gustafsson, E., Peterson, L. *et al.* (1980) Quadriceps function and training after knee ligament surgery. *Medical Science in Sport and Exercise*, **12**, 70–75.

Hakkinen, K. and Komi, P.V. (1983) Electromyographic changes during strength training and detraining. *Medicine and Science in Sports and Exercise*, **15**, 6, 455–460.

Higgins, J.R. (1972) Movements to match environmental demands. *Research Quarterly*, **43**, 312–336.

Holding, D.H. (1965) *Principles of Training*, Pergamon Press, New York.

Holding, D.H. (1970) Learning without errors. In *Psychology of Motor Learning* (ed. L.E. Smith), Athletic Institute, Chicago.

Holding, D.H. (ed.) (1989) *Human Skills*, 2nd edn, John Wiley and Sons, Chichester.

Imms, F.J. (1980) The use of physiological techniques for monitoring of progress during rehabilitation following fractures of the lower limb. *International Rehabilitation Medicine*, **2**, 181–188.

Imms, F.J., Hacett, A.J., Prestidge, S.P. *et al.*(1977) Voluntary isometric muscle strength of patients undergoing rehabilitation following fractures of the lower limb. *Rheumatology and Rehabilitation*, **16**, 161–171.

Ingemann-Hansen, T. and Halkjaer-Kristensen, J. (1980) Computerised tomography determination of human thigh components. *Scandinavian Journal of Rehabilitation Medicine*, **12**, 27–31.

Jacobson, E. (1932) Muscular phenomenon during imagining. *American Journal of Psychology*, **49**, 677–694.

Johnson, P. (1984) The acquisition of skill. In *The Psychology of Human Movement* (eds M.M. Smyth and A.M. Wing), Academic Press, London, pp. 215–240.

Jones, B. (1965) Motor learning without demonstration of physical practice, under two conditions of mental practice. *Research Quarterly*, **36**, 270–276.

Jones, D.A. and Rutherford, O.M. (1987) Human muscle strength training: the effects of three different regimes and the nature of the resultant changes. *Journal of Physiology*, **391**, 1–11.

Kanehisa, H. and Miyashita, M. (1983) Specificity of velocity in strength training. *European Journal of Applied Physiology and Occupational Physiology*, **52**, 104–106.

Keele, S.W. and Summers, J.J. (1976) The structure of motor programs. In *Motor Control: Issues and Trends* (ed. G.E. Stelmark) Academic Press, New York.

Kitai, T.A. and Sale, D.G. (1989) Specificity of joint angle in isometric training. *European Journal of Applied Physiology*, **58**, 744–748.

Knapik, J.J., Mawdsley, R.H. and Ramos, N.U. (1983) Angular specificity and test mode specificity of isometric and isokinetic strength training. *Journal of Orthopaedic Sports Physical Therapy*, **5**, 58–65.

Knott, M. and Voss, D.E. (1968) *Proprioceptive Neuromuscular Facilitation*, Harper and Row, New York.

Knuttgen, H.G., Bonde-Petersen, F. and Klausen, K. (1971) Oxygen uptake and heart rate response to exercise performed with concentric and eccentric muscle contractions. *Medical Science in Sports*, **3**, 1–5.

Komi, P.V. (1986) The stretch-shortening cycle and human power output. In *Human Muscle Power* (eds N.L. Jones, N. McCartney and A.J. McComas), Human Kinetics Publisher, Champaign, IL, pp. 27–39.

Komi, P.V. (1973) Relationship between muscle tension, EMG and velocity of contraction under concentric and eccentric work. In *New Developments in Electromyography and Clinical Neurophysiology* (ed. J.E. Desmedt) Karger, Basel, pp. 596–606.

Komi, P.V. and Buskirk, E.R. (1972) Effects of eccentric and concentric muscle conditioning on tension and electrical activity of human muscle. *Ergonomics*, **15**, 417–434.

Komi, P.V., Kaneko, M. and Aura, O. (1987) EMG activity of the leg extensor muscles with special reference to mechanical efficiency in concentric and eccentric exercise. *International Journal of Sports Medicine*, Supplement, **8**, 22–29.

Kuo, A.D. and Zajac, F.E. (1993) A biomechanical analysis of muscle strength as a limiting factor in standing posture. *Journal of Biomechanics*, **26**, 137–150.

Larsson, L. (1982) Physical training effects on muscle morphology in sedentary males at different ages. *Medicine and Science in Sports and Exercise*, **14**, 203–206.

Leont'ev, A.N. and Zaporozhets, A.V. (1960) *Rehabilitation of Hand Function*, Pergamon Press, London.

Lindh, M. (1979) Increase of muscle strength from isometric quadriceps exercises at different knee angles. *Scandinavian Journal of Rehabilitation Medicine*, **11**, 1, 33–36.

Logigian, M.K., Samuels, M.A., Falconer, J. *et al.* (1983) Clinical exercise trial for stroke patients. *Archives of Physical Medicine and Rehabilitation*, **64**, 364–367.

Loomis, J.E. and Boersma, F.J. (1982) Training right brain-damaged patients in a wheelchair task: case studies using verbal mediation. *Physiotherapy Canada*, **34**, 204.

Lord, S.R. and Castell, S. (1994) Physical activity program for older persons: effect on balance, strength, neuromuscular control, and reaction time. *Archives of Physical Medicine and Rehabilitation*, **75**, 648–652.

Lord, S.R., Clark, R.D. and Webster, I. W. (1991) Postural stability and associated physiological factors in a population of aged persons. *Journal of Gerontology*, **46**, M69–76.

McCartney, N., Moroz, D., Garner, S.H. *et al.* (1987) The effects of strength training in patients with selected neuromuscular disorders. *Medicine and Science in Sports and Exercise*, **20**, 362–368.

MacConaill, M.A. and Basmajian, J.V. (1969) *Muscles and Movements. Basis for Human Kinesiology*, Williams and Wilkins, Baltimore, MD.

McDonald, P.V., van Emmerick, R.E.A. and Newell, K.M. (1989) The effects of practice on limb kinematics in a throwing task. *Journal of Motor Behavior*, **21**, 245–264.

MacDougall, J.D., Ward, G.R., Sale, D.G. *et al.* (1977) Biochemical adaptation of human skeletal muscle to heavy resistance training and immobilisation. *Journal of Applied Physiology*, **43**, 700–703.

MacDougall, J.D., Elder, G.C.B., Sale, D.G. *et al.* (1980) The effects of strength training and immobilisation on human muscle fibres. *European Journal of Applied Physiology*, **43**, 25–34.

Matyas, T.A., Galea, M.P. and Spicer, S.D. (1986) Facilitation of maximum voluntary contraction in hemiplegia by concomitant cutaneous stimulation. *American Journal of Physical Medicine*, **65**, 125–134.

Mehrabian, A. (1969) Significance of posture and position in the communication of attitude and status relationships. *Psychological Bulletin*, **71**, 359–372.

Milner-Brown, H.S. and Miller, R.G. (1988a) Muscle strengthening through high-resistance weight training in patients with neuromuscular disorders. *Archives of Physical Medicine and Rehabilitation*, **69**, 14.

Milner-Brown, H.S. and Miller, R.G. (1988b) Muscle strengthening through electric stimulation combined with low-resistance weights in patients with neuromuscular disorders. *Archives of Physical Medicine and Rehabilitation*, **69**, 20.

Milner-Brown, H.S., Mellenthin, M. and Miller, R.G. (1986) Quantifying human muscle strength, endurance and fatigue. *Archives of Physical Medicine and Rehabilitation*, **67**, 530.

Milner-Brown, H.S., Stein, R.B. and Lee, R.G. (1975) Synchronization of human motor units: possible roles of exercise and supra-spinal reflexes. *Electroencephalography and Clinical Neurophysiology*, **38**, 245.

Moffried, M. and Whipple, R.H. (1970) Specificity of speed of exercise. *Physical Therapy*, **50**, 1692–1700.

Moritani, T. and DeVries, H. (1979) Neural factors versus hypertrophy in the time course of muscle strength gain. *American Journal of Physical Medicine*, **58**, 3, 115–130.

Mulder, T. (1991) A process-oriented model of human motor behavior: toward a theory-based rehabilitation approach. *Physical Therapy*, **71**, 157–164.

Mulder, T. and Hulstijn, W. (1985) Sensory feedback in the learning of a novel task. *Journal of Motor Behavior*, **17**, 110–128.

Mulder, T. and Hulstijn, W. (1988) From movement to action: the learning of motor control following brain damage. In *Complex Movement Behaviour: The Motor-Action Controversy* (eds O.G. Meijer and K. Roth) Elsevier Science, New York, pp. 247–259.

Narici, M.V., Roi, G.S., Landoni, L. *et al.* (1989) Changes in force, cross-sectional area and neural activation during strength training and detraining of the human quadriceps. *European Journal of Applied Physiology and Occupational Physiology*, **59**, 310–319.

Nashner, L.M., Woollacott, M. and Tuma, G. (1979) Organization of rapid responses to postural and locomotor-like perturbations of standing man. *Experimental Brain Research*, **36**, 463–476.

Nativ, A. (1993) Kinesiological issues in motor retraining following brain trauma. *Critical Review of Physical Rehabilitation Medicine*, **5**, 3, 227–246.

Newell, K.M. (1976) Knowledge of results and motor learning. *Exercise in Sport Science Review*, **4**, 195–227.

Newell, K.M. (1981) Skill learning. In *Human Skills* (ed. D.H. Holding), John Wiley and Sons, New York, pp. 203–226.

Newell, K.M. and Walter, C.B. (1981) Kinematic and kinetic parameters as information feedback in motor skill acquisition. *Journal of Human Movement Studies*, **7**, 235–254.

Nugent, J.A., Schurr, K.A. and Adams, R.D. (1994) A dose-response relationship between amount of weight-bearing exercise and walking outcome following cerebrovascular accident. *Archives of Physical Medicine and Rehabilitation*, **75**, 399–402.

Olsen, T.S. (1990) Arm and leg paresis as outcome predictors in stroke rehabilitation. *Stroke*, **21**, 247–251.

Olesen, J., Simonsen, K., Norgaard, B. *et al.* (1988) Reproducibility and utility of a simple neurological scoring system for stroke patients (Copenhagen Stroke Scale). *Journal of Neurologic Rehabilitation*, **2**, 59–63.

O'Sullivan, S.B. (1988) Stroke. In *Physical Rehabilitation Assessment and Treatment* (eds S.B. O'Sullivan and T.J. Schmitz), 2nd edn, F.A. Davis, Philadelphia, p. 335.

Oxendine, A. (1984) *Psychology of Motor Learning*, 2nd edn, Prentice-Hall, Englewood Cliffs, NJ.

Pai, Y-C. and Rogers, M.W. (1991) Segmental contributions to total body momentum in sit-to-stand. *Medicine and Science in Sports and Exercise*, **29**, 2, 225–230.

Pavone, E. and Moffat, M. (1985) Isometric torque of the quadriceps femoris after concentric, eccentric and isometric training. *Archives of Physical Medicine and Rehabilitation*, **66**, 168–170.

Poole, J.L. (1991) Application of motor learning principles in occupational therapy. *American Journal of Occupational Therapy*, **45**, 6, 531–537.

Posner, J.D., Gorman, K.M., Gitlin, L.N. *et al.* (1990) Effects of exercise training in the elderly on the occurrence and time to onset of cardiovascular diagnoses. *Journal of American Geriatric Society*, **38**, 205–210.

Proteau, L. (1992) On the specificity of learning and the role of visual information for movement control. In *Vision and Motor Control* (eds L. Proteau and D. Elliott), Elsevier Science, New York, pp. 67–103.

Rasch, P.T. and Morehouse, L.E. (1957) Effect of static and dynamic exercise on muscular strength and hypertrophy. *Journal of Applied Physiology*, **11**, 29–34.

Roland, P.E., Larsen, B., Lassen, N.A. *et al.* (1980a) Supplementary motor area and other cortical areas in organization of voluntary movements in man. *Journal of Neurophysiology*, **43**, 118–136.

Roland, P.E., Skinhoj, E., Lassen, N.A. *et al.* (1980b) Different cortical areas in man in organization of voluntary movements in extrapersonal space. *Journal of Neurophysiology*, **43**, 137–150.

Rooney, K.J., Herbert, R.D. and Balnave, R.J. (1994) Fatigue contributes to the strength training stimulus. *Medicine and Science in Sports and Exercise*, **26**, 1160–1164.

Rosenbaum, D.A. (1991) *Human Motor Control*, Academic Press, New York.

Rutherford. O.M. (1988) Muscular coordination and strength training. Implications for injury rehabilitation. *Sports Medicine*, **5**, 196–202.

Rutherford, O.M. and Jones, D. (1986) The role of learning and coordination in strength training. *European Journal of Applied Physiology and Occupational Physiology*, **55**, 100–105.

Rutherford, O.M., Grieg, C.A., Sargeant, A.J. *et al.*(1986) Strength training and power output-transference effects in the human quadriceps muscle. *Journal of Sports Science*, **4**, 101–107.

Rutherford, O.M., Jones, D.A. and Round, J.M. (1990) Long-lasting unilateral muscle wasting and weakness following injury and immobilization. *Scandinavian Journal of Rehabilitation Medicine*, **22**, 33–37.

Sabari, J.S. (1991) Motor learning concepts applied to activity-based intervention with adults with hemiplegia. *American Journal of Occupational Therapy*, **45**, 6, 523–530.

Sachs, D., Talley, E. and Boley, K. (1976) A comparison of feedback and reinforcement as modifiers of a functional motor response in a hemiparetic patient. *Journal of Behavioural Therapy and Experimental Psychiatry*, **1**, 7, 171.

Sale, D.G. (1987) Influence of exercise and training on motor unit activation. *Exercise and Sports Science Reviews*, **15**, 95–151.

Sale, D.G. (1988) Neural adaptation to resistance training. *Medical Science and Sports Exercise*, **20**, S135-S145.

Sale, D.G. and MacDougall, D. (1981) Specificity in strength training: a review for the coach and athlete. *Canadian Journal of Applied Sport Science*, **6**, 2, 87–92.

Sale, D.G., MacDougall, J.D., Upton, A.R.M. *et al.* (1983) Effect of strength training upon motoneuron excitability in man. *Medicine and Science in Sports and Exercise*, **15**, 57–62.

Sargeant, A.J., Davies, C.T.M., Edwards, R.H.T. *et al.* (1977) Functional and structural changes after disuse of human muscle. *Clinical Science and Molecular Medicine*, **52**, 337–342.

Schenkman, M., Berger, R.A., O'Riley, P. *et al.* (1990) Whole-body movements during rising to standing from sitting. *Physical Therapy*, **70**, 10, 638–651.

Schmidt, R.A. (1988) *Motor Control and Learning*, 2nd edn, Human Kinetics Publishers, Champaign, IL.

Schwartzman, R.J. (1972) Somatesthetic recovery following primary somatosensory projection cortex ablations. *Archives of Neurology*, **27**, 340.

Seligman, M. (1975) In *Helplessness on Depression, Development and Death*, W.H. Freeman, San Francisco, pp. 21–41, 180–188.

Semans, S. (1967) The Bobath concept in treatment of neurological disorders. *American Journal of Physical Medicine*, **46**, 1, 732–785.

Shephard, R. (1972) *Alive Man*, Thomas, Springfield, IL.

Shepherd, R.B. and Gentile, A.M. (1994) Sit-to-stand: functional relationship between upper body and lower limb segments. *Human Movement Science*, **13**, 817–840.

Shumway-Cooke, A., Anson, D. and Haller, S. (1988) Postural sway biofeedback: its effect on reestablishing stance stability in hemiplegic patients. *Archives of Physical Medicine and Rehabilitation*, **69**, 395–400.

Singer, R.N. (1980) *Motor Learning and Human Performance*. Macmillan, New York.

Sjostrom, M., Fugl-Meyer, A.R., Nordin, G. *et al.* (1980) Post-stroke hemiplegia: crural muscle strength and structure. *Scandinavian Journal of Rehabilitation Medicine*, **19** (Suppl. 7), 53–61.

Smith, J., Henriques, M. and Parsonson, B. (1985) The use of reinforcement procedures in training hand movement of CVA hemiplegic. *Behavioural Change*, **2**, 52.

Sparrow, W. A. (1983) The efficiency of skilled performance. *Journal of Motor Behaviour*, **15**, 237–261.

Sparrow, W.A. and Irizarry-Lopez, V.M. (1987) Mechanical efficiency and metabolic cost as measures of learning a novel gross motor task. *Journal of Motor Behaviour*, **19**, 240–264.

Stanish, W.D., Rubinovich, R.M. and Aurwin, S. (1986) Eccentric exercise in chronic tendinitis. *Clinical Orthopaedics*, **208**, 65–68.

Stockmeyer, S.A. (1967) An interpretation of the approach of Rood to the treatment of neuromuscular dysfunction. *American Journal of Physical Medicine*, **46**, 900–956.

Sullivan, S.J., Richer, E. and Laurent, F. (1990) The role of and possibilities for physical conditioning in the rehabilitation of traumatically brain-injured persons. *Brain Injury*, **4**, 407.

Sunderland, A., Tinson, D., Bradley, L. *et al.* (1989) Arm function after stroke. An evaluation of grip strength as a measure of recovery and a prognostic indicator. *Journal of Neurology, Neurosurgery and Psychiatry*, **52**, 1267–1272.

Tax, A.A.M., Denier van der Gon, J.J. and Erkelens, C.J. (1990) Differences in coordination of elbow flexors in force tasks and in movement. *Experimental Brain Research*, **81**, 567–572.

Thepaut-Mathieu, C., Van Hoecke, J. and Maton, B. (1985) Length specificity of strength and myoneural activation improvements following isometric training. In *Biomechanics I-A* (ed. B. Johnson), Human Kinetics Publishers, Champaign, IL, pp. 513–517.

Thepaut-Mathieu, C., Van Hoecke, J. and Maton, B. (1988) Myoelectrical and mechanical changes linked to length specificity during isometric training. *Journal of Applied Physiology*, **64**, 1500–1505.

Thorndike, E.L. (1927) The law of effect. *American Journal of Psychology*, **39**, 212–222.

Thorstensson, A., Hulten, B., Von Dobeln, W. and Karlsson, J. (1976) Effect of strength training on enzyme activities and fibre characteristics in human skeletal muscle. *Acta Physiologica Scandinavia*, **96**, 392–398.

Tinetti, M.E. (1987) Factors associated with serious injury during falls by ambulatory nursing home residents. *Journal of American Geriatrics Society*, **35**, 644–648.

Trowbridge, E.L. and Cason, H. (1932) An experimental study of Thorndike's theory of learning. *Journal of General Psychology*, **7**, 245–258.

van der Weel, F.R., van der Meer, A.L. and Lee, D.N. (1991) Effect of task on movement control in cerebral palsy: implications for assessment and therapy. *Developmental Medicine and Child Neurology*, **33**, 419–426.

Van Deusen Fox, J. (1964) Cutaneous stimulation: effects on selected tests of perception. *American Journal of Occupational Therapy*, **18**, 53–55.

Vincken, M.H. (1984) Control of limb stiffness. Unpublished doctoral thesis, University of Utrecht.

van Rossum, J.H.A. (1990) Schmidt's schema theory: the empirical base of the variability of practice hypothesis. A critical analysis. *Human Movement Science*, **9**, 387–435.

Wade, D.T. and Hewer, R.L. (1987) Functional abilities after stroke: measurement, natural history and prognosis. *Journal of Neurology, Neurosurgery and Psychiatry*, **50**, 177–182.

Wallace, S.A. and Hagler, R.W. (1979) Knowledge of performance and the learning of a closed motor skill. *Research Quarterly*, **50**, 265–271.

Weese, G.D., Neimand, D. and Finger, S. (1973) Cortical lesions and somesthesis in rats: effects of training and overtraining prior to surgery. *Experimental Brain Research*, **16**, 542–550.

Weinberg, J., Diller, L., Gordon, W.A. *et al.* (1979) Training sensory awareness and spatial organization in people with right brain damage. *Archives of Physical Medicine and Rehabilitation*, **60**, 491.

Westing *et al.* (1990) Effects of electrical stimulation on eccentric and concentric torque-velocity relationships during knee extension in man. *Acta Physiologica Scandinavia*, **140**, 17–22.

White, M.J. and Davies, C.T.M. (1984) The effects of immobilisation, after lower leg fracture, on the contractile properties of human triceps surae. *Clinical Science*, **66**, 277–282.

Whiting, H.T.A. and den Brinker, B.P.L.M. (1982) Image of the act. In *Theory and Research in Learning Disabilities* (eds J.P. Das, R.F. Mulcahy and A.E. Wall), Plenum Press, New York.

Whiting, H.T.A., Bijlard, M.J. and den Brinker, B.P.L.M. (1987) The effect of the availability of a dynamic model on the acquisition of a complex cyclical action. *Quarterly Journal of Experimental Psychology*, **39A**, 43–59.

Wilson, D.J., Baker, L.L. and Craddock, J.A. (1984) Functional test for the hemiparetic upper extremity. *American Journal of Occupational Therapy*, **38**, 159–164.

Winstein, C.J. and Schmidt, R.A. (1989) Sensori-motor feedback. In *Human Skills* (ed. D.H. Holding), 2nd edn, John Wiley and Sons, Chichester, pp. 17–47.

Winstein, C.J., Pohl, P.S., Cardinale, C. *et al.* (1996) Learning a partial-weight-bearing skill: effectiveness of two forms of feedback. *Physical Therapy*, **76**, 9, 985–993.

Wise, S.P. and Desimone, R. (1988) Behavioral neurophysiology: insights into seeing and grasping. *Science*, **242**, 736–741.

Wolf, S.L. and Binder-MacLeod, S.A. (1982) Use of the Krusen Limb Load Monitor to quantify temporal and loading measurements of gait. *Physical Therapy*, **61**, 976–982.

Wolf, S.L., Baker, M.P. and Kelly, J.L. (1979) EMG biofeedback in stroke: effect of patient characteristics. *Archives of Physical Medicine and Rehabilitation*, **60**, 96–103.

Wolf, S.L., Baker, M.P. and Kelly, J.L. (1980) EMG biofeedback in stroke: a one-year follow-up of the effect on patient characteristics. *Archives of Physical Medicine and Rehabilitation*, **61**, 351–355.

Wood, C.A., Gallagher, J.D., Martime, P.V. *et al.* (1992) Alternate forms of knowledge of results: interaction of augmented feedback modality on learning. *Journal of Human Movement Studies*, **22**, 213–230.

Wynn-Parry, C.B. and Salter, M. (1975) Sensory re-education after median nerve lesions. *The Hand*, **8**, 250–257.

Yekutiel M. and Guttman E. (1993) A controlled trial of the retraining of the sensory function of the hand in stroke patients. *Journal of Neurology, Neurosurgery and Psychiatry*, **56**, 241–244.

Young, A., Hughes, I., Round, J.M. *et al.* (1982) The effect of knee injury on the number of muscle fibres in the human quadriceps femoris. *Clinical Science*, **62**, 227–234.

Yue, G. and Cole, K.J. (1992) Strength increases from the motor program: comparison of training with maximal voluntary and imagined muscle contractions. *Journal of Neurophysiology*, **67**, 1114–1123.

Further reading

Annett, J. (1986) On knowing how to do things. In *Generation and Modulation of Action Patterns* (eds H. Heuer and C. Fromm), Springer, Berlin, pp. 187–200.

Annett, J. (1993) The learning of motor skills: sports science and ergonomics perspectives. *Ergonomics*, **37**, 5–16.

Barnes, G.R. (1993) Visual-vestibular interaction in the control of head and eye movement: the role of visual feedback and predictive mechanisms. *Progress in Neurobiology*, **41**, 435–472.

Edgerton, V.R., Roy, R.R., Gregor, R.J. *et al.* (1986) Morphological basis of skeletal muscle power output. In *Human Muscle Power* (eds N.L. Jones and N. McCartney), Human Kinetics Publishers, Champaign, IL, pp. 43–64.

Halsband, U. and Freund, H-J. (1993) Motor learning. *Current Opinion in Neurobiology*, **3**, 940–949.

Harms-Ringdahl, K. (ed.) (1993) *Muscle Strength*, Churchill Livingstone, Edinburgh.

Jacobs, R. and van Ingen Schenau, G.J. (1992) Control of an external force in leg extensions in humans. *Journal of Physiology*, **457**, 611–626.

Jeannerod, M. (1994) The representing brain: neural correlates of motor intention and imagery. *Behavioral and Brain Sciences*, **17**, 187–245.

Lincoln, N.B. and Sackley, C.M. (1992) Biofeedback in stroke rehabilitation. *Critical Reviews in Physical and Rehabilitation Medicine*, **4**, 37–47.

Magill, R.A. (1989) *Motor Learning*, 3rd edn, W.C. Brown, Dubuque, IA.

Moritani, T. (1993) Neuromuscular adaptations during the acquisition of muscle strength, power and motor tasks. *Journal of Biomechanics*, **26**, Suppl. 1, 95–107.

Mulder, T. (1985) The use of artificial sensory feedback in the rehabilitation of physical disabilities: a critical review. In *The Learning of Motor Control following Brain Damage: Experimental and Clinical Studies* (ed. T. Mulder), Swets and Zeitlinger, Lisse, pp. 4–28.

Mulder, T. (1993) Current topics in motor control: implications for rehabilitation. In *Neurological Rehabilitation* (eds R. Greenwood *et al.*). Churchill Livingstone, Edinburgh, pp. 125–134.

Rundgren, A., Ariansson, A., Ljunberg, P. *et al.* (1984) Effects of a training programme for elderly people on mineral content of the heel bone. *Archives of Gerontology and Geriatrics*, **3**, 243–248.

Taunton, J.E., Martin, A.D., Rhodes, E.C. *et al.* (1997) Exercise for the older woman; choosing the right prescription. *British Journal of Sports Medicine*, **3**, 5–10.

Young, D.E. and Schmidt, R.A. (1992) Augmented kinematic feedback for motor learning. *Journal of Motor Behavior*, **24**, 261–273.

Zajac, F.E. (1993) Muscle coordination of movement: a perspective. *Journal of Biomechanics*, **26**, Suppl. 1, 109–124.

3

Measurement

Global measures
    Barthel ADL Index
    Functional Independence Measure
Measures of motor performance
    Motor Assessment Scale for Stroke
    Gait
    Balance
    Upper limb function
    Biomechanical measures
Other measures of motor function
    Rivermead Motor Assessment
    Brunnstrom–Fugl–Meyer Assessment
Specific measures of impairment
    Muscle strength
    Joint range of motion
    Tone
    Cardiorespiratory fitness/exercise capacity
Tests of discrete sensation
    Tactile sensation
    Stereognosis
    Kinaesthetic sensation
Measures of perception–cognition
    Mini-Mental State Examination
        Rivermead Behavioural Memory Test
        Rivermead Perceptual Assessment Battery
        Behavioural Inattention Test
Environmental analysis
    Behaviour mapping
    Behaviour stream analysis
Measures of anxiety and depression
Diagnosis-specific measures
    Parkinson's disease
    Traumatic brain injury or post-brain surgery coma
Self-assessment and self-efficacy scales
Clinical audit

The assessment or evaluation of an individual with a neurological diagnosis involves reference to relevant medical and surgical notes, including results of X-rays, brain scans, EMG investigations, neurological examination, other relevant medical tests, psychology assessments and current medication. Reports of social (particularly family) and work situations may provide information which makes it unnecessary to ask certain questions. Individuals in hospital typically have to answer the same questions asked by large numbers of staff, often because staff have not acquired the information from the records. Where a patient is unconscious or unable to communicate, information from relatives may help the therapist's understanding of the patient's personality and preferences.

The major role of physiotherapy is the evaluation and training of everyday motor function so that the individual can return to the leisure, household and work-related activities they normally perform and to independent function in the community. Physiotherapy practice therefore involves gaining accurate and objective (i.e., measurement-generated) information about the individual's performance abilities in the motor tasks most critical to the person's everyday life. This information is critical to the design and ongoing modification and variation of the individual's training programme and is collected on entry to physiotherapy, at regular periods during hospital- or community-based rehabilitation and on discharge and follow-ups. The information collected, therefore, provides the knowledge necessary to plan appropriate exercise and practice, but also can be used to collate data on particular patient groups within a centre and between centres or countries. It is an important means of establishing best practice and making changes to best practice as more effective methods of intervention are developed.

Information is also collected by observation, which is subjective and open to error and bias, but which can be made more reliable if it is structured in some way and if the observer is well-informed with an up-to-date and relevant knowledge base. Check-lists are useful to give structure to an observational assessment and there is some evidence that such simplification may improve reliability (Kemer and Alexander 1981). One advantage of objective functional scales which measure performance on important functions like standing up and walking is that they can provide objective input into the more subjective observational analysis and some confirmation of the accuracy of observations which have formed the basis of training that particular function or task.

There are several textbooks that either discuss issues related to measurement or contain information related to the large number of tests available in neurological rehabilitation (for example, see Wade 1992a). This chapter outlines details of a small selection of the tests available which have been shown to be reliable and valid measures and which could be used clinically by physiotherapists. There are many reliable and valid tests of specific tasks and actions which are not mentioned here because they require laboratory facilities. However, a computer literature search will guide the clinician to the tests available.

Global measures

Details of these tests are not provided, since they are more likely to be administered by a physician or nurse than a physiotherapist, who would concentrate on the motor performance measures described in more detail below. Therapists should make themselves aware of the details of these tests by referring to the articles recommended and to texts such as Wade (1992a). The two global measures below tend to be used as measures of dependence.

Barthel ADL Index

The test is considered valid but it has not been shown to be reliable. Whether or not it is a valid measure may depend on the questions being asked. There have been concerns expressed by therapists about its insensitivity to change due to the broad nature of the mobility categories. It is not likely to be a valid indicator of change in the sensorimotor tasks usually addressed in rehabilitation but it was not designed to be.

It is said to be the most widely used index. There are several variations. Wade (1992a) includes a simple version in his text. Its categories consist of:

- Bowels
- Bladder
- Grooming
- Toilet use
- Feeding
- Transfer
- Mobility
- Dressing
- Stairs
- Bathing

These items are scored from 0 to 3, with 0 meaning total dependence on others and 3 independence (although in walking, aids can be used). The scores are summed. This test is very broad indeed and provides no indicators of value to planning intervention. Nevertheless, the Index does provide a general overview of a person's status, although to attach any meaning to the total score, individual items need to be identified for their particular contributions to the overall score.

References: Mahoney and Barthel (1965), Wade (1992b)

A superficially similar test is the **Katz Activities of Daily Living Index**. It was developed some time ago and shows its age. Its reliability and validity are not established. Wade (1992a) considers the Barthel to be superior.

Other ADL tests, such as the **Rivermead ADL Index** (Lincoln and Edmans 1989), the **Nottingham Extended ADL Index** (Nouri and Lincoln 1987) and the **Frenchay Activities Index** (Holbrook and Skilbeck 1983), may be more suitable for occupational therapists to perform. They are not necessarily reliable, however, the information available provides the therapist with general information about the patient's ability to perform daily activities.

Functional Independence Measure (FIM)

FIM is widely used in some countries. It is intended as a standard measure to enable comparisons to be made amongst rehabilitation centres. Its 6 categories comprise:

Personal care
  Feeding
  Grooming
  Bathing
  Dressing
  Toileting
Sphincter control
  Bladder management
  Bowel management
Mobility
  Transfers
Locomotion
  Walking/using wheelchair
  Stairs
Communication
  Comprehension
  Expression
Social cognition
  Social interaction
  Problem-solving
  Memory

Each category is scored from 1 to 4, 1 indicating complete dependence and 4 complete independence. It has been reported as reliable and valid in its current state.

References: Granger *et al.* (1986), Keith *et al.* (1987).

Measures of motor performance

Despite the fact that intervention is generally aimed broadly at improving performance on functional tasks in individuals with motor impairments, the measurement of performance has received scant attention.

Clinicians usually rely on their own subjective impressions. That is to say, non-standardized observational analysis of movement has long been the method of analysis of choice amongst therapists. An observational analysis using biomechanical details in a check-list is a useful way for evaluating motor performance, and in the hands of an observer who understands the biomechanical components of the action, the information gathered is probably of considerable value in the planning of intervention. The human observer can be reliable under reasonable conditions, although this does not seem to be supported in gait analysis (Krebs *et al.* 1985). However, many physiotherapists have little or no understanding of biomechanics and the 'normal' range of performance in able-bodied individuals, a situation which will rapidly change once this subject becomes a required area of study for undergraduate and graduate physiotherapists on university courses. In the meantime, therapy may be based on an erroneous appreciation of able-bodied performance. It has been pointed out in relation to gait analysis that there is a discrepancy between the therapists' assessment of their own capabilities and their real ability (Malouin 1995).

Although objective tests of movement are not frequently used by therapists, there are several reliable and valid tests available for use in the clinic.

Motor Assessment Scale (MAS) for Stroke

A decade ago, in an attempt to provide some reliable and valid method for testing the more task-related interventions we were investigating, we developed and tested this scale (Carr *et al.* 1985). The recently updated version consists of eight items:

- Supine to side lying on to intact side
- Supine to sitting over the side of bed
- Balanced sitting
- Sitting to standing
- Walking
- Upper-arm function
- Hand movements
- Advanced hand activities

It is a seven-point ordinal scale, so these items are scaled from 0 to 6. Criteria for scoring are provided together with general rules for administering the scale. Reliability of physiotherapists is tested, after practice sessions with five patients, by rating individual physiotherapist's scores made while observing videotapes of patients against a criterion rating.

In the original version, muscle tone was included. In a recently modified version, we omitted this unreliable item (see Poole and Whitney 1988). This deletion is also appropriate given the probability that such tests are more likely to examine muscle length and stiffness rather than reflex hyperexcitability.

The scale has test-retest and inter-rater reliability (Carr *et al.* 1985; Poole and Whitney 1988; Loewen and Anderson 1988). It is a valid instrument (Malouin *et al.* 1994; Lennon and Hastings 1996), and the validity of the Sitting to Standing item is supported by several biomechanical studies of the action, which indicate that improvement on the scale occurs in conjunction with increasing normalization of certain biomechanical parameters (Ada and Westwood 1992; Ada *et al.* 1993).

Individual items from the scale have been shown to be good predictors of stroke outcome (Loewen and Anderson 1990), with scores at 1 week and 1 month being predictors of functional arm recovery at discharge. Interestingly, one study which compared MAS scores with scores on the Fugl-Meyer Assessment (FMA) (Malouin *et al.* 1994) showed good correlations between the two except for the sitting balance item. This may not be surprising, given that the FMA assesses the ability to sit still, whereas the MAS assesses the ability to balance while moving about (reaching in different directions) in sitting and may, therefore, be the better indicator of balance.

An advantage of the test is that it takes a short time to administer (10–15 minutes) in experienced hands (Carr *et al.* 1985; Malouin *et al.* 1994). It is intended to be used to measure each item as a separate entity since they bear no particular relationship to each other but are separate actions. Therefore, individual items can be used or all 8 items, depending on what information is needed. It has been used in at least one clinical trial with a summative score, which is inappropriate since it is an ordinal scale. The items do not have to be tested in any order; they are not in any way hierarchically organized.

The MAS is routinely used in some Australian hospitals and elsewhere for clinical audits and in clinical trials (Dean and Mackey 1992; Wales 1994). Its major advantage seems to be in providing information related to the performance of actions which patients have a vested interest in improving, such as standing up and sitting down, walking and hand use. It is useful in clinical audits since it enables particular functions, e.g., walking, to be selected for scrutiny. An audit of walking outcome in one Sydney hospital found, at the end of 6 months, an outcome considered by the therapists to be unsatisfactory. They mobilized resources and planned changes to walking training in an attempt to improve outcome on a subsequent group of patients.

The MAS appears to be a useful measure of functional ability both in clinical data collection and for laboratory research. It has been shown to be predictive of stroke recovery and has been suggested as a means of prioritizing rehabilitation management (Loewen and Anderson 1990). It should be noted that the so-called Modified MAS referred to by Loewen and Anderson is the MAS with minor editorial modifications made by Loewen and Anderson. We have made our own modifications, omitting the muscle tone item and making minor changes to the text, which are awaiting publication.

References: Carr *et al.* (1985).

Several tests directed as specific tasks provide a means of testing a specific aspect of a task (e.g., Timed Walking Tests) or of testing patients who achieve a higher level of performance than can be tested with a scale such as the Motor Assessment Scale (e.g., Nine-hole Peg Test, Frenchay Arm Test).

Gait

The walking item of the MAS can be used as a measure of gait function. Particularly in patients who achieve the highest score, it is often useful to perform some other measure, of, for example, speed, distance walked or stride length. There are several tests suitable for clinical use that measure critical aspects of gait and are simple to use. They require, of course, that particular attention is paid to standardization issues.

Timed walking test

This test can be carried out over any reasonable distance, say 5–50 metres. The patient is asked to walk at their preferred pace or can be asked to walk 'as fast as possible'. The distance to be walked is marked out clearly on the floor. Time taken from when the patient crosses a starting line (on the floor) to the finishing line is measured with a stopwatch. Note is taken of any aids (such as a cane) used. The patient's performances are compared over time and displayed by graph for feedback and kept as a record of progress. The result can be expressed as time taken (seconds) or as speed (metres/second). This test should be reliable provided it is standardized and a careful record is kept of details.

No importance is attached to what therapists like to call the 'quality' of movement. However, progressive decreases in time taken, appear to be a valid and reliable indicator of improvement in biomechanical parameters and muscle power and control, at least following stroke (Wade, Wood *et al.* 1987).

References: Wade, Wood *et al.* (1987), Wolfson *et al.* (1990).

Cadence and stride length measures

Several methods of quantifying these gait parameters in the clinic have been reported. Although they may not be reliable unless standardized rigorously, such tests can provide useful information to guide training. Some are very simple and inexpensive. For example, a procedure requiring a stopwatch, two felt-tip marking pens with washable ink and a walkway of suitable length has been described (Cerny 1983; Ada and Canning, 1990). Foot switches are available (e.g., Perry *et al.* 1980), also grid systems (Wall *et al.* 1976). Another reliable measurement of these gait parameters involves a computerized stride analyser.

References: Robinson and Smidt (1981).

Balance

Balance, or more accurately postural adjustments, are tested in the laboratory using accelerometry (Bouisset and Zattara 1981), EMG (Lee *et al.* 1980; Hansen *et al.* 1988), force platform (Hayes 1982) and video (Friedl *et al.* 1988). The self-initiated actions tested include arm raising, pointing and reaching (see Chapter 6). Other aspects of balance tested include the person's response to an unexpected support surface perturbation (Nashner 1977; Nashner *et al.* 1982) and the ability to remain relatively still, in which the extent of postural sway is usually measured on a force platform.

One needs to be clear in selecting a method of testing balance what question one is asking, since different tests measure different aspects of balancing and there is little indication as yet about generalizability. For clinical purposes, balance can be classified under three broad classes of action: whenever we make a volitional movement, when the support surface moves unexpectedly and when we maintain a posture against external interference (Carr and Shepherd 1987). In our view the most important test of balance in the clinic is testing of the person's ability to balance during a self-initiated action. Postural adjustments throughout actions such as walking, standing up, stair climbing and descent, when reaching for an object in sitting and standing, looking around the room, are critical to the performance of these actions. Without appropriate postural muscle activations and segmental rotations the person would fail to achieve the goal or fall; if the person thinks they will fall, they will be reluctant to move.

The testing of balance in the clinic, although very important to evaluating the effects of different interventions, has been difficult to quantify. The

MAS has a sitting balance item which is reliable and valid, requiring the patient to reach in different directions (see above). The Fugl–Mayer Scale has a balance section but the ability of the patient to perform a parachute reaction or withstand a push by the examiner are tested which may not be valid measures of ability to balance while moving about.

A set of measures using a moveable platform has been devised that measures response to support surface perturbation under different sensory input conditions (Horak 1987). These measures appear to test principally the ability of individuals to balance under reduced sensory input conditions which may be useful for diagnostic purposes. The relevance of measures which test only the person's response to unexpected support surface movement or to perturbation (pushes) initiated by the examiner to balance under the dynamic conditions of self-initiated movement is not known. Similarly, the reliability and validity of measures of postural sway (e.g. centre of pressure) are not understood, and there is some criticism of postural sway as a measure of functional balance (e.g., Goldie *et al.* 1989).

Below are some tests of ability to balance in standing which can be used easily in the clinic.

Functional reach test

This test measures the difference between arm's length and maximum reach forward in standing. It is relatively simple and inexpensive, and appears to be reliable. The test is valid in that it measures an action which is very common in everyday life and because reach distance scores correlate with biomechanical change (centre of pressure excursion). It is therefore a more dynamic test than tests of ability to stand still. The test is performed with the patient standing next to a wall to which a yardstick is attached. The starting position is with the feet a standard few centimetres apart and the arm flexed forward to a horizontal position in line with the yardstick but not touching the arm. The

Table 3.1 Functional reach test: age-related norms

Norms	Men (in inches)	Women (in inches)
20–40 yrs	16.73+1.94	14.64+2.18
41–69 yrs	14.98+2.21	13.81+2.20
70–87 yrs	13.16+1.55	10.47+3.53

Table 3.2   Scoring of standard balance test

Grade	Description
0	Unable to stand (i.e. worse than next grade)
1	Able to stand with feet apart, but less than 30 sec
2	Stand with feet apart for 30 sec, but not with feet together
3	Stand with feet together, but less than 30 sec
4	Stand with feet together, 30 sec or more

patient makes a fist and the position of the 3rd metacarpal relative to the yardstick is noted. The patient is then asked to reach forward as far as possible without taking a step and the position of the 3rd metacarpal is again noted. The distance reached is compared to age-related norms (see Table 3.1). The test has been found to be predictive of falls in the elderly.

Reference: Duncan *et al.* (1990).

Standing balance

This is a simple ordinal scale in which patients stand with eyes open (Table 3.2). It is said to be reliable. Its validity including its generalizability to more dynamic situations is uncertain and the ability to stand still may not be a suitable goal for all patients with brain lesions.

References: Bohannon (1989), Bohannon *et al.* (1993).

'Get-up and go' test and timed 'up and go' test

The test was originally developed as a clinically possible method of detecting balance difficulties in elderly patients. The authors noted that many elderly people fall when rising from a chair, walking, turning and sitting down and the test provides a method of measuring performance of these actions. The patient is required to stand up from a chair, walk 3 m (10 ft), turn around and return. Performance is scored as:

1 Normal
2 Very slightly abnormal
3 Mildly abnormal
4 Moderately abnormal
5 Severely abnormal

An increased risk of falling is associated with those who scored 3 or more. The test is reported as reliable between raters and its validity is supported by high correlations between it and laboratory tests

of postural sway, and gait parameters such as speed and stride width.

The modified version of the test has a timing component and depends less on qualitative judgements. Able-bodied adults are able to perform the test in less than 30 seconds. Its validity is supported by its high correlation with functional capacity as measured on the Barthel Index.

References: Mathias *et al.* (1986), Podsialo and Richardson (1991).

There have been many other measures of balance developed. The *Berg Scale* (Berg *et al.* 1989, 1992), for example, measures balance during 14 tasks (including sitting and standing unsupported, sitting to standing, retrieving object from floor in standing, turning 360°, transfers). It has been reported to be reliable and appears to have content validity. However, it is very long and would take considerable time to administer. The shorter balance tests mentioned above may give sufficient information.

Forceplates, bathroom scales and limb-load monitors are used, under standardized conditions, to measure postural sway and symmetrical weight-bearing. Tests of postural control under different visual and support surface conditions have been proposed (e.g., Shumway-Cook and Horak 1986) but in many patients these very specific tests may not add any information to aid the patient's rehabilitation. Interestingly, although many clinicians carry out observational analyses of righting and equilibrium reactions (e.g., Davies, 1990; Ryerson, 1995; Edwards 1996), no studies that we know of have investigated whether any relationship exists between these relatively automatic responses to perturbations and the ability to balance under other conditions. It is important in clinical assessment that a test is chosen that answers a question that is valid in terms of the patient's needs. Test of responses to therapist-produced perturbations may not constitute a valid measure.

Upper limb function

Nine-hole peg test (NHPT)

This is a useful test to use in patients who have a relatively high level of performance since it tests dexterity and speed in a task which requires movement of the arm and hand. It is a suitable test to administer to patients who have achieved top scores in the upper-arm function and hand movements items of the Motor Assessment Scale.

The apparatus consists of nine wooden pegs and a wood base with nine holes. The time taken by the patient to place all the dowels in the holes is measured with a stop-watch. This may be varied by testing how many pegs can be placed in a given time, say 50 seconds. The result is expressed as time to place one peg (in seconds).

The test is reliable and valid. The able-bodied take approximately 18 seconds to complete the task. There is also a Ten-hole Peg Test (Turton and Fraser 1986).

Reference: Mathiowetz *et al.* (1985), Sunderland *et al.* (1989).

Frenchay Arm Test

This short test consists of five tasks to be performed with the affected hand:

1 Stabilize a ruler while drawing a line with a pencil held in the other hand. To pass, the ruler must be held firmly.
2 Grasp a cylinder (12 mm diam., 5 cm long) set on its end approximately 15 cm from the table edge, lift it about 30 cm and replace it without dropping.
3 Pick up a glass half-full of water positioned 15–30 cm from the table edge, drink some water and replace the glass without spilling any water.
4 Remove and replace a spring clothes peg from a 10 mm diameter dowel, 15 cm long, set in a 10 cm square base, placed 15–30 cm from the table edge. The peg must not be dropped or the dowel knocked over.

5 Comb the hair (or imitate); the hair must be combed across the top, down the back and down each side of the head.

The test is performed in sitting with the hands in the lap, with each task starting from this position. A score of 1 is given for successful performance, zero for failure.

The test is valid and reliable. It is simple and quick to carry out. Tests such as this appear to be rarely used in clinical practice, perhaps because it would be perceived by therapists to be too difficult for most patients. In our view, it would be a useful test to use routinely, as are the upper limb items in the Motor Assessment Scale.

References: DeSouza *et al.* (1980), Sunderland *et al.* (1992).

Another reliable and valid test of upper limb function is the **Action Research Arm Test** (Carroll 1965; Crow *et al.* 1989). However, it takes 30 minutes to administer and we would argue that the upper limb items of the MAS, which take only a few minutes, may be more functionally valid.

The **Spiral Test** (Verkerk *et al.* 1990) was developed as a measure of coordination and tested on two patients, one with cerebellar ataxia, the other with Parkinson's disease (Fig. 3.1). Two spirals are printed on a sheet of paper, with 1 cm between the lines. The subject must draw a line from a starting position (the arrow) to the central point as quickly as possible and without touching the lines. The subject is scored on time taken to perform the test in seconds. Each time a line is touched, 3 seconds is added to the time taken, and 5 seconds every time a line is crossed. The test appears reliable and is a valid measure of accuracy and speed on an accuracy task. It is also a useful way of providing qualitative feedback to a patient.

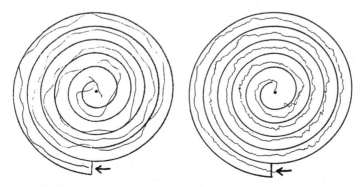

Fig. 3.1 Spiral test results of individuals with cerebellar ataxia (L) and Parkinson's disease (R) (Reprinted from Verkerk *et al.* (1990) by kind permission of Elsevier Science, Amsterdam, The Netherlands)

Biomechanical measures

Increasingly it is becoming possible for simple biomechanical tests to be carried out on specific tasks or actions. Physiotherapists are using stop-frame video equipment to perform simple yet accurate measures of angular and linear displacement and velocity (see Wall and Crosbie 1995). Biomechanical tests are useful both as pre- and post-intervention measures of change in performance. They are also useful in providing a means of validating functional tests such as the MAS.

Departments with a forceplate system and computer are able to test ground reaction forces produced by the patient in standing, sitting and walking. A commercially available stride analyser enables measurement of spatial and temporal characteristics of foot step pattern (Morris *et al.* 1994). It consists of foot switches, a start–stop controller and data storage unit.

Rehabilitation departments with easy access to motion analysis laboratories are those with the greatest potential to produce reliable and meaningful biomechanical data for clinical research. Such laboratories can also assist the clinician to identify more accurately the nature of motor performance dysfunction.

Smith (1990) describes some simple biomechanical measures.

Other measures of motor function

Rivermead Motor Assessment

This scale is a measure of 'motor function' after stroke. Its three sections include both impairments and disabilities: Gross Function, Leg and Trunk, Arm. Each section contains 10–15 items. For example, Gross Function includes walking, sitting to standing, lying to sitting over side of the bed. Each item is scored 0 or 1 and the total for each section is summed.

The scale has a number of problems which raise the question of validity. Each section is based on a hierarchy of actions, which since they are unrelated to each other in a biomechanical or a functional sense, cannot be considered to reflect a progression. The scale is extremely long and we are not aware that it has been formally tested for reliability (Lincoln and Leadbitter 1979; Collin *et al.* 1990). A recent prospective study concludes that much of the scale is outdated (Adams *et al.* 1997).

Brunnstrom–Fugl–Meyer Assessment (BFMA or FMA)

This assessment tool is popular in some centres, particularly in North America where many therapists use Brunnstrom's methods of treatment. It has been criticised for being too lengthy and difficult to understand (e.g., Wade 1992a). The test has been shown to have moderate inter-rater reliability (Sanford *et al.* 1993) but its validity is questionable given that it is based on what appears to be an inaccurate view of the pattern of recovery from stroke (e.g., Malouin *et al.* 1994). The FMA has been found to discriminate better in the early stage of recovery, probably because it assesses isolated joint movement rather than task-related actions. The MAS has been suggested as a replacement for the FMA (Poole and Whitney 1988). As there are other shorter and more valid tests available, details are not included here.

References: Fugl-Meyer *et al.* (1975).

Several other scales exist which have been shown to be valid for the purposes for which they were designed, as well as reliable, for example, the Elderly Mobility Scale (Smith 1994). There have been several other scales developed, of questionable validity, and untested for reliability (e.g., the Motor Club Assessment, Ashburn 1982).

Specific measures of impairment

These typically are measures of specific factors related to movement such as muscle power, muscle tone, ataxia, involuntary movement (e.g., tremor), joint range, and strength. Other measures useful to the therapist are associated with fitness or intensity of exercise.

Muscle strength

The Medical Research Council (MRC) grades

These are used mostly for peripheral nerve lesions as an indication of the strength of muscle. Strength is graded on an ordinal scale from 0 to 5.

0 No contraction
1 Palpable contraction
2 Movement without gravity
3 Movement against gravity

4 Movement against resistance lower than the resistance overcome by the healthy side
5 Movement against resistance equal to the maximum resistance overcome by the healthy side

These grades provide a subjective impression of the ability to contract a muscle under certain conditions. In no sense do they provide an objective measure. The reliability and validity of the tests are doubtful for a number of reasons, one of which is that the ability of a target muscle to contract is diminished if its synergists are inactive. Since grades 4 and 5 require a 'normal' side, this presents difficulties following stroke, where muscles on the unaffected side may also be affected by the lesion.

References: Medical Research Council (1976).

A **Motricity Index** has been devised based on the MRC grades. It appears to be reliable and valid for stroke patients (Collin and Wade 1990). The Index sums scores for one limb and for one side of the body.

References: Demeurisse *et al.* (1980), Wade (1992a).

Muscle force

Muscle force is measured using a dynamometer (Bohannon and Andrews 1987a,b). A **hand dynamometer** is used to measure grip or pinch force. Given the possible variability between devices, it is wise to use the same device for pre- and post-tests. The provision of normative age-related values for the dynamometer (see Mathiowetz *et al.* 1985) increases usefulness. Isokinetic dynamometers are primarily used to measure dynamic muscle strength, although they are sometimes used to measure static force. Such devices need to be checked for reliability (see Tripp and Harris 1991).

References: Sunderland *et al.* (1989), Collin and Wade (1990); Bohannon *et al.* (1993).

Joint range of motion

It is often important to record *passive* joint range, before and after intervention to stretch short calf muscles, for example. To standardize the test a known force must be used. A hand-held dynamometer is used to apply force and a standard goniometer (or electro-goniometer) to measure range. Body weight in standing or walking can also be used as a means of standardization (see Ada and Canning 1990; Moseley and Adams 1991). Testing of joint range using a goniometer should always be standardized in terms of factors such as anatomical landmarks and force application otherwise the test is unreliable (see Gajdosik and Bohannon 1987).

Active joint range is best measured during some relevant action, for example, during stance or swing phase of walking, during sit-to-stand. In a motion analysis laboratory the test is done using a computerized motion analysis system. In the clinic, range can be measured at a particular point during an action using video camera or still photography under standardized conditions.

Tone

Many therapists and physicians set great store by the assessment of tone, since they would also believe that spasticity is the major impairment following acute lesion such as stroke. These views have not, however, resulted in the development of any objective measures suitable for use in the clinic (Wade 1992a). Given the evidence that what clinicians regard as increased tone or spasticity is more likely to be muscle stiffness coupled with muscle length changes, it is likely that methods of assessment currently in use are actually testing these mechanical factors. There is recent evidence that this may be so from a study of the **pendulum test** (Fowler *et al.* 1998). In attempting to develop methods of assessing tone, clinicians are focusing their attention on what McLellan (1977) called an 'epiphenomenon'. The **Modified Ashworth Scale** (Ashworth 1964; Bohannon and Smith 1987) is a good example of a scale that sets out to test one impairment (spasticity) but really tests another (muscle stiffness etc.). In this scale 'tone' is graded according to the amount of resistance to passive movement.

References: Ashworth (1964), Bohannon and Smith (1987).

Cardiorespiratory fitness/exercise capacity

Fitness is typically tested using a treadmill or bicycle ergometer. Aerobic testing is performed sub-maximally or maximally. The former involves calculating target heart rate, which is a percentage of estimated maximal heart rate for that individual. Maximal aerobic testing is carried out using a methodology such as the Bruce Protocol (Bruce *et al.* 1973). Maximal testing requires simultaneous electrocardiograph monitoring and is typically carried out by specially trained staff. Tests of VO_2 peak and O_2 consumption per kilogram body weight at a given power output in walking, treadmill walking, bicycle ergometry and using mechanical stairs provide means of evaluating exercise capacity or efficiency (Hunter *et al.* 1990; Jankowski and Sullivan 1990).

The use of heart rate measures, however, is a simple method of ensuring that exercise is sufficiently vigorous (where vigorous exercise and improved fitness are the goals) and to test whether or not a patient's cardiovascular system is adapting to exercise. Such testing should probably become a standard tool in the attempt to build up the fitness of patients in neurological rehabilitation (e.g., following head injury, brain surgery and stroke, and in Parkinson's disease).

Heart rate (HR)

A measure of heart rate provides an indication of intensity of exercise and is typically used when it is necessary to monitor the level of exercise. This test may be used to monitor fitness in any patient with a brain lesion. This measure also provides a means of measuring functional improvement on a motor action such as sit-to-stand or walking.

To exercise at the appropriate level to improve cardio-vascular fitness, the target HR is determined using a heart rate monitor. To determine target HR:

Calculate maximum age-predicted HR by subtracting the patient's age from 220, i.e.,

Maximum age-predicted HR = 220 − age

Calculate target HR as between 60–80% of maximum age-predicted HR, i.e.

Target HR range = 60–80% maximum age-predicted HR

E.g., for a 50-year-old person

Maximum age-predicted HR = (220−50)
= 170

Target HR range = (60–80% of 170)
= 102–136

Another test which may be suitable as a measure is the **6-** or **12-minute walk test** (McGavin *et al.* 1976), which requires the individual to walk as far as possible in the 6 or 12 minutes.

Tests of discrete sensation

The typical tests performed clinically by physicians and therapists, such as light touch, pin-prick, heat and cold, sense of passive and position, have been shown to be subjective and unreliable (Garraway *et al.* 1976; Tomasello *et al.* 1982).

The subjectivity of sensory tests and their relevance to functional sensory discrimination in patients with central lesions (and, therefore, their validity) has come under considerable scrutiny recently (e.g., Lincoln *et al.* 1989; Carey 1995). At best, if standardized, they will give the clinician an impression of the patient's ability to discriminate sensory inputs, despite a lack of reliability between examiners. In addition, the patient is often able to give insight to the impairment by describing the difference between what is felt by each hand.

The common clinical tests, in a standardized version (Lincoln *et al.* 1989), are described below. During these tests, the patient is blindfolded. Lincoln and colleagues have shown even the standardized versions of these tests to have doubtful reliability. Furthermore, their validity in terms of relevance to function is not clear.

Tactile sensation

The patient is asked to indicate when they feel the test sensation. The skin is touched with the test object. Body part and side are tested in random order. Responses are scored: 0 Absent, 1 Impaired and 2 Normal. Six aspects of tactile sensation can be tested: temperature, light touch, pressure, pain, tactile localization, bilateral simultaneous touch and 2-point discrimination.

The entire battery of tests put together by Lincoln and colleagues (1991) (including the kinaesthetic tests below), can take an hour to administer. We would suggest that each test is administered on a need-to-know basis, rather than routinely. Some of the tactile tests are outlined below as standardized by Lincoln and colleagues:

● Light Touch
Touch, not brush, the skin lightly with cotton wool ball.
● Pressure
Applied by the index finger, sufficient to just deform the skin contour.
● Tactile localization
Pressure test repeated with index finger tip coated with powder to mark the spot touched. Patient is asked to point, describe or indicate on

a drawing the exact spot touched; 2 cm of error is allowed.

- Bilateral simultaneous touch
  Corresponding sites on both sides of the body are touched simultaneously using finger tips. Patient is asked which side has been touched or indicate as above.
- 2-point discrimination
  Using blunt dividers, 1 or 2 points are applied simultaneously to the skin in an irregular order for approximately 0.5 sec. Patient is asked to say whether one or both points are in skin contact. Normally an 8 mm space can be detected on the palm, 3 mm on the fingertip.

Stereognosis

In this test of the ability to recognize common objects by touch alone (i.e., blindfolded), as described by Lincoln *et al.* (1989), a common object is placed in the patient's hand for a maximum time of 15 seconds. The patient identifies the object by naming it, describing it or by pair-matching with an identical object. Objects include: coins, ball-point pen, pencil, toothbrush, comb, scissors, large safety pin, sponge and flannel. Note that objects are chosen for their different shapes and/or textures. Scoring is 0 Absent, 1 Impaired, 2 Normal.

Kinaesthetic sensation

In the tests standardized by Lincoln and colleagues (1991), appreciation of movement, direction of movement and joint position sense are tested simultaneously. Responses are scored as above 0 to 2 for each modality.

The affected limb, only one joint at a time, is moved by the examiner. The patient is asked to mirror the movement with the other limb. If they cannot they are asked to indicate whether or not a movement has occurred. Three practice movements are performed before blindfolding. When the examiner moves the joint, the following are tested simultaneously:

- Appreciation of movement
  Patient indicates that a movement takes place but in incorrect direction.
- Direction of movement
  Patient is able to mirror direction of movement but its new position is incorrect.
- Joint position
  Patient mirrors test movement to within 10° of new position.

The above tests were standardized by Lincoln and colleagues in an attempt to increase inter-rater reliability, which is notoriously poor for sensory testing. They were shown, however, to have poor inter-rater reliability despite their standardization. There was better consistency over time on some items when they were assessed by the same therapist.

More quantitative tests are available (see Carey 1995 for some details), for research purposes but are not generally used in the clinic. Their relevance to function has been questioned.

Carey (1995) reviews methods of testing and describes two quantified and standardized tests recently developed, which have been shown to be reliable and able to identify the presence of impairment relative to normative standards: the **Tactile Discrimination Test** and the **Proprioceptive Discrimination Test** (Carey *et al.* 1993; Carey 1995).

A simple test, **Find-the-Thumb**, can be used to give an indication of a patient's ability to locate this body part in space. The patient is blindfolded, the arm is moved passively and the patient asked to find the thumb (Prescott *et al.* 1982; Smith *et al.* 1983).

Measures of perception–cognition

Mini-Mental State Examination (MMSE)

This is a widely used test of cognitive impairment. It is scored out of 30 with 24 being used to distinguish normal from abnormal. It is said to be reliable and valid. The items tested are:

- Orientation
- Registration
- Attention and calculation
- Recall
- Language
- Copying

A modified version of this is also used (Galasko *et al.* 1990).

References: Folstein and Luria (1973); Beatty and Goodkin (1990).

Rivermead Behavioural Memory Test

This test is easy to administer and may be carried out by a therapist in the absence of a psychologist It is scored out of 24 on these items:

1 First name of person in photograph
2. Second name (surname) of person in photograph

3. Remembering hidden belongings
4. Remembering to ask about appointment
5. Picture (object) recognition (selecting 10 from 20 shown)
6a. Prose recall – immediate (21 ideas)
6b. Prose recall – delayed (20 min)
7. Face recognition (recognizing 5 from 10 shown)
8a. Route – immediate (5 places)
8b. Route – delayed (about 20 min)
9. Route – message (envelope to be left)
10. Date (correct)

Reference: Wilson *et al.* (1985, 1989).

There are several tests used to test perceptual-cognitive function. Commonly used are:

Rivermead Perceptual Assessment Battery (RPAB)

This test is used to test different perceptuo-cognitive tasks such as picture matching, figure-ground discrimination, body image and letter cancellation. The entire test takes approximately one hour to administer and a reliable shortened version has been published (Lincoln and Edmans 1989) which comprises picture matching, object matching, size recognition, animal halves, right/left word and shape copying, three-dimensional copying and cube copying. The RPAB has been shown to have some predictive ability in terms of functional outcome following stroke.

References: Lincoln and Edmans (1989), Barer *et al.* (1990).

Behavioural Inattention Test (BIT)

Another means of detecting and testing visuospatial neglect, this test includes six conventional tests:

● Line crossing (Albert's test)
● Letter cancellation
● Star cancellation
● Figure and shape copying
● Line bisection
● Representational drawing

and nine behavioural tests:

● Picture scanning
● Telephone dialling
● Menu reading
● Article reading
● Telling and setting the time (digital clock)
● Coin sorting
● Address and sentence copying
● Map navigation
● Card sorting

Individual tests can be taken from this battery. For example, the Star Cancellation Test has been reported to be the most sensitive at detecting neglect (Halligan *et al.* 1989) and the Letter Cancellation Test has also been used in clinical trials (e.g., Dean and Shepherd 1997).

References: Albert (1973), Wilson *et al.* (1987a,b), Halligan *et al.* (1989).

Environmental analysis

Behaviour mapping

A behaviour map represents the distribution of behaviour in a particular setting, and the methodology involves sampling predetermined behaviours at regular intervals. This is basically a time-sampling technique for studying environmental influences on behaviour. Data can be collected relating various aspects of behaviour to the physical spaces in which they are observed. The necessary features are descriptions of behaviour and participants and statements relating the behaviour to its physical locus, for example, in ward areas or in the rehabilitation department. The picture that emerges is an indication of where patients spend their day and the effects on their behaviour of the environmental features in these settings.

There have been several studies of rehabilitation environments using behaviour mapping (Keith 1980; Kennedy *et al.* 1988; Lincoln *et al.* 1989; Tinson 1989). The results of some are discussed in Chapter 1. Methodology involves determining the activities to be monitored, the venues and the patient group. For example, Keith (1980) divided activities into treatment, social interaction and solitary behaviour in his study of stroke patients. Tinson (1989), in his more recent study, examined such behaviours as recreation, therapy, own exercise, travel and waiting. Recording sheets are used for data collection. The results can be presented in graphic form as a pie diagram or histogram, which may help staff take the next step following the mapping process, which is to plan and carry out any necessary changes.

References: Ittelson *et al.* (1976); Keith (1980).

Behaviour stream analysis

A behaviour stream is a detailed sequential record of a segment of a person's behaviour. The purpose is to capture an individual's behaviour in narrative form with as little distortion as possible, with no predetermined categories. One study of patients with spinal cord injuries (Willems 1972) set out to seek answers to these questions: how do patients spend their time and in what settings? With whom do they interact? Is the distribution of the patient's time in keeping with the aims of therapy?

In this study, a patient was followed for one waking day from 5.00 am to 11 pm while the observer dictated a description of activities into a tape recorder. Observers were rotated every 2 hr. After typing up, the information was coded into episodes with categories of time, activity, who was involved and ratings of initiation of behaviour (see Keith 1988).

Modifications to this basic method, which was originally described by Barker and Wright (1971), include random sampling and setting categories in advance, according to what questions one is seeking to answer. The method of collecting information has been used to find out how much time a person spends in bed (pressure sensors under the mattress), how far a patient travels by wheelchair (with an odometer) (Halstead 1976; Halstead *et al.* 1979), and what potentially damaging events occur to a patient. Another use is to discover to what extent patients initiate behaviour without assistance over an extended period (Keith 1988). This latter may provide information relevant to a person's ability to cope in a less assistive environment, i.e., at home.

References: Willems (1972); Keith (1988).

Measures of anxiety and depression

There are many tests available which are used in hospital or rehabilitation settings, including the Wakefield Self-Assessment Depression Inventory (Snaith *et al.* 1971; Wade, Legh-Smith *et al.* 1987); the Beck Questionnaire (Beck *et al.* 1961; House *et al.* 1989), the General Health Questionnaire (Goldberg 1972; Wade *et al.* 1986) and the Modified Self-Report Measure of Social Adjustment (Weissman and Bothwell 1976). Such scales may be useful in giving an indication of how people feel during rehabilitation. Wade (1992a) points out that some of these scales are indicators of misery and distress rather than clinical depression; hence their

usefulness for showing rehabilitation and hospital staff how their patients feel. They are not necessarily reliable for use with neurological patients, however, because they give an indication of how people feel, they enable staff to set about instituting changes in environment and staff and family attitudes.

Diagnosis-specific measures

Parkinson's disease

Degree of Disability Scale (Hoehn and Yahr Scale)

Stage I   Unilateral involvement only, usually with minimal or no functional impairment.

Stage II   Bilateral or midline involvement, without impairment of balance.

Stage III   First sign of impaired righting reflexes. This is evident by unsteadiness as the patient turns or is demonstrated when he is pushed from standing equilibrium with the feet together and eyes closed. Functionally the patient is somewhat restricted in his activities but may have some work potential depending upon the type of employment. Patients are physically capable of leading independent lives, and their disability is mild to moderate.

Stage IV   Fully developed, severely disabling disease; the patient is still able to walk and stand unassisted but is markedly incapacitated.

Stage V   Confinement to bed or wheelchair unless aided.

This scale was an initial attempt to classify Parkinson's disease. It is included for historical reasons since it is of little use for measurement.

Reference: Hoehn and Yahr (1967).

Parkinson's Disease Rating Scale (Webster Scale)

Bradykinesia of hands – including handwriting
  0 No involvement.
  1 Detectable slowing of the supination-pronation rate evidenced by beginning difficulty in handling tools, buttoning clothes and with handwriting.
  2 Moderate slowing of supination-pronation rate, one or both sides, evidenced by moderate

impairment of hand function. Hand writing is greatly impaired, micrographia present.

3 Severe slowing of supination-pronation rate. Unable to write or button clothes, marked difficulty in handling utensils.

Rigidity

0 Non-detectable.

1 Detectable rigidity in neck and shoulders. Activation phenomenon is present. One or both arms show mild, negative, resting rigidity.

2 Moderate rigidity in neck and shoulders. Resting rigidity is positive when patient not on medication.

3 Severe rigidity in neck and shoulders. Resting rigidity cannot be reversed by medication.

Posture

0 Normal posture. Head flexed forward less than 10 cms (4 in).

1 Beginning poker spine. Head flexed forward up to 12 cms (5 in).

2 Beginning arm flexion. Head flexed forward up to 15 cm (6 in). One or both arms raised but still below waist.

3 Onset of simian posture. Head flexed forward more than 15 cm (6 in). One or both hands elevated above the waist. Sharp flexion of hand, beginning interphalangeal extension. Beginning flexion of knees.

Upper extremity swing

0 Swings both arms well.

1 One arm definitely decreased in amount of swing.

2 One arm fails to swing.

3 Both arms fail to swing.

Gait

0 Steps out well with 45–75 cm (18–30 in) stride. Turns about effortlessly.

1 Gait shortened to 30–45 cm (12–18in) stride. Beginning to strike one heel. Turn around time slowing. Requires several steps.

2 Stride moderately shortened – now 15–30 cm (6–12 in). Both heels beginning to strike floor forcefully.

3 Onset of shuffling gait, steps less than 8 cm (3 in). Occasional stuttering-type or blocking gait. Walks on toes – turns around very slowly.

Tremor

0 No detectable tremor found.

1 Less than 2 cm (1 inch) of peak-to-peak tremor movement observed in limbs or head at rest or in either hand while walking or during finger-to-nose testing.

2 Maximum tremor envelope fails to exceed 10 cm (4 in). Tremor is severe but not constant and patient retains some control of hands.

3 Tremor envelope exceeds 10 cm (4 in). Tremor is constant and severe. Patient cannot get free of tremor while awake unless it is a pure cerebellar type. Writing and feeding self are impossible.

Facies

0 Normal. Full animation. No stare.

1 Detectable immobility. Mouth remains closed. Beginning features of anxiety or depression.

2 Moderate immobility. Emotion breaks through at markedly increased threshold. Lips parted some of the time. Moderate appearance of anxiety or depression. Drooling may be present.

3 Frozen facies. Mouth open 0.06cm ($\frac{1}{4}$ in) or more. Drooling may be severe.

Seborrhea

0 None.

1 Increased perspiration, secretion remaining thin.

2 Obvious oiliness present. Secretions much thicker.

3 Marked seborrhea, entire face and head covered by thick secretion.

Speech

0 Clear, loud, resonant, easily understood.

1 Beginning of hoarseness with loss of inflection and resonance. Good volume and still easily understood.

2 Moderate hoarseness and weakness. Constant monotone, unvaried pitch. Beginning of dysarthria, hesitancy, stuttering, difficult to understand.

3 Marked harshness and weakness. Very difficult to hear and to understand.

Self-care

0 No impairment.

1 Still provides full self-care but rate of dressing definitely impeded. Able to live alone and often still employable.

2 Requires help in certain critical areas, such as turning in bed, rising from chairs, etc. Very slow in performing most activities but manages by taking much time.

3 Continuously disabled. Unable to dress, feed self, or walk alone.

There are no formal studies of reliability. The scale is quite widely used in either its lengthy form or in an amended version.

Reference: Webster (1968).

Step-second test

The patient is asked to stand up from a chair, walk 5 m, turn, return to the chair, and sit down. The patient is timed from the start to end and counts the number of steps taken. The two numbers are multiplied to obtain step-seconds. The able-bodied are said to score between 50 and 100.

Reference: Webster (1968).

Other recommended measures for Parkinson's disease are the Nine-Hole Peg Test and the Ten-metre Walk Test.

Traumatic brain injury or post-brain surgery coma

Glasgow outcome scale

This is a widely used scale to measure outcome from head injury. It comprises five states:

1 Death
2. Vegetative state
3. Severe disability; conscious but dependent
4. Moderate disability; independent but disabled
5. Good recovery

There is also an 8-point version. This 5-point version has been shown to be reliable. This scale is considered useful as a global measure of outcome for these patients and its value lies in the general vision it gives of their status.

References: Jennett and Bond (1975), Maas *et al.* (1983).

Glasgow Coma Scale

This is a method of testing state of arousal, and is particularly in common use after head injury. It is reported to be valid, reliable and sensitive. It has three sections:

Eye opening
None | Even to pain
To pain | Pain from stimulus to limbs
To speech | Opens eyes on verbal approach
Spontaneous | Opens eyes spontaneously

Motor Response
None | To any pain; limbs remain flaccid
Extension | Shoulder adducted/internally rotated, forearm pronated
Abnormal flexion | Shoulder flexes/adducts

Withdrawal | Arm withdraws from pain, shoulder abducts
Localizes pain | Arm attempts to remove supraorbital/chest pain
Obeys commands | Follows simple commands

Verbal Response
None | As stated
Incomprehensible | Moans/groans; no words
Inappropriate | Intelligible, exclamatory or random
Confused | Responds with conversation, but confused
Oriented | Aware of time, place, person

The scale varies in detail from centre to centre; the above is an example. It is usually reported as separate scores and as a summed score. In general, a score of <8 is taken to separate a comatose state from non-coma (Wade 1992a).

References: Teasdale and Jennett (1974), Teasdale *et al.* (1979).

Westmead Post-Traumatic Amnesia (PTA) Scale

The designers of this scale use as an operational definition of PTA the inability to lay down memories reliably from one day to the next (Shores *et al.* 1986). Patients are said to be in a state of PTA if they cannot get a perfect score for three consecutive days. The validity of the scale was tested by comparing scores on the scale with results on a test of verbal new learning. It should be noted that, although patients may not be in a state of PTA as defined, they may still suffer from amnesia to some extent.

Reference: Shores *et al.* (1986).

Self-assessment and self-efficacy scales

It is helpful to the rehabilitation process to elicit input from the patient (and from relatives) about such issues as self-perception of handicap, quality of life, ability to perform the required actions at home, work and leisure. Self-efficacy scales enable patient input regarding outcome of the rehabilitative process. It is heartening to see a patient questionnaire being included as a measurement tool in research investigations of the effects of rehabilitation (e.g., Dean and Shepherd 1997). Questionnaire measures used to provide data about rehabilitation outcome, for example, require to be reliable and valid as does any other measure. However, there is also a need to have input from the patient in order to guide the rehabilitative process. Gathering such information should not be done without consultation with other relevant staff, lest an individual be swamped with questionnaires. There are many reliable and valid measures published. Choice will depend on the questions to be asked. Examples are the **Self-Assessment Parkinson's Disease Disability Scale** (Brown *et al.* 1989), the **Sickness Impact Profile** (Bergner *et al.* 1981), the **Multiple Sclerosis Self-Efficacy Scale (MSSE)** and the **Fatigue Severity Scale** (Krupp *et al.* 1989) specifically for individuals with multiple sclerosis.

Clinical audit

The collection of information in a clinical audit is a valuable first step to a realistic appraisal of what is the outcome of the rehabilitative process and the possible contribution of physiotherapy. The results can be used to guide future interventions and to provide a benchmark for overtaking in subsequent measurements. As an example, a group of physiotherapists in Sydney developed a set of nine clinical indicators for neurological patients (Wales 1994). Seven of the measures have been demonstrated to be reliable; the two that have not were shoulder subluxation (usually unreliable) and the equal weight-bearing test. Table 3.3 shows these indicators, five of which were dependent upon MAS scores. The clinical indicators were trialled in the stroke unit of one Sydney hospital, data being collected from 192 patients admitted in one 6-month period. The logical next step is to attempt to identify for a particular functional outcome, say, walking performance, a more effective method of training.

Table 3.3 Neurological clinical indicators

---

1 A score of 5 or greater on the sitting balance item of the MAS
2 A score of 3 or greater on the standing up item of the MAS
3 A score of 4 or greater on the walking item of the MAS
4 A score of 5 or greater on the upper arm function item of the MAS
5 A score of 5 or greater on the hand movements item of the MAS
6 Able to walk with a velocity of 1 m/sec or greater
7 Able to achieve equal weight-bearing in unsupported standing for 1 min or more
8 Dorsiflexion range of 100° or less
9 Shoulder subluxation of 1 cm or more

Courtesy of A. Wales

In conclusion, assessment of the motor performance of patients with neurological impairments provides information upon which training and therapy are based. For such assessment to be accurate requires that the therapist develops the knowledge base to enable subjective observational analysis and comparison to have a rational basis. Therapists need an education which encompasses biomechanics and kinesiology taught by those who study these sciences. At the moment much of the 'knowledge' of movement in neurological therapy appears to have evolved from pseudoscientific and often erroneous views of movement handed down in the therapy literature over the past few decades. We have suggested earlier that observational assessment can utilize check-lists made up of information from biomechanics and other fields of movement, which are updated as necessary.

Clinical measurement is another facet of physiotherapy which provides objective information of value in determining the direction and detail of training and therapy but which also provides information about the broader issues of, for example, recovery, change in performance and outcome. It is interesting to note that recent textbooks aimed at physiotherapists continue to omit reference to the use of objective measures in the clinic (e.g., Umphred 1995; Edwards 1996). Even a recent text on gait analysis which sets out to provide clinical guidelines (Craik and Oatis 1995) contains little direct information on methods of measuring gait in the clinic, although it refers to the results of many laboratory biomechanical studies of gait. It seems that in many rehabilitation situations the gulf between measurement, particularly of movement, and the clinic remains. On the other hand, there is a risk that an excessive use of measurement in the clinic can bring its own problems. Experience in rehabilitation units where the physiotherapists are enthusiastic about the principle of measurement suggests that, once the idea takes on, it holds such interest that more time can be spent in assessment and measurement than in training.

Measurement carries with it a number of responsibilities. Therapists need to consider carefully, with their medical colleagues and the patients, what questions need answers.

Patient-oriented measurement should be directed to answering questions that have meaning for the patient, for example, relating to the performance of everyday actions such as walking, standing up and reaching to grasp an object; changes to performance over time. Such measures could be performed on a weekly basis, recorded and graphed for all to see. If particular information is sought which would impact upon therapy or training given, then this is measured on a need-to-know basis; examples are shoulder or ankle joint range of motion or amount of time spent in active training. It is a mistake to consider that every aspect of motor function needs to be measured.

Terminology makes more sense if standardized across professional boundaries. Many physiotherapists (and others) use the terms subjective and objective in relation to assessment in a misleading way, subjective referring to information obtained by patient report, objective meaning the assessment performed by the therapist. Of course, the therapist's evaluation of the patient is as subjective as the patient's, although the patient's evaluation may be more reliable! Both patient and therapist will bring their own biases, beliefs and attitudes to such an evaluation, hence, both are being subjective. The terms, as far as we can find out, originated in medicine and have made their way recently, via manipulative physiotherapy into neurological physiotherapy (cf. Mawson 1993). It is to minimize the effects of subjectivism that methods of measurement have been developed.

Finally, we agree with Wade (1992a) that good measures exist for evaluating outcome and that clinicians must agree on measures, collect data routinely and reliably and act on the results of evaluation. Nevertheless, in the search for the 'perfect' scale clinicians keep developing new functional scales to address their own particular concerns (e.g., Badke *et al.* 1993), and it may be that more time and money is spent in this endeavour and in the continuing testing of reliability and validity than in using available tests actually to evaluate patient performance. Critical papers emerge in large numbers pointing out that scales exist which have not been tested for reliability and validity (e.g., Lyden and Lau 1991). Surely by now we have all got the message. We know which scales do what and whether or not they are reliable and valid and we should be using them. Clinicians do, however, have to make a decision as to what questions they want answered in order to choose which (out of the many) scales they should use. For example, if physiotherapists set out to train a patient to improve performance on some functional task(s), then a method of measuring those tasks needs to be identified (e.g., MAS, Frenchay Arm Test, Timed Walk Test, Nine-hole Peg Test); if calf muscle length is the issue then a different type of measure is used. However,

therapists also need to be able to cope with the results of their measurement and face up to the possibility sometimes of a less than positive outcome. Was poor outcome on a walking test due to the effects of the lesion (not all patients will be able to regain optimal function) or was it due to inappropriate and ineffective physiotherapy? It really is rewarding to sort this out. There is often the possibility that an improved physiotherapy programme may be more beneficial to patients. Surely we ought to be finding out, rather than searching for a measurement tool which will show our methods are effective!

References

Ada, L. and Canning, C. (1990) Anticipating and avoiding muscle shortening. In *Key Issues in Neurological Physiotherapy* (eds L. Ada and C. Canning), Butterworth Heinemann, Oxford, pp. 219–236.

Ada, L. and Westwood, P. (1992) A kinematic analysis of recovery of the ability to stand up following stroke. *Australian Journal of Physiotherapy*, **38**, 135–142.

Ada, L., O'Dwyer, N.J. and Neilson, P.D. (1993) Improvement in kinematic characteristics and coordination following stroke quantified by linear systems analysis. *Human Movement Science*, **12**, 137–153.

Adams, S.A., Pickering, R.M., Ashburn, A. *et al.* (1997) The scalability of the Rivermead Motor Assessment in nonacute stroke patients. *Clinical Rehabilitation*, **11**, 52–59.

Albert, M.L. (1973) A simple test of visual neglect. *Neurology*, **23**, 658–664.

Ashburn, A. (1982) A physical assessment for stroke patients. *Physiotherapy*, **68**, 109–113.

Ashworth, B. (1964) Preliminary trial of carisoprodol in multiple sclerosis. *Practitioner*, **192**, 540–542.

Badke, M.B., DiFabio, R.P., Leonard, E. *et al.* (1993) Reliability of a functional mobility assessment tool with application to neurologically impaired patients: a preliminary report. *Physiotherapy Canada*, **45**, 15–20.

Barer, D.H., Edmans, J.A. and Lincoln, N.B. (1990) Screening for perceptual problems in acute stroke patients. *Clinical Rehabilitation*, **4**, 1–11.

Barker, R. and Wright, H.F. (1971) *One Boy's Day*, Harper and Row, New York.

Beatty, W.W. and Goodkin, D.E. (1990) Screening for cognitive impairment in multiple sclerosis. An evaluation of the Mini-Mental State Examination. *Archives of Neurology*, **47**, 297–301.

Beck, A.T., Ward, C.H., Mendelson, M. *et al.* (1961) An inventory for measuring depression. *Archives of General Psychiatry*, **4**, 561–571.

Berg, K., Wood-Dauphinee, S., Williams, J.I. *et al.* (1989) Measuring balance in the elderly: preliminary development of an instrument. *Physiotherapy Canada*, **41**, 304–311.

Berg, K.O., Maki, B.E., Williams, J. *et al.* (1992) Clinical and laboratory measures of postural balance in an elderly population. *Archives of Physical Medicine and Rehabilitation*, **73**, 1073–1080.

Bergner, M., Bobbitt, R.A., Carter, W.B. *et al.* (1981) The Sickness Impact Profile: developmental and final revision of a health status measure. *Medical Care*, **19**, 789–805.

Bohannon, R.W. (1989) Correlation of lower limb strengths and other variables with standing performance in stroke patients. *Physiotherapy Canada*, **41**, 198–202.

Bohannon, R.W., Walsh, S. and Joseph, M.C. (1993) Ordinal and timed balance measurements: reliability and validity in patients with stroke. *Clinical Rehabilitation*, **7**, 9–13.

Bohannon, R.W. and Andrews, A.W. (1987a) Interrater reliability of hand-held dynamometry. *Physical Therapy*, **67**, 931–933.

Bohannon, R.W. and Andrews, A.W. (1987b) Relative strength of seven upper extremity muscle groups in hemiparetic stroke patients. *Journal of Neurological Rehabilitation*, **1**, 161–165.

Bohannon, R.W. and Smith, M.B. (1987) Interrater reliability of a modified Ashworth scale of muscle spasticity. *Physical Therapy*, **67**, 206–207.

Bouisset, S. and Zattara, M. (1981) A sequence of postural movements precedes voluntary movement. *Neuroscience Letters*, **22**, 263–270.

Brown, R.G., MacCarthey, B., Jahanshahi, M. *et al.* (1989) Accuracy of self-reported disability in patients with parkinsonism. *Archives of Neurology*, **46**, 955–959.

Bruce, R.A., Kusumi, F. and Hosmer, D. (1973) Maximal oxygen intake and nomographic assessment of functional aerobic impairment in cardiovascular disease. *American Heart Journal*, **85**, 546–562.

Carey, L.M. (1995) Somatosensory loss after stroke. *Critical Reviews in Physical and Rehabilitation Medicine*, **7**, 51–91.

Carey, L.M., Matyas, T.A. and Oke, L.E. (1993) Sensory loss in stroke patients: effective tactile and proprioceptive discrimination training. *Archives of Physical Medicine and Rehabilitation*, **74**, 602–611.

Carr, J.H., Shepherd, R.B., Nordholm, L. *et al.* (1985) Investigation of a new motor assessment scale for stroke patients. *Physical Therapy*, **65**, 175–180.

Carr, J.H. and Shepherd, R.B. (1987) *A Motor Relearning Programme for Stroke*, Butterworth Heinemann, Oxford.

Carroll, D. (1965) A quantitative test of upper extremity function. *Journal of Chronic Diseases*, **18**, 479–491.

Cerny, K. (1983) A clinical method of quantitative gait analysis. *Physical Therapy*, **63**, 1125–1126.

Collin, C. and Wade, D. (1990) Assessing motor impairment after stroke: a pilot reliability study. *Journal of Neurology, Neurosurgery, and Psychiatry*, **53**, 576–579.

Collin, F.M., Wade, D.T. and Bradshaw, C.M. (1990) Mobility after stroke: reliability and measures of impairment and disability. *International Disability Studies*, **12**, 6–9.

Craik, R.L. and Oatis, C.A. (eds) (1995). *Gait Analysis. Theory and Application*, Mosby, St Louis.

Crow, J.L., Lincoln, N.N.B., Nouri, F.M. *et al.* (1989) The effectiveness of EMG biofeedback in the treatment of arm function after stroke. *International Disability Studies*, **11**, 155–160.

Davies, P.M. (1990) *Right in the Middle*, Springer-Verlag, Berlin.

Dean, C. and Mackey, F. (1992) Motor assessment scale scores as a measure of rehabilitation outcome following stroke. *Australian Journal of Physiotherapy*, **38**, 31–35.

Dean, C.M. and Shepherd, R.B. (1997) Task-related training improves performance of seated reaching tasks following stroke: A randomised controlled trial. *Stroke*, **28**, 1–7.

Demeurisse, G., Demol, O. and Robaye, E. (1980) Motor evaluation in vascular hemiplegia. *Journal of European Neurology*, **19**, 381–389.

DeSouza, L.H., Langton Hewer, R. and Miller, S. (1980) Assessment of recovery of arm control in hemiplegic stroke patients. Arm function test. *International Rehabilitation Medicine*, **2**, 3–9.

Duncan, P.W., Weiner, D.K., Chandler, J. *et al.* (1990) Functional reach: a new clinical measure of balance. *Journal of Gerontology*, **45**, M192–197.

Edwards, S. (1996) *Neurological Physiotherapy. A Problem-Solving Approach*, Churchill Livingstone, London.

Folstein, M.F. and Luria, R. (1973) Reliability, validity and clinical application of the visual analogue mood scale. *Psychological Medicine*, **3**, 479–486.

Fowler, V., Canning, C.G., Carr, J.H. *et al.* (1998) The effect of muscle length on the pendulum test. *Archives of Physical Medicine and Rehabilitation* (in press).

Friedl, W.G., Cohen, L., Hallett, M. *et al.* (1988) Postural adjustments associated with rapid voluntary arm movements. II Biomechanical analysis. *Journal of Neurology, Neurosurgery, and Psychiatry*, **51**, 232–243.

Fugl-Meyer, A.R., Jaasko, L. Leyman, I. *et al.* (1975) The post-stroke hemiplegic patient. 1. A method of evaluation of physical performance. *Scandinavian Journal of Rehabilitation Medicine*, **7**, 13–31.

Gajdosik, R.L. and Bohannon, R.W. (1987) Clinical measurement of range of motion: review of goniometry emphasizing reliability and validity. *Physical Therapy*, **67**, 1867–1872.

Galasko, D., Klauber, M.R., Hofstetter, R. *et al.* (1990) The Mini-Mental State Examination in the early diagnosis of Alzheimer's disease. *Archives of Neurology*, **47**, 49–52.

Garraway, W.M., Akhtar, A.J., Gore, S.M. *et al.* (1976) Observer variation in the clinical assessment of stroke. *Age and Ageing*, **5**, 233–239.

Goldberg, D.P. (1972) *The Detection of Psychiatric Illness by Questionnaire*, Monograph 21, Oxford University Press, Oxford.

Goldie, P.A., Bach, T.M. and Evans, O.M. (1989) Force platform measures for evaluating postural control: reliability and validity. *Archives of Physical Medicine and Rehabilitation*, **70**, 510–517.

Granger, C.V., Hamilton, B.B. and Sherwin, F.S. (1986) *Guide for the Use of the Uniform Data Set for Medical Rehabilitation*, Project Office, Buffalo General Hospital, New York.

Halligan, P.W., Marshall, J.C. and Wade, D.T. (1989) Visuospatial neglect: underlying factors and test sensitivity. *Lancet*, **ii**, 908–910.

Halstead, L.S. (1976) Longitudinal unobtrusive measurements in rehabilitation. *Archives in Physical Medicine and Rehabilitation*, **57**, 189–193.

Halstead, L.S., Willems, E.P. and Frey, S. (1979) Spinal cord injury: time out of bed during rehabilitation. *Archives in Physical Medicine and Rehabilitation*, **60**, 590–595.

Hansen, P.D., Woollacott, M.H. and Debu, B. (1988) Postural responses to changing task conditions. *Experimental Brain Research*, **73**, 627–636.

Hayes, K.C. (1982) Biomechanics of postural control. *Exercise and Sports Sciences Review*, pp. 363–391.

Hoehn, M.M. and Yahr, M.D. (1967) Parkinsonism: onset, progression, and mortality. *Neurology*, **17**, 427–442.

Holbrook, M. and Skilbeck, C.E. (1983) An activities index for use with stroke patients. *Age and Ageing*, **12**, 166–170.

Horak, F.B. (1987) Clinical measurement of postural control in adults. *Physical Therapy*, **67**, 1881–1885.

House, A., Dennis, M., Hawton, K. *et al.* (1989) Methods of identifying mood disorders in stroke patients: experience in the Oxfordshire Community Stroke Project. *Age and Ageing*, **18**, 371–379.

Hunter, M., Tomberlin, J.A., Kirkikis, C. *et al.* (1990) Progressive exercise testing in closed head-injured subjects: comparison of exercise apparatus in assessment of a physical conditioning program. *Physical Therapy*, **70**, 363–371.

Ittelson, W.H., Rivlin, L.G. and Proshansky, H.M. (1976) Use of behavioral maps in environmental psychology. In *Environmental Psychology: People and their Physical Settings* (ed. H.M. Proshansky, W.H. Ittelson and L.G. Rivlin), Rinehart and Winston, New York, pp. 340–351.

Jankowski, L.W. and Sullivan, S.J. (1990) Aerobic and neuromuscular training: Effect on the capacity, efficiency, and fatiguability of patients with traumatic brain injuries. *Archives of Physical Medicine and Rehabilitation*, **71**, 500–504.

Jennett, B. and Bond, M. (1975) Assessment of outcome after severe brain damage. A practical scale. *Lancet*, **i**, 480–484.

Keith, R.A. (1980) Activity patterns in a stroke rehabilitation unit. *Social Science and Medicine*, **14A**, 575–580.

Keith, R.A. (1988) Observations in the rehabilitation hospital: twenty years of research. *Archives of Physical Medicine and Rehabilitation*, **69**, 625–631.

Keith, R.A., Granger, C.V., Hamilton, B.B. *et al.* (1987) The Functional Independence Measure: a new tool for rehabilitation. In *Advances in Clinical Rehabilitation* (ed. M.G. Eisenberg), Springer-Verlag, New York, pp. 6–18.

Kemer, J.F. and Alexander, J. (1981) Activities of daily living: reliability and validity of gross vs specific ratings. *Archives of Physical Medicine and Rehabilitation*, **62**, 161–166.

Kennedy, P., Fisher, K. and Pearson, E. (1988) Ecological evaluation of a rehabilitative environment for spinal cord injured people: behavioural mapping and feedback. *British Journal of Clinical Psychology*, **27**, 239–246.

Krebs, D.E., Edelstein, J.E. and Fishman, S. (1985) Reliability of observational kinematic gait analysis. *Physical Therapy*, **65**, 1027–1033.

Krupp, L.B., LaRocca, N.G., Muir-Nash, J. *et al.* (1989) The Fatigue Severity Scale. *Archives of Neurology*, **46**, 1121–1123.

Lee, W. (1980) Anticipatory control of postural and task muscles during rapid arm flexion. *Journal of Motor Behaviour*, **12**, 185–196.

Lennon, S. and Hastings, M. (1996) Key physiotherapy indicators for quality of stroke care. *Physiotherapy*, **82**, 655–664.

Lincoln, N.B. and Edmans, J.A. (1989) A re-validation of the Rivermead ADL scale for elderly patients with stroke. *Age and Ageing*, **19**, 9–24.

Lincoln, N. and Leadbitter, D. (1979) Assessment of motor function in stroke patients. *Physiotherapy*, **65**, 48–51.

Lincoln, N.B., Gamlen, R. and Thomason, H. (1989) Behavioural mapping of patients on a stroke unit. *International Disability Studies*, **11**, 149–154.

Loewen, S.C. and Anderson, B.A. (1988) Reliability of the Modified Motor Assessment Scale and the Barthel Index. *Physical Therapy*, **68**, 1077–1081.

Loewen, S.C. and Anderson, B.A. (1990) Predictors of stroke outcome using objective measurement scales. *Stroke*, **21**, 78–81.

Lyden, P.D. and Lau, G.T. (1991) A critical appraisal of stroke evaluation and rating scales. *Stroke*, **22**, 1345–1352.

Maas, A.I.R., Braakman, R., Schouten, H.J.A. *et al.* (1983) Agreement between physicians on assessment of outcome following severe head injury. *Journal of Neurosurgery*, **58**, 321–325.

McGavin, C.R., Gupta, S.P. and McHardy, G.J. (1976) Twelve-minute walking test for assessing disability in chronic bronchitis. *British Medical Journal*, **1**, 822–823.

McLellan, D.L. (1977) Co-contraction and stretch reflexes in spasticity during treatment with baclofen. *Journal of Neurology, Neurosurgery, and Psychiatry*, **40**, 30–38.

Mahoney, R.I. and Barthel, D.W. (1965) Functional evaluation: the Barthel Index. *Maryland Medical Journal*, **14**, 61–65.

Malouin, F. (1995) Observational gait analysis. In *Gait Analysis. Theory and Application* (ed. R.L. Craik and C.A. Oatis), Mosby, St Louis, pp. 112–124.

Malouin, F., Pichard, L., Bonneau, C. *et al.* (1994) Evaluating motor recovery early after stroke: comparison of the Fugl-Meyer Assessment and the Motor Assessment Scale. *Archives of Physical Medicine and Rehabilitation*, **75**, 1206–1212.

Mathias, S., Nayak, U.S.L. and Isaacs, B. (1986) Balance in elderly patients: the 'Get-up and Go' test. *Archives of Physical Medicine and Rehabilitation*, **67**, 387–389.

Mathiowetz, V., Weber, K., Kashman, N. *et al.* (1985) Adult norms for the nine-hole peg test of finger dexterity. *Occupational Therapy Journal of Research*, **5**, 24–37.

Mawson, S.J. (1993) Measuring physiotherapy outcome in stroke rehabilitation. *Physiotherapy*, **79**, 762–765.

Medical Research Council (1976) *Aids to the Examination of the Peripheral Nervous System*, Her Majesty's Stationery Office, London.

Morris, M.E., Iansek, R., Matyas, T.A. *et al.* (1994) The pathogenesis of gait hypokinesia in Parkinson's disease. *Brain*, **117**, 1169–1181.

Moseley, A. and Adams, R. (1991) Measurement of passive ankle dorsiflexion procedure and reliability. *Australian Journal of Physiotherapy*, **37**, 175–181.

Nashner, L.M. (1977) Fixed patterns of rapid postural responses among leg muscles during stance. *Experimental Brain Research*, **30**, 13–24.

Nashner, L.M., Black, F.O. and Wall, C. (1982) Adaptation to altered support surfaces and visual conditions in patients with vestibular deficits. *Journal of Neuroscience*, **2**, 536–544.

Nouri, F.M. and Lincoln, N.B. (1987) An extended activities of daily living scale for stroke patients. *Clinical Rehabilitation*, **1**, 301–305.

Perry, J., Fox, J.M., Boitano, M.A. *et al.* (1980) Functional evaluation of the pes anserinus transfer by electromyography and gait analysis. *Journal of Bone and Joint Surgery*, **62A**, 973–980.

Podsialo, D. and Richardson, S. (1991) The timed 'Up & Go': a test of basic functional mobility for frail elderly persons. *Journal of American Geriatric Society* **39**, 142–148.

Poole, J.L. and Whitney, S.L. (1988) Motor Assessment Scale for stroke patients: concurrent validity and interrater reliability. *Archives of Physical Medicine and Rehabilitation*, **69**, 195–197.

Prescott, R.J., Garraway, W.M. and Akhtar, A.L. (1982) Predicting functional outcome following acute stroke using a standard clinical examination. *Stroke*, **13**, 641–647.

Robinson, J.L. and Smidt, G.L. (1981) Quantitative gait evaluation in the clinic. *Physical Therapy*, **61**, 351–353.

Ryerson, S.D. (1995) Hemiplegia. In *Neurological Rehabilitation* (ed. D.A. Umphred), Mosby, St. Louis, pp. 681–721,

Sanford, J., Moreland, J., Swanson, L.R. *et al.* (1993) Reliability of the Fugl-Meyer assessment for testing motor performance in patients following stroke. *Physical Therapy*, **73**, 447–454.

Shores, E.A., Marosszeky, J.E., Sandanam, J. *et al.* (1986) Preliminary validation of a clinical scale for measuring the duration of post-traumatic amnesia. *The Medical Journal of Australia*, **144**, 569–572.

Shumway-Cook, A. and Horak, F. (1986) Assessing the influence of sensory interaction on balance. *Physical Therapy*, **66**, 1548–1550.

Smith, A. (1990). The measurement of human performance. In *Key Issues in Neurological Physiotherapy* (eds L. Ada and C. Canning), Oxford, Butterworth Heinemann, pp.51–80.

Smith, D.L., Akhtar, A.J. and Garraway, W.M. (1983) Proprioception and spatial neglect after stroke. *Age and Ageing*, **12**, 63–69.

Smith, R. (1994) Validation and reliability of the Elderly Mobility Scale. *Physiotherapy*, **80**, 744–747.

Snaith, R.P., Ahmed, S.N., Mehta, S. *et al.* (1971) Assessment of severity of primary depressive illness: Wakefield self assessment depression inventory. *Psychological Medicine*, **1**, 143–149.

Sunderland, A., Tinson, D., Bradley, L. *et al.* (1989) Arm function after stroke. An evaluation of grip strength as a measure of recovery and a prognostic indicator. *Journal of Neurology, Neurosurgery, and Psychiatry*, **52**, 1267–1272.

Sunderland, A., Tinson, D.J., Bradley, E.L. *et al.* (1992) Enhanced physical therapy improves recovery of arm function after stroke. A randomised controlled trial. *Journal of Neurology, Neurosurgery, and Psychiatry*, **55**, 530–535.

Teasdale, G. and Jennett, B. (1974) Assessment of coma and impaired consciousness. A practical scale. *Lancet*, **ii**, 81–83.

Teasdale, G., Murray, G., Parker, L. *et al.* (1979) Adding up the Glasgow Coma Scale. *Acta Neurochirurgica*, Suppl 28, 13–16.

Tinson, D.J. (1989) How stroke patients spend their days. *International. Disability Studies*, **11**, 45–49.

Tomasello, F., Mariani, F., Fieschi, C. *et al.* (1982) Assessment of interobserver differences in the Italian multicenter study on reversible cerebral ischaemia. *Stroke*, **13**, 32–34.

Tripp, E.J. and Harris, S.R. (1991) Test-retest reliability of isokinetic knee extension and flexion torque measurements in persons with spastic hemiparesis. *Physical Therapy*, **71**, 390–396.

Turton, A.J. and Fraser, C.M. (1986) A test battery to measure the recovery of voluntary movement control following stroke. *International Rehabilitation Medicine*, **8**, 74–78.

Umphred, D. (ed.) (1995) *Neurological Rehabilitation* (ed. D.A. Umphred), Mosby, St. Louis.

Verkerk, P.H., Schouten, J.P. and Oosterhuis, H.J.G.H. (1990) Measurement of the hand coordination. *Clinical Neurology and Neurosurgery*, **92** (2), 105–109.

Wade, D.T. (1992a) *Measurement in Neurological Rehabilitation*, Oxford University Press, Oxford.

Wade, D.T. (1992b) Evaluating outcome in stroke rehabilitation. *Scandinavian Journal of Rehabilitation Medicine*, Suppl 26, 97–104.

Wade, D.T., Legh-Smith, J. and Langton Hewer, R. (1986) Effects of living with and looking after survivors of a stroke. *British Medical Journal*, **293**, 418–420.

Wade, D.T., Legh-Smith, J. and Langton Hewer, R. (1987) Depressed mood after stroke. A community study of its frequency. *British Journal of Psychiatry*, **151**, 200–205.

Wade, D.T., Wood, V.A., Heller, A. *et al.* (1987). Walking after stroke. *Scandinavian Journal of Rehabilitation Medicine*, **19**, 25–30.

Wales, A. (1994) Neurological clinical indicators. *Efferents*, **14**, 16–18.

Wall, J.C. and Crosbie, J. (1995) Measurement of the temporal parameters of gait from slow motion video using a personal computer. In *Proceedings of the XXth Congress of World Confederation for Physical Therapy*, Washington, DC, p. 360.

Wall, J.C., Dhanendran, M. and Klenerman, L. (1976) A method of measuring the temporal/distance factors of gait. *Biomedical Engineering*, **11**, 409–412.

Webster, D.D. (1968) Critical analysis of the disability in Parkinson's disease. *Modern Treatment*, **5**, 257–282.

Weissman, M.M. and Bothwell, S. (1976) Assessment of social adjustment by patient self-report. *Archives of General Psychiatry*, **33**, 1111–1115.

Willems, E.P. (1972) The interface of the hospital environment and patient behaviour. *Archives of Physical Medicine and Rehabilitation*, March, 115–122.

Wilson, B.A., Cockburn, J. and Baddeley, A.D. (1985) *The Rivermead Behavioural Memory Test*, Thames Valley Test Company, Titchfield, Hants.

Wilson, B.A., Cockburn, J. and Halligan, P. (1987a) *Behavioural Inattention Test*, Thames Valley Test Company, Titchfield, Hants.

Wilson, B.A., Cockburn, J. and Halligan, P. (1987b) Development of a behavioural test of visuospatial neglect. *Archives of Physical Medicine and Rehabilitation*, **68**, 98–102.

Wilson, B.A., Cockburn, J., Baddeley, A.D. *et al.* (1989) The development and validation of a test battery for detecting and monitoring everyday memory problems. *Journal of Clinical Experimental Neuropsychology*, **11**, 855–870.

Wolfson, L., Whipple, R., Amerman, P. *et al.* (1990) Gait assessment in the elderly: a gait abnormality rating scale and its relation to falls. *Journal of Gerontology*, **45**, 12–19.

Further reading

Bohannon, R.W. (1995) Measurement, nature, and implications of skeletal muscle strength in patients with neurological disorders. *Clinical Biomechanics*, **10**, 283–292.

Goldie, P.A., Matyas, T.A., Spencer, K.I. et al. (1990) Postural control in standing following stroke: test-retest reliability of some quantitative clinical tests. *Physical Therapy*, **70**, 234–243.

Schwartz, C.E., Coulthard-Morris, L., Zeng, Q. *et al.* (1996) Measuring self-efficacy in people with multiple sclerosis: a validation study. *Archives of Physical Medicine and Rehabilitation*, **77**, 394–398.

Vanclay, F. (1991) Functional outcome measures in stroke rehabilitation. *Stroke*, **22**, 105–108.

Wade, D.T. (1993) Measurement in neurologic rehabilitation. *Current Opinion in Neurology*, **6**, 778–784.

Part Two
Task-Related Exercise and Training

4

Standing up and sitting down

The ability to stand up (STS) and sit down (SIT) are in themselves essential to independence. STS is in addition a prerequisite to the independent performance of other actions such as walking which require the ability to get into the standing position (Carr and Shepherd 1989, 1990). To put it simply, performing actions in standing and walking has to be preceded by the action of standing up. There is some evidence that STS is one of the most demanding everyday tasks we perform regularly (Berger *et al.* 1988), and lack of independence in this action has been reported to be one of the most likely factors associated with risk of institutionalization (Branch and Meyers 1987).

STS requires the ability to move the body mass forward from over a large base of support (thighs and feet) to a small base of support (feet) and to extend the lower limb joints (knees, hips and ankles) to raise the body mass over the feet. The ability to use the lower limbs to balance the body mass while propelling it away from the support surface is an important feature of standing up.

Support, propulsion and balance are major attributes of the lower limbs. STS is one of a class of actions in which the lower limbs extend and flex over the feet, which form a fixed base of support. These actions include standing up and sitting down, the stance phase of walking, walking up and down stairs, squat or crouch-to-stand and the initial phase of jumping and hopping. Lack of practice of this movement pattern is eventually associated with weakness of the lower limb extensor muscles and short calf muscles, a situation which may make it mechanically impossible to perform the actions. As an exercise, standing up from a seat, if considered solely from a mechanical point of view, provides an active stretch to the calf muscles, a muscle group which tends, in relatively immobile/inactive individuals, to become short and stiff.

Standing up requires the ability to maintain balance while pivoting the body mass over the feet. Generating angular and linear momentum sufficient to perform this translatory movement is potentially destabilizing. The individual who first attempts this action after a brain lesion has to learn not only how to generate and control muscle forces but also how to harness the interactional effects of segment rotations so that the action eventually becomes well-balanced and energy-efficient.

Standing up: description of the action

For ease of description, STS can be divided into a pre-extension and an extension phase (Carr and Gentile 1994; Shepherd and Carr 1994; Shepherd and Gentile 1994), the change occurring at the time the thighs leave the seat (thighs-off). There are other methods of identifying particular phases of the action (Kralj *et al.* 1990; Pai and Rogers 1990; Schenkman *et al.* 1990) but this may be the simplest classification for clinical purposes and it also has some mechanical validity.

In the pre-extension phase, in which the initial or starting posture is formed, one critical component is movement of the feet backward to a position behind an imaginary perpendicular line drawn down from the knees. This positions the feet so that the activation of lower limb extensor muscles in the extension phase will generate the backward horizontal component of ground reaction

forces essential to propel the body mass forward. Having positioned the feet, the upper body (head, arms and trunk) is rotated forward at the hips. The velocity of trunk flexion, by reactive forces, causes the thighs to move forward (Fig. 4.1). Since the feet are fixed, the shanks rotate forward at the ankles, with movement taking place at the knee (flexion) and ankle (dorsiflexion) joints. This movement of thighs and shanks may augment the active ankle dorsiflexion that, together with the trunk rotation, provides the horizontal momentum that moves the body mass forward.

The shoulder marker traces a path horizontally, then vertically, with some overlap around the time the thighs leave the seat (Fig. 4.2). The overlap between horizontal and vertical movement of the shoulder path shows that the horizontal movement of the body mass is transferred into vertical movement with no pause, the pre-extension and extension phases forming one continuous forward and upward movement. This means that the movement forward of the body, by angular displacement at the hip (flexion) and ankle (dorsiflexion) in the pre-extension phase, can have a dynamic effect on the upcoming extension phase.

Over the past decade there has been an increasing interest in examining the dynamics of STS and SIT. Results of investigations performed in the laboratory provide insight into the nature of the control of these actions and provide guidelines,

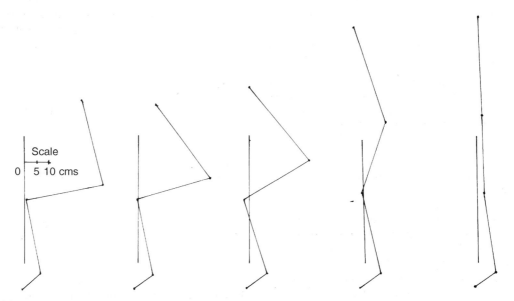

Fig. 4.1 Stick figures drawn from XY coordinates illustrating movement of the thigh forward (ankle dorsiflexion) as the trunk flexes. Note: the foot is on the floor. Middle figure represents thighs-off

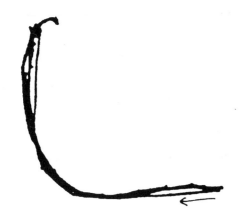

Fig. 4.2 Note the smooth continuous and curvilinear path of the shoulder marker (n = 10 trials)

which, if implemented, have the potential to improve clinical practice in terms of this significant action.

Kinematics

The everyday performance of STS is flexible, details varying in adaptation to task and environmental demands. However, optimal performance in the execution of STS involves a mechanically efficient movement pattern and a basic underlying coordination, regardless of the goal or the environmental context.

From experimental evidence so far, the critical kinematic features appear to be:

1 the generation of horizontal linear momentum of the body mass to move the body mass forward over the new base of support and
2 the translation of horizontal momentum to vertical momentum which propels the body mass upward to the standing position.

The action requires a propulsive impulse in the horizontal direction at the beginning of the movement to initiate forward momentum which changes to a braking impulse to decelerate the horizontal body movement to terminate the movement (Pai and Rogers 1990). Horizontal movement of the body mass is brought about principally by clockwise rotation of the trunk at the hips and of the shank segments at the ankles (Fig. 4.3). Vertical movement of the body mass is brought about by extension at the hips, knees and ankles, i.e.,

counter-clockwise rotation of the trunk and shank segments and clockwise rotation of the thigh (Fig. 4.3). Hip extension is, therefore, brought about both by counter-clockwise rotation of the trunk (at hips) and clockwise rotation of the thigh (at hip and knee). The latter also extends the knee together with counter-clockwise rotation of the shank. The horizontal and vertical movements of the body mass overlap, reflecting the typical sequential onsets of knee, hip and ankle, the knee starting to extend before the hip. That is, the knee starts to extend while the hip is still flexing (e.g., Canning *et al.* 1985). It should be noted that the trunk (pelvis, spine and head) appears to behave as a single 'virtual' segment, maintained erect as it rotates forward in the pre-extension phase and then backward at the hips in the extension phase. Although some movement is likely to occur at spinal joints, biomechanical analysis indicates that this is of relatively small excursion.

The extent of angular displacements in STS will vary depending on the starting position of the trunk and feet, the height of the stool in relation to leg length, the type of seat (e.g., slanted backward), the presence or not of a back rest, and the position of the upper limbs (whether folded across the chest or free to move naturally). In spite of this, under constrained laboratory conditions, we (and others) have found remarkable and repeatable consistency in performance variables. Although the key features are preserved, variation in the motor pattern has been shown to occur as a result of different foot placements, initial body positions and speeds. It is very likely that the timing relationship

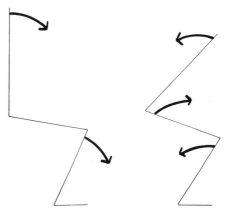

Fig. 4.3 Stick figures, drawn from the R side, indicating the direction of segmental movement during STS

between horizontal movement of the body mass and lower limb extension is critical to optimal performance.

Kinetics

Segmental rotations are brought about by muscle forces, together with gravitational, inertial and interactive forces. Winter (1987), however, has suggested that inertial forces may be negligible in everyday activities. Major force generation in STS occurs around the time the thighs are lifted off the seat in order to accelerate the body mass vertically into the standing position. When conditions demand it, able-bodied subjects can stand up with weight relatively evenly distributed between both lower limbs. In everyday life, however, the distribution of weight borne through the two lower limbs depends on the goal of the action and the environmental demands.

We have used support moment of force (Fig.4.4), an algebraic summation of the moments of force or torques at the three lower limb joints (Winter 1980), as a global measure to examine kinetic function (Carr and Gentile 1994; Shepherd and Gentile 1994). Similar to the stance phase of walking, moments of force at individual joints in STS can vary cooperatively to produce the overall force necessary to support the body mass and propel it vertically. That is, a decrease in force at one joint is compensated for by an increase at the other joints to ensure the limb does not collapse. For example, the knee moment at thighs-off can be flexor, however, this results in an increase in extensor moment at the ankle with the magnitude of the overall support moment remaining virtually the same (Khemlani *et al.* 1995). On average, peak support moments of force range from 4.00 to 5.50 Nm/kg in young able-bodied subjects standing up at their preferred speed (Carr and Gentile 1994; Shepherd and Gentile 1994).

Since the feet are on the floor, ground reaction forces play an important part in the movement. Figure 4.5 illustrates the rapid rise in amplitude of vertical ground reaction forces, peaking around the time the thighs are lifted off the seat, when able-bodied subjects stand up at their preferred speed.

Muscle activity

STS occurs as a result of force generation in many monoarticular and biarticular muscles spanning hip, knee and ankle joints. In addition, trunk muscles are active to stabilize the upper body.

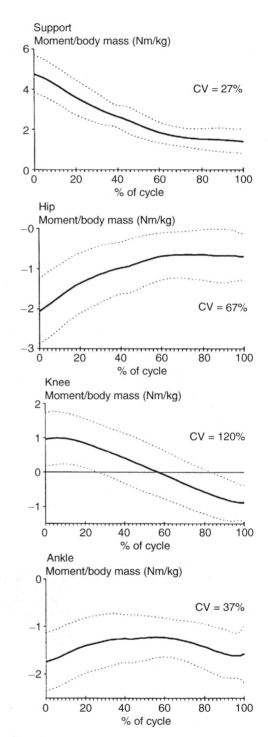

Fig. 4.4 Ensemble-averaged normalized support moment and moments at the hip, knee and ankle (Nm/kg) as able-bodied subjects stand up at their preferred speed. 0: thighs-off; – ve values; extensor at hip and ankle, flexor at knee

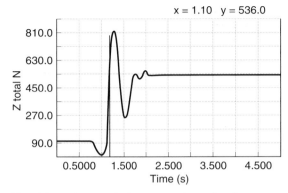

x = 1.10   y = 536.0

Fig. 4.5 Typical vertical (z) ground reaction force profile of an able-bodied subject standing up at a preferred speed. Vertical line indicates thighs-off

Several investigators have used EMG to examine muscle activations during STS (e.g., Kelley et al 1976; Munton et al. 1984; Richards 1985; Arborelius *et al.* 1992; Millington *et al.* 1992; Khemlani *et al.* 1995). Muscles investigated have included trunk muscles – erector spinae, rectus abdominus – and lower limb muscles – gluteus maximus, biceps femoris, semitendinosis, rectus femoris, vastus lateralis, vastus medialis, tibialis anterior, gastrocnemius and soleus.

Tibialis anterior is reported to be one of the first muscles to be activated, reflecting its role in foot placement backward, its contribution both to stabilizing the shank on the foot early in the action and to forward movement of the shank on the foot (Fig. 4.6). Onsets of hip extensors (gluteus maximus, biceps femoris), and knee extensors (rectus

femoris, vastus lateralis, vastus medialis) tend to occur almost simultaneously. Hip and knee extensor muscles demonstrate peak activity around the time the thighs are lifted off the seat. Variable patterns of EMG activity have been found in gastrocnemius and soleus muscles probably reflecting their additional role in balancing the body mass.

Two studies that have monitored rectus femoris (Kelley *et al.* 1976; Millington *et al.* 1992) and one which monitored rectus abdominus (Millington *et al.* 1992) concluded that neither of these muscles was activated early enough to initiate trunk segment flexion. Iliopsoas by its action on the pelvis and thigh would be expected to be an initiator of trunk flexion, however, this relatively deep muscle is difficult to monitor. The simultaneous onsets of the biarticular rectus femoris and biceps femoris may be related to their contributions to the control of hip flexion, with rectus femoris contributing to flexion and biceps femoris exerting a braking force at the hip and thus serving to slow down hip flexion at the hip prior to the beginning of lower limb extension.

Factors influencing performance

This section looks at some factors which appear to be critical to optimizing performance.

Contribution of initial foot position to lower limb extension

It could be assumed that a critical component for the ease of standing up would be related to foot

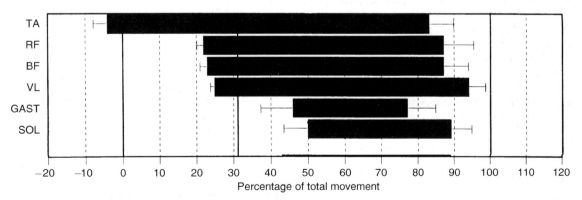

Fig. 4.6 Means and standard deviations of time-normalized onsets and durations of six lower limb muscles as able-bodied subjects stand up at their preferred speed. TA: tibialis anterior; RF: rectus femoris; BF: biceps femoris; VL: vastus lateralis; GAST: gastrocnemius; SOL: soleus. 0: movement onset, 31:thighs-off, 100: movement end (from Khemlani *et al.*, 1995)

placement given that it affects the distance the body mass must be moved forward. Put simply, the further forward the feet, the further forward the body mass has to be moved. Performance is normally flexible, and able-bodied individuals appear to be able to stand up from a range of foot placements with varying degrees of ease. Stevens and colleagues (1989) had subjects stand up from a standardized position in which the thighs were horizontal and shanks vertical, and a preferred position when subjects were able to place their feet in any position. Notably in the preferred foot condition, all subjects moved their feet backward.

Two recent studies had as their major objective the examination of the effects of different foot placements on the mechanics of standing up in healthy elderly men (Saravanamuthu and Shepherd 1994) and healthy young women (Shepherd and Koh, 1996). There were three foot placements: feet back, feet preferred, feet forward (shank vertical). Preferred foot placement was calculated as the mean position each subject used over three practice trials.

The effects of varying foot placement were similar for both age groups. In both young and elderly subjects, as the feet were placed further forward, flexion of the trunk at the hips increased progressively as did flexion velocity. Although the peak value of support moment remained relatively constant, the pattern of moments of force at hip, knee and ankle varied according to placement. Hip extensor moments increased and knee and ankle extensor moments decreased as feet were placed further forward, so that the extensor moment at the hip contributed almost all the total extensor force produced at thighs-off when the feet were furthest forward. One reason for the lack of extensor force produced at the ankle when the feet were forward was the need for the shank segment to dorsiflex actively at least half way into the extensor phase as a means of getting the body mass the additional distance forward.

The results indicate that standing up with the feet relatively forward does not allow for optimal performance in either young or elderly subjects and may prove difficult for certain patient populations who have poor muscle strength and coordination. The need for increased force generation at the hip at thighs-off may be difficult or impossible for individuals with weak hip extensor muscles (e.g., following stroke). The increased amplitude of trunk flexion at the hips and increased extensor moment at the hips may aggravate joint disease, or may cause a loosening of the endoprosthesis

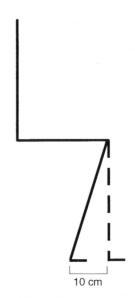

10 cm

Fig. 4.7 Preferred foot placement is, on average, 10 cm from a vertical line drawn from the middle of the knee joint (approximately 75° dorsiflexion)

following hip surgery (Fleckenstein *et al.*, 1988). For preferred foot placement in both young and elderly subjects, it seems that an optimal foot position involves the feet being placed approximately 10 cm behind a line drawn vertically from the centre of the knee joint (Fig. 4.7).

Contribution of trunk segment to lower limb extension

Several studies have pointed to the importance of trunk flexion in setting up the conditions for ascent into standing. The results of two studies (Canning *et al.* 1985; Schenkmann *et al.* 1990) have suggested that a timing relationship between trunk flexion and lower limb extension may be a critical feature in the movement's organization. For example, peak acceleration of the flexing trunk segment has been found to occur simultaneously with the onset of lower limb extension at the knee (Carr 1987). Schenkmann and colleagues (1990) have proposed that forward momentum of the trunk may facilitate the lower limb extension action which raises the body to the standing position. Pai and Rogers (1991) have shown that the trunk is a major contributor to horizontal linear momentum of the body mass, with the thigh segment being the major contributor to vertical momentum. These authors have also found that peak horizontal momentum of the body mass occurs at the same time in the action regardless of speed, probably reflecting the balance constraints of the task (Pai and Rogers 1990).

Shepherd and Gentile (1994) investigated the relationship between the trunk and lower limb segments by varying the initial position of the trunk segment. Subjects stood up from three different starting positions (Fig. 4.8): trunk erect, and trunk flexed forward at the hips 30° and 60°. The results indicated that a high level of overall muscle force (support moment) had to be produced over a longer period of time when subjects stood up from the fully flexed position of the trunk, i.e., when subjects stood up without active upper body flexion and in the absence of horizontal momentum of the body mass.

The results suggest that the generation of extension force to raise the body mass vertically in STS can be optimized by:

- Starting active trunk flexion from the erect position in order to optimize horizontal momentum of the body mass since the distance over which the trunk can be accelerated is greater.
- Encouraging the individual to swing the trunk forward at a reasonable speed.
- Ensuring that the extension phase does not commence with the trunk stationary and flexed forward.

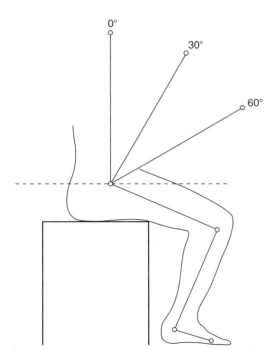

Fig. 4.8 Diagram illustrating the three starting positions of the trunk

Attempts to stand up with the trunk stationary and flexed forward would present problems for individuals with lower limb muscle weakness. Increased duration of a high level of overall force by lower limb extensors for a relatively long period of time may be difficult for people with weak lower limb extensor muscles.

Speed of movement

Although able-bodied individuals stand up at different speeds depending on the environment and goal of the action, the aged population (Alexander *et al.*, 1991; Saravanamuthu and Shepherd 1994) and individuals with movement dysfunction have been found to stand up relatively more slowly (Yoshida *et al.* 1983; Ada and Westwood 1992; Hesse *et al.* 1994). In a recent study, when healthy young subjects stood up at three different speeds (slow, preferred, fast), it was apparent that increased velocity of trunk segment flexion had a potentiating effect on extensor force production in the extension phase of the action (Carr and Ow 1994). That is, with increased velocity of trunk flexion there was a relatively short burst of overall extensor force to propel the body mass vertically rather than the more sustained effort when subjects moved slowly.

Individuals with movement dysfunction who move very slowly may need to be encouraged to move a little faster, in particular, to swing the trunk forward more quickly in order to potentiate the effect of trunk flexion on lower limb extension. Since increasing the speed of movement is not simply a matter of speeding up a slower version of the action, practice of a range of speeds is probably critical to optimize performance for the varying demands of daily life.

Contribution of upper limbs to balance and propulsion

It could be assumed that balance would be critical to STS during the period that the relatively large upper body pivots over the fixed feet (extension phase). It has been shown that, at thighs-off, the centre of body mass has moved forward over the feet (Carr 1992). This position may ensure that the relative position of body segments at thighs-off enables lower limb extensor forces to accelerate the body vertically into the standing position.

A study designed to examine the intersegmental relationship between upper and lower limbs during STS, varied the extent of arm movement (Carr and

Gentile 1994). Subjects stood up with arm movement occurring naturally, functionally restricted, and augmented. Although subjects had no difficulty standing up while pointing or when arm movement was restricted, variations in extent of arm movement did have an effect on the dynamics of the action. The results indicated that when the arms were constrained, there was increased time spent producing a high level of extensor force throughout the lower limbs, decreased horizontal displacement and horizontal and vertical linear momentum of the centre of body mass, and the shank continued to move forward on the foot for approximately 28% of the extension phase.

These results suggest that subjects were less likely to risk projecting their body mass as far forward or move it as fast as when the arms were free to move. This may have been a strategy to increase stability. The finding that the shank continued to move forward on the foot in the early part of the extension phase suggests a major role of forward rotation of the shank at the ankle in moving the body mass forward when arms were restrained from moving forward.

It is a common clinical practice to have a patient hold the affected arm in front of the body with the intact arm when standing up (Bobath, 1990; Davies, 1990; Ryerson 1995). It has been suggested that supporting the affected upper limb during STS encourages 'even weight shift through the lower extremity' (Ryerson 1995, p. 713). This technique effectively restricts movement of both arms and, since the extension phase now has to start with the upper body inclined forward at the hips, restricting arm use in this way will interfere with the natural momentum of the movement.

Seelen and colleagues (1995) compared the amplitude of normalized ground reaction forces and EMG activity in biceps femoris, rectus femoris and vastus lateralis when able-bodied and stroke subjects stood up under three different STS conditions: free STS, NDT/STS, and asymmetrical STS (ASTS), in which one foot was placed posterior to the other foot. In the stroke patients in ASTS, the paretic foot was placed posteriorly. All subjects were familiar with the NDT (neurodevelopmental) STS technique which Bobath clinicians assume facilitates weight-bearing on and muscle activity in the paretic leg. For the NDT/STS condition, subjects were instructed to move the clutched hands in an anterior direction as far as possible while bending the trunk forward, moving in the mediosagittal plane. From this position they were asked to stand up. In all three STS conditions, peak ground reaction forces were greater in the non-paretic leg than in the paretic leg in the stroke subjects.

Interestingly, the NDT/STS condition did not lead to more weight being borne on the paretic leg either during the action or in the standing position. Furthermore, there was no significant difference in muscle activity in the paretic leg in the NDT/STS manoeuvre compared with the other two STS conditions. Muscle activity in the paretic leg, however, did increase in the ASTS condition.

Sitting down (SIT)

There appears to be an assumption in the literature that STS and SIT are fundamentally the same action only in reverse. Certainly, angular displacements at the hip, knee and ankle joints are similar (e.g., Kralj *et al*. 1990; Shepherd and Hirschhorn 1997). However, SIT is controlled by extensor moments at hip, knee and ankle while the joints are flexing, i.e., the lower limb extensor muscles spanning these joints are lengthening rather than shortening as in STS. Since SIT lacks the facilitating effect of vigorous trunk flexion, the part of the movement just before the body mass is lowered on to the seat requires considerable muscle strength and control, particularly at the knee.

Movement duration in SIT has been found to be longer than in STS (Krajl *et al*. 1990; Shepherd and Hirschhorn 1997). This, however, was attributable to the increased time spent in the seat contact phase for SIT compared with STS, since there was no difference in the durations of the non-seat contact phase (Shepherd and Hirschhorn 1997). These authors suggest that the balance mechanism for SIT may differ from STS since the pattern of horizontal momentum was found to be discontinuous in SIT suggesting that SIT may be under relatively more feedback control than STS.

Changes in the elderly

Undoubtedly, pain, muscle stiffness, decreased range of joint motion and muscle weakness can affect the performance of both STS and SIT. Several investigators have examined the STS action in healthy elderly subjects (e.g., Yoshida *et al*. 1983; Wheeler *et al*. 1985; Ikeda *et al*. 1991; Schultz *et al*. 1992; Saravanamuthu and Shepherd 1994).

Under standardized procedures, for example, when the starting position is standardized and moments of force are normalized to subject's body mass, there is a tendency toward an increase in movement duration and decreased amplitude in kinematic and kinetic variables but these are not significant (Ikeda *et al.* 1991; Saravanamuthu and Shepherd 1994). These findings may reflect relatively decreased vigour in performance. Interestingly, however, a group of elderly subjects were able to increase their movement speed when asked to do so (Vander Linden *et al.* 1994).

Schultz and colleagues (1992) examined a group of healthy elderly people, a group of elderly subjects who could not stand up without using their arms and a group of young healthy adults. Their results suggest that hands may not be used to reduce joint moments, at least when the thighs are lifted off the seat, but rather they may be used to gain more postural stability particularly at thighs-off. This may reflect the need to balance the relatively large upper body, particularly when displacement at the hip is reversed, in order to propel the body mass vertically and finish the action in a balanced upright position. However, using the hands at thighs-off may also be a strategy to decrease force requirements at the knee in individuals with substantial joint pain.

Comparisons between values of joint moments necessary to achieve STS and published average values of joint moments achieved by subjects in an age range of 60–80, suggest that, with the possible exception of very frail individuals or those who have joint pain, inability to produce joint moments of sufficient magnitude may not be a factor limiting the ability to stand up in healthy elderly subjects (Schultz *et al.* 1992).

Motor dysfunction

There are several motor control impairments, including difficulty activating muscles, and generating, timing and sustaining muscle force, which may interfere with the ability to stand up and sit down. As a result of neural dyscontrol, together with enforced immobility, another factor that dictates what motor behaviours emerge as the individual attempts to stand up is the state of the musculoskeletal system, i.e., the effector apparatus. Enforced immobility causes structural changes to occur in muscle and soft tissue, with muscles held at a shortened length developing contracture and generating tension at a shorter length. Contracture of the soleus muscle is the most common musculoskeletal adaptation likely to impose severe

constraints on STS and SIT. Hip and knee flexion contracture following a prolonged period of coma associated with traumatic brain injury can also interfere with performance of the action.

Individuals with neural dysfunction tend to stand up more slowly (e.g., Yoshida *et al.* 1983; Ada and Westwood 1992). For example, Ada and Westwood reported that individuals following stroke took on average 2.3 secs to complete the extension phase (thighs-off to movement end), whereas able-bodied elderly subjects standing up at their preferred speed can complete this phase in a range of 0.7–1.4 secs (Saravanamuthu and Shepherd 1994). Engardt and Olsson (1992) also found that movement duration for SIT was longer than STS in stroke subjects.

Since the action of STS itself constrains the number of possible ways to combine hip, knee and ankle displacements, it is not surprising that Ada and Westwood (1992) found little change in the spatial characteristics of the action after training compared with changes in the temporal aspects of the action.

Individuals with hemiplegia spontaneously stand up with more weight on the non-paretic, and therefore stronger leg compared with the paretic leg (Yoshida *et al.* 1983; Engardt *et al.* 1993). Vertical ground reaction force traces of STS following stroke (Fowler and Carr 1996) also typically show either no discernible peak or the peak occurs later in the action (Fig. 4.9). Note also the fluctuations in the vertical force, as previously reported (Yoshida *et al.* 1983).

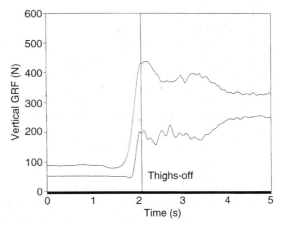

Fig. 4.9 Typical vertical ground reaction force (GRF) profile in Newtons (N) of STS performed by a stroke patient. Lower trace shows the hemiparetic leg

Common observable deficits

The major primary problems in performing STS which arise directly out of the sensorimotor impairments are typically:

- *Difficulty generating and timing sufficient force in the lower limb extensor muscles to propel the body mass vertically.* If severe, it is impossible for the individual to stand up from a seat independently.

- *Failure to place one or both feet backward (decreased amplitude of dorsiflexion at the ankles).* This may be due to weakness of ankle dorsiflexors and hamstring muscles. Inability to place the foot back can also be due to contracture of the soleus muscle which mechanically restrains ankle dorsiflexion. Even a small amount of soleus shortening can create a problem in STS as the ankles must dorsiflex well beyond the plantigrade position. Since the extensibility of soleus determines whether or not individuals are able to position their feet back, preservation of the length of the soleus, through both active and passive means, is essential to allow optimal performance of the action.

- *Failure to move the body mass sufficiently far forward at thighs-off.* This may be due to lack of vigour, loss of the stabilizing effect of a paretic lower limb and fear of falling forward. Failure to move the body mass far enough forward at thighs-off may prevent the action being achieved or may cause any extensor force generated to propel the body backward instead of forward (Fig. 4.10).

    If the ankle dorsiflexors and knee extensors are weak, the foot is not stabilized on the floor. This prevents the shank from moving forward on the foot, which is necessary to move the body mass horizontally. Inability to stabilize the foot (feet) on the floor through muscle weakness will interfere with the pre-extension phase of the action since the feet are used both passively and actively to balance the body in this phase.

    If the individual flexes the upper body forward then pauses before the extension phase, the natural effect of the momentum created by the relatively large upper body segment is lost and the extension phase will start from the fully flexed trunk position. There is evidence that there may be some energy cost in this case, as the extension phase is prolonged and a high value of extensor force is produced throughout a large proportion of the phase (Shepherd and

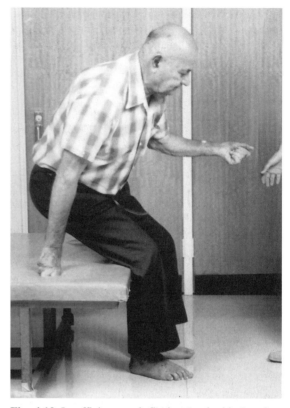

Fig. 4.10 Insufficient trunk flexion (at the hips) and ankle dorsiflexion to move the body mass forward. Note, the adaptive use of arms

Gentile 1994). This may make the action difficult or impossible for patients with weakness of lower limb extensor muscles.

- *Difficulty balancing the body mass, particularly at the point in the action when horizontal momentum must be controlled (at or after thighs-off).* This may be due to difficulty generating and timing force, particularly the lower limb extensor muscles as well as those that attach the shank to the foot.

Adaptive motor behaviour

Whenever individuals have difficulty activating muscles and generating and timing force, certain adaptive movements emerge as they try to stand up. The individual utilizes typical adaptive motor behaviours:

- *Weakness of lower limb extensors.* There are several adaptations that can be observed when the lower limb extensors are weak. If muscle

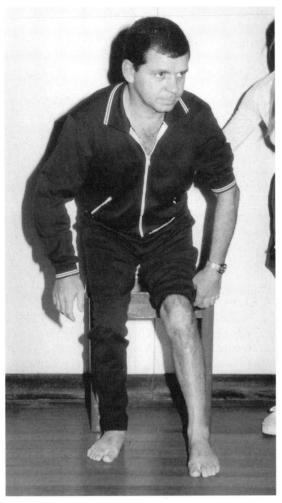

Fig. 4.11 Weight concentrated on his stronger and more easily controlled R leg. Note that he has not moved his L foot back – wide base of support

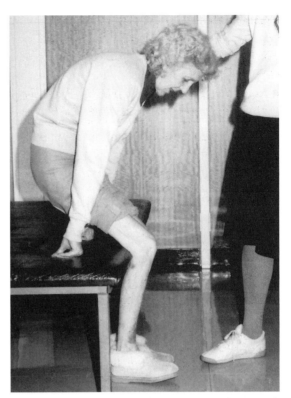

Fig. 4.12 Following a lengthy hospital stay for a medical condition, it is difficult for this frail woman to stand up. She has not moved her body mass forward over her feet. She is flexing her lumbar spine instead of flexing at her hips and uses her arms for support, balance and to assist initial propulsion

weakness is unilateral, the individual stands up by generating force through the stronger and more easily controlled intact leg. The body mass is seen to shift laterally toward the stronger leg at thighs-off (Fig. 4.11). Adduction and internal rotation at the hip of the paretic leg may be a way of gaining more effective lower limb extension, possibly by using adductor muscles to increase extensor force, by stabilizing one leg against the other.

The foot of the stronger leg may be positioned behind the weaker. This posterior position of the foot relative to the other means that more force will be generated through this leg (see Seelen *et al.* 1995).

Another, usually unsuccessful, adaptation to weakness of lower limb extensors and ankle dorsiflexors is that the trunk segment continues to flex forward (Carr *et al.* 1997) and the spine, instead of remaining erect, tends to flex (Fig. 4.12). The shoulder path, therefore, moves downward from the horizontal instead of upward. This adaptation has also been described in children with diplegia (Shepherd and McDonald 1995).

Hands may be used to assist at thighs-off (Fig. 4.12), in an attempt to push the body mass up from the arms of a chair. Alternatively, the arms may be swung forward and upward to aid the horizontal and vertical propulsion (Fig. 4.13).

- *Lack of balance and stability.* Hands may be used to increase stability, particularly around the time the thighs are lifted off the seat. The individual may widen the base of support to increase stability and move slowly.

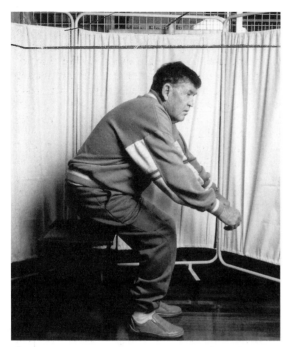

Fig. 4.13 Difficulty generating and timing lower limb extensor force. Arms are swung forward to aid horizontal momentum

To optimize performance of STS and SIT, these adaptive movements or fundamentally inappropriate movements to use Newell's term (Newell 1981), need to be discouraged through training and modification of the environment, since they do not have a positive effect on motion and reduce flexibility of performance.

Essential components

These are key kinematic details of the action observable as angular displacements and linear paths of body parts and are reflective of the underlying momentum and force characteristics. Outlined below is a synthesis of biomechanical (kinematic) findings which we have found consistently in healthy subjects across different age groups (Carr and Shepherd, 1987):

- Initial foot placement backward (approximately 10 cm from an imaginary vertical line drawn from the knee joint).
- Flexion of the erect trunk segment at the hips and dorsiflexion at the ankle.
- A sequence of lower limb extensions (knee, hip and ankle).

Through an appreciation of these observable components, and an understanding of the biomechanics of the action, physiotherapists are better able to analyse the motor deficits and to apply biomechanically based training strategies. An understanding of the underlying momentum and force requirements of the action enables physiotherapists to make inferences about the causative mechanisms underlying their kinematic observations. Periodic measurement with a force plate, motion analysis system and EMG can confirm or not some of the therapist's inferences. Understanding the critical features of the action also assists nursing staff and relatives, not only to provide appropriate assistance which enables the patient to participate actively, but also makes the task easier for the helper.

Training

Safe and effective performance of STS and SIT is essential to independence and may influence whether or not the person is able to participate in everyday activities and go home. Successful training of STS also obviates the necessity for a patient to be hauled up into the standing position by others, with the likelihood of damage to the soft tissues around the shoulder (Wanklyn *et al.* 1996). A critical factor in the ease of STS is foot placement backward (approximately 75° ankle

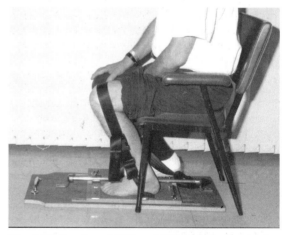

Fig. 4.14 Practice of STS and SIT with the feet back puts an active stretch on the soleus muscle. This stretcher provides a passive stretch on the soleus muscle. (Conceived and developed by Karl Schurr and Julie Nugent, Physiotherapists, Bankstown-Lidcombe Hospital, Sydney, Australia)

dorsiflexion). This highlights the need for maintaining the length of soleus by both active (multiple repetitions of STS and SIT) and passive means (Fig. 4.14).

Modification of the environment

Modification of the environment principally involves increasing the height of the seat to decrease force requirements. Standing up is trained and practised from a seat which is of appropriate height for the individual's ability. The seat should be flat and not sloped backward, as the initial flexed hip position imposed by a backward slanting seat increases any difficulty the individual has in standing up by increasing the distance upward the body mass must be moved. Initially, the height of the seat should be chosen depending on the individual's ability to generate the necessary force with lower limb extensor muscles. If the individual is very weak or is unable to stand up from a 'normal' seat height without gross adaptation, a higher than normal seat should be used both during practice with the therapist and throughout the day. A higher than normal seat is known to require less force production (e.g., Burdett *et al.* 1985; Rodosky *et al.* 1989). As ability to generate force through the affected limb(s) improves, the seat is lowered. In this way, seat height is used to add progressive resistance to the leg extensor muscles and strengthen them.

Since practice is usually required in order to develop the necessary strength in the muscles involved and also to enable the individual to learn the movement pattern, the seat should not have arms. The presence of chair arms tends to encourage habitual use of the hands.

It is important during training that practice of an action encourages *flexibility*, as the goal of training is for the individual to be able to perform the action from a variety of different seats and in combination with other goals or actions, such as standing up while holding on to an object, while carrying on a conversation, or standing up to walk. However, with individuals who have a great deal of difficulty controlling the action, it is probably inevitable that the action be practised first in a relatively closed environment.

Appropriate *chair design* (Fig. 4.18) can make a large contribution to a person's well-being and independence, particularly for the less mobile who may spend long periods of the day seated. Chair design, however, seldom takes into account the ease of getting out of it. For example, Wheeler and colleagues (1985), when comparing a standard chair and a chair designed for comfort in sitting, found that standing up from the specially designed chair appeared to be more difficult than standing up from the standard chair. The depth and slant of the seat and the barrier to foot placement back necessitated greater trunk flexion at the hips and knee flexion, with increased EMG activity in the vastus lateralis.

In a survey, elderly individuals from Day Centres or Rehabilitation Clinics were asked to rank in order of importance the five factors they considered important in terms of chair design (Munton *et al.* 1981). 'Easy to get out of' was considered to be the most important factor when choosing a chair and 'high seat' was ranked third, before comfort, although these individuals spent a great deal of their time sitting. The most important factors in chair design to assist rising are the height of seat and the need to be able to place the feet back. Seats need to be high enough to allow STS to be performed without gross adaptations but not so high that legs are left unsupported and the edge of the seat restricts circulation. Other factors which need to be considered are texture of seat covering and slant of the seat and back rest. A deep seat increases the distance the body mass has to be moved forward and requires a lot of effort merely to get to the edge of the chair before starting to stand up.

Practice

Training is aimed at giving the individual practice of STS and SIT with a prescribed number of repetitions. Repetition is necessary for two principal reasons: to strengthen the muscles for this action, and to optimize learning. The individual is learning again, with an altered CNS, how to utilize the characteristics of the segmental linkage in order to optimize the intersegmental transfer of power and to minimize the energy requirements. Prescribing the number of repetitions at the start of the session also provides a motivating goal. It is necessary for the individual to practise the whole action in order to develop the necessary sequencing and timing of segmental rotations to both generate and utilize momentum. With practice, timing and coordination between segments becomes more precise.

Strengthening exercises

The major route to learning how to stand up and sit down is through practice of the action with a sufficient number of repetitions in order to improve the strength and control of lower limb extensors and the timing characteristics of the action. However, many individuals, following acute brain lesion in particular, need exercises designed to address specific problems. For example, placing the foot on a towel on a low friction surface and practising moving it backwards and forwards may enable the person to activate ankle dorsiflexors and hamstring muscles. Lines on the floor can provide a concrete goal and visual cue of the extent of the movement required.

Of critical importance to the action of STS and SIT is the strength and control of the lower limb extensor muscles (hip extensors, quadriceps and ankle plantarflexors). If an individual has difficulty sustaining extensor muscle activity throughout the action, stopping the movement at various points in the extension phase may be useful. As strength and control improve, placing one foot (of the weaker leg, in hemiplegia) posteriorly to the other during practice can force the posteriorly placed limb to generate greater force.

Stopping the movement and reversing for a few degrees can help the individual develop control over changing from concentric to eccentric muscle activity. Engardt and colleagues (1993) have suggested that the reason stroke subjects following a training programme did not perform SIT as well as STS in terms of amplitude of vertical force may have been a reluctance to activate lower limb extensor muscles for adequate eccentric work.

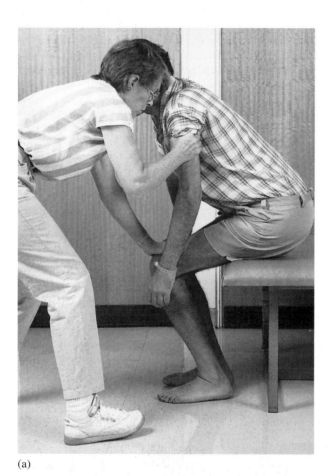

(a)

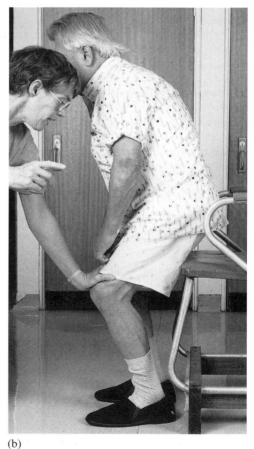

(b)

Fig. 4.15 (*a*) The therapist stabilizes the foot on the floor by pushing down along the line of the shank. Note that the shanks are angled at approximately 75°. The therapist needs to understand the biomechanics of the action and take care not to prevent the thigh from moving forward (see Fig. 4.1). (*b*) Standing up from a high seat in relation to lower leg length reduces the force requirements of STS and SIT. This man requires manual guidance to stabilize his tibia for him to be able to activate his quadriceps sufficiently to extend thigh on shank

This finding highlights the need to emphasize the training of SIT as well as STS. It may be that individuals with motor impairment (and physiotherapists) perceive SIT as being 'easier' than STS since SIT can be achieved by 'collapsing' into a chair, using the arms of the chair or an assistant to brake the movement. Functional scales used for assessing motor performance also tend to place greater importance on STS than SIT. Yet, there are several differences between the two actions. Not only does SIT involve controlled lengthening of muscles, there is a major timing difference with simultaneous onset of flexion at the hips, knees and ankles in SIT. In addition, ankle flexion changes to extension to shift the body mass backward prior to the thighs being placed on the seat, while the hips and knees continue to flex until seat contact.

Repetitive stepping exercises using steps of different heights can be practised to increase strength in the lower limb extensor muscles (see Fig. 5.22). This exercise and practice of STS with the feet positioned back place an active stretch on the soleus muscle. The calf muscles may need to be stretched passively to enable the feet to be placed far enough back for ease of standing up. Exercises and passive stretches are followed immediately by practice of STS and SIT, with, if necessary, the environment modified to optimize practice conditions. A patient may need to do other lower limb exercises as part of a general programme of strengthening.

Manual guidance

Individuals who are weak may require some manual guidance initially. Two types of manual guidance have been described in the motor learning literature to improve skill (Holding 1965; Newell 1981) (see Chapter 2). One involves *passive movement* in order either to place a limb in a position so that movement can take place from an appropriate segmental alignment or to give the person the idea of the movement to be performed. In the first instance, if the patient cannot activate the ankle dorsiflexor muscles to move the foot backward, the physiotherapist places it back to enable the person to practise STS from an optimal starting position. In the second instance, the shoulders can be moved passively along the normal path by the therapist to give the patient the idea of how far the body mass must move forward. The patient then

actively attempts the action with modification of the environment such as raising the seat height, if needed.

The other type of manual guidance described (Holding 1965; Newell 1981) is *physical restriction* of a segment to constrain the action spatially while the patient performs part of the action actively. For example, with the feet placed back, the foot (or feet) can be held in contact with the ground by the therapist, who exerts an external force by giving pressure down and back along the line of the shank (Fig. 4.15*a,b*). Stabilizing the foot on the ground may be necessary to ensure that when the quadriceps muscles are activated, the thigh will be moved on the shank and not the reverse. In other words, if the foot is not fixed to the floor, either by muscle activation or by physical restriction (by the therapist), quadriceps activation can extend the shank on the thigh, the foot sliding forward and lifting off the floor. This movement has been described as being due to spasticity of the knee extensors. It is, however,

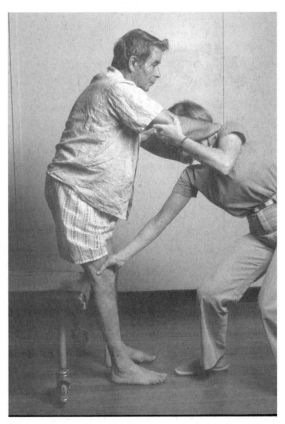

Fig. 4.16 Passive extension of the knee by the therapist pushes this man off balance backward

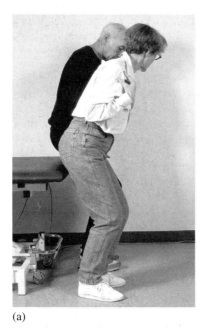

(a)

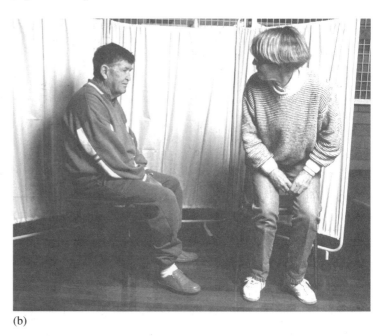

(b)

Fig. 4.17 The therapist demonstrates the extent of trunk flexion at the hips (*a*) beside the patient so he can line his trunk up with hers, (*b*) providing a sagittal plane view to show him how far forward shoulders are moved

more likely to be due to an inability both to stabilize the foot on the floor and to time extensor muscle contraction. By stabilizing the shank, any activity generated by the quadriceps is utilized, along with hip and ankle extensor force, to generate ground reaction forces and to propel the body mass vertically.

The therapist can use manual guidance not only to stabilize the shank but also as a means of ensuring the body mass is sufficiently forward. When manual guidance is given in this way, care has to be taken that the knee is not passively extended by the therapist too early in the movement sequence (Fig. 4.16). The knee does not fully extend until the individual is in the upright standing position. To put it another way, the ankles remain in dorsiflexion (shank rotated forward) until after the thighs leave the seat in order to keep the body mass centred over the base of support.

This type of manual guidance can be used during training with the physiotherapist and can also be used by others to assist the person to stand up and sit down during the rest of the day. As strength and control improves, the physiotherapist reduces manual guidance and organizes practice to train flexibility.

Demonstration and augmented feedback

In initial training sessions, the individual may benefit from a demonstration of the action. The plane of motion demonstrated will depend on the problem to be addressed. For example, if the patient is not moving the body mass far enough or fast enough forward, the demonstrator can present a sagittal plane view to the patient to indicate the position of the shoulders forward of the knees (Fig. 4.17*a,b*).

Video replay is a useful way to explain to a patient where performance needs improvement and what to concentrate on. Concurrent video or computerized feedback about performance and matching the 'shape' of the movement against an ideal may well be one of the most effective learning tools, however, such devices have yet to be developed for the clinic.

Augmented feedback, utilizing either auditory or visual signals from electronic devices such as a force plate, pressure sensitive foot pad, or Balance Performance Monitor* (Fig. 7.11) plates under one or both feet, can provide information about the magnitude and timing of force production. In a

* SMS Healthcare

recent study, two groups of subjects following stroke participated in a 3 week training programme of STS (Fowler and Carr 1996). Both groups received training of STS. One group practised with feedback from an auditory signal from a pressure-sensitive foot pad. In general, all subjects increased the magnitude of vertical force produced through the affected lower limb to approximately 50% at the end of the study. It appeared that the feedback subjects, who also performed fewer repetitions in their self-monitored practice sessions, increased force production through the affected lower limb more than the control subjects. Feedback subjects, however, had more difficulty producing vertical force close to thighs-off than control subjects. This may be due, in part, to the characteristic of the feedback signal as previously suggested by Yates (1980). Since the auditory signal is produced after the target force is applied to the footpad, subjects may wait to see if the force applied is sufficent to activate the signal, causing them to focus on producing force later in the movement, rather than at the critical time of thighs-off. A visual signal from

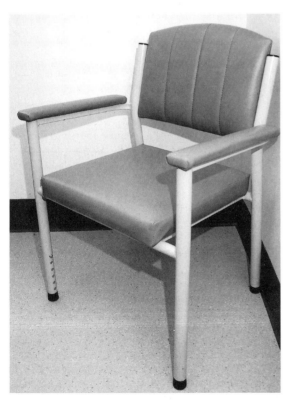

Fig. 4.18 An 'easy to get out of' chair with adjustable seat height

the limb load monitor may have a more positive training effect in the timing of force productions.

Self-monitored practice

Self-monitored or unsupervised practice is typically not considered to be part of neurological rehabilitation. Yet it is well known for the able-bodied population that, as a general rule, skill in performance increases as a direct result of the amount of practice. Kottke (1974) suggested that thousands of repetitions are required to improve performance during neurological rehabilitation. To our knowledge, there is only one study that has attempted to record the number of repetitions required to improve performance on STS. Canning (1987) found that, on average, stroke patients stood up and sat down approximately 1000 times as they progressed from 2 on the Standing Up item of the Motor Assessment Scale (Chapter 3) to 4,5 or 6 on the scale. This number of repetitions was achieved during practice with the therapist, but perhaps more importantly, also during practice without the therapist.

It is often possible for patients to practise STS without the therapist present even when they need some assistance. For example, placing the arms on a table in front provides some support so the individual can concentrate on practising concentric and eccentric lower limb extensions to move the body mass vertically and lower it repetitively and not have to attend also to the need to move the upper body forward and balance (Fig 4.19a). As soon as possible, the individual should practise without using the hands for support, since an essential feature of STS is the concurrent postural adjustment that occurs throughout the action. The muscles which make these adjustments are particularly those distal muscles that link the shank to the foot, i.e., ankle plantar- and dorsiflexors. Patients can also practise this exercise using a set of weighing scales under the weaker leg for self-monitoring of extent of weight-bearing (Fig. 4.19b), with a block of the same height under the other leg.

Physical assistance

Although the rehabilitation literature emphasizes teaching the patient to '*transfer*', we would argue that training this manoeuvre is in conflict with the training of STS and SIT. To our knowledge, this term was first used in the management of spinal cord injured individuals who, because of bilateral lower limb paresis, have to learn an alternative

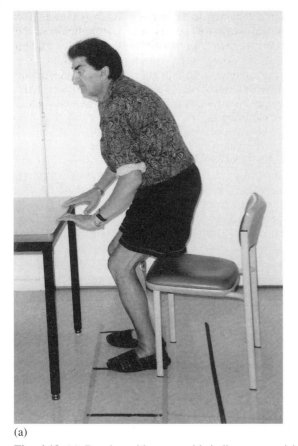

(a)

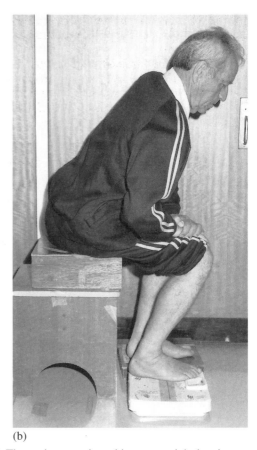

(b)

Fig. 4.19 (*a*) Practice without or with indirect supervision. (*b*) The patient monitors his own weight-bearing ability as he practises shifting his weight on to his feet

way of getting from one surface to another. It is probable that more attention and time in neurological rehabilitation have been placed on teaching 'stand-pivot-sit transfer', weight-bearing through the non-affected leg, than on training STS and SIT. It has been suggested that teaching transfers from chair, bed, toilet 'will promote symmetry through weight shift, weight-bearing and rotation to each side' (Ryerson 1995, p.712), an unlikely assumption given that these manoeuvres normally require asymmetrical weight-bearing!

Independence in daily life does not require the ability to move from one seat to another but the ability to get into standing. To have as a primary objective the teaching of transfers is not to prepare the patient for independent life, but for a dependent life in which assistance from others in an altered environment is critical. If for some reason a person is not going to be able to stand up and walk (e.g., spinal injury, severe arthritis, severely debili-

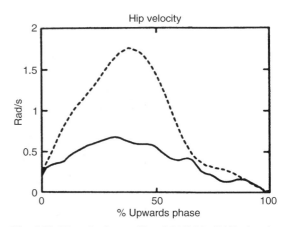

Fig. 4.20 Hip velocity profile at MAS 2 (solid line) and MAS 6 (broken line). Note the flattened profile at MAS 2 and the bell-shaped curve at MAS 6. (From Ada, L. and Westwood, P. (1992) A kinematic analysis of recovery of the ability to stand up following stroke. *Australian Journal of Physiotherapy*, **38**, 135–142, by permission)

tated), then transfers may be relevant. However, a person who is training to walk needs to be trained to stand up.

Any physical assistance involves the therapist becoming part of the patient's environment and there are several ways in which the therapist's presence can constrain the patient's performance in an unhelpful way which may necessitate the patient having to be being lifted into standing. A useful way for nurses and physiotherapists to improve their skill in assisting a person to stand up and sit down is to videotape the session. The sagittal view of the patient and helper, for example, provides feedback about whether or not the helper's position impedes the forward movement of the body mass.

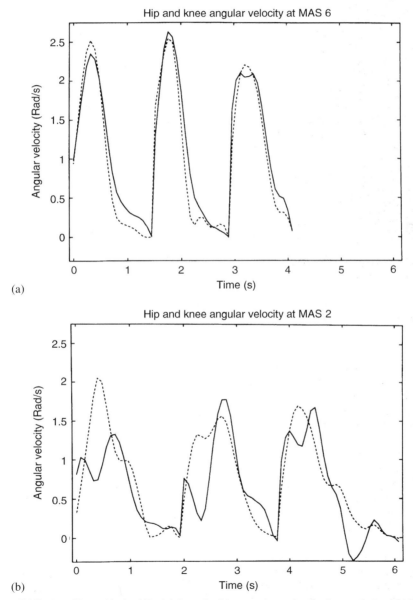

Fig. 4.21 Hip (solid line) and knee (dashed line) joint velocities are almost perfectly coupled at MAS 6 (*a*) whereas there was significant independent activity at MAS 2 (*b*). (From Ada, L., O'Dwyer, N.J. and Neilson, P.D. (1992) Improvement in kinematic characteristics and coordination following stroke quantified by linear systems analysis. *Human Movement Science,* **12**, 137–153, by kind permission of Elsevier Science, Amsterdam, The Netherlands)

Measurement of outcome

It seems evident that understanding the critical biomechanical features of standing up enables one to analyse the reasons why an individual is having difficulty with the action and provides a guide to training. Physiotherapists also need to take advantage of biomechanical measures to test the effectiveness of training. Several investigators have done this (Ada and Westwood 1992; Engardt *et al.* 1993; Fowler and Carr 1996). For example, Ada and Westwood demonstrated that, as stroke patients progressed from to 2 to 6 on the Motor Assessment Scale (MAS), a score of 6 indicating that subjects can stand up and sit down three times in 10 seconds with no observable asymmetry (Carr *et al.* 1985), movement time decreased by one-third and amplitude of peak hip and knee angular velocity also increased. Furthermore, the velocity profiles became smooth and bell-shaped whereas initially they had multiple peaks (Fig. 4.20). Smooth, bell-shaped velocity curves are said to be typical of well-coordinated movements and have been reported at hip and knee joints when able-bodied subjects stand up (Carr 1987). Further analysis revealed that, with a score of MAS 6, the hip and knee joints became almost perfectly coupled, whereas previously there was significant independent activity at each joint (Fig. 4.21). Ada and colleagues (1993) proposed that the kinematic changes observed in the stroke patients as the synergic couplings across joints became stronger show that processes similar to normal skill acquisition are operative in adults with acquired brain damage. The subjects in this study had participated in a training programme (mean duration 29 days) based on a biomechanical model of the action similar to that described here. It is encouraging for all therapists involved in movement rehabilitation to note the high level of skill achievable by these patients, at least in the task of STS.

In a retrospective study of all inpatients diagnosed as having cerebrovascular accident and discharged during a calendar year in a rehabilitation centre, Dean and Mackey (1992) found that overall performance of the STS item on the MAS was 4.5. Fifty-four per cent of patients reached MAS 6 on discharge. Of the remainder, 10% reached 5 and another 10% reached 4 on the scale.

In conclusion, lack of independence in standing up limits full participation in everyday activities and ensures an overall deterioration of lower limb muscle function. STS is, therefore, an important action to emphasize in rehabilitation, not only for increasing the individual's independence but also for its role in increasing muscle strength in the lower limbs. In support of this suggestion, it is interesting to note that Engardt and colleagues (1993) found that the more stroke patients loaded their paretic leg in STS and SIT the better they scored on the Barthel Index and the lower extremity Fugl-Meyer Assessment as well as the Motor Assessment Scale items.

References

Ada, L. and Westwood, P. (1992) A kinematic analysis of recovery of the ability to stand up following stroke. *Australian Journal of Physiotherapy*, **38**, 135–142.

Ada, L., O'Dwyer, N. and Neilson, P.D. (1993) Improvement in kinematic characteristics and coordination following stroke quantified by linear systems analysis. *Human Movement Science*, **12**, 137–153.

Alexander, N.B., Schultz, A.B. and Warwick, D.N. (1991) Rising from a chair: effects of age and functional ability on performance biomechanics. *Journal of Gerontology: Medical Sciences*, **46**, M91–98.

Arborelius, U.P., Wretenberg, P. and Lindberg, F. (1992) The effects of armrests and high seat heights on lower-limb joint load and muscular activity during sitting and rising. *Ergonomics*, **35**, 1377–1391.

Berger, R.A., Riley P.O., Mann R.W. *et al.* (1988) Total body dynamics in ascending stairs and rising from a chair following total knee arthroplasty. In *Proceedings of the 34th Annual Meeting of the Orthopedic Research Society,* Atlanta, GA.

Bobath, B. (1990) *Adult Hemiplegia: Evaluation and Treatment*, 3rd edn, Heinemann, Oxford.

Branch, L.G. and Meyers, A.R. (1987) Assessing physical function in the elderly. *Clinical Geriatric Medicine*, **3**, 29–51.

Burdett, R.G., Habasevich, R., Pisciotta, J.*et al.* (1985) Biomechanical comparison of rising from two types of chairs. *Physical Therapy*, **65**, 1177–1183.

Canning, C. (1987) Training standing up following stroke – a clinical trial. In *Proceedings of the Tenth International Congress of the World Confederation for Physical Therapy*, Sydney, Australia, pp. 915–919.

Canning, C.G., Carr, J.H. and Shepherd, R.B. (1985) A kinematic analysis of standing up. *Proceedings of the Australian Physiotherapy Association National Congress,* Brisbane.

Carr, J.H. (1987) Analysis and training of standing up. In *Proceedings of the Tenth International Congress of the World Confederation for Physical Therapy*, Sydney, Australia, pp. 383–388.

Carr, J.H. (1992) Balancing the centre of body mass during standing up. *Physiotherapy Theory and Practice,* **8**, 159–164.

Carr, J.H. and Gentile, A.M. (1994) The effect of arm movement on the biomechanics of standing up. *Human Movement Science*, **13**, 175–193.

Carr, J.H. and Shepherd, R.B. (1987) *A Motor Relearning Programme for Stoke*, 2nd edn, Heinemann, Oxford, pp. 100–111.

Carr, J.H. and Shepherd, R.B. (1989) A motor learning model for stroke rehabilitation. *Physiotherapy*, **75**, 372–380.

Carr, J.H. and Shepherd, R.B. (1990) A motor learning model for rehabilitation of the movement-disabled. In *Key Issues in Neurological Physiotherapy* (eds L. Ada and C. Canning), Butterworth Heinemann, Oxford, pp. 1–24.

Carr, J.H. and Ow, J. (1994) The effects of speed of sit-to-stand movement on force production in the lower limbs. In *Second World Congress of Biomechanics Abstracts* (eds L. Blankevoort and J.G.M. Kooloos) Stichting World Biomechanics, Nijmegen.

Carr, J.H., Monger, C. and Fowler, V. (1997) The effect of task-specific training on a group of chronic stroke patients. *Proceedings XVIth International Society of Biomechanics Congress*, Tokyo.

Carr, J.H., Shepherd, R.B., Nordholm, L. *et al.* (1985) Investigation of a new motor assessment scale for stroke patients. *Physical Therapy*, **65**, 175–180.

Davies, P.M. (1990) *Right in the Middle. Selective Trunk Activity in the Treatment of Adult Hemiplegia.* Springer-Verlag, Berlin.

Dean, C. and Mackey, F. (1992) Motor assessment scale scores as a measure of rehabilitation outcome following stroke. *Australian Journal of Physiotherapy*, **38**, 31–35.

Engardt, M. and Olsson, E. (1992) Body weight-bearing while rising and sitting down in patients with stroke. *Scandinavian Journal of Rehabilitation Medicine*, **24**, 67–74.

Engardt, M., Ribbe, T. and Olsson, E. (1993) Vertical ground reaction force feedback to enhance stroke patients' symmetrical body-weight distribution while rising/sitting down. *Scandinavian Journal of Rehabilitation Medicine*, **25**, 41–48.

Fleckenstein, S.J., Kirby, R.L. and MacLeod, D.A. (1988) Effect of limited knee-flexion range on peak hip moments of force while transferring from sitting to standing. *Journal of Biomechanics*, **21**, 915–918.

Fowler, V. and Carr, J. (1996) Auditory feedback: effects on vertical force production during standing up following stroke. *International Journal of Rehabilitation Research*, **19**, 265–269.

Hesse, S., Schauer, M., Malezic, M. *et al.* (1994) Quantitive analysis of rising from a chair in healthy and hemiparetic subjects. *Scandinavian Journal of Rehabilitation Medicine*, **26**, 161–166.

Holding, D.H. (1965) *Principles of Training*, Pergamon, London, pp. 17, 63, 206, 211, 218, 219.

Ikeda, E.R., Schenkman, M.L., O'Riley, P. *et al.* (1991) Influence of age on dynamics of rising from a chair. *Physical Therapy*, **71**, 473–481.

Kelley, D.L., Dainis, A. and Wood, G.K. (1976) Mechanics and muscular dynamics of rising from a seated position. In *Biomechanics V-B* (ed. P.V. Komi) University Park Press, Baltimore, MD, pp. 127–134.

Khemlani, M., Carr, J.H., Crosbie, W.J. *et al.* (1995) The contribution of six lower limb muscles to segmental rotations in standing up under two different initial foot positions. In *Proceedings of the Twelfth International Congress of the World Confederation for Physical Therapy*, Washington, USA.

Kottke, F.J. (1974) Historia obscura hemiplegiae. *Archives of Physical Medicine and Rehabilitation*, **55**, 4–13.

Kralj, A., Jaeger, R.J. and Munih, M. (1990) Analysis of standing up and sitting down in humans: definitions and normative data presentation. *Journal of Biomechanics*, **23**, 1123–1138.

Millington, P.J., Myklebust, B.M. and Shambes, G.M. (1992) Biomechanical analysis of the sit-to-stand motion in elderly persons. *Archives of Physical Medicine and Rehabilitation*, **73**, 609–617.

Munton, J.S., Ellis, M.I., Chamberlain, M.A. *et al.* (1981) An investigation into the problems of easy chairs used by the arthritic and the elderly. *Rheumatology and Rehabilitation*, **20**, 164–173.

Munton, J.S., Ellis, M.I. and Wright, V. (1984) Use of electromyography to study leg muscle activity in patients with arthritis and in normal subjects during rising from a chair. *Annals of the Rheumatic Diseases*, **43**, 63–65.

Newell, K.M. (1981) Skill learning. In *Human Skills* (ed. D. Holding), John Wiley, New York, pp. 203–226.

Pai, Y. and Rogers, M.W. (1990) Control of body mass transfer as a function of speed of ascent in sit-to-stand. *Medicine and Science in Sports and Exercise*, **22**, 378–384.

Pai, Y. and Rogers, M.W. (1991) Segmental contributions to total body momentum in sit-to-stand. *Medicine and Science in Sports and Exercise*, **23**, 225–230.

Richards, C.L. (1985) EMG activity level comparisons in quadriceps and hamstrings in five dynamic activities. In *International Series on Biomechanics. IX-A* (eds D.A. Winter, R.W. Norman, R.P. Wells *et al.*), Human Kinetics Publishers, Champaign, IL, pp. 313–317.

Rodosky, M.V., Andriacchi, T.P. and Andersson, G.B.J. (1989) The influence of chair height on lower limb mechanics during rising. *Journal of Orthopedic Research*, **7**, 266–271.

Ryerson, S.D. (1995) Hemiplegia. In *Neurological Rehabilitation* (ed. D.A. Umphred), Mosby, St Louis, pp. 681–721.

Saravanamuthu, R. and Shepherd, R.B. (1994) The effect of foot placement on the movement pattern of sit-to-stand in the elderly. In *Second World Congress of Biomechanics Abstracts* (eds L. Blankevoort and J.G.M. Kooloos), Stichting World Biomechanics, Nijmegen.

Schenkman, M., Berger, R.A., O'Riley, P. *et al.* (1990) Whole-body movements during rising to standing from sitting. *Physical Therapy*, **70**, 638–651.

Schultz, A.B., Alexander, N.B. and Ashton-Miller, J.A. (1992) Biomechanical analyses of rising from a chair. *Journal of Biomechanics*, **25**, 1383–1391.

Seelen, H.A.M., van Wiggen, K.L., Halfens, J.H.G. *et al.* (1995) Lower limb postural responses during sit-to-stand transfer in stroke patients during neurorehabilitation. In *Book of Abstracts of the XVth Congress of the International Society of Biomechanics* (eds K. Hakkinen, K.L. Keskinen, P.V. Komi et al.), University of Jyvaskyla, Jyvaskyla, Finland, pp. 826–827.

Shepherd, R.B. and Carr, J.H. (1994) Reflections on physiotherapy and the emerging science of movement rehabilitation. *Australian Journal of Physiotherapy*, 40th Jubilee Issue, pp. 39–47.

Shepherd, R.B. and Gentile, A.M. (1994) Sit-to-stand: functional relationships between upper body and lower limb segments. *Human Movement Science*, **13**, 817–840.

Shepherd, R.B. and Hirschhorn, A.D. (1997) Standing up and sitting down at two different seat heights. *Proceedings XVIth International Society of Biomechanics Congress*, Tokyo.

Shepherd, R.B. and Koh, H.P. (1996) Some biomechanical consequences of varying foot placement in sit-to-stand in young women. *Scandinavian Journal of Rehabilitation Medicine*, **28**, 79–88.

Shepherd, R.B. and McDonald, C.M. (1995) A biomechanical analysis of sit-to-stand in children with diplegic cerebral palsy. In *Book of Abstracts of the XVth Congress of the International Society of Biomechanics* (eds K. Hakkinen, K.L. Keskinen, P.V. Komi *et al.*), University of Jyvaskyla, Jyvaskyla, Finland, pp. 834–835.

Stevens, C., Bojsen-Moller, F. and Soames, R.W. (1989) The influence of initial posture on the sit-to-stand movement. *European Journal of Applied Physiology*, **58**, 687–692.

Vander Linden, D.W., Brunt, D. and McCulloch, M.U. (1994) Variant and invariant characteristics of the sit-to-stand task in healthy elderly adults. *Archives of Physical Medicine and Rehabilitation*, **75**, 653–660.

Wanklyn, P., Forster, A. and Young, J. (1996) Hemiplegic shoulder pain (HSP): natural history and investigation of associated features. *Disability and Rehabilitation*, **18**, 497–501.

Wheeler, J., Woodward, C., Ucovich, R.L. et al. (1985) Rising from a chair. Influence of age and chair design. *Physical Therapy*, **65**, 22–26.

Winter, D.A. (1980) Overall principle of lower limb support in normal walking. *Journal of Biomechanics*, **13**, 923–927.

Winter, D.A. (1987) *The Biomechanics and Motor Control of Human Gait*, University of Waterloo Press, Waterloo, Ontario.

Yates, A.J. (1980) *Biofeedback and the Modification of Behaviour*, Plenum Press, New York.

Yoshida, K., Iwakura, H. and Inoue, F. (1983) Motion analysis in the movements of standing up from and sitting down on a chair. *Scandinavian Journal of Rehabilitation Medicine*, **15**, 133–140.

Further reading

Engardt, M. (1994) Long term effects of auditory feedback training on relearned symmetrical body weight distribution in stroke patients. A follow-up study. *Scandinavian Journal of Rehabilitation*, **26**, 65–69.

Kerr, K.M., White, J.A., Mollan, R.A.B. *et al.* (1991) Rising from a chair: a review of the literature. *Physiotherapy*, **77**, 15–19

Kotake, T., Dohi, N., Kajiwara, T. *et al.* (1993) An analysis of sit-to-stand movements. *Archives of Physical Medicine and Rehabilitation*, **74**, 1095–1099.

Pai, Y and Lee, W.A. (1994) Effect of a terminal constraint on control of balance during sit-to-stand. *Journal of Motor Behaviour*, **26**, 247–256.

Roebroeck, M. (1994) Biomechanics and muscular activity during sit-to-stand transfer. In *Clinical Assessment of Muscle Function* (ed. M. Roebroeck), CIP-Gegevens Koninklijke Bibliotheck, Den Haas, pp. 69–88.

5

Walking

Introduction

Just as standing up is essential to independence so also is walking. The ability to walk independently is a life-enriching activity and the most efficient way of getting from one place to another in the course of our daily lives. The principle substitute for walking is propelling a wheelchair and, although this is preferable to not being able to get about at all, individuals who must use this substitution miss out on the considerable versatility of behaviour and experience associated with walking.

There is a large body of literature on the biomechanics and control of walking in able-bodied subjects and in different age groups (e.g., Saunders *et al*. 1953; Bernstein 1967; Inman *et al*. 1981; Forssberg 1982; Grillner 1985; Winter 1987; Patla 1991). There have been numerous studies investigating the characteristics of gait in the presence of neuromusculoskeletal dysfunction in different patient populations. Recent developments in technology and in mathematical modelling have the potential to provide greater insights into the mechanics of gait and of pathological gait problems.

Walking is one of the most consistent yet flexible actions we perform, individuals displaying the same qualitative pattern of movement, presumably geared to optimum efficiency, from one cycle to the next (e.g., Murray *et al*. 1964; Bernstein 1967). Individuals have the same joint angular displacements over a wide range of cadences, all we do is accomplish that same pattern in less or more time (Winter 1989).

Although the kinematics of 'normal' gait remain relatively stable between subjects, the pattern of muscle use may vary, not only from subject to subject, but also with speed and fatigue in a single subject. In other words, there is considerable redundancy in the muscle/motor system such that if a particular muscle cannot be used, another muscle or group of muscles may take over the function (e.g., Winter 1987; Whittle 1991). For example, the knee angle during stance phase is under control of at least three joint moments and many muscles, both mono- and biarticular (Winter *et al*. 1991). It is, therefore, virtually impossible to identify 'normal' patterns of muscle usage with the methods of measurement available at the present time.

The major requirements for successful walking are: the production of a basic locomotor rhythm; support and propulsion of the body in the intended direction; dynamic balance control of the moving body; and the ability to adapt the movement to changing environmental demands and goals (Forssberg 1982).

Description of the action: The gait cycle

For ease of analysis, the gait cycle is divided into a stance phase, which commences at heel contact, and a swing phase which commences at toe-off. Each leg in turn has a stance phase when the upper body moves forward from behind the foot on the ground to in front of the foot, and a swing phase when the leg swings forward from behind the pelvis (and upper body). There is also a brief double support phase when both feet are in contact with the support surface. Stance and swing times as reported for natural cadences are: stance

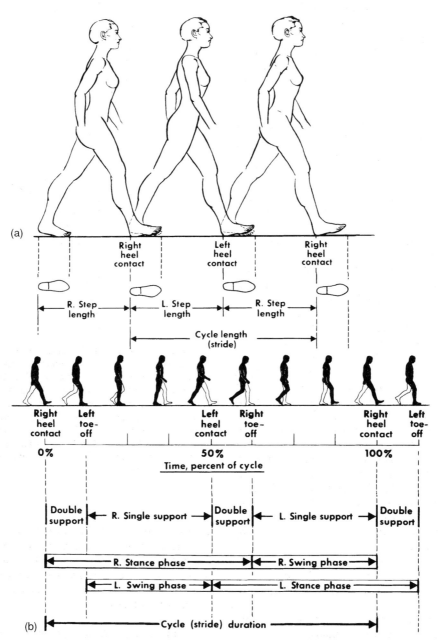

Fig. 5.1 Time dimensions of the walking cycle. (From Inman, V.T., Ralston, H.J. and Todd, F. (1981) *Human Walking*. Baltimore: Williams & Wilkins, by permission)

58–61%; swing 42–39%. Stance percentages increase at slower walking velocities. If symmetry is assumed, two double support periods of 8–11% of the stride occur. The short double support phase is critical in transferring weight from one limb to the other and in the control of balance and posture of the upper body (Winter 1989). As walking velocity increases, double support times decrease progressively and, in running, double support is replaced with a free flight phase.

For the purpose of description, stance can be subdivided into weight/load acceptance, mid-stance and push-off, while swing is divided into lift-off (early swing) and reach (late swing) (Winter 1987). The terms used to describe foot placements on the ground are shown in Fig. 5.1. Natural cadences vary from 101–122 steps/min with gender differences of 6–11 steps higher in females compared with males. Walking velocity (stride length × cadence/120) is the average speed of forward progression of the body and is typically reported in metres per second (m/s) or centimetres per second (cm/s). Stride length may be correlated with stature and, therefore, walking speed tends to increase with stature (Grieve 1968), although there is contemporary debate about this.

The pathway described by the total body centre of gravity in the plane of progression as the body moves forward is a smooth, sinusoidal curve. The centre of gravity is displaced twice in the vertical direction from heel contact of one foot to subsequent heel contact of the same foot. The centre of gravity is also displaced laterally in the horizontal plane in a smooth sinusoidal curve, the summits of which move to the right and to the left in relation to support of the stance leg. By keeping the walking base narrow, lateral movement of the body mass to preserve balance is also reduced (e.g, Whittle 1991). Figure 5.2 is a translational plot showing the path of the body's centre of gravity for one walking stride (Winter *et al.* 1991). Note that the body's centre of gravity does not fall within the perimeter of the foot during progression forward, indicating that, except during double support, walking is an inherently unstable movement.

In the *stance phase* of walking, the lower limb's principal functions are support, balance and propulsion, together with absorbtion of energy:

1 *Support*: the upper body is supported by the prevention of lower limb collapse.
2 *Balance*: maintenance of upright posture over the base of support.

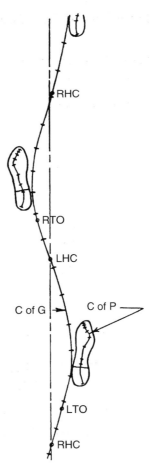

Fig. 5.2 A translational plot showing the body's centre of gravity (C of G) and foot centre of pressure (C of P) for one walking stride. Note: the C of G never passes over the foot, indicating that walking is an inherently unstable movement except during double support. TO: toe-off; HC: heel contact. (From Winter, D.A., McFadyen, B.J. and Dickey, J.P. (1991) Adaptibility of the CNS in human walking. In *Adaptability of Human Gait*. Amsterdam, Elsevier Science by permission)

3 *Propulsion (acceleration of the body in space)*: generation of mechanical energy to enable the appropriate forward motion of the body.
4 *Absorption*: of mechanical energy for both shock absorption and to decrease the body's forward velocity.

In the *swing phase*, the lower limb's main function is to clear the foot from the ground and to prepare the foot for its landing on the support surface: the foot moves on a smooth path through swing from toe-off to heel contact.

These functions are, according to Winter (1987), the main functions that must be performed in effective walking.

Kinematics

Kinematics is the term used to describe movement itself independent of internal and external forces. A wide variety of measurement techniques have been used to quantify kinematic variables and include video-based motion analysis systems and electrogoniometry.

The *stance phase* begins at heel contact and, after the foot is flat on the supporting surface (called foot flat), is characterized by extension of the hip and dorsiflexion at the ankle as the body moves forward over the fixed forward-placed foot. This ensures an erect posture. At heel contact, the ankle plantarflexes to bring the forefoot in contact with the ground and the shank starts to pivot over the fixed foot. This is generally known as the load acceptance phase of gait. Early in the phase, there is a small flexion movement at the knee, the so-called 'yield' of the knee. The knee functions in this way to smooth the path of the centre of gravity thus conserving energy (Saunders *et al*. 1953). Knee flexion occurs with eccentric quadriceps activity.

Movement of the upper body forward over the stance hip is associated with some internal rotation at the hip until full weight-bearing, when there is a reversal of the direction into external rotation as the foot is about to leave the ground. At mid-stance the hip is more than half-way into extension with a typical angle about zero (Whittle 1991). At this point in the cycle, as the lateral horizontal shift of the pelvis towards the stance leg reaches its maximum of about 4–5 cm (Saunders *et al*. 1953), excessive adduction of the hip is prevented by activity of the hip abductors, particularly gluteus medius. Activation of the hip abductors also prevents the pelvis from tilting down more than a few degrees (on average 5°, according to Saunders *et al*. 1953) on the swing side, along with lateral flexion of the lumbar spine. Knee extension during mid-stance seems an important factor in preventing excessive horizontal pelvic shift, due to the abduction of the tibia relative to the femur which occurs when the knee is extended and the femur is adducting at the hip (Saunders *et al*. 1953; Whittle 1991).

About two-thirds of the way through the stance phase, while the hip is still extending, the knee

starts to flex and the ankle to plantarflex (heel-off). Between heel-off and toe-off the hip reaches its peak extension (10–15° with respect to the trunk/pelvis, according to Whittle 1991) and starts to flex prior to the termination of stance. Extension of the hip appears to be essential in setting up the conditions both for the propulsive push-off and for the initiation of the swing phase of that leg allowing a smooth transition from one phase to the other (Pearson 1976).

In the *transition from stance to swing phase*, kinematic events which occur in pre-swing, i.e., at the end of stance, appear to set up the conditions for swing. Extension of the hip at the end of stance is critical to optimize the propulsive push-off and for the initiation of the swing phase of that leg. Hip extension and the large initial hip flexion angular velocity appear to be critical to subsequent flexion in the swing phase. The hip flexors at the end of stance are stretched, probably facilitating the swinging forward of the leg by the hip flexors together with the plantarflexor contraction necessary for toe-off. Knee flexion, occurring about two-thirds of the way through stance, contributes to shortening the leg for swing.

The *swing phase* begins at toe-off, with the ankle plantarflexed, knee flexed and hip extended, and is characterized initially by hip flexion and knee flexion then by extension at the knee and dorsiflexion at the ankle prior to heel contact. Swing phase can be divided into an acceleratory phase before mid-swing and a deceleratory phase from mid-swing to heel contact. The swing phase is executed with considerable precision, with average toe clearance of about 1 cm (e.g., Winter 1987).

By the time the toes are lifted off the supporting surface, the knee is already flexed to an angle of 40–50° and flexes rapidly to a maximum of 63° early in swing. The pelvis lists down slightly on the swing side and this can only be achieved if the swing phase leg is shortened sufficiently to clear the ground despite the lowering in the height of the hip joint (Whittle 1991). Flexion at the knee effectively 'shortens' the swinging leg, enabling the foot to take a forward path without contacting the ground (Eberhart *et al*. 1965). Knee flexion continues after toe-off, partly as a mechanical result of the continued forward movement of the thigh. Muscle activity is necessary at the end of the swing phase when the knee flexors contract to decelerate the extension at the knee for heel contact. Extension of the knee at the end of swing serves to lengthen the leg again before heel contact so as to place the leg in a more stable configuration and minimize lowering of the trunk.

Some rotation of the pelvis at the hips occurs in the horizontal plane (cephalocaudal axis), its maximum excursion occurring at heel contact. This pelvic rotation is countered by thoracic rotation. The magnitude of the pelvic rotation is typically small, some 4° on either side of the central axis (Saunders *et al.* 1953). Murray and colleagues (1964) reported an absence of pelvic rotation in some subjects and also suggested that it may vary with stride length. The variability between subjects suggested to these authors that pelvic rotation may not be an 'obligatory element of normal gait, but rather a convenient excursion, available when walking and, perhaps, attitude demand it' (p. 358). In a recent study, Crosbie and colleagues (1997a) also reported a restricted and somewhat variable inter-subject range of pelvic rotation, with limited overall contribution to increased step length. When walking speed is increased, the component of movement most responsible for increased step length appears to be more accurately described in terms of increased pelvic tilt and list although there appear to be some gender differences.

Sagittal plane rotation of the pelvis (anterior and posterior pelvic tilting) occurs through a mean excursion of 3° with the maximum anterior tilt occurring just before heel contact and the maximum posterior tilt early in the stance phase (Murray *et al.* 1964). The velocity of walking depends to a large extent on the efficiency of the swing phase, since the stride length depends on how far the foot can be moved forward during this time (Whittle 1991).

Kinetics

The forces producing displacements of the segments of the lower limb are muscular, gravitational and interactive, the latter being the result of dynamic interactions between segments. The ability to propel oneself forward manifests itself in the generation of appropriate forces on the support surface, i.e., the limbs have to produce forces that act downward and backward to propel the body mass forward and upward (Patla 1991). Kinetics is concerned with individual muscle forces, the net moments generated by those muscles at each joint, and the mechanical power pattern (i.e., rate of generation or absorption of mechanical energy by muscles or the rate of transfer between segments).

Ground reaction forces, measured by a force plate, are the simplest kinetic variables to record.

They reflect the vertical and horizontal acceleration and deceleration of the body's centre of mass during weight-bearing (Winter 1987). The vertical force plot (Fig. 5.3) illustrates the characteristic double hump indicating that the body is being accelerated upward at the end of weight acceptance. In mid stance there is downward acceleration and during push-off there is a net upward acceleration. The magnitudes of the peaks and valleys vary with cadence (Winter 1987).

There are many combinations of muscle forces that can result in the same movement pattern and many combinations of muscle activity that can produce the same moments of force at a given joint. Indeed, muscles act cooperatively to prevent collapse of the limb. Winter (1980, 1984) has

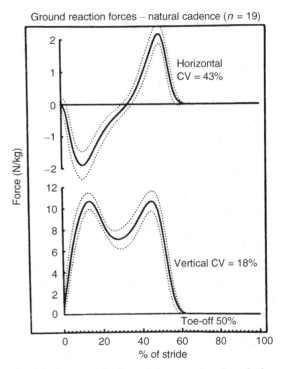

Fig. 5.3 Averaged horizontal (top trace) and vertical (bottom trace) ground reaction forces. The horizontal force has a negative phase during the first half of stance, indicating a slowing down of the body and a positive phase, indicating forward acceleration of the body, during the latter half of stance. The vertical force has the characteristic double hump, the first related to weight-acceptance and the second to push-off. CV: coefficient of variation. (From Winter, D.A. (1987) *The Biomechanics and Motor Control of Human Gait.* Waterloo, Canada: University of Waterloo Press, by permission)

shown that collapse of the lower limb in stance is prevented by an overall extensor moment of force called a support moment (SM). This SM is consistently extensor despite variability which occurs at hip, knee and ankle joints (Fig. 5.4).

While the ankle moment of force remains relatively consistent under different speeds, trial-by-trial and subject-by-subject, hip and knee moments covary or cooperate, a decrease in extensor moment at the knee, for example, being countered by an increase in moment at the hip. It has been shown that, on a given stride, the quadriceps may be dominant in supporting the lower limb (by preventing knee collapse) and, therefore, contributing to support moment. On a subsequent stride for the same subject, the quadriceps may be inactive, the control of the knee resulting primarily from hamstring and gluteus maximus action. Whatever the relative muscle contributions, the net support moment remains the same. In effect, there is a flexible stride-to-stride

trade-off between the muscles crossing the hip and knee joints. Although the pattern of SM is rather consistent trial-by-trial and subject-by-subject, it does vary according to speed.

An analysis of *mechanical power* provides information about which muscles are generating energy and which are absorbing energy (Winter 1987). Power (measured in watts) is the rate at which energy is generated and absorbed and is the product of the net moment at the joint and the angular velocity. Negative power results from eccentric contraction and positive power from concentric contraction. Power profiles of the three lower limb joints for healthy subjects are shown in Figure 5.5. These profiles describe the magnitude and direction of the flow of energy in and out of muscles and reveal that: the major energy generation (>80%) takes place at push-off by plantar-flexor activity; the knee extensors are primarily absorbing energy during stance; and the second most important source of power is from the hip

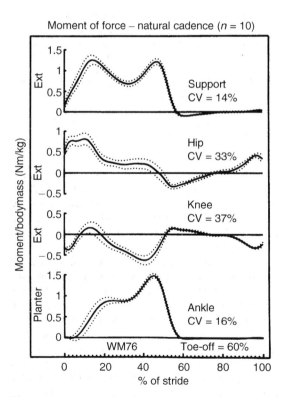

Fig. 5.4 Support moment of force, an algebraic summation of the moments of force at the hip, knee and ankle. CV: coefficient of variation. (From Winter, D.A. (1987) *The Biomechanics and Motor Control of Human Gait.* Waterloo, Canada: University of Waterloo Press, by permission)

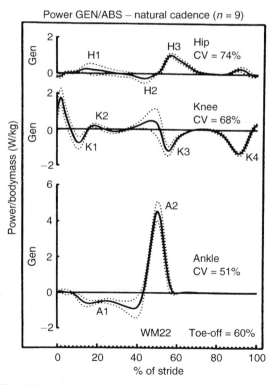

Fig. 5.5 Typical power profiles of hip (H), knee (K) and ankle (A) indicating the most important power phases. CV: coefficient of variation. (From Winter, D.A. (1987) *The Biomechanics and Motor Control of Human Gait.* Waterloo, Canada: University of Waterloo Press, by permission)

flexors during late stance and early swing which serves to pull the leg forward (Winter 1983). Winter has also shown that power patterns over the stride remain constant in shape but increase in amplitude as cadence increases. An understanding of power patterns can be used to guide the development of training strategies. For example, power analysis at the knee indicates that the major role of the quadriceps muscle group in stance is to lengthen actively (knee flexion) and absorb energy.

Muscle activity

In natural quiet walking it is thought that the muscles themselves produce rather a small amount of the total force required to propel the body mass forward. Muscles appear to act over relatively short periods of time and, during large intervals in the cycle, the limb is carried forward by its own inertia. The major role of muscles in walking is to provide the appropriate burst of power at the appropriate time in the walking cycle (Fig. 5.6) (Winter 1985). Muscles act to initiate the movement, which is carried through by the body's momentum, then to brake the movement or momentum. Additional force is required when walking fast or when climbing up a slope or stairs.

Since the body is moving over the relatively fixed foot in stance phase, it is not surprising that the muscles linking the foot to the shank play a critical role in body translation. The tibialis anterior and long toe flexors show increased activity at the start of stance phase. Although this muscle activity controls the plantarflexion which places the foot on the floor after heel contact, it also subsequently rotates the shank forward over the heel. At the start of single support, dorsiflexion at the ankle accounts for the forward progression of the body/shank over the foot. This is controlled by eccentric activity in the plantarflexors, particularly the soleus muscle. The restraining action of the plantarflexors as they prevent the collapse of the shank forward makes an essential contribution to stability of the ankle, the tension required to prevent collapse being two to three times body weight (Skinner *et al.* 1985).

The effect of muscle activation when linked segments rotate over a fixed distal segment is quite different from what one might expect from reading anatomical texts in which lower limb muscle function is described in relation to segmental rotations when the foot is free to move. For

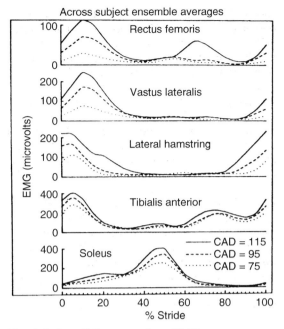

Fig. 5.6 Overall linear envelope EMG pattern changes associated with three different walking cadences (n=11). Stride time was normalized across subjects and speeds. Note the change in EMG pattern is primarily in amplitude, the shape remaining similar. The degree of amplitude change was muscle-specific. (From Yang, J.F. and Winter, D.A. (1985) Surface EMG profiles during different walking cadences in humans. *Electroencephalography and Clinical Neurophysiology*, **60**, 485–491 by permission)

example, the quadriceps are active early in the stance phase to prevent the limb from collapsing into flexion but also to move the thigh forward over the shank (Skinner *et al.* 1985) and, therefore, to aid in the progression of the whole body forward over the foot.

Although the knee is extended in mid-stance, the extension is not necessarily brought about by the quadriceps since they may be inactive at this stage. It has been suggested that extension is maintained both by forward movement of the thigh on the shank and by slowing down of the forward movement of the shank. The plantarflexors, particularly soleus, by contributing to the deceleration of the forward movement of the shank, can also prevent knee as well as ankle collapse. This mechanism may make an essential contribution to the stability of the knee as well as to the ankle (Sutherland *et al.* 1980).

Investigation of push-off towards the end of the stance phase shows that a concentric contraction of calf muscle, between about 10° of dorsiflexion and 20° of plantarflexion, causes a rapid ankle plantarflexion which generates a major propulsive power burst just before toe-off (Winter 1987). Concentric calf muscle activity during push-off occurs when the alignment of the foot, shank and thigh are in an ideal position to push the body upward and forward. There remains no doubt that the major power generation during the natural walking cycle is caused by the ankle plantarflexors during push-off (Winter 1983).

Stair walking

The biomechanics of walking up and down stairs or steps is described by several authors (e.g., Joseph and Watson 1967; Townsend *et al.* 1978; Andriacchi *et al.* 1980). Although it is discussed briefly in this section as an action involving the lower limbs in support, balance and propulsion, it is mechanically different from level walking, in terms of range of joint movement, muscle activity and magnitude of joint forces (Andriacchi *et al.* 1980). The major problem in walking up stairs is the conservation of energy while that of descending is principally that of ensuring safety.

Lower limb function in stair climbing and descending differs from level walking due to the necessity for a greater raising and lowering of the body mass while progressing forward to another stair level. This results in increased demands on both duration and intensity of muscle activity and increased ranges of motion at the lower limb joints (Andriacchi *et al.* 1980). Greater demands are also made on balance, particularly during the period of single stance (James and Parker 1989). Stair descent has been found to have a shorter double support phase than stair ascent, probably reflecting different mechanical demands and greater inherent stability (Zachazewski *et al.* 1993).

An essential feature of walking up stairs is the ankle dorsiflexion which occurs after the foot has been placed on the stair. The forward transport of the body mass takes place at the ankle, while the body remains in the same relative alignment. The back leg pushes the body forward and upward diagonally over the front foot while this leg lifts the body along a vertical inclination. In contrast, when descending, the body mass is kept back over the supporting leg which flexes at the hip, knee and ankle to lower the body mass and place the foot on to the next step. Displacement at the knee joint in stance phase of stair walking is greater than in

level walking, being from full extension to approximately 90° in both climbing and descending (Shinno 1971).

In walking up stairs, concentric lower limb extensor activity raises the body mass vertically; in walking down stairs, the body mass is lowered by eccentric muscle activity. Extensor muscles have to generate much larger forces in both than in level walking. Extensor muscle strength is, therefore, particularly critical to this activity since the body mass must be raised or lowered essentially by one limb.

Changes to walking in the elderly

Since many adults with lesions of the CNS, particularly following stroke, are in an older age group, it is of interest to consider the effect of ageing on gait. Payton and Poland (1983) summarize the physiological adaptations that take place with ageing. How many of the changes observed in older individuals are due to an ageing process and how many to the reduced activity that may accompany getting older, however, is not understood.

It is a common observation that the walking pattern changes with increasing age. Investigators have described age-related decreases in aerobic capacity, joint flexibility, muscle strength and bone mass. Interestingly, these decrements are similar to those associated with extended periods of bed rest and even with relative inactivity (Bortz 1982). It is also of note that certain aspects of physical performance are strongly influenced by both the level and type of activity. For example, in a longitudinal study of aerobic capacity in elite athletes aged between 50 and 82 years, Pollock and colleagues (1987) found that those who continued training maintained their aerobic capacity irrespective of their age.

Murray and colleagues (1969) reported that, providing individuals with pathology were excluded, the walking performance of older men was a 'slowed down' version of the gait of younger men. A subsequent study confirmed this observation on women subjects (Murray *et al.* 1970). More recently Winter and colleagues (1990) studied a group of active and healthy men and women with an age range of 62–78 and compared their performance with younger subjects. The authors reported the following findings: walking velocity was decreased (stride length was decreased); duration of double support was increased; push-off power decreased; and there was a more flat-footed heel contact. The nature of these adaptations suggests they are made to improve stability. It appears also that elderly subjects increase their walking speed by increasing step frequency to a greater extent than increasing stride length (Imms and Edholdm 1981). Changes in gait as a function of age may also be due to changes in muscle strength (Nigg *et al.* 1994) associated with motor unit adaptation, for example, a decrease in the number of motor units and a slowing of recruitment. Capacity to increase speed is also reduced in the elderly.

In terms of energy expenditure, it appears that individuals of any age normally have a small range of walking speeds in which they are able to walk most economically (Smidt 1990). In a study in which oxygen uptake was measured in three different age groups (19–29, 39–49, 55–66) walking at four different speeds, Cunningham and colleagues (1982) concluded that self-selected walking velocity was associated with maximal aerobic power independent of age.

Motor dysfunction

Biomechanical data related to the kinematics, kinetics and muscle activations of gait help elucidate the performance and control deficits in individuals with neural lesions. This section considers movement dysfunction associated with acute brain lesions, such as stroke and head injury. However, the information is applicable to other neurological conditions in which the upper motor neuron is involved. Walking dysfunction in Parkinson's disease and ataxia are discussed in Chapters 13 and 9 respectively.

The major primary impairments following an upper motor neuron (UMN) lesion (see Chapter 8) are muscle weakness or paralysis, hyperreflexia, loss of both dexterity (i.e., skill) and ability to fractionate movement (Burke 1988). Weakness is a loss of strength of voluntary muscle action, i.e., a depression of motor function. There is insufficient motor unit activity and a slowing of the rate and amplitude of recruitment.

Compared with the large body of data-based studies of gait in healthy subjects, there are relatively few investigations of walking performance in individuals following stroke and even fewer related to head injury. The majority of these studies have focused on temporal variables. One of the most consistent differences reported between able-bodied subjects and individuals following stroke is in walking velocity (e.g., Bogardh and Richards 1981; Olney *et al.* 1986; Lehmann *et al.* 1987; Bohannon 1987). For individuals who walk slowly, it is important to determine the extent to which the deficits seen in gait are a result rather than a cause of the slow speed. There is evidence that some of the characteristics of the gait of disabled subjects, such as decreased angular excursion and decreased stride, are readily evident in healthy subjects walking at comparable speeds (O'Brien *et al.* 1983; Lehmann *et al.* 1987).

Subjects with hemiplegia who have significantly reduced walking speeds typically demonstrate decreased stride length, shorter stance phase and longer swing phase in the affected limb. To compensate for these changes, the stance/swing ratio in the unaffected leg shifts to an increased stance and decreased swing phase. Consistent with these findings is an increase in the duration of double support. It is sometimes suggested that individuals following stroke deliberately reduce stance time on the affected leg and rely on the unaffected leg. One biomechanical explanation for increased time on the unaffected leg, however, is that the affected leg will take more time to swing through because less power is put into the limb during late stance and early swing (Olney *et al.* 1991).

Although the majority of studies of walking in patients following stroke have used temporal measures, others have studied joint angle excursions, kinetics and mechanical power. In general, joint angular displacements are decreased (e.g., Bogardh and Richards 1981; Lehmann *et al.* 1987), with evidence of decreased ankle dorsiflexion at initial foot contact (e.g., Richards and Knutsson 1974; Basmajian *et al.* 1975), decreased knee flexion in swing (e.g., Knutsson 1981) and lack of knee flexion in stance (e.g., Knutsson 1981). In terms of decreased amplitude of hip extension in stance associated with decreased velocity, Lehmann and colleagues (1987) reported that stroke patients exhibited 14° less hip extension at late mid-stance and push-off than healthy subjects.

Knee moments of force have been reported to be abnormal in stance (Lehmann *et al.* 1987) but this is difficult to interpret without more data on moments of force at the hip and ankle joint, considering the cooperative nature of support moments of force (Winter 1980). Vertical force traces suggest that individuals following stroke lack the peak vertical force associated with push-off (Carlsoo *et al.* 1974).

An abnormal coactivation of leg muscles is reported as a characteristic of abnormal gait in individuals following stroke (e.g., Peat *et al.* 1976; Brandstater *et al.* 1983; Dietz and Berger 1983). It has been suggested that inappropriate coactivation may alter the biomechanical characteristics of a limb, as well as its capacity for absorbing and storing energy (Harrison and Kruze 1987). It is interesting to speculate that inappropriate coactivation of muscles may emerge as the individual attempts to generate sufficient muscle activity in weak muscles to load the limb, balance and progress forward. This may be the source of many clinical observations of 'extensor spasticity'.

Recently Olney and colleagues (1994), using multiple regression analyses, assessed the relationship between temporal, kinematic and kinetic variables in an attempt to identify those variables that may be most helpful in understanding the major impairments contributing to temporal deficits in stroke patients. The most useful variables in predicting stride speed for the affected side were hip flexion moment, ankle moment, knee moment and proportion of time spent in double support.

Although muscle power patterns at the three lower limb joints of the affected limb have been found to be similar in shape to normal, they are reduced in amplitude, with the muscles of the affected side providing about 40% of the positive work (Olney *et al.* 1991). Energy cost of walking has been found to be higher in individuals following stroke than for able-bodied subjects (Winter 1978; Olney *et al.* 1986).

Considerable investigative attention has been directed to the deficits occurring at the ankle joint in stance phase, i.e., between shank and foot segments (e.g., Berger *et al.* 1984; Olney *et al.* 1991; Thilmann *et al.* 1991). One study of power curves (Olney *et al.* 1991) reported a low level of power generated by the ankle plantarflexors in stance phase in individuals following stroke. Berger and colleagues (1984) found that adult hemiplegic subjects showed an increase in tension in the Achilles tendon that did not equate with plantarflexor activation. This increased tension was said to be due to mechanical changes in muscle fibres themselves. They found no influence of pathological reflex activity (spasticity) in the gastrocnemius. In animal experiments, it has been shown that immobilization (i.e., inactivity) can lead to significant stiffening of the muscle and soft tissue (e.g., Akeson *et al.* 1973) (see Chapter 8). These findings illustrate the importance of understanding the mechanism

underlying motor performance deficits in planning intervention.

The Berger study (1984) suggests that intervention would involve training control of the foot-shank segment during the stance phase of walking, exercises to increase the force output of calf muscles at the length where this output is required for the action and to stretch the short calf muscles, with the addition of serial casting in the case of more severe calf muscle contracture.

Common observable gait deficits

Since walking has a remarkable consistency, a clearly identifiable pattern and prescribed ranges for the kinematic variables, the major spatio-temporal deficits can be identified from observation. However, observational analysis requires much practice and understanding of biomechanics. Without the necessary knowledge, observation of walking can be very inaccurate and erroneous conclusions can be drawn (Malouin 1995).

Non-observable deficits, such as segmental coordination, force generation and timing of muscle activity, can only be inferred from observation and require confirmation with appropriate instrumentation. Some findings of interest to the physiotherapist, from studies of specific patient populations, are described later in this section. There are, however, several mechanical problems that commonly interfere with the ability to walk, irrespective of the age of the individual and the underlying pathological mechanisms.

It is essential at this point to refer back to the principal functions of the lower limbs in stance and swing phases. In general, it is problems associated with the *stance phase* that interfere most with progression forward. *Support* in the erect position for stance requires extensor muscle activity to prevent the limb from collapsing and to maintain segmental alignment as the body mass is moved forward. Extensibility of muscles, particularly hip flexor and calf muscles, is also critical to allow the body to move forward over the foot. The ability to generate force, particularly in calf muscles for push-off, is critical to *propulsion* of the body mass forward and upward. *Balance* of the body mass over a relatively small and changing base of support, with two-thirds of the body mass high above the ground, demands preparatory and ongoing postural adjustments throughout, particularly in single limb support.

Certain gait abnormalities arise as a consequence of the lesion, which are in part the result of muscle weakness/paralysis and in part due to the person's attempts to walk despite the muscle strength and balance impairments. Due to the complexity of gait, it is difficult to establish with certainty which deficits are primary and which are secondary. Adaptations to the gait cycle resulting from secondary adaptive changes of soft tissue are, however, easier to identify. Therapists need to attempt to distinguish between the two in order for training to focus on the primary impairments and on preventing (or treating) secondary musculoskeletal impairments/deficits.

Stance phase

As a consequence of the lesion, it is typical for individuals to have difficulty in the stance phase supporting the body mass through the affected leg and balancing, due to decreased and poorly timed muscle force, particularly of gluteal muscles, hamstrings, quadriceps and calf muscles. Movement in the frontal plane is particularly dependent

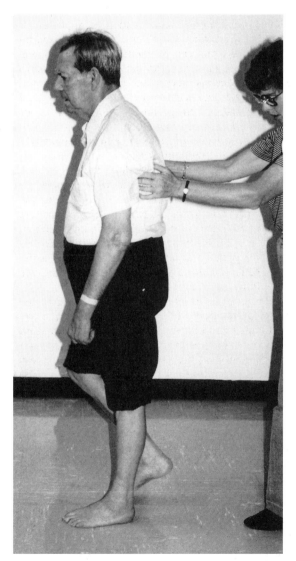

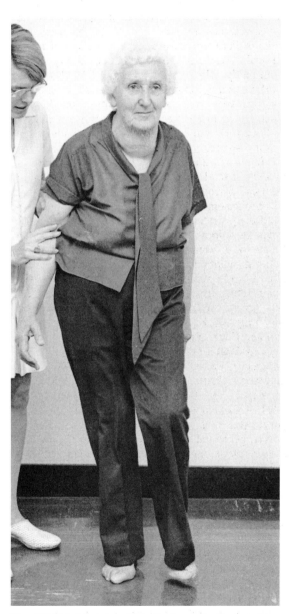

Fig. 5.7 L mid stance. Lack of hip extension (pelvis moving on hip) and ankle dorsiflexion mean body mass has not advanced forward. Knee is too extended

Fig. 5.8 R mid stance. Note the excessive horizontal pelvic shift to the R and downward list of pelvis on the L

on abductor/adductor control and movement in the plane of progression (sagittal) is dependent on the lower limb extensors.

Observations of attempts to walk may show:

- *Decrease in extension at the hip and in transport of the trunk and pelvis forward over the stance foot (Fig. 5.7).*
- *Excessive lateral horizontal shift of the pelvis, associated with an excessive downward tilt on the side of the swinging leg (Fig. 5.8).*
- *Absence of knee flexion at the beginning of stance.*
- *Lack of knee extension in mid-stance.*
- *Absence of knee flexion toward the end of stance (Fig. 5.9a).*
- *Decreased plantarflexion at the ankle joint for push-off (Fig. 5.9a).*

Swing phase

Since the stance phase sets up the optimal conditions for swing, many of the problems in the *swing leg* may be related to problems observed in the stance phase. However, there may also be:

- *Decreased flexion at the hip.*
- *Decreased flexion at the knee to 'shorten' the leg for toe clearance as the leg swings forward (Fig. 5.9b).*

These may be related to decreased amplitude of extension at the hip in stance and lack of push-off at the ankle. Lack of knee flexion may also be due to contracture or increased stiffness of rectus femoris, a two-joint muscle which flexes the hip as well as extends the knee. A short or stiff rectus femoris may interfere with flexion of the knee at the stance/swing interchange.

- *Decreased dorsiflexion at the ankle as a contribution to toe clearance.* It is interesting to note that this problem, commonly observed by clinicians, may be due to slowness in flexing the knee rather than decreased amplitude of dorsiflexion (Whittle 1991).
- *Decreased extension at the knee and dorsiflexion at the ankle for heel contact. The foot is set down flat or toe first and step length is decreased/short.* This is often secondary to contracture of calf muscles, although it will also occur when ankle dorsiflexors are weak or paralysed. When the foot is set down in this

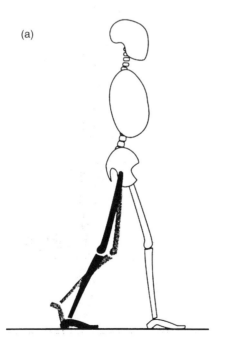
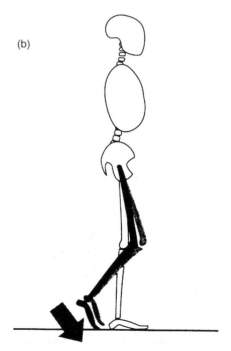

Fig. 5.9 Bold limb shows (*a*) Inadequate knee flexion, excessive ankle dorsiflexion and prolonged contact in pre-swing (*b*) inadequate knee flexion at the beginning of swing with toe drag as foot is not lifted sufficiently. (From Perry, J. (1992) *Gait Analysis Normal and Pathological Function.* Thorofare, NJ: Slack, by permission)

way, the body's centre of gravity is relatively posterior on foot contact. Contacting the floor with the forefoot first tends to stretch the calf muscles earlier in the cycle, particularly when there is contracture or reflex hyperactivity of these muscles. This mechanism may underlie the knee hyperextension in many individuals (Fig. 5.10).

In addition, individuals with sensorimotor impairment (e.g., muscle paralysis or weakness, ataxia) commonly have difficulty *balancing* over the stance foot during single support and over both feet in double support. Fear of falling and a feeling of instability often result in a widening of the walking base. Walking base or stride-width in the side-to-side direction, usually measured at the mid-point of the heel, is normally approximately 50–100 mm between the line of the two feet (Whittle 1991).

Rhythm, sequencing and timing of segmental rotations may be abnormal even when muscle activity is present. There may be a difference in timing between the two legs, but with the same pattern repeated on each cycle, or, conversely,

there may be an irregular timing disturbance. In the latter, the timing tends to vary from step-to-step and is typically seen in individuals with ataxia.

Secondary gait adaptations

In response to primary sensorimotor impairment and secondary muscle contracture, certain adaptive motor behaviours emerge as the individual attempts to walk. These can be summarized as:

- *Decreased amplitude of movement, i.e., decreased angular displacement.*
- *Decreased stride length.*
- *Decreased step length.*
- *Uneven step and stride lengths.*
- *Increased stride width.*
- *Increased time spent in double support.*
- *Decreased walking velocity.*
- *Use of arms for support and balance (as with walking aids).*

Some movement abnormalities, which are typically considered by clinicians to be due to primary impairments, may instead be the result of secondary adaptations. It is important to attempt to

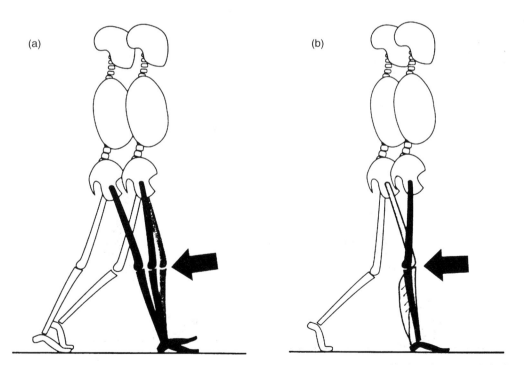

(a)   (b)

Fig. 5.10 (*a*) Normally the knee flexes at start of stance. Compare the lack of knee flexion (*b*). Instead the knee hyperextends. (After Perry, J. (1992) *Gait Analysis Normal and Pathological Function*. Thorofare, NJ: Slack, by permission)

differentiate between those impairments of gait which arise as a consequence of the lesion and those that emerge as adaptive motor patterns or compensation. Short step length, for example, may be due to weak push-off prior to swing, weak hip flexion at toe-off and early swing or it may be an adaptation to fear of falling. Weak push-off may be due to weakness of calf muscles or a secondary contracture of calf muscles.

It is also important to consider that lower limb movements provide the driving force in gait. Movements of the pelvis and lower trunk appear to occur in response to lower limb movements, and it has further been suggested that thoracic spine movements occur principally in response to arm swing (Crosbie and Vachalathiti 1997).

It is not possible at the present time to do other than make an educated guess about the underlying mechanism associated with adaptive movements (see Latash and Anson 1996, and commentaries). The complexity of muscle action in a multisegment system, particularly when the foot is fixed, and the role of the mono-, bi- and multiarticular muscles, is referred to in few anatomy texts (e.g., in Kapandji 1970), and it is only relatively recently that investigations have been carried out into muscle function and segmental interactions in multijoint actions such as jumping (e.g., Gregoire *et al.* 1984; van Ingen Schenau 1989).

Some examples of mechanisms underlying typical *adaptations* which need to be considered in the analysis of gait are:

- The ability to move the body mass forward over the foot is essentially dependent on the extent of displacement at hip and ankle joints (Fig. 5.7). *Decreased hip extension and ankle dorsiflexion* may be the result of contracture of the soleus muscle which can constrain movement of the body mass forward and result in a shorter step length of the swing leg.
- *Lack of control of the knee in stance* may result in one of two adaptive behaviours: the knee may extend ('hyperextend') and remain extended throughout stance (Fig. 5.11), or it may be held in a few degrees of flexion (Fig. 5.12). Clearly, when the lower limb extensor muscles are very weak, hyperextension of the knee enables the individual to prevent collapse of the lower limb and still walk independently. It is also possible, if the plantarflexors are weak, that hyperextension of the knee may provide some push-off at the end of stance (Whittle 1991). Contracture of soleus muscle holds the shank back

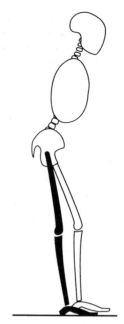

Fig. 5.11 Knee hyperextension and lack of forward movement of the shank on the foot (ankle dorsiflexion) is compensated for by forward movement of the trunk at the hip (hip flexion). (From Perry, J. (1992) *Gait Analysis Normal and Pathological Function.* Thorofare, NJ: Slack, by permission)

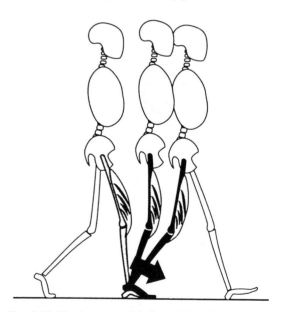

Fig. 5.12 The knee remains flexed throughout stance. Soleus weakness fails to stabilize the tibia. As a result, without a stable base the quadriceps cannot extend the flexed knee. (After Perry, J. (1992) *Gait Analysis Normal and Pathological Function.* Thorofare, NJ: Slack, by permission)

(i.e., prevents dorsiflexion at the ankle) and, because of the segmental linkage, the knee is held extended, preventing knee flexion.

● If the knee is not flexed at the end of stance-beginning of swing, *the pelvis may be 'hitched' up* on the side of the swinging leg in order to clear the foot from the ground. Alternatively, *the leg may be abducted and externally rotated*. The leg is swung forward by tilting the pelvis backwards (Fig. 5.13).

● Difficulties with balance (i.e., postural adjustments) may result in an increased stride width in *double support*, and, therefore, an increased side-to-side excursion of the body. There are two ways of increasing the base of support: the swing foot may be set down too far to the side (Fig. 5.14); and/or the foot is set down with the hip in external rotation. The arms may be held abducted as an additional method of maintaining and restoring balance. If an individual feels unable to walk without overbalancing, the hands are used (via walking aids) to gain stability and to compensate for the lack of postural muscle activations in the lower limbs.

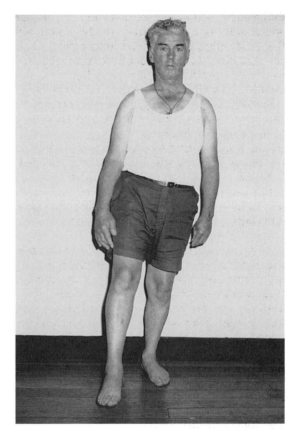

Fig. 5.14 A frontal view showing increased stride width. The L leg is externally rotated

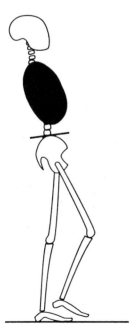

Fig. 5.13 Backward trunk movement with posterior pelvic tilt can advance the thigh in swing. (From Perry, J. (1992) *Gait Analysis Normal and Pathological Function*. Thorofare, NJ: Slack, by permission)

● Although decreased speed of muscle contraction and a slowness in reaching peak amplitude are probably major contributors to the *decreased walking speed*, walking may also be slowed down in response to feelings of instability or unsteadiness. Alternatively, some individuals may walk rather fast, the increased speed probably making it easier to balance (Winter 1987). This can often be seen in young adults with ataxia following head injury.

Task related training

The major emphasis in training for independent walking is on methods of training support and propulsion of the lower limbs, balance of the body mass over one or both feet, and control of the foot and knee paths through swing. The use of the hands for support should be discouraged to enable the regaining of dynamic balance and the ability to support the body through the lower limbs.

Intervention aims to:

- Prevent soft tissue adaptive shortening.
- Elicit muscle activity; increase muscle strength and control (mode and velocity of contraction) to provide support, propulsion, balance and toe clearance.
- Train rhythm and coordination.

These aims are addressed by a combination of *weight-bearing and stretching exercises* and *walking practice*.

Muscle extensibility and length must be maintained since muscle shortening restricts movement and imposes abnormal segmental alignment throughout the walking cycle. For example, a contracted soleus muscle not only prevents ankle dorsiflexion and hip extension in standing but also interferes with progression forward of the body mass in stance, as well as dorsiflexion for heel contact at the end of swing.

In general, it is the tendency for the stance limb to collapse and a lack of forward momentum that interfere most with gait. Since support (loading of the limb) is a prerequisite for upright stance, and push-off sets up the conditions for propulsion and swing, training focuses initially on this phase. Note that balance, weight-bearing and stepping are trained simultaneously when the individual practises walking itself.

Essential components

Despite the complexity of walking, it is possible to identify critical components. A simplification is convenient for the clinic since it gives clues to analysis and intervention. In the classic article by Saunders and colleagues (1953), the authors comment that

> the synthesis of all the elements which simultaneously participate in locomotion, although an ideal worthy of achievement, is a task of such magnitude and difficulty that its early attainment cannot be expected. Therefore, it is our purpose . . . to consider . . . what we have called the primary determinants of human locomotion . . . It is our expectation that, by an appreciation of these fundamental determinants, the orthopaedic surgeon [read physiotherapist] will be able to analyse disorders of locomotion with greater precision and to apply corrective measures with a fuller understanding of the interrelationships which exist between the various segments of the locomotor mechanism. (p. 543, reprinted with permission)

We have described in an earlier publication (Carr and Shepherd 1987) what we termed the essential components of walking. These form an observable kinematic pattern of walking (joint angle rotations and linear paths of body parts) that can be used as a basis for evaluating an individual's walking performance. We understand that only limited interpretation of motor control deficits can be made based on kinematic data alone. However, angular displacements and linear paths do form a repeatable, invariant pattern of walking and, therefore, enable comparisons to be made at that level.

The components (Fig. 5.15) listed below have been developed out of an updated synthesis of data-based findings (see references throughout).

Stance phase

- Extension at the hip (with dorsiflexion at ankle) to move body forward.
- Lateral horizontal shift of pelvis to the stance side.
- Flexion at the knee (approximately 15°) initiated on heel contact, followed by extension in mid-stance, then flexion prior to push-off.
- Plantarflexion at heel contact, followed by dorsiflexion then plantarflexion at the ankle (push-off).

Swing phase

- Flexion at the hip.
- Flexion at the knee.
- Lateral pelvic list downwards (approximately 5°) toward swing side in horizontal plane at toe-off.
- Rotation of pelvis forward on swing side.
- Extension at the knee plus dorsiflexion at the ankle immediately prior to heel contact.

Evaluation of motor performance

Observational evaluation involves comparing the individual's performance against a list of essential components or critical kinematic features of walking. Observational analysis without such a formalized structure tends to be arbitrary. In an observational analysis, discrepancies in the plane of progression are best observed from the side while frontal plane discrepancies, for example, lateral horizontal pelvic shift, pelvic list and stride width are best observed from the front or back.

There has been a tendency in physiotherapy to observe movement from a diagnosis- or lesion-specific set of gait abnormalities or from an erroneous view of what constitutes 'normal' gait. These observations do not necessarily have any biomechanical basis and may not take into account the adaptations that emerge from mechanical necessity in the presence of muscle weakness or paralysis, timing impairments and/or secondary muscle contracture. It has been found that pathology tends to bias raters' observations and that there is a lack of inter-rater reliability between therapists in assessing gait, despite confidence in their own ability (Malouin 1995). Using a proforma for recording observations during gait analysis, therefore, not only provides readily accessible data but also avoids mistakes inherent in relying on memory of previous observations.

Analysis of an individual's walking pattern is very complex, yet physiotherapists must do this in the clinic in order to be able to plan an appropriate training programme for individuals with movement dysfunction. Although instrumented gait analysis techniques are widely used in research, in most clinics, physiotherapists make their evaluation via observation, since both instrumentation and technical know-how are not readily available. It is our view that physiotherapists working in movement rehabilitation, in addition to becoming familiar with the published literature on biomechanics, need to have access to quantitative biomechanical measures from movement analysis laboratories attached to rehabilitation centres in order to measure both kinematic and kinetic aspects of performance, plan appropriate intervention and evaluate outcome. These procedures confirm (or not) observational analyses, and can also lead to improved observational skills.

There are, however, simple methods of measuring some biomechanical variables without sophisticated and expensive instrumentation (Smith 1990). For example, freeze-frame videotapes and still photography can be used to measure angular displacements, i.e., segmental alignment, at different points in time throughout the gait cycle (e.g., van Vliet 1988). These measures can be used to confirm (or not) the therapist's observations and subsequent measures are used to test the effects of training. In addition, a tape measure, stop watch and marking pens attached to the heels can be used to measure step and stride lengths in order to calculate cadence and velocity. Objective and reliable functional scales (e.g., Motor Assessment Scale, timed walking tests) that either include walking as a separate item or combine walking with other functional activities are described in Chapter 3.

Many intervention strategies currently in common use in the clinic do not take into account neuroscience, biomechanical and behavioural advances over the past few decades. We have been arguing the importance of eliciting and strengthening synergistic muscle activity and ensuring task-related practice for over a decade. Nevertheless, common physiotherapy practice emphasizes preparation for walking rather than walking itself. Furthermore, active exercises to lengthen and strengthen muscles are typically not described.

Individuals following an upper motor neuron (UMN) lesion have impairments of muscle action

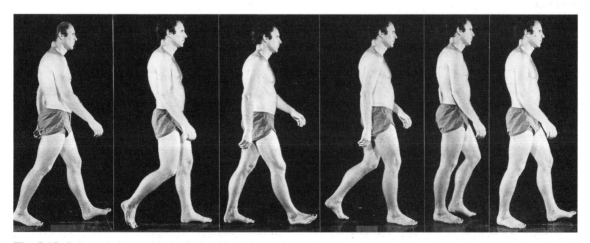

Fig. 5.15 Gait cycle in an able-bodied subject illustrating major components

leading to difficulty with support, propulsion and balance. Training to improve force-generation and the speed of muscle contraction is usually essential, in the early stages in particular, and task-related exercises can be directed toward these deficits. Functional improvement, however, depends on regaining the appropriate timing of segmental rotations, and this requires practice of walking.

There are many reasons, including mechanical, physiological and behavioural, why practice of walking itself is critical to improving performance. Walking requires multiple levels of neural control to support the body against gravity and propel it forward. This necessitates control of many joints and coodination of multiple muscles, both mono- and biarticular. At the same time the nervous system must exercise active control to balance the moving body as well as adapt the walking pattern to the environmental and social demands. Although sensory input does not appear to be essential for the generation of a rhythmic walking pattern, speed and coordination are reduced in the absence of peripheral input. To a large extent, the ease with which we walk can be attributed to intrinsic spinal circuits that take care of the details of the complex coordination of

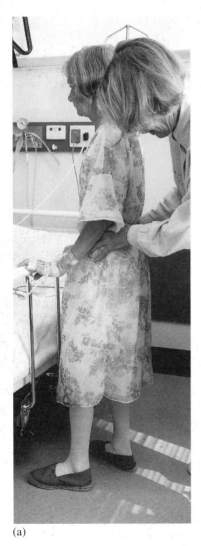

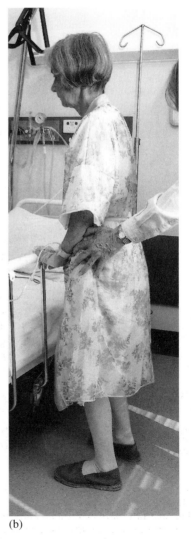

(a)   (b)

Fig. 5.16 This woman with L hemiplegia practises walking sideways. (*a*) Note she steps forward with her L leg rather than holding her hip extended while abducting it. She is successful on her next attempt

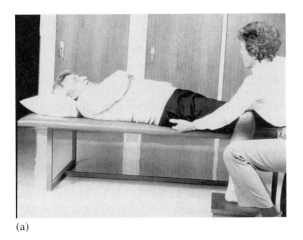

(a)

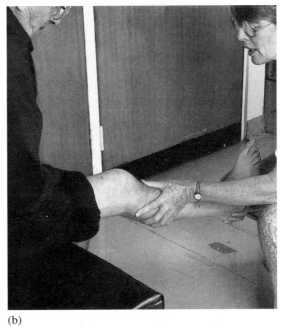

(b)

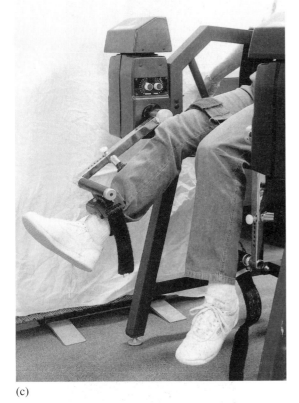

(c)

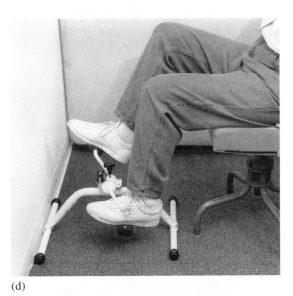

(d)

Fig. 5.17 (*a*) Getting the idea of eliciting activity in the hip extensor muscles by pushing down through the foot. (*b*) The therapist applies a flexor torque at the hip and knee to enable practise of extension (shortening contraction) and flexion (lengthening contraction) of the knee in the range required in the stance phase of walking. Note, force must be constant and the shank kept stable for the quadriceps to be able to function in both modes. (*c*) Exercising on an ioskinetic dynamometer. (*d*) This individual is able to exercise unsupervised on a pedal machine. The foot/feet can be bandaged on to the pedal/s if necessary

muscle contraction needed to generate rhythmic stepping of the legs (Gordon 1991). Animal research has demonstrated the existence of spinal circuits capable of generating sustained rhythmic outputs without input from either supraspinal structures or sensory receptors (Brown 1914; Grillner and Shik 1973). Spinal cat, for example, can produce stepping movements on a moving treadmill with external support. Although spinal circuits or central pattern generators have not been shown to exist in man, it seems likely that they, or a similar mechanism, may be capable of generating a rhythmic pattern and thus simplifying the control of walking.

This concept may help to provide a physiological reason for the reported effectiveness of treadmill walking in individuals with UMN lesions. A treadmill (with supportive harness if necessary) provides an opportunity to practise under challenging and interesting conditions. The moving belt maximizes the extent of hip extension and ankle dorsiflexion, thereby setting up two of the necessary conditions for the swing phase of that leg. Another possible mechanism underlying effectiveness may be the fact that loading of the lower limbs during weight-bearing in a harness can take place without fear of the leg collapsing and provoking a fall. A harness enables patients to bear weight and walk.

The opportunity for weight-bearing seems critical for promoting muscle function in the lower limbs. In animal experiments in which rat's back

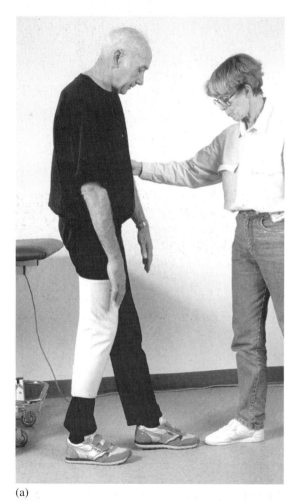 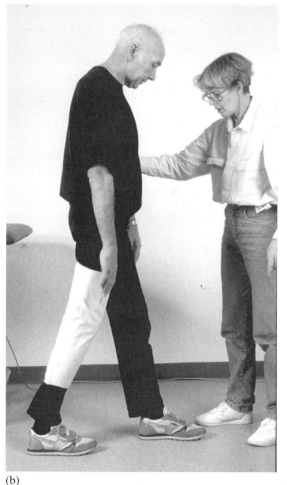

(a)   (b)

Fig. 5.18 This man was unable to generate sufficient lower limb extensor force through his R leg for support. The calico splint constrains his knee and he is now able to load the leg and step forward and back with the L leg. Note in (*a*) he did not advance his body mass forward but in (*b*) he was able to achieve this

legs are suspended (i.e., the animal is deprived of weight-bearing and loading the limb), it has been observed that the animal ceases to move the suspended limbs. Examination of gastrocnemius muscle revealed evidence of muscle atrophy within seven days although gastrocnemius was free to contract (Musacchia *et al.* 1980). This finding supports the critical importance of enabling such weight-bearing.

Although the individual has to be given the opportunity to walk early after a brain lesion, it is usually necessary to have an additional programme of specific exercises designed to increase strength and control in the muscle groups required to generate force at particular stages in the gait cycle and to maintain appropriate segmental alignment for balance. Timing relationships between segmental rotations is critical to effective and efficient gait and can only be learned through practice of the action itself or of similar actions. Walking practice is also critical to improve the exchange between kinetic and potential energy (Olney *et al.* 1988). Walking sideways simplifies the number of joint rotations to be controlled (Fig. 5.16) and is useful when the patient has limited muscle activity.

Weight-bearing and strengthening exercises

Emphasis in exercise is on the extensor muscles of hip, knee and ankle, since these muscles provide the basic support, balance and propulsive functions. Exercises may have to be practised to elicit contraction of a muscle or to strengthen a weak muscle group (Figs. 5.17*a–d*). The position in which muscles are activated may not be of any consequence in the early stage of training, since such exercises are designed to get weak or inactive muscles to twitch and generate force. However, for muscles to be able to both generate and time the necessary muscle force in the synergy required for walking or stair walking, it is clear that closed chain (foot on support surface) actions must be practised repetitively, frequently and under different environmental and speed conditions.

Practising loading the leg

In the initial stages, if the patient cannot support the body mass with hips and knees extended, standing and stepping can still be practised. A

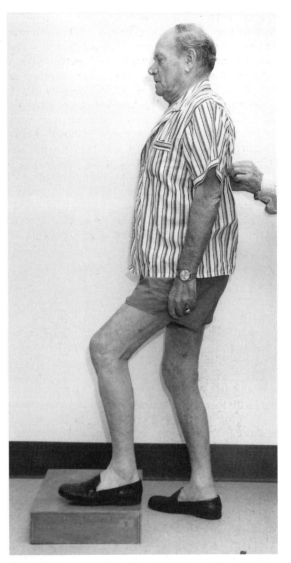

Fig. 5.19 Practice of loading the R leg while placing the L leg on and off the step

simple calico splint prevents the knee from collapsing and enables the individual to get the idea of loading the limb and moving the body mass forward over the stance foot (Fig. 5.18) (by extending at the stance hip and dorsiflexing at the ankle). The splint enables practice of stepping forward (Fig. 5.18*b*) or up on to a step with the opposite leg similar to the exercise in Fig 5.19. External constraint using tape prevents the knee from hyperextending during exercises and for walking (Fig. 5.20*a,b,c*).

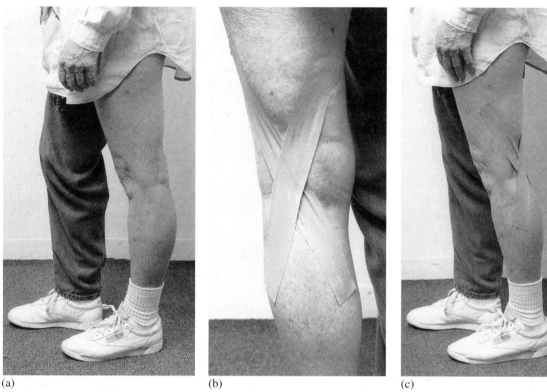

(a)   (b)   (c)

Fig. 5.20 (*a*) The knee hyperextends when lower limb extensors are unable to generate sufficient force to load the limb. Note plantarflexion at the ankle. (*b*) Tape at back of knee. (*c*) Note the improved alignment of lower limb segments with muscles at an appropriate length for function

Since it appears that stance sets up the conditions for swing, in the initial stages of practice the individual is trained to step off with the stronger and more easily controlled leg, thus allowing the first step with the weaker leg to be executed under more optimal conditions. It should be noted that the therapist can interfere with progression forward by standing too close to the patient (Fig. 5.21) or by holding the person back which can prevent the continuous displacement of the body forward in the plane of progression.

Stepping up and down exercises

Exercises designed to address specific impairments (difficulty activating a muscle, activating sufficient motor units to generate necessary force, timing muscle activity, sustaining a muscle contraction/force) will usually have to be practised. Strength and control for support, propulsion and balance over a fixed foot can be practised by step up and down exercises (Fig. 5.22) These exercises require the ability to generate concentric force with the lower limb extensors while keeping the body mass over the foot (dorsiflexion at the ankle), then the ability to switch from a concentric to an eccentric mode of contraction to lower the body mass. Stepping up and down in different directions strengthens different synergic relationships between hip, knee and ankle extensors and hip abductors/adductors to train the flexibility in muscle activity patterns needed in daily life. For example, stepping up and down in the frontal plane produces a greater knee extensor moment than stepping in the sagittal plane (Shepherd *et al.* 1996). Stepping in the frontal plane also requires adductor and abductor muscle force. Practice of walking sideways and backwards similarly involves different patterns of muscle activation and also trains flexible walking performance.

Calf muscle exercises

It appears that the contribution of the plantar-flexors to progression forward and to balance in walking is little understood by some clinicians

angular position of the foot, shank and thigh are in an ideal alignment to push the body upward and forward. Standing on a block, the individual can practise lowering the heels (which stretches the calf muscles) and raising the heels to the planti-grade position. This strengthens the calf muscles from their fully extended length to mid-length, the length at which force is produced at the end of stance (Fig. 5.23). This exercise and other similar exercises ensure optimal muscle length as well as training the muscles to generate force in the range from 8–10° dorsiflexion to 16–19° plantarflexion necessary for push-off (Winter 1983). The exercise should probably be practised routinely by anyone in whom shortness and stiffness due to immobility and disuse can be predicted. At the very least, prevention of this peripheral mechanical compo-nent of hypertonus is possible, and it is also likely that optimal muscle length enables the individual to improve performance.

Walking practice

There appears to be some confusion in the clinic with regard to walking practice. At one end of the spectrum there are reports of therapists being reluctant to allow patients to practise walking on their own in case they should practise an abnormal synergy. At the other end, patients are supplied with a quadripod stick (four-point cane), an orthosis and possibly a leg splint and are 'walked' by the therapist or nurse, with little regard for the fact that there may be negligible muscle activity in the limb. In between the two extremes of current clinical practice is the training of walking by a therapist who understands the biomechanics and muscle activity of walking and can apply exercise and learning strategies.

Treadmill walking

As long ago as 1982, we proposed treadmill walking as a means of providing walking training (Carr and Shepherd 1982, 1987), based on findings from investigations of the spinal cat (Barbeau and Rossignol 1967; Rossignol *et al.* 1986). Finch and Barbeau (1985) also supported this dynamic approach to gait training in humans. Their proposal was to walk the patient on a treadmill with a percentage of body weight supported (BWS) by an overhead harness in order to reduce the amount of active support through the weak limb/s. Subse-quently, Finch and colleagues (1991) examined EMG data from one leg, foot switch signals and

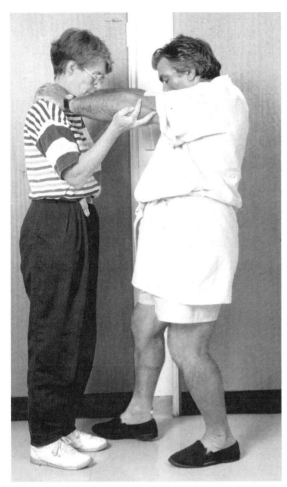

Fig. 5.21 By standing too close, the therapist is preventing the patient from advancing his body mass forward when stepping

when one considers both the prevalence of calf muscle contracture and frequently an absence of training. There appears to be a reluctance to strengthen calf muscles although there is no evidence to support this reluctance (Olney *et al.* 1988). Their dominant role in push-off and in energy generation (Winter 1989), as well as their contribution to walking velocity (Olney *et al.* 1986), make it critical that plantarflexors are exercised. It is interesting to note that Marks as long ago as 1953, following a biomechanical analysis of walking in subjects following stroke, recommended the inclusion of training gastroc-nemius for a forceful push-off.

Every attempt should be made to elicit concen-tric plantarflexor activity during push-off when the

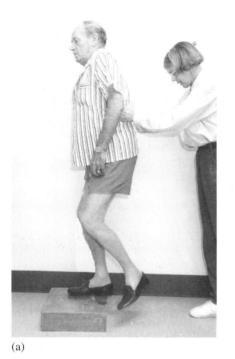
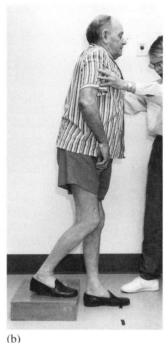
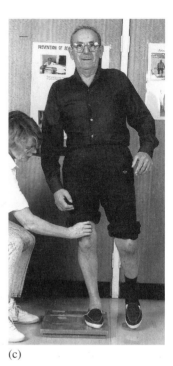

(a)   (b)   (c)

Fig. 5.22 Stepping exercises. Starting with the foot of the affected leg on a small step (*a*) stepping up and down (extending and flexing R hip, knee and ankle). (*b*) Stepping down forwards. (*c*) Lateral stepping exercises. Note he is raising and lowering body mass repetitively without putting his foot on the step

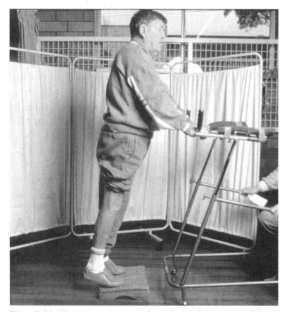

Fig. 5.23 Calf muscle exercise. Lowering the heels (lengthening contraction of plantarflexors) then rasising them to plantigrade (shortening contraction) to train specifically the muscles in the range and mode for push-off. Note: hips should remain extended

joint rotations as healthy subjects walked on a treadmill while the percentage of BWS was varied. The adaptations to BWS were few and did not produce an abnormal gait. (For additional information see Further Reading.)

Treadmill walking (Fig. 5.24) is increasingly being shown to be an effective means of promoting rhythmical vigorous walking and appears a useful method of task-related training. Recent results investigating the effectiveness of treadmill walking training with and without BWS, in chronic and acute individuals following stroke, are very encouraging (e.g., Waagfjord *et al.* 1990; Richards *et al.* 1993; Hesse *et al.* 1994a, 1995a).

In one study, nine stroke patients (mean time since stroke: 4 months), who could not walk at all or who required extensive support, and who had been treated by an experienced physiotherapist for at least 3 weeks prior to entering the study (with Bobath therapy), participated in a treadmill training study supported by a body harness (Hesse *et al.* 1994a). Mean BWS was 31% initially and was decreased as soon as possible to enable full loading of the lower limbs. The criterion used for the amount of BWS was the

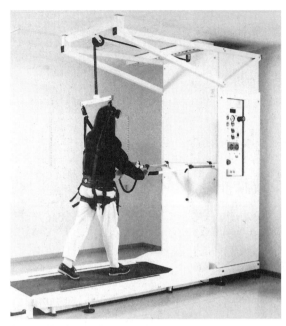

Fig. 5.24 Treadmill walking with supportive harness (Courtesy of TR Equipment, S-57322 Tranag, Sweden)

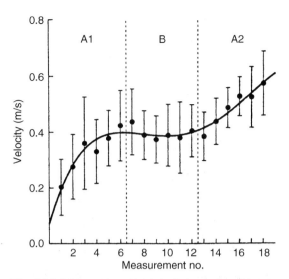

Fig. 5.25 Mean and standard deviations of walking velocity over time. Walking velocity increased during treadmill training (A1 and A2) but did not increase during conventional therapy (B: Bobath). (From Hesse, S., Bertelt, C., Jahnke, M.T. *et al.* (1995) Treadmill training with partial body weight support compared with physiotherapy in nonambulatory hemiparetic patients. *Stroke*, **26**, 976–981, with permission)

individual's ability to support the remaining load on the affected leg during the single support phase. At the end of the study (25 treadmill sessions), all but one individual could walk by themselves and gait velocity was approximately three times faster. Other motor functions for the legs and trunk, measured on the Rivermead Motor Assessment (Lincoln and Leadbitter 1979), improved steadily during the study.

In a subsequent A–B–A study design – 30 minutes of treadmill walking (phase A); 45 minutes of conventional physiotherapy based on Bobath (phase B); followed by another 30 minute period of treadmill training (phase A) – treadmill training was found to be significantly more effective than conventional physiotherapy in terms of walking speed (Hesse et al. 1995a). At the end of the study, all seven subjects could walk independently. It is interesting to note that improvement in walking speed occurred only in the treadmill phases and that, during the physiotherapy phase, the score on walking velocity remained static (Fig. 5.25). Hesse and colleagues (1997) have also investigated the effect of varying BWS (full body weight to 60% BWS) on gait parameters in stroke subjects using video analysis and EMG. The reduction in muscle activity in

antigravity muscles suggests that BWS of 30% is optimal and should not be exceeded.

The results of the two training studies seem to indicate the importance of task-related training, and providing the opportunity for walking under conditions which 'force' the action and increasing intensity of practice. Hesse and colleagues (1994b) noted that Bobath therapists spend a relatively long period in 'preparatory' activities, walk the patient in a slow controlled manner and are reluctant to encourage patients to walk on their own for fear of stereotyped mass synergies, as suggested and described by Davies (1985) and Bobath (1990). Chapters in two recent textbooks on neurological physiotherapy, one from North America and one from Europe, confirm that this view is commonly held by physiotherapists (Ryerson 1995; Carter and Edwards 1996).

Environmental modification

The environment can be modified in other ways to facilitate a particular outcome and prevent unwanted (i.e., non-functional) adaptations from becoming habitual. For example, if an individual has difficulty flexing the hip and knee to shorten the leg and swing it forward, walking can be practised over an obstacle course, with obstacles placed so the individual has to step over them. If an individual walks with a wide base, practice can be encouraged ('forced') with a narrower base by walking within a boundary outlined on the floor. Walking under obstacles provides a challenge since this imposes the need for controlled flexion of the lower limbs (by eccentric activity of extensors) followed by extension. Such modifications also assist by giving feedback about error. Their main benefit, however, is probably in forcing or driving the required action (Chapter 1).

Practice of ascending and descending stairs is necessary to both increase strength and familiarity with this and other similar activities such as stepping up a curb. It has been reported that more falls occur on stairs than in level walking, indicating the importance of training this activity.

Cueing

The significance of *visual cues* during walking training in individuals with Parkinson's disease is discussed in Chapter 13. Rhythmical *auditory (musical) cuing* versus noncuing during walking trials in stroke subjects has been found to increase the time spent on the affected stance leg and to increase rhythmicity (Thaut *et al.* 1993). Interestingly, rhythmic cuing not only modified the amplitude and timing of muscle activation of the gastrocnemius with a high degree of task specificity in the affected leg, but also decreased the amplitude of muscle activity on the intact side indicating 'cooperation' between both lower limbs. Variability in EMG amplitude also decreased, suggesting an improvement in motor unit recruitment. It would be interesting to explore whether the improved performance would carry over into other environments.

Walking velocity

On average, 'normal' walking speed is approximately 1.2 m/sec (Olney *et al.* 1986). Not surprisingly, walking velocities have been found to vary in able-bodied subjects depending on location (Finley and Cody 1970; Gifford *et al.* 1977) and intention (strolling for pleasure vs hurrying to work), with women reaching the same velocity as men by shortening their steps and increasing cadence (Eke-Okoro and Sandlund 1984). The literature suggests that an average walking velocity of 1.1–1.5 m/sec is probably fast enough to be functional as a pedestrian in different environmen-

tal and social contexts. Walking velocities required to cross a street safely using pedestrian lights vary considerably (Robinett and Vondran 1988) depending on many factors, including whether in rural or urban settings. Walking speeds compatible with stepping on or off a moving footway, crossing a street with and without pedestrian lights, getting in or out of a lift, walking up and down a curb all need to be practised to enable the individual to walk in the community. Lerner-Frankiel and colleagues (1986) found that actual distances required for independence in an urban area were far greater than those typically used as criteria by physiotherapists for assessing independence in community ambulation. Their findings also suggest that independent community ambulation requires a near 'normal' walking speed and ability to negotiate curbs.

Walking velocity as an indicator of improved performance

It is an interesting observation that having patients increase their speed of walking can have the effect of changing a slow, asymmetrical and relatively ineffective walking pattern into more vigorous and effective walking.

There is an ongoing discussion in the literature about what gait parameters are the most functionally meaningful for measuring outcome. In a large number of gait studies on able-bodied subjects, significant relationships have been found between speed and gait parameters (see Wagenaar and Beek 1992) This raises the question of whether gait speed is a valid measure for assessing outcome in individuals with movement dysfunction, following stroke, for example. One problem in treatment studies is the fact that kinetic data and symmetry ratios depend on gait velocity (Andriacchi *et al.* 1977; Brandstater *et al.* 1983) and walking speed tends to increase with recovery (e.g., Wade *et al.* 1987).

In an attempt to test the hypothesis that walking speed influences the pattern of gait in stroke subjects and is, therefore, a useful variable for measuring outcome, Wagenaar and Beek (1992) had a group of healthy subjects and a group of stroke subjects walk at a wide range of different velocities on a treadmill and showed that stride length and stride frequency changed with walking speed for individuals following stroke in a similar way to healthy subjects.

Richards and colleagues' (1991) findings also support the view that gait velocity reflects both functional and physiological changes in individuals following stroke. Improvements in gait velocity, however, did not correlate with the Fugl-Meyer scale (Fugl-Meyer *et al.* 1975), Barthel's ambulation scale (Mahoney and Barthel 1965) or the Berg balance test (Berg *et al.* 1989) scores, with speeds greater than about 0.3 m/sec.

At our present level of understanding, these results suggest that walking speed is an important independent variable to use as a basis for the evaluation of gait outcome; i.e., increased speed appears to bear a positive relationship to improvement in functional walking. Since distance as well as walking speed is important for independent mobility outside the home, the addition of distance and endurance may be particularly useful in determining effectiveness of intervention. Hesse and colleagues (1994b) have used walking endurance (self-adopted speed: limit 600 m) and stair climbing (self-adopted speed with or without hand rails: limit 90 stairs of 16 cm each) to measure outcome.

These findings may present a dilemma for those physiotherapists who believe that objective measures, such as walking velocity and stride length, are not sensitive enough to measure the qualitative changes they perceive in the clinic. An interesting series of studies highlights the dilemma when physiotherapy aims related to the quality of movement, i.e., what are believed by therapists to be important in the movement, are achieved but without a significant improvement in functional measures (Hesse *et al.* 1994b; Jahnke *et al.* 1995). A group of stroke patients, who were already walking independently, participated in a 4 week rehabilitation programme based on the Bobath (NDT) concept which concentrated on 'normalizing' tone and on symmetry of gait but did not emphasize functional ability such as increasing walking speed. At the end of the study Hesse and colleagues (1993) found no positive correlations between changes in symmetry and spontaneous walking speed. It is very likely, however, that rather than having the patient practise symmetrical stepping, having them increase speed may have increased both symmetry *and* walking speed.

An increase in velocity in natural walking has been found to be associated with an improved walking pattern, i.e., the patient's walking in terms of critical biomechanical features improves. For example, with an increase in velocity, Olney and colleagues (1991) found a tendency toward greater hip extension at the end of stance and a larger burst of work by the hip flexors at the initiation of swing, both critical components of an effective walking pattern. In a subsequent study, the greater the angle of hip extension in late stance, the greater was the speed of walking and a strong relationship existed between walking speed and maximum hip flexion moment (Olney *et al.* 1994). These findings support the suggestion that the hip muscles play a major role in balancing the upper body segment (Winter 1987). Bohannon (1987) has also reported a positive relationship between speed of walking and strength of the affected lower limb in stroke patients.

Functional electrical stimulation (FES)

Hesse and colleagues (1995b) combined FES with treadmill training with BWS for a group of severely affected non-ambulatory chronic stroke patients. FES to the lower extremity, trunk and upper extremity muscles was modified during the study according to the individual's needs and included stimulation of ankle dorsiflexors, hamstrings, quadriceps, gluteus medius and minimus in the lower limb. A single-case A–B–A design was used: 15 treadmill/FES sessions (A phase), 15 days of Bobath (NDT) physiotherapy (B phase), followed by 15 sessions of treadmill/FES (A phase). Average time since stroke was 25 weeks (range 11 weeks to 6 years). Although 'spontaneous' recovery cannot be controlled for in this study, it is generally considered that the major recovery occurs in the first 3 months following stroke (Kelly-Hayes 1990) and the distinction between outcomes for the three phases was quite unequivocal.

The seven subjects who participated in the study (patient characteristics are reported) showed a marked increase in stride length, cadence and velocity during the first treadmill/FES phase. The variables remained stable or decreased during phase B and increased again in the final treadmill/FES phase. At the end of the study, all patients could walk independently with three needing help on stairs and three needing verbal assistance. Other reports of gait training in individuals following stroke using FES to improve gait are inconclusive.

Feedback

Feedback (see Chapter 2), variously described as biofeedback, augmented feedback or sensory feedback, utilizing devices including pressure-sensitive footpads, EMG, videotape and joint angle monitors has been used in gait training. The effectiveness of feedback may well depend on the physiotherapist's ability to analyse the disability and organize training in a task-related way.

EMG biofeedback has been used to assist individuals to activate weak or paralysed muscles or to reduce unnecessary muscle activity. There is little evidence of carryover into improved functional performance. However, in some instances feedback about muscle activity has been given out of context, i.e., unrelated to the action of walking, despite the evidence of the superiority of learning a movement component within a task-related context (e.g., Mulder *et al.* 1986).

In an attempt to overcome some of these shortcomings, a computer-assisted feedback system, developed by Colborne and colleagues (1993), was used in a study designed to compare the effectiveness of (1) EMG feedback from soleus, (2) sagittal plane ankle joint angular feedback with electrogoniometers of the affected leg during walking practice and (3) conventional physiotherapy. A three-period crossover design in which subjects received all three treatments was used. Physiotherapy was either the first or the last treatment. Feedback treatment from both electrogoniometers and EMG resulted in significant increases in stride length and walking velocity. Overall, conventional physiotherapy treatment produced no significant results, although changes in function were in the same direction. Knee and ankle joint kinematics changed as a result of all three treatments. There were increases in knee flexion during swing, in knee flexion at foot contact and in ankle range of motion. Interestingly, electrogoniometric feedback resulted in the greatest increase in knee joint flexion and ankle range on the affected side, probably reflecting the specificity of the feedback. Similar to the signal provided by a pressure-sensitive footpad, it is unclear whether subjects had time to use the feedback information on the actual stride or whether feedback was used in organizing a subsequent stride.

Aids and orthoses

Walking aids (parallel bars, walking frame, three/four point stick – tripod/quadripod – an assistant's arm) have a number of predictable drawbacks and all rely on upper limb support. Although all aids tend to impose some mechanical constraint, a simple walking stick interferes least with balance and walking yet provides some assistance.

Orthoses The International Society for Prosthetics and Orthotics has defined an orthosis as an externally applied device used to modify structural and functional characteristics of the neuromuscular system. A major factor in determining the use of an orthosis is the evaluation from a mechanical and muscular perspective, since constraint of any joint necessitates mechanical adaptation in both the ipsilateral and contralateral limbs and may reduce the need for muscles to contract at appropriate times and with appropriate intensity throughout the gait cycle. Although orthoses impose an external constraint, they also have the capacity to affect neural networks (Jenkins and Merzenich 1987).

The issue of whether or not some form of orthosis enables independent walking to be practised is controversial. It is possible that there may be an incongruity between the goals of training and the design of some orthoses. For example, an orthosis designed to aid ankle dorsiflexion may be less effective in helping an individual produce an effective and efficient walking pattern than exercises and walking training designed to lengthen shortened calf muscles and train control of the lower limb as it moves over the fixed foot. The effect of an orthosis on walking can be measured in terms of physiological parameters such as heart rate (e.g., Mossberg *et al.* 1990), oxygen consumption (Hirschberg and Ralston 1965), or biomechanical variables (Balmaseda *et al.* 1988). Physiotherapists need to become familiar with such measures so as to be able to prescribe an orthosis (or walking aid) or not, based on some knowledge of the potential mechanical and physiological effects.

Balmaseda and colleagues (1988) studied a group of healthy subjects who wore either a narrow or wide semi-rigid plastic ankle-foot orthosis (AFO) set in neutral position. When walking with the AFO there was a decrease in the duration of stance of the ipsilateral leg, centre of pressure was shifted to a more lateral position throughout stance, probably in an attempt to increase stability by inverting the foot, and the point of impact at heel contact was more posterior. This alignment may tend to hyperextend the knee in individuals with poor control over knee extensors. Probably due to relative rigidity of the AFO, there was an increase in the magnitude of vertical force at the end of push-off, since more force was required to propel the body forward.

More recently, hinges have been incorporated into the AFO to allow dorsiflexion and/or plantarflexion. The effect of this modification needs to be studied to establish the imposed mechanical and muscular adaptations in both the ipsilateral and contralateral legs. The use of 'smart' orthoses to enable walking practice and to 'force' a segmental alignment appropriate for the activation of certain critical muscle groups remains for future development (Shepherd (1997).

In conclusion, if physiotherapists are to be part of neurological rehabilitation in the twenty-first century, it is time for a paradigm shift to a more scientifically based walking rehabilitation. The authors have been proposing for over a decade training guidelines designed to increase lower limb muscle strength and optimize walking performance in neurological patients. We agree with Olney that such treatment guidelines must be enunciated if information from research findings is to be transferred to improve clinical practise, which is one of the major goals of biomechanical research (Olney *et al.* 1988). We would add that such guidelines, having been enunciated, need to be implemented in order to improve rehabilitation outcomes.

References

Akeson, W.H., Woo, S.L-Y., Amiel, D. *et al.* (1973) The connective tissue response to immobility: biomechanical changes in periarticular connective tissue of the immobilized rabbit knee. *Clinical Orthopaedics and Related Research*, **93**, 356–362.

Andriacchi, T.P., Andersson, G.B.J., Fermier, R.W. *et al.* (1980) A study of lower-limb mechanics during stair-climbing. *Journal of Bone and Joint Surgery*, **62A**, 749–757.

Andriacchi, T.P., Ogle, J.A. and Galante, J.O. (1977) Walking speed as basis for normal and abnormal gait measurements. *Journal of Biomechanics*, **10**, 261–268.

Balmaseda, M.T., Koozekanani, S.H., Fatehi, M.T. *et al.* (1988) Ground reaction forces, center of pressure, and duration of stance with and without an ankle-foot orthosis. *Archives of Physical Medicine and Rehabilitation*, **69**, 1009–1012.

Barbeau, H. and Rossignol, S. (1967) Recovery of locomotion after chronic spinalization in the adult cat. *Brain Research*, **412**, 84–95.

Basmajian, J.V., Kukulka, C.G., Narayan, M.G. *et al.* (1975) Biofeedback treatment of foot-drop after stroke compared with standard rehabilitation technique: effects on voluntary control and strength. *Archives of Physical Medicine and Rehabilitation*, **56**, 231–236.

Berg, K., Wood-Dauphinee, S., Williams, J.I. *et al.* (1989) Measuring balance in the elderly: preliminary development of an instrument. *Physiotherapy Canada*, **41**, 304–311.

Berger, W., Horstmann, G. and Dietz, V. (1984) Tension development and muscle activation in the leg during gait in spastic hemiparesis: independence of muscle hypertonia and exaggerated stretch reflexes. *Journal of Neurology, Neurosurgery, and Psychiatry*, **47**, 1029–1033.

Bernstein, N. (1967) *Coordination and Regulation of Movement*, Pergamon, New York.

Bobath, B. (1990) *Adult Hemiplegia Evaluation and Treatment*, 3rd edn. Butterworth Heinemann, Oxford.

Bogardh, E. and Richards, C.L. (1981) Gait analysis and relearning of gait control in hemiplegic patients. *Physiotherapy Canada*, **33**, 223–230.

Bohannon, R.W. (1987) Gait performance of hemiparetic stroke patients: selected variables. *Archives of Physical Medicine and Rehabilitation*, **68**, 777–781.

Bortz, W.M. (1982) Disuse and aging. *Journal of the American Medical Association*, **248**, 1203–1208.

Brandstater, M.E., de Bruin, H., Gowland, C. *et al.* (1983) Hemiplegic gait: analysis of temporal variables. *Archives of Physical Medicine and Rehabilitation*, **64**, 583–587.

Brown, T.G. (1914) On the nature of the fundamental activity of the nervous centres; together with an analysis of the conditioning of rhythmic activity in progression, and a theory of the evolution of function in the nervous system. *Journal of Physiology, London*, **48**, 18–46.

Burke, D. (1988) Spasticity as an adaptation to pyramidal tract injury. In *Advances in Neurology, 47: Functional Recovery in Neurological Disease* (ed. S.G. Waxman), Raven Press, New York, pp. 401–423.

Carlsoo, S., Dahllof, A. and Holm, J. (1974) Kinetic analysis of gait in patients with hemiparesis and in patients with intermittent claudication. *Scandinavian Journal of Rehabilitation Medicine*, **6**, 166–179.

Carr, J.H. and Shepherd, R.B. (1982) *A Motor Relearning Programme for Stroke*, Butterworth Heinemann, Oxford, pp. 138.

Carr, J.H. and Shepherd, R.B. (1987) *A Motor Relearning Programme for Stroke*, 2nd edn, Butterworth Heinemann, Oxford, pp. 125–148.

Carr, J., Shepherd, R.B., Nordholm, L. *et al.* (1985) A motor assessment scale for stroke. *Physical Therapy*, **65**, 175–180.

Carter, P. and Edwards, S. (1996) General principles of treatment. In *Neurological Physiotherapy: A Problem-Solving Approach* (ed. S. Edwards), Churchill Livingstone, London, pp.87–113.

Colborne, G.R., Olney, S.J. and Griffin, M.P. (1993) Feedback of ankle joint angle and soleus electromyography in the rehabilitation of hemiplegic gait. *Archives of Physical Medicine and Rehabilitation*, **74**, 1100–1106.

Crosbie, J., Vachalathiti, R. and Smith, R. (1997a) Age, gender and speed effects on spinal kinematics during walking. *Gait and Posture*, **5**, 13–20.

Crosbie, J. and Vachalathiti, R. (1997) Synchrony of pelvic and hip joint motion during walking. *Gait and Posture*, **5**, 6–12.

Cunningham, D.A., Rechnitzer, P.A., Pearce, M.E. *et al.* (1982) Determinants of self-selected walking pace across ages 19 to 66. *Journal of Gerontology*, **37**, 560.

Davies, P.M. (1985) *Steps to Follow. A Guide to the Treatment of Adult Hemiplegia*, Springer-Verlag, Berlin.

Dietz, V. and Berger, W. (1983) Normal and impaired regulation of muscle stiffness in gait: a new hypothesis about muscle hypertonia. *Experimental Neurology*, **7**, 680–687.

Eberhart, H.D., Inman, V.T. and Bresler, B. (1965) The principal elements in human locomotion. In *Human Limbs and their Substitutes* (eds P.F. Klopstag and D.P. Wilson), McGraw-Hill, New York, pp. 437–471.

Eke-Okoro, S.T. and Sandlund, B. (1984) The effects of load, shoes, sex and direction on the gait characteristics of street pedestrians. *Journal of Human Movement Studies*, **10**, 107–114.

Finch, L. and Barbeau, H. (1985) Influences of partial weight-bearing on normal human gait: the development of a gait retraining strategy. *Canadian Journal of Neurological Science*, **12**, 183.

Finch, L., Barbeau, H. and Arsenault, B. (1991) Influence of body weight support on normal human gait: development of a gait retraining strategy. *Physical Therapy*, **71**, 842–856.

Finley, F.R. and Cody, K.A. (1970) Locomotive characteristics of urban pedestrians. *Archives of Physical Medicine and Rehabilitation*, **51**, 423–426.

Forssberg, H. (1982) Spinal locomotor functions and descending control. In *Brain Stem Control of Spinal Mechanisms* (eds B. Sjolund and A. Bjorklund) Elsevier Biomedical Press, New York.

Fugl-Meyer, A.R., Jaaskd, L., Leyman, I. *et al.* (1975) The post-stroke hemiplegic patient. A method for evaluation of physical performance. *Scandinavian Journal of Rehabilitation Medicine*, **7**, 13–31.

Gifford, R., Ward, J. and Dahms, W. (1977) Pedestrian velocities: a multivariate study of social and environmental effects. *Journal of Human Movement Studies*, **3**, 66–68.

Gordon, J. (1991) Spinal mechanisms of motor coordination. In *Principles of Neural Science*, 3rd edn (eds E.R. Kandel, J.H. Schwartz and T.M. Jessell), Appleton and Lange, Norwalk, CT, pp.582–595.

Gregoire, L., Veeger, H.E., Huijing, P.A. *et al.* (1984) Role of mono- and biarticular muscles in explosive movements. *International Journal of Sports Medicine*, **5**, 301.

Grieve, D.W. (1968) Gait patterns and the speed of walking. *Biomedical Engineering*, **3**, 119–122.

Grillner, S. (1985) Neurobiological bases of rhythmic motor acts in vertebrates. *Science*, **228**, 143–149.

Grillner, S. and Shik, M.L. (1973) On the descending control of the lumbosacral spinal cord from the 'mesencephalic locomotor region'. *Acta Physiologica Scandinavia*, **87**, 320–333.

Harrison, A. and Kruze, R. (1987) Perturbation of a skilled action II. Normalising the responses of cerebral palsied individuals. *Human Movement Science*, **6**, 133–159.

Hesse, S., Bertelt, C., Jahnke, M.T. *et al.* (1995a) Treadmill training with partial body weight support compared with physiotherapy in nonambulatory hemiparetic patients. *Stroke*, **26**, 976–981.

Hesse, S., Bertelt, C., Schaffrin, A. *et al.* (1994a) Restoration of gait in nonambulatory hemiparetic patients by treadmill training with partial body-weight support. *Archives of Physical Medicine and Rehabilitation*, **75**, 1087–1093.

Hesse, S., Helm, B., Krajnik, J. *et al.* (1997) Treadmill training with partial body weight support: influence of body weight release on the gait of hemiparetic patients. *Journal of Neurological Rehabilitation*, **11**, 15–26.

Hesse, S.A., Jahnke, M.T., Bertelt, C.M. *et al.* (1994b) Gait outcome in ambulatory hemiparetic patients after a 4-week comprehensive rehabilitation program and prognostic factors. *Stroke*, **25**, 1999–2004.

Hesse, S.A., Jahnke, M.T., Schreiner, C. *et al.* (1993) Gait symmetry and functional walking performance in hemiparetic patients prior to and after a 4-week rehabilitation programme. *Gait and Posture*, **1**, 166–171.

Hesse, S., Malezic, M., Schaffrin, A. *et al.* (1995b) Restoration of gait by combined treadmill training and multichannel electrical stimulation in non-ambulatory hemiparetic patients. *Scandinavian Journal of Rehabilitation Medicine*, **27**, 199–204.

Hirschberg, G.G. and Ralston, H.J. (1965) Energy cost of stair-climbing in normal and hemiplegic subjects. *American Journal of Physical Medicine*, **44**, 165–168.

Imms, F.J. and Edholdm, O.G. (1981) Studies of gait mobility in the elderly. *Age and Ageing*, **10**, 147–156.

Inman, V.T., Ralston, H.J. and Todd, F. (1981) *Human Walking*, Williams and Wilkins, Baltimore, MD.

Jahnke, M.T., Hesse, S., Schreiner, C. *et al.* (1995) Dependences of ground reaction force parameters on habitual walking speed in hemiparetic subjects. *Gait and Posture*, **3**, 3–12.

James, B. and Parker, A.W. (1989) Electromyography of stair locomotion in elderly men and women. *Electromyography Clinical Neurophysiology*, **29**, 161–168.

Jenkins, W.M. and Merzenich, M.M. (1987) Reorganization of neocortical representations after brain injury: a neurophysiological model of the basis of recovery from stroke. In *Progress in Brain Research* (eds F.J. Seil, E. Herbert and B.M. Carlson), Elsevier Science, New Rork, pp. 249–266.

Joseph, J. and Watson, R. (1967) Telemetering electromyography of muscles used in walking up and down stairs. *Journal of Bone and Joint Surgery*, **49B**, 774–780.

Kapandji, I.A. (1970) *The Physiology of the Joints*, vol. 1: *Upper Limb*, Churchill Livingstone, Edinburgh, pp. 146–203.

Kelly-Hayes, M. (1990) Time intervals, survival, and destination three crucial variables in stroke outcome research. *Stroke,* Suppl. 11, **21**, 24–26.

Knutsson, E. (1981) Gait control in hemiparesis. *Scandinavian Journal of Rehabilitation Medicine*, **13**, 101–108.

Latash, M.L. and Anson, J.G. (1996) What are 'normal movements' in atypical populations? *Behavioural and Brain Sciences*, **19**, 55–106.

Lehmann, J.F., Condon, S.M., Price, R. *et al.* (1987) Gait abnormalities in hemiplegia: their correction by ankle-foot orthoses. *Archives of Physical Medicine and Rehabilitation*, **68**, 763–771.

Lerner-Frankiel, M.B., Vargas, S., Brown, M. *et al.* (1986) Functional community ambulation: what are the criteria? *Clinical Management*, **6**, 12–15.

Lincoln, N. and Leadbitter, D. (1979) Assessment of motor function in stroke patients. *Physiotherapy*, **65**, 48–51.

Mahoney, F.D. and Barthel, D.W. (1965) Functional evaluation: the Barthel Index. *Maryland State Medical Journal*, **14**, 61–65.

Malouin, F. (1995) Observational gait analysis. In *Gait Analysis. Theory and Application* (eds R.L. Craik and C.A. Oatis) Mosby, St. Louis, pp. 112–124.

Marks, M. (1953) Gait studies of the hemiplegic patient and their clinical applications. *Archives of Physical Medicine and Rehabilitation*, **34**, 9–25.

Mossberg, K.A., Linton, K.A. and Friske, K. (1990) Ankle-foot orthoses: effect on energy expenditure of gait in spastic diplegic children. *Archives of Physical Medicine and Rehabilitation*, **71**, 490–494.

Mulder, T., Hulstijn, W. and Van der Meer, J. (1986) EMG feedback and the restoration of motor control. *American Journal of Physical Medicine*, **65**, 173–188.

Murray, M.P., Drought, A.B. and Kory, R.C. (1964) Walking patterns of normal men. *Journal of Bone and Joint Surgery*, **46A**, 335–360.

Murray, M.P., Kory, R.C. and Clarkson, B.H. (1969) Walking patterns in healthy old men. *Journal of Gerontology*, **24**, 169–178.

Murray, M.P., Kory, R.C. and Sepic, S.B. (1970) Walking patterns of normal women. *Archives of Physical Medicine and Rehabilitation*, **51**, 637–650.

Musacchia, X.J., Daniel, R., Deavers G.A. *et al.* (1980) A model for hypokinesia: effects on muscle atrophy in the rat. *American Physiological Society*, pp. 479–486.

Nigg, B.M., Fisher, V. and Ronsky, J.L. (1994) Gait characteristics as a function of age and gender. *Gait and Posture*, **2**, 213–220.

O'Brien, M., Power, K., Sanford, S. *et al.* (1983) Temporal gait patterns in healthy young and elderly females. *Physiotherapy Canada*, **35**, 323–326.

Olney, S.J., Griffin, M.P. and McBride, I.D. (1994) Temporal, kinematic, and kinetic variables related to gait speed in subjects with hemiplegia: a regression approach. *Physical Therapy*, **74**, 872–885.

Olney, S.J., Griffin, M.P., Monga, T.N. *et al.* (1991) Work and power in gait of stroke patients. *Archives of Physical Medicine and Rehabilitation*, **72**, 309–314.

Olney, S.J., Jackson, V.G. and George, S.R. (1988) Gait re-education guidelines for stroke patients with hemiplegia using mechanical energy and power analyses. *Physiotherapy Canada*, **40**, 242–248.

Olney, S.J., Monga, T.N. and Costigan, P.A. (1986) Mechanical energy of walking of stroke patients. *Archives of Physical Medicine and Rehabilitation*, **67**, 92–98.

Patla, A.E. (1991) Understanding the control of human locomotion: a prologue. In *Adaptability of Human Gait* (ed. A.E. Patla), Elsevier Science, Amsterdam, pp. 3–17.

Payton, O.D. and Poland, J.L. (1983) Aging process: implications for clinical practice. *Physical Therapy*, **63**, 41–48.

Pearson, K. (1976) The control of walking. *Scientific American*, **24**, 72–86.

Peat, M., Dubo, H.I.C., Winter, D.A. *et al.* (1976) Electromyographic temporal analysis of gait: hemiplegic locomotion. *Archives of Physical Medicine and Rehabilitation*, **57**, 421–425.

Pollock, M.L., Foster, C., Knapp, D. *et al.* (1987) Effect of age and training on aerobic capacity and body composition of master athletes. *Journal of Applied Physiology*, **62**, 725–731.

Richards, C. and Knutsson, E. (1974) Evaluation of abnormal gait patterns by intermittent-light photography and EMG. *Scandinavian Journal of Rehabilitation Medicine*, Suppl 3, 61–68.

Richards, C.L., Malouin, F., Dumas, F. *et al.* (1991) New rehabilitation strategies for the treatment of spastic gait disorders. In *Adaptability of Human Gait* (ed. A.E. Patla) Elsevier Science, Amsterdam, pp. 387–411.

Richards, C.L., Malouin, F., Wood-Dauphinee, S. *et al.* (1993) Task-specific physical therapy for optimization of gait recovery in acute stroke patients. *Archives of Physical Medicine and Rehabilitation*, **74**, 612–620.

Robinett, C.S. and Vondran, M.A. (1988) Functional ambulation velocity and distance requirements in rural and urban communities. *Physical Therapy*, **68**, 1371–1373.

Rossignol, S., Barbeau, H. and Julien, C. (1986) Locomotion of the adult chronic spinal cat and its modifications by monoaminergic agonists and antagonists. In *Development and Plasticity of the Mammalian Spinal Cord* (eds M. Golberger, M. Gorio and M. Murray) Liviana Editrice Spat, Padua, pp. 323–346.

Ryerson, S.D. (1995) Hemiplegia. In *Neurological Rehabilitation* (ed. D.A. Umphred), 3rd edn, Mosby, St Louis, pp. 681–721.

Saunders, J.B., Inman, V.T. and Eberhart, H.D. (1953) The major determinants in normal and pathological gait. *Journal of Bone and Joint Surgery*, **35A**, 543–558.

Shepherd, R.B. (1997) Optimising motor performance following brain lesions. In *Proceedings of the Annual Scientific Meeting of ISPO, Australia*, Nov., Melbourne.

Shepherd, R.B., Westwood, P. and Agahari, I. (1996) A comparative evaluation of lower limb forces in two variations of the step exercise in able-bodied subjects. In *Proceedings of the First Australasian Biomechanics Conference* (eds. M. Lee, W. Gilleard, P. Sinclair *et al.*), Sydney, pp. 94–95.

Shinno, N. (1971) Analysis of knee function in ascending and descending stairs. *Medicine and Sport*, **6**, 202–207.

Skinner, D.R., Antonelli, D., Perry, J. *et al.* (1985) Functional demands on the stance limb in walking. *Orthopedics*, **8**, 355–361.

Smidt, G.L. (1990) Aging and gait. In *Gait in Rehabilitation* (ed. G.L. Smidt), Churchill Livingstone, New York, pp.185–198.

Smith, A. (1990) The measurement of human motor performance. In *Key Issues in Neurological Physiotherapy* (eds L. Ada and C. Canning), Butterworth Heinemann, Oxford, pp. 51–79.

Sutherland, D.H., Cooper, L. and Daniel, D. (1980) The role of the ankle plantar flexors in normal walking. *Journal of Bone and Joint Surgery*, **62A**, 354–363.

Thaut, M.H., McIntosh, G.C., Prassas, S.G. *et al.* (1993) Effect of rhythmic auditory cuing on temporal stride parameters and EMG patterns in hemiparetic gait of stroke patients. *Journal of Neurological Rehabilitation*, **7**, 9–16.

Thilmann, A.F., Fellows, S.J. and Ross, H.F. (1991) Biomechanical changes at the ankle joint after stroke. *Journal of Neurology, Neurosurgery and Psychiatry*, **54**, 134–139.

Townsend, M.A., Lainhart, S.P. and Shiavi, R. (1978) Variability and biomechanics of synergy patterns of some lower-limb muscles during ascending and descending stairs and level walking. *Medical and Biological Engineering and Computing*, **16**, 681–688.

van Ingen Schenau, G.J. (1989) From rotation to translation: constraints on multijoint movements and the unique action of bi-articular muscles. *Human Movement Science*, **8**, 423–442.

van Vliet, P. (1988) Kinematic analysis of videotape to measure walking following stroke: a case study. *Australian Journal of Physiotherapy*, **34**, 48–51.

Waagfjord, J., Levangle, P.K. and Certo, C.M.E. (1990) Effects of treadmill training on gait in a hemiparetic patient. *Physical Therapy*, **70**, 549–558.

Wade, D.T., Wood, V.A., Heller, A. *et al.* (1987) Walking after stroke. *Scandinavian Journal of Rehabilitation Medicine*, **19**, 25–30.

Wagenaar, R.C. and Beek, W.J. (1992) Hemiplegic gait: a kinematic analysis using walking speed as a basis. *Journal of Biomechanics*, **25**, 1007–1015.

Whittle, M.W. (1991) *Gait Analysis: An Introduction*, Butterworth Heinemann, Oxford.

Winter, D.A. (1978) Energy assessment in pathological gait. *Physiotherapy Canada*, **30**, 183–191.

Winter, D.A. (1980) Overall principle of lower limb support during stance phase of gait. *Journal of Biomechanics*, **13**, 923–927.

Winter, D.A. (1983) Biomechanical motor patterns in normal walking. *Journal of Motor Behaviour*, **15**, 302–330.

Winter, D.A. (1984) Kinematic and kinetic patterns of human gait: variability and compensating effects. *Human Movement Science*, **3**, 51–76.

Winter, D.A. (1985) Concerning the scientific basis for the diagnosis of pathological gait and for rehabilitation protocols. *Physiotherapy Canada*, **37**, 245–252.

Winter, D.A. (1987) *The Biomechanics and Motor Control of Human Gait*, University of Waterloo Press, Waterloo, Ontario.

Winter, D.A. (1989) Coordination of motor tasks in human gait. In *Perspectives on the Coordination of Movement* (ed. S.A. Wallace) North-Holland, New York, pp. 329–363.

Winter, D.A., Patla, A.E., Frank, J.S. *et al.* (1990) Biomechanical walking pattern changes in the fit and healthy elderly. *Physical Therapy*, **70**, 340–347.

Zachazewski, J.E., Riley, P.O. and Krebs, D.E. (1993) Biomechanical analysis of body mass transfer during stair ascent and descent of healthy subjects. *Journal of Rehabilitation Research and Development*, **30**, 412–422.

Further reading

Chan, C.W. and Rudins, A. (1994) Foot biomechanics during walking and running. *Mayo Clinic Proceedings*, **69**, 448–461.

Harburn, K.L., Hill, K.M., Kramer, J.F. *et al.* (1993) An overhead harness and trolly system for balance and ambulation assessment and training. *Archives of Physical Medicine and Rehabilitation*, **74**, 220–223.

Malouin, F., Potvin, M., Prevost, J. *et al.* (1992) Use of an intensive task-oriented gait training program in a series of patients with acute cerebrovascular accidents. *Physical Therapy*, **72**, 781–793.

Morris, M.E., Matyas, T.A., Bach, T.M. *et al.* (1992) Electrogoniometric feedback: its effect on genu recurvatum in stroke. *Archives of Physical Medicine and Rehabilitation*, **73**, 1147–1153.

Norman, K.E., Pepin, A., Ladouceur, M. *et al.* (1995) A treadmill apparatus and harness support for evaluation and rehabilitation of gait. *Archives of Physical Medicine and Rehabilitation*, **76**, 772–778.

Perry, J. (1992) *Gait Analysis: Normal and Pathological Function*. Slack, Thorofare, NJ.

Pillar, T., Dickstein, R. and Smolinski, Z. (1991) Walking reeducation with partial relief of body weight in rehabilitation of patients with locomotor disabilities. *Journal of Rehabilitation Research and Development*, **28**, 47–52.

Rose, J. and Gamble, J.G. (eds) (1994) *Human Walking*, 2nd edn., Williams and Wilkins, Baltimore, MD.

Smidt, G.L. (1990) Aging and gait. In *Gait in Rehabilitation* (ed. G.L. Smidt), Churchill Livingstone, New York, pp. 185–198.

Van Ingen Schenau, G.J. (1980) Some fundamental aspects of the biomechanics of overground versus treadmill locomotion. *Medicine and Science in Sports and Exercise*, **12**, 257–261.

Visintin, M. and Barbeau, H. (1989) The effects of body weight support on the locomotor pattern of spastic paretic patients. *Canadian Journal of Neurological Sciences*, **16**, 315–325.

Winter, D.A. (1985) Concerning the scientific basis for the diagnosis of pathological gait and for rehabilitation protocols. *Physiotherapy Canada*, **37**, 245–252.

6

Reaching and manipulation

Introduction

The arm functions principally in order to place the hand in the appropriate position and orientation in space to interact with the environment. Reaching movements are, therefore, the major actions of the arm, and interaction with the environment the major purpose of the hand. The upper limb is involved in a large variety of tasks which require the limb to produce different joint configurations and different timing and sequencing of joint movements.

It is evident from research findings that the arm and hand function as a single unit in reaching and manipulation, enabling the individual to interact with objects and people. The individual both responds to environmental demands and imposes intentions upon the environment. In many activities involving reaching, the upper body or the entire body also become part of the single coordinated unit (Ada *et al.* 1994).

The fact that the arm and hand function as a single coordinated unit is remarkable given the number of components in the unit and the complexity of human manipulative actions. The unit is made up of many joints and muscles (mono-articular, biarticular and multiarticular), with many degrees of freedom which must be constrained or utilized if reaching and manipulative activities are to be coordinated.

The function of the hands is as much sensory as it is motor (Hogan and Winters 1990). Tactile and pressure sensors give us information that helps us identify objects, classify them according to properties such as texture and density and to gauge the potential for slippage. In addition, due to the important informational role of vision in reaching and manipulation, eye and head movement play a critical part in enabling a coordinated movement to take place (Biguer *et al.* 1982). Coordination between eye and hand movements has also been noted in pointing actions (Biguer *et al.* 1982; Beaubaton and Hay 1986). Vision is obviously critical to the gathering of information related to the object, particularly its distance from the body and orientation. Vision enables precision. However, in the dark we can still manipulate objects successfully by substituting tactile senses, although reaching and grasping movements will be slower and less precise.

The arms are also yoked into the postural system (Gentile 1987). When balance is compromised, the arms play a stabilizing and supportive function and, if balance is lost, the hands are used to form a new base of support. If an object is beyond arm's length, body movement toward the object provides an extension of the reach, effectively enlarging the attainable part of the surroundings. Unless the body is in a fully supported position, any reaching action in sitting or standing is preceded and accompanied by postural adjustments. These ensure that the body segment alignment is appropriate to the upcoming perturbation which will be caused by the arm movement.

Postural adjustments occurring prior to and during arm movement are brought about by muscle activation and usually result in some alteration in segmental alignment (e.g., Bouisset and Zattara 1981). As well as numerous studies performed in standing, postural activity before and during arm movement has also been reported in sitting, during fast pointing (Crosbie *et al.* 1995) and in self-paced reaching to pick up an object (Dean and Shepherd 1997).

Most commonly performed tasks are carried out not with one hand but with two. In bimanual actions, the two upper limbs have to function in concert, and since the object being grasped and manipulated becomes the connection between the two limbs, the interactions are complex. The requirement for coordination of the two limbs needs to be kept in mind particularly during rehabilitation of individuals with a hemiplegic distribution of motor impairments, since training needs to involve the practice of bimanual actions as well as exercises to regain muscle activity in the affected limb.

Reaching to grasp: description of the activity

Many studies of reaching are of one- or two-joint movements carried out in the horizontal plane and under highly constrained conditions (e.g., Karst and Hasan 1990; Flanagan *et al.* 1993). There are, however, an increasing number of studies of more 'natural' reaching or pointing movements in which the subject interacts with an everyday object. It is these studies which are of particular relevance to clinical practice since they provide essential information from which analysis and intervention can be planned and carried out.

According to Jeannerod's investigations (Jeannerod, 1984), reaching to grasp an object can be divided into two components: a *transportation component* in which the hand moves quickly to the vicinity of the target, and a slower *manipulation component* when, under visual control, final

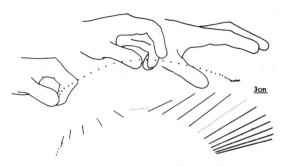

Fig. 6.1 A cinematographic study by Jeannerod of reaching toward an object. Dots represent successive positions of the hand every 20 ms and illustrate fast movement of the hand toward the object, slowing down on approach. Lines represent the size of the grasp aperture (between thumb and index finger tip) every 40 ms. Note that aperture formation starts when movement starts and that the aperture reaches a maximum of 3 cm then decreases until it is the size necessary for grasping. (We thank the International Association for the Study of Attention and Performance for permission to reprint from Long and Baddeley 1981)

adjustment to the grasp apertures is made just prior to grasp. The relationship between these two components has also been investigated (e.g., Jeannerod 1981, 1984; Marteniuk *et al.* 1990; Hoff and Arbib 1993).

Evidence that the arm and hand function as a single unit comes from the finding that the hand starts to open for the grasp at the start of the reaching action (Jeannerod 1981). Jeannerod filmed his subjects as they reached for objects of various sizes lying on the surface of a table. The grasp aperture (the distance between thumb and index finger) increased throughout the transport phase, reaching a maximum before contact and around the time the transport movement started to decelerate. The grasp size then decreased as the hand neared the object (Fig. 6.1). When under visual control, the distance between the two grasp components (thumb and index finger), although a little greater than necessary for the size of the object, reflected the size of the object. The aperture was greater when visual control was removed.

A study of a single subject (Wing and Fraser 1983) suggests that the thumb plays a role in guiding the transport component of reaching (Fig. 6.2). They noted that during the final approach phase in a reaching task, the closing of the hand from peak aperture was largely due to movement

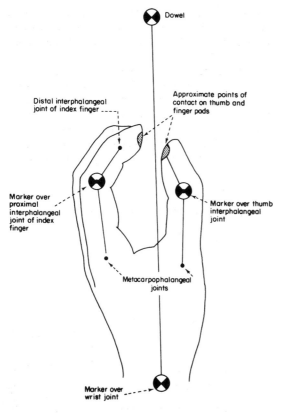

Fig. 6.2 Drawing to illustrate position of markers used in digitizing transport and grasp components of reaching to an object. (From Wing and Fraser 1983, by permission)

of the index finger with little thumb movement. The authors suggested that, since the position of the thumb relative to the line of approach to the object remained invariant, thumb stabilization may have provided a focus for visual monitoring of the relationship between grasp aperture and object size.

It seems to make a difference to the organization of both transport and manipulation components of the movement whether subjects reach to grasp with the whole hand or with a precision grip (Castiello *et al.* 1992). The object and what is to be done with it certainly affects the shape of the grasp. In reaching to grasp a mug, for example, the hand is pre-shaped into a configuration suitable for grasping the handle. Evidence of the effect of both object and the individual's goal on reaching and grasping also comes from a study in which the orientation of the hand was shown to vary according to what was to be done with the object once it was grasped (Iberall *et al.* 1986). When subjects were asked to tap the end of the dowel on the table top, approach and grasp were different from when they were asked to shake the dowel up and down (Fig. 6.3). The grasp and hand orientation that develops during transportation of the hand toward the object also reflects the final position desired for the object (see Rosenbaum *et al.* 1992; van Vliet 1993), i.e., whether the mug is to be raised to the lips or moved from table to floor. Knowledge of the properties of the object to be

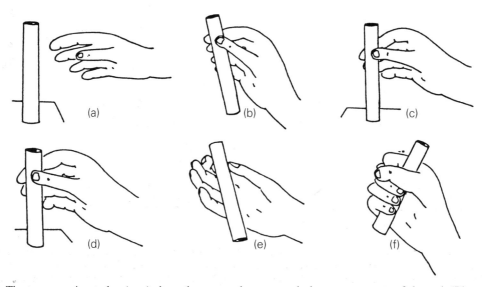

Fig. 6.3 The two grasping tasks. (*a–c*) show the approach, grasp and place components of the task 'Place Cylinder'. (*d–f*) show the grasp and lift, the transition from initial to a firmer grasp and the shake components of the task 'shake cylinder'. (From Iberall *et al.* 1986, by permission)

grasped (e.g., degree of fragility) has been shown to affect the transport phase, i.e., the reach itself, with an increase in length of the deceleration phase when the object is perceived to be fragile compared to when it is not (Marteniuk *et al.* 1987).

There has recently been considerable experimental interest in bimanual actions which illustrate the cooperative manner in which the two hands interact with objects to achieve a goal (e.g., Kelso *et al.* 1979; Marteniuk *et al.* 1984; Castiello *et al.* 1993). One experiment showed that when a subject holds a ball and lets it drop into a cup held by the other hand, the grip force of the cup hand increases in anticipation of the ball's impact (Johansson and Westling 1988).

Speed of hand movement is also affected. If a task requires that one limb has to perform a more complex action than the other, which requires a longer movement time, the other limb slows down also so that both hands arrive simultaneously (Kelso *et al.* 1979). In many bimanual reaching-to-grasp tasks, the two hands usually perform different

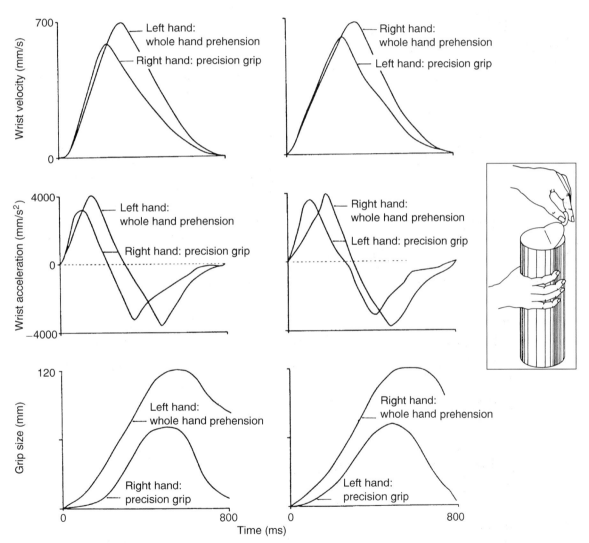

Fig. 6.4 A single trial of the bilateral task. Three traces on R: wrist velocity (*top*), wrist acceleration (*middle*) and grip size (*lower*) during the reach to grasp (R hand) and pull tab (L hand) tasks. Traces on L are for a trial in which the tasks for each hand were reversed. Note that in both cases peak velocity, acceleration and deceleration occur earlier for the precision grip hand. The 'can' (*inset*) used in the experiment. (Reprinted from Castiello *et al.* The bilateral reach to grasp movement, *Behavioural Brain Research*, **56**, 43–57 1993, with kind permission of Elsevier Science, Amsterdam, The Netherlands)

actions in order to interact with the object. Nevertheless, both limbs tend to be constrained as a single unit while engaged in the one task. For example, in using the hands to open a can, one hand holds the tin to stabilize it while the fingers of the other grasp the ring in order to pull. In the former, the whole hand forms the grasp; in the latter only the ends of fingers and thumb are used. A recent kinematic study of this task (Castiello *et al.* 1993) illustrates very well the difference between unimanual and bimanual reaching to grasp. The results show that, in unimanual reaching, reaches to the ring (the more complex precision task) are performed more slowly than reaches to the can (the whole-hand task). However, in bimanual reaching to grasp the can with one hand and pull the tab to open it with the other, although the kinematic details differed according to the task, there was no difference in movement duration between the two limbs (Fig. 6.4). The speed-accuracy trade-off would suggest that the accuracy requirement of the more precise task requires the decrease in speed. In this bimanual task, the accuracy requirement of one hand's contribution therefore demands that both hands slow down so that they reach the target at the same time.

Reaching to various parts of the workspace can be achieved by a great variety of movement combinations (Fig. 6.5). For example, reaching to an object placed within arm's length involves principally the shoulder, elbow, wrist, forearm and hand joints, although the upper body, if it is not supported, may also move to a small extent at the hips (Dean and Shepherd 1997). Reaching beyond arm's length, however, involves movement at all these joints and, theoretically, with a multitude of possible configurations, as shown in Figure 6.5. In reality, however, it is likely that only the most cost-efficient (parsimonious) options are used. Two recent studies have shown a remarkable consistency in movement pattern both for individuals and groups of individuals when they reached forward in sitting to an object beyond arm's reach (Kaminski *et al.* 1995; Dean and Shepherd 1997).

The upper limbs are also involved in *throwing and striking actions*. These actions have their own patterns of coordination, reflecting the different interactions required, the intentions of the performer and the type of object. Most of these actions are characterized by sequential motions of the segments comprising the linkage, with movements of proximal segment preceding more distal segments (Zajak and Winters 1990; Putnam 1993). Such a sequence maximizes the speed of the distal segment (holding the ball or the bat).

Manipulation: description of the activity

The hand is the principal means by which the individual interacts with people and objects in the external environment. The anatomical structure of the hand and the nature of cortico-motor neuronal connections to hand muscles (Landsmeer 1976; Smith 1981; Muir 1985; Lemon *et al.* 1990; Lemon *et al.* 1991) allow a large number of combinations of joint rotations and a vast array of movement possibilities. Even in relatively simple tasks, there may be a variety of different configurations of hand segments. It has been shown in the limited number of studies available that the intention as well as the

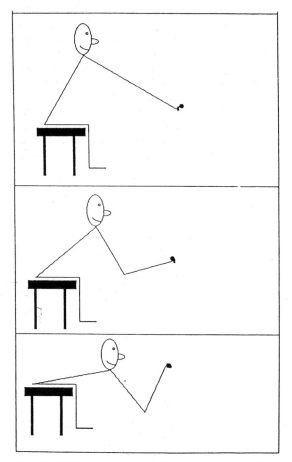

Fig. 6.5 Different patterns of the reach action made to a target in the same part of the workplace by a stick figure with 3 degrees of freedom. (From Rosenbaum *et al.* 1993, by permission)

object itself affect the approach and grasp as well as the manipulation (see Fig. 6.3). The organization of cortico-motor neuronal input involves axons directly facilitating motor neurons supplying hand muscles. These axons diverge intraspinally, making functional contact with a small number of different target muscles making up the 'muscle field' of the cortico-motor neuronal cell (Lemon *et al.* 1991).

Lemon and colleagues point out (1991) that, during natural manipulative or prehension tasks, many different muscles are active. When the fingers move to manipulate an object, the dominant pattern is one of fractionation of muscle activity. When force is required in gripping, a pattern of co-contraction emerges, with the number of muscles involved depending on the degree of force exerted.

Grip is typically categorized as either precision or power (Napier 1956), the former involving pads of digits and sometimes only thumb and index finger, the latter the whole hand. This general distinction between accuracy and power remains despite the more recent acknowledgement of the task- and object-relatedness of grasp configurations (Fig. 6.6) (Iberall and Lyons 1984; Castiello *et al.* 1993).

The hand takes on various configurations in order to perform grasping and manipulative tasks. The large number of small bones which make up the hand are moulded into the necessary shapes by

an interplay between passive and active properties of hand and forearm muscles. Despite the tendency for interaction between the components of the hand, due to its articulated anatomy, the various components can also function relatively independently, producing more fractionated movement of individual fingers or thumb (as in playing a musical instrument, typing on a keyboard or pressing a button).

Many tasks involve interactions between an object and thumb and index finger as the object is grasped and manipulated. These actions require the thumb to abduct and rotate and the index finger to flex so that their pulps contact the object. Force is effectively exerted on the object primarily by the long flexor muscles of thumb and index finger, and stabilization of each bone is achieved by both joint geometry and intrinsic musculature (Spoor 1983). The force produced on the index finger by the thumb is countered by the first dorsal interosseus muscle. The force produced on the mobile carpometacarpal joint of the thumb is constrained by activity of all the thenar muscles (Chao *et al.* 1989). As in any other part of the body's segmental linkage, force applied to one segment can affect segments at some distance from the original force, and motor control mechanisms must take these segmental interactions into account. With the hand, the combination of small mobile segments and a rich array of muscles

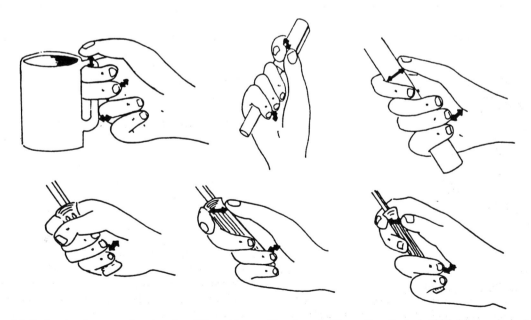

Fig. 6.6 Task-related grasps showing the different 'oppositions' used. (From Iberall *et al.* 1986, by permission)

means that the complexity of these interactional forces, even though they may be small, is considerable. The lumbrical and interossei muscles, for example, exert axial rotary moments of force which are balanced by other appropriate muscles (Lemon *et al.* 1991). Not surprisingly, it appears that for a given task, although similar muscle groups are active, the degree of activity and the relative contributions of muscles differ and are task-related.

It is necessary to understand the significance of the fifth metacarpal and little finger, together with the fourth metacarpal and finger, to some grasping tasks. Tasks such as holding a knife or fork to eat or carrying a tray or a plate require these segments of the hand, in the first example, to lock the implement into the palm to allow manipulation, in the second and third examples, to provide a support surface. These two grasps have been characterized as the 'locking grip' and the 'supporting grip' (Bendz 1993). Bendz has described these grasps in some detail and the following description is from his journal article. It is evident that the metacarpals are flexed at the carpometacarpal joints, actively in the case of the fifth metacarpal, passively for the fourth because of the intercapitular ligament's attachments. For the locking grip, all the joints of the two fingers are flexed and rotated at the metacarpophalangeal (MCP) joints. The fifth metacarpal is flexed by the hypothenar muscles. Opponens digiti minimi acts directly on the metacarpal, while the abductor digiti minimi and flexor brevis act indirectly to flex the metacarpal through their common attachment

to the proximal phalanges of the little finger (see Forrest and Basmajian 1965). Flexor brevis and the abductor also flex the little finger at the MCP joint and the abductor also rotates the finger at this joint. The fourth interosseus and long finger flexors act similarly on the fourth finger (see Eyler and Markee 1954).

Bendz stresses that the major function of the abductor digiti minimi is in the application of flexing and rotational force to the proximal phalanx of the fifth finger at the MCP joint. The force provided by this muscle is augmented by the action of the flexor carpi ulnaris via their common attachment to the pisiform bone. Using electrogoniometry and electromyography in two tasks, holding a knife and a plate, Bendz showed the effect of a loaded (grip knife firmly; lift plate) and an unloaded condition on the action of hypothenar muscles and flexor carpi ulnaris. Only in the loaded conditions, when more strength was required, was the latter strongly active, illustrating this muscle's augmenting effect on hypothenar muscle activity.

There are several grip variations used by individuals when they manipulate food with cutlery. Most involve some interaction with the implement of the fourth and fifth fingers. For example, in the grip used in Fig. 6.7, the wrist is held flexed and deviated to the ulnar side. Since the long finger extensors are fully lengthened in this position, it is likely that the muscles flexing the fourth and fifth fingers to hold the base of the knife and fork firmly in the palm also act to counteract some extending force. Flexor carpi

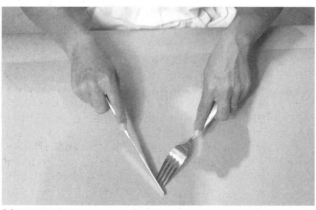

(a)

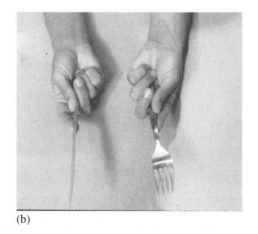

(b)

Fig. 6.7 Using a knife and fork: (*a*) superior view – force is used through index fingers to hold and cut food; (*b*) inferior view – 4th and 5th fingers exert force to stabilize the cutlery in the palm. (From Carr and Shepherd 1987, by permission)

ulnaris would also be acting in this position, not only to augment the action of abductor digiti minimi but also to flex the wrist and deviate the hand to the ulnar side.

Shaping the hand to an object is critical for manipulation of that object. The carpal and meta-carpal bones take on a concave shape through the combined actions of thenar, hypothenar and inter-ossei muscles. It is suggested that such shaping constitutes a 'postural set' for the promotion of precision movements (Lemon *et al.* 1991). A similar notion, that of a 'virtual finger' (Arbib *et al.* 1985), is that a group of fingers acts as a single functional unit. These are useful simplifications when it comes to evaluating patient performance on manipulative tasks and planning intervention. Figure 6.6 illustrates how in a mug task three independent functional units operate cooperatively to effect a stable effective grasp.

While reaching for an object appears to be carried out under visual control, once the hand comes into contact with the object, major sensory inputs contributing to movement control have been shown to come from tactile and pressure inputs. Tactile cutaneous inputs in the skin of the palm give information critical to our ability to localize stimuli and appreciate fine details. It is clear that motor commands are precisely tuned to relevant physical properties of objects. Tactile information is used to monitor the weight of an object (the vertical lifting force) and the frictional character-istics of the object in relation to slip (the slip-triggered grip force) enabling motor output (mus-cle force) to be adjusted accordingly (Johansson and Westling 1984, 1990; Westling and Johansson 1984).

While perceived fragility can affect the reaching phase of the reach to grasp action, object weight affects only the time after hand contact. As object weight increases, the time spent in contact with the object prior to lifting it increases (Weir *et al.* 1991b). The pause before lift probably reflects the time needed to generate functionally effective forces. As the friction offered by an object decreases, grip force decreases (Weir *et al.* 1991a) and reaching to grasp a slippery object results in slower movement times (Fikes *et al.* 1994). Moving the hand while holding an object produces inertial forces and these are compensated for by simultaneous changes in grip force (Flanagan and Wing 1993). A general function of all reaching-to-grasp tasks is that, once grasped, the object should not be dropped, whether it is light or heavy, slippery or not.

Recovery of upper limb function

Sadly, most reports of upper limb function after acute brain lesion suggest that recovery is minimal in patients with an initially severely affected limb (Basmajian *et al.* 1982; Wade *et al.* 1983; Nakayama *et al.* 1994a). It is not known how well patients with a less severely affected limb recover. Overall, reports of recovery of functional use vary from 5% (Gowland 1982) to 52% (Dean and Mackey 1992). Basmajian and colleagues (1982) put the percentage of patients regaining full arm and hand function after stroke at 5% and the percentage with no functional use, at 20%. Another study reports that, of those patients who started rehabilita-tion with marked impairment of function, only about 15% regained useful function (Sunderland *et al.* 1992). It is typically reported that most potential recovery of the upper limb takes place within 3 months (Wade *et al.* 1983; Parker *et al.* 1986; Olsen 1990; Nakayama *et al.* 1994b). However, studies of training and forced use commenced more than 1 year after stroke have shown substantial recovery considerably beyond the 3-month period (e.g., Ostendorf and Wolf 1981).

The complex nature of hand use requiring coordination of many muscles and segments and the nature of the lesion itself may be significant factors in poor recovery. However, there are other factors which may impact negatively upon out-come following stroke. One is the view that all recovery of arm function is intrinsic (Wade *et al.* 1983; Heller *et al.* 1987), inferring that what the person does, what happens to the individual post-lesion, including therapy, has little effect upon recovery. (The issue of recovery and adaptation is discussed in Chapter 1.) It should be noted that most studies of upper limb recovery have exam-ined patients receiving the commonly used neu-rotherapies (mostly Bobath therapy) and the results are also likely to reflect the effects of these therapies on recovery processes. The studies which show more positive results (e.g., Dean and Mackey 1992; Butefisch *et al.* 1995; Mudie and Matyas 1996) were carried out with patients whose rehabilitation was active and task-related. In the Dean and Mackey study (1992), the extent of functional recovery was indicated by the highest score in the Upper Limb items of the Motor Assessment Scale (Carr *et al.* 1985). According to this criterion, 52% of all stroke patients seen over a 1-year period were able to comb their hair at the back of the head using the affected hand by the time of discharge.

It is our view that poor recovery may reflect not only the direct effects of the lesion itself but also inappropriate and insufficient therapeutic intervention for the upper limb, the ease with which patients manage their limited responsibilities with one hand when they are in hospital and rehabilitation centre, and the effects of immobility on soft tissue adaptability.

The evidence, from reading modern physiotherapy texts (Davies 1990; Ryerson 1995; Edwards 1996) is that active upper limb function is neglected in rehabilitation. Where intervention is mentioned in these texts, it typically consists of passive interventions, including inhibition (by the therapist) of spasticity, facilitatory movements (performed by the therapist) and splinting for the shoulder and hand (see Edwards 1996). Hand function, specifically voluntary activation of distal arm and hand musculature, is typically not addressed in commonly used traditional physiotherapy approaches (see Butefisch *et al.* 1995, for comments). Guidelines for training of reaching and manipulation have, however, been in the clinical literature for some time (e.g., Carr and Shepherd 1987a,b; Ada *et al.* 1990).

It is clear that a very small percentage of the day is spent in intervention relevant to the upper limb when one examines the total time spent in therapy (Tinson 1989). Although therapists may consider they are addressing their interventions to the affected limb, the patient is still able to use the unaffected limb for functional activities both during and after treatment sessions, and most actions are, therefore, carried out by the relatively unaffected limb. One-arm drive wheelchairs and the use of slings are two factors mitigating against any potential for recovery of the affected upper limb. Instead of learning to use the affected limb and to regain some ability to activate muscles in a coordinated manner, many stroke patients learn instead to become more proficient with their unaffected arm (Ostendorf and Wolf 1981).

Rehabilitation is also hampered by common beliefs in the rehabilitation community which govern the intervention given. Three views – one that recovery takes place from proximal to distal (e.g., de Souza *et al.* 1980); the second, that stability and control of the shoulder are necessary before the hand is used; and the third, that spasticity must be inhibited before active use of the limb – are still expressed in the literature (e.g., Bobath 1990; Davies 1990). These beliefs result in any early therapeutic endeavours concentrating on

the shoulder (in passive support through the arm not in active reaching actions) and neglecting the hand.

A fourth belief is that there is a 'natural' recovery pattern in the upper limb. This pattern was first described by Twitchell (1951) from clinical observations, and it continues to be used to guide (see Brunnstrom 1970) and test (see Fugl-Meyer Scale, p. 54) interventions despite the lack of any investigation beyond observation. This pattern of recovery – proximal to distal, 'gross flexor and extensor synergies' before functional motor patterns – has led to the expectation that these recovery patterns are 'natural' and to be expected. This view does not take account of the patient's adaptive patterns of use in response to muscle weakness and functional imbalance, or of the position in which the immobile arm is kept during the day. The clinical observations of Twitchell and Brunnstrom may well have reflected the effects of these two factors and there is likely to be a close relationship between flexion activity (the 'flexion synergy'; cf Twitchell, 1951; Brunnstrom 1970) and the presence of short flexor muscles with shifted length-tension curves. In other words, a gross flexion synergy may be dependent upon an adaptive pattern performed repetitively by a patient attempting to use the limb, and/or the persistent maintenance of flexion and consequent muscle shortening (see Figs 6.8, 6.9) rather than a 'natural' and immutable recovery pattern.

More recent evidence supports the view that use and context have an effect on the motor pattern, that the pattern of muscle activity reflects the biomechanical demands of the task and the distribution of muscle weakness rather than a stereotyped neurological linkage (Trombly 1993). There are several studies which report recovery patterns that vary considerably from those observed by Twitchell (Bourbonnais *et al.* 1989; Wing *et al.* 1990; Trombly 1993) and which result from factors other than those proposed by Twitchell and Brunnstrom. A group of patients following stroke, for example, showed different sequences of recovery of movement at the elbow with no evidence that flexion 'recovered' before extension (Wing *et al.* 1990).

Linked in with the idea of mass pathological synergies is the persistent belief that spasticity (hyperreflexia) of muscles is the major impairment interfering with recovery, which underlies the Bobath and Brunnstrom approaches. Several studies of stroke patients have found few signs of hyperreflexia in the upper limb (Sahrmann and

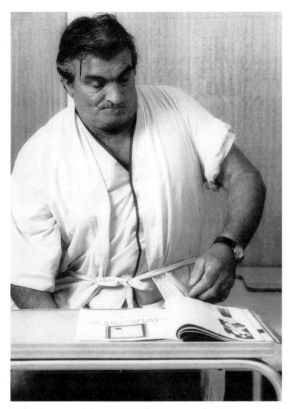

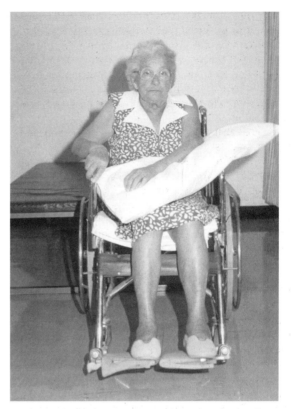

Fig. 6.8 Post-stroke, adaptations to weakness or paralysis of shoulder flexors and external rotators in this case include shoulder girdle elevation, lateral flexion of spine with some rotation allowing him to swing his arm forward

Fig. 6.9 Typical post-stroke resting posture with internal rotation, adduction of GH joint, elbow flexion, forearm pronation and wrist flexion. In the absence of movement, the muscles held short will develop adaptive changes

Norton 1977; Wing *et al.* 1990; O'Dwyer *et al.* 1996), but all have reported weakness (Bourbonnais *et al.* 1989; Sahrmann and Norton 1977). (See Chapter 8 for discussion of this issue.) Nevertheless, many physiotherapists persist in the belief that spasticity is the major impairment, that muscles are not weak and that repetitive and intensive exercise is contraindicated. Bobath therapists believe there is a relationship between spasticity-inhibiting techniques directed at trunk and proximal arm muscles and the voluntary activation of hand muscles, but a recent study shows that this relationship is doubtful (Butefisch *et al.* 1995). Emphasis on facilitation of the patient's automatic response to therapist-induced perturbations (Davies 1985; Bobath 1990) means that the person gets little practice of actively engaging with the environment using vision and hands. It is becoming evident that the hypertonus (resistance to passive movement, usually by the

flexors) which is considered by many clinicians to be a manifestation of spasticity, is in most patients typically due to muscle shortening and increased stiffness. The rather rapid development of these adaptive soft tissue changes may be a major factor interfering with recovery from acute brain lesion.

A common method said to inhibit spasticity and used by Bobath (NDT) therapists is weight-bearing through the upper limb. There is, however, no evidence that reducing reflex hyperactivity is associated with any increase in functional performance so it is unclear what would be the point of such exercise, except as a means to preserve soft tissue extensibility. In addition, monitoring with EMG suggests that weight-bearing through the limb is not necessarily associated with muscle activity in able-bodied subjects. A recent study using transcranial magnetic stimulation (Brouwer and Ambury 1994) suggests that upper limb weight-bearing might affect the excitability of corticospinal neurons projecting to spinal motor neurons. As the authors point out, it is necessary to establish in future studies whether or not this change is associated with any functional gain for the patient. Given that it has been demonstrated experimentally that localized changes to muscle or neural system from non-task-related stimuli are not linked to functional change, further studies should also address the issue of whether or not more dynamic task-related practice might be more effective.

There is increasing evidence that specific, intensive and task-related training, with repetitive practice of relevant movements, has a more positive outcome on upper limb motor function (e.g., Dean and Mackay 1992; Butefisch *et al.* 1995; Mudie and Matyas 1996) than some therapies in current use. In addition, specific training of sensory awareness in the hand has shown significant gains in the treated group and none in the untreated group (Yekutiel and Guttman 1993). One study showed the effects of superimposing behavioural methods to encourage active learning, and self-directed exercises based on published guidelines for task-related training (Carr and Shepherd 1987a,b), on orthodox (Bobath) therapy (Sunderland *et al.* 1992). The enhanced therapy group spent approximately twice the time in therapy and independent exercise than the Bobath only group. The results showed that the greatest recovery occurred in the first month (particularly for the enhanced therapy group) and that the group of patients who received the more intensive rehabilitation did significantly better in the short term than the group who did not.

Reports of recovery of upper limb function do not present information related to the physical condition of the limb, i.e., whether muscles have shortened and become stiff or whether there is shoulder pain. One major factor interfering with recovery, particularly in the early stages after an acute lesion, would be the adaptive length-associated changes that occur in muscles when a limb is immobile. Another factor would be a shoulder which is painful constantly, at night or on movement. We argue that such adaptive musculoskeletal changes are probably preventable and that, if they are allowed to occur, they are treatable. The Appendix of Chapter 11 describes in some detail the causes of these changes (including inadequate therapy methods, learned non-use and pre-existing pathological conditions), the underlying mechanisms and methods of prevention and treatment.

Motor dysfunction

This section considers the major impairments and movement dysfunctions associated with acute brain lesions, such as CVA and traumatic brain injury (see also Chapter 8). Specific aspects of upper limb dysfunction in ataxia and Parkinson's disease are discussed in Chapters 9 and 13.

Muscle weakness

The major impairment underlying the functional disability of the upper limb following an acute lesion affecting the upper motor neuron, such as stroke or head injury, is muscle weakness apparently due to diminished motor unit recruitment. The neurophysiological evidence (Colebatch and Gandevia 1989) is supported by clinical studies (e.g., Bourbonnais *et al.* 1989; Gowland *et al.* 1992).

Colebatch and Gandevia (1989) studied the muscle strength of 16 patients with hemiplegia from stroke. The authors reported partial sparing of shoulder and elbow muscles, particularly of shoulder adductors, which were minimally affected. Overall, wrist and finger muscles, particularly the flexors, were the most affected. There was no evidence that extensor muscles were weaker than flexor muscles, as has been a common clinical assumption. In other studies, reduced EMG activity has been reported to be greater in muscles such as biceps brachii than in triceps brachii (Colebatch *et al.* 1986; Bourbonnais *et al.* 1989). Grip-force control during grasping and lifting objects is a common problem and has been described, in association with cerebral and cerebellar lesions and Parkinson's disease, by several authors (Jeannerod 1984; Wing 1988; Muller and Dichgans 1994; Hermsdorfer and Mai 1996). Force produced when gripping can be slow to build up, difficult to stabilize at the required level for a particular task, and characterized by irregular force change (Hermsdorfer and Mai 1996).

In addition to muscle weakness, a disturbance of motor unit activation patterns has been reported (Tang and Rymer 1981). However, whether or not this is directly the result of the lesion or of the development of maladaptive motor patterns is not clear. Co-contraction of muscles is often observed clinically and has been reported from investigations. This seems to reflect poor control of synergic muscle activity as well as a tendency to stiffen a limb to compensate for poor control.

A common adaptive motor action in the presence of arm muscle weakness following stroke is elevation of the shoulder often with some retraction of the arm/shoulder girdle when the individual attempts to reach (Fig. 6.8). We have suggested that this pattern reflects the best the person can do given the pattern of muscle paralysis and the dynamics of the musculoskeletal linkage (Carr and Shepherd 1996). It has been suggested that these movements may also be a strategy for activating biceps (Bourbonnais *et al.* 1989).

Proximal muscles are often reported to be less severely affected by stroke than distal muscles (Colebatch and Gandevia 1989). It is clinically observed that activity in shoulder adductors is frequently present early after a lesion but that the abductors (particularly deltoid) are typically inactive. This observation is supported by evidence of bilateral innervation of some proximal muscles (Colebatch and Gandevia 1989; Jones *et al.* 1989). A recent study of corticospinal influences on two antagonistic shoulder muscles, deltoid and pectoralis major, by Colebatch and colleagues (1990) appears to confirm a bilaterally distributed cortical motor outflow, since inputs from both hemispheres appeared to be particularly marked for the shoulder adductors.

The belief that direct (monosynaptic) corticospinal projections exist only to hand muscles and not to more proximal muscles has also been used to provide an explanation for the relatively poor recovery of distal movements compared to proximal. However, the above study provides some evidence that there are also direct corticospinal projections to proximal muscles. The findings further suggest that these projections may be muscle-specific and are greater to the deltoid, for example, than to the pectoralis major.

Hence the fact that there is relative sparing of some proximal upper limb muscles (particularly adductor muscles such as pectoralis major) compared to others may be partially explained by (1) the existence of bilateral innervation, more marked for adductor muscles, and (2) by the stronger monosynaptic corticospinal inputs to some muscles (e.g., deltoid) than to others (adductors). These findings help to explain the relatively severe involvement of deltoid following stroke and the relative ease with which patients can be trained to activate the adductor muscles.

It should be noted that there is increasing evidence that individuals with hemiplegia also have impairments of the ipsilateral upper limb (e.g., Colebatch and Gandevia 1989). These muscles have been shown to generate less force than in able-bodied subjects.

Muscle stiffness and muscle length changes

The relationship between spasticity (hyperreflexia) and upper limb dysfunction has until recently been considered to be strong. There is increasing evidence, however, that this is not the case, particularly following stroke (O'Dwyer *et al.* 1996). It is likely with this group of patients, and perhaps with many individuals following other acute lesions, that what appears clinically as spasticity is actually increased muscle stiffness and muscle contracture. This is a critical point to contemplate since the belief that spasticity is the dominant impairment results in relatively passive interventions involving inhibition. On the other hand, once it becomes clear to the clinical community that weakness and incoordination are major impairments, therapy may shift to more active exercise and training.

Secondary adaptations occurring post-lesion, principally as a result of disuse, frequently include length-associated changes in muscles and other soft tissues. Muscles held short for long periods of immobilization (Fig. 6.9) shorten and become stiffer, and, when these muscles are activated, they generate tension at shorter lengths. The muscles which typically shorten are the shoulder adductors and internal rotators, elbow flexors, pronators, wrist and finger flexors and thumb adductors (Fig. 6.10). This consequence of muscle paralysis and disuse is in our view preventable by intensive active exercise of the limb and by passive stretching carried out during the day while muscles remain paralysed. The Appendix of Chapter 11 reviews the issue of soft tissue adaptations around the shoulder with guidelines for prevention.

There are now numerous studies which report abnormal mechanical properties in so-called spastic muscles (see Chapter 8 for discussion), including one indicating mechanical abnormalities in elbow flexor muscles (Lee *et al.* 1987). As a result of changes associated with weakness and disuse, the typical picture for many patients following acute brain lesion is of a stiff, immobile and sometimes painful upper limb. Failure to recover the ability to use the limb is said to result in depression and withdrawal (Balliet *et al.* 1986). When one limb is affected, the very large number of tasks usually performed bimanually can only be attempted with difficulty, if at all.

There have been relatively few investigations of the performance deficits in reaching and manipulation in brain-injured individuals. Kinematic

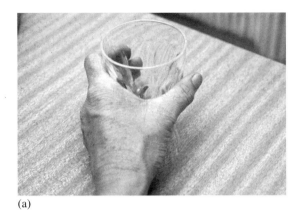

(a)

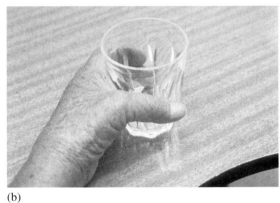

(b)

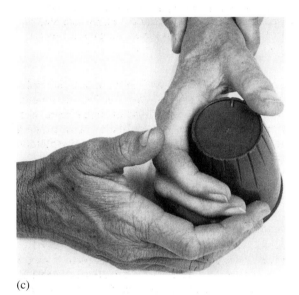

(c)

Fig. 6.10 (*a*) Grasping the glass is normally made possible by the extensible web space between thumb and index metacarpals. (*b*) Shortening of web space soft tissues (including thumb adductor muscle) forces an abnormal posture at the MCP joint. (*c*) When combined with weakness of abductor pollicis brevis muscle, attempts at moving the thumb away from the cylinder result in thumb extension

analyses of reaching tasks and analyses of force production between hand segments and the object being manipulated increase our understanding of the motor dysfunction in individuals with lesions. The use of non-invasive methods of examining brain function has also resulted in findings which help clarify some issues raised in the clinic about the nature of impairments.

Observable problems with reaching to an object include deviations from a normal path, extreme slowness of movement and inability to pre-shape the hand prior to grasp. The hand may not open until it nears the object and it may not be oriented to grasp the object appropriately in terms of its characteristics (e.g., shape) or what is to be done with it. Hand path deviations may be caused by inability to combine, for example, glenohumeral joint flexion with external rotation and a deficiency

in supination. Poor timing of hand contact may result in the hand knocking into the object or closing before the object is reached.

Observable problems with hand use include an apparently greater ability to flex the fingers and wrist than to extend them (although finger flexors are typically weak); a tendency for finger flexion to be associated with wrist flexion rather than extension (probably reflecting lack of synergistic wrist extensor activity); thumb extension in releasing grip rather than abduction; and inability to cup the hand by rotating thumb and little finger inwards (Fig. 6.11). It has been suggested that lesions affecting the motor cortex or cortico-motor neuronal projections seem to be followed by a loss or clumsiness of fine finger control (Lough *et al.* 1984) and patients who have some ability to activate hand muscles may still have

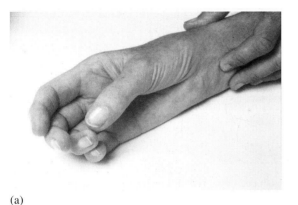 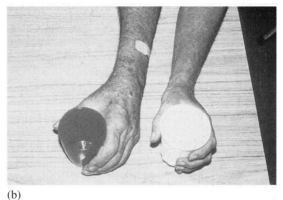

(a)   (b)

Fig. 6.11 (*a*) Weakness of hand muscles means the hand is unable to assume a cupping posture of palm and fingers and the thumb and 4th and 5th digits cannot be opposed. (*b*) It is difficult to hold and manipulate objects if wrist extension and forearm supination are absent. Note the difference in hand and forearm alignment between the arm with weak muscles and short long finger flexors and pronators compared to normal (on R)

great difficulty gaining the ability to move fingers independently, as in finger tapping.

Abnormal posturing of the hand (Fig. 6.12) is seen in a few patients some time after stroke, for example, and may represent dystonic movement or an acquired motor pattern. Inadequate posturing of the hand in patients with posterior parietal lobe lesion is described by Jeannerod (1986), with palmar grasping of an object rather than grasping with finger tips. He ascribes this to a mismatch between visual and proprioceptive inputs.

An individual with hemiplegia may not use the affected hand unless the other hand is immobilized (Taub *et al.* 1993). There is considerable evidence from monkey experiments and from studies and

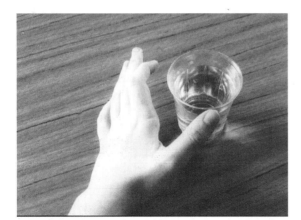

Fig. 6.12 Post-stroke: dystonic movement is evident as the hand reaches to pick up the glass. Note that grasp aperture is formed by thumb and side of index finger

observations of adults and children with hemiplegia that constraint of the unaffected arm is associated with increased use of the affected arm. Forced-use will be discussed below as a training strategy in patients with a hemiplegic distribution of muscle weakness.

Training

A major factor in early training of the upper limb is the need to modify what is to be practised in order to take into account the individual's motor impairments. For example, a person may appear to have a paralysed limb under certain circumstances (e.g., when asked to lift the arm). However, when conditions have been modified so that the amount of muscle force which needs to be generated in order to achieve movement is minimal, the person may be able to achieve some movement of the limb. Practice of simple actions using muscles which are active may have a positive motivational effect on the initially severely impaired patient. For example, most patients can contract their shoulder adductor muscles and several simple movements can be performed using these muscles (Fig. 6.13).

The absence of sitting balance should not be a deterrent to early training of upper limb function. Practice of reaching to objects or pointing in sitting and standing can be a means of improving a person's balance in these positions (see Chapter 7). Similarly, absence of or poor control of the shoulder for reaching should not be considered a deterrent to early training of hand function. Sitting

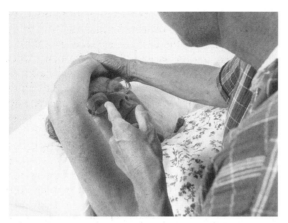

Fig. 6.13 Post-stroke: in lying, the person attempts to move the elbow to the therapist's finger. This action is carried out by pectoralis major muscle

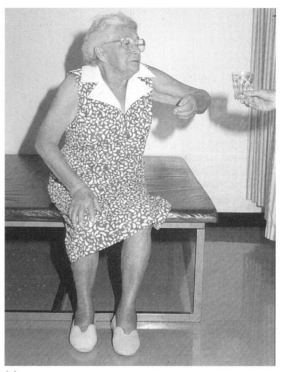

(a)

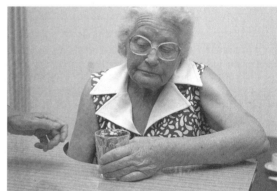

(b)

Fig. 6.14 Post-stroke: (*a*) Reaching is attempted. Biceps brachii works as a GH flexor but also flexes elbow in the absence of triceps brachii activation. (*b*) With her arm on a table, she concentrates on eliciting activity in the triceps. She was instructed not to flex her elbow since her attempts at extension resulted at first in flexion

at a table with the arm(s) supported enables the person to practise hand tasks and exercises even when control over reaching and balance are poor. In lying and with the arm supported in sitting, reaching and pointing can also be practised before the individual is able to raise the arm from the side actively to the horizontal (Fig. 6.14).

In developing control over the linked segments of the upper limb, individuals with motor impairments must regain the ability to match their motor performance to the characteristics of objects within their environment. They learn again to judge how the hand should be oriented to match the object and what is to be done to it; whether all or only some of the fingers are needed in order to grasp the object. In reaching, individuals have to learn to control for direction and distance. They have to regain the ability to judge the distance over which they can successfully reach, which means knowing the length of the arm and the distance over which other body segments can extend the reach. This means that the individual must learn to incorporate the necessary postural adjustments into reaching and manipulation in upright positions such as sitting and standing.

First, however, patients with muscle paralysis have to be able to activate their muscles. After an acute lesion such as stroke, voluntary activation of muscles even for simple one-joint movements may be impossible. The first step, therefore, is to provide a means of exercise that enables the person to practise muscle activation and regain the ability to generate the necessary force. We have suggested that patients practise major movement components as a means of getting muscles active (Carr and

Shepherd 1987a). By proposing such 'essential components' we are presenting a simplification strategy designed to train the individual to contract muscles in components of movement which are likely to lead to generalization into more complex interactions of hand(s) with objects in the environment. Recent studies seem to support this view (Butefisch *et al*. 1995; Mudie and Matyas 1996).

Essential components

Part of the complexity of hand movement arises out of the large number of degrees of freedom potentially available in the multi-segmental physical structure of the hand and from the different possibilities inherent in the physical interaction between intention and object. It is, however, possible to identify certain components of movement, or combinations of components which are present in many otherwise different tasks. Such a simplification has been developed out of our understanding of the literature available and the evidence for task- and activity-related groupings of fingers. We have hypothesized that intensive training and repetitive practice of the muscle actions involved in these components have the potential for generalization into the tasks they are components of, and that this is enhanced by practice of these tasks (Carr and Shepherd 1987a).

- **Reaching**
  Forward: Flexion at shoulder
  Sideways: Abduction at shoulder
  Backward: Extension at shoulder
     with
     Shoulder girdle elevation
     Elbow extension and varying amount of shoulder external rotation
     Opening of hand aperture between thumb and fingers
     Extension of wrist
     Pronation-supination appropriate to object orientation
- **Grasping:**
     Extension of wrist and fingers with abduction and conjoint rotation of the carpometacarpal joint of thumb and fifth finger
     Closure of fingers and thumb around object
- **Holding**
     Flexion and extension of wrist holding object
     Lifting, placing and rotating objects of different sizes and weights
- **Manipulation and finger dexterity**
     Flexion and extension of fingers
     Flexion and conjunct rotation at carpometacarpal joints of the fifth finger and thumb (e.g., cupping)
     Independent finger flexion and extension (e.g., tapping)

Figure 6.15 illustrates some examples of how some of these components might be trained.

These movement components are essential at some stage and in varying degrees in many tasks. Despite the apparently limitless variety of tasks we perform daily with our hands, apparently different tasks appear to represent ways of putting together in various combinations a relatively small number of component parts (see the different grips in Fig. 6.6; see also Kapandji 1992 on thumb oppositions). These components can be visualized as configurations, i.e., ways of putting together fingers and thumb to fit with an object and what is to be done with it. This may of course appear to be a gross over-simplification of real dexterity. Such a simplification does, however, offer a guide to intervention, particularly when a patient has little muscle activity.

It is often necessary in the clinic to determine what critical component(s) are missing or interfering with performance of a complex task. For example, in holding a knife and fork (see Fig. 6.7), apart from the position of the index fingers on the implements enabling force to be directed downward and the flexed wrist position, a palmar view of the grasp makes it clear that crucial to any pressure downward through the knife and fork with the index finger is the ability to hold the implements firmly into the palm. Cooperation between functional groupings of fingers thus produces the appropriate levels of opposing forces. Although probably critical to effective use of this particular grip, the palmar component requires the long finger flexor muscles to generate force while held at a shortened length at which the muscle's capacity to generate force is limited by its structure and by the need to counteract the extending force produced by the finger extensors. This component requires, therefore, that the long finger extensors are able to lengthen to the extent necessary.

Task-related practice

When patients have little or no apparent muscle activity in the early stages following a brain lesion, as in stroke, it may be impossible for them to practise meaningful tasks, i.e., those which are essential for independence. Nevertheless, practice of even simple actions can involve objects. In an earlier publication (Carr and Shepherd 1987a) we outlined simple actions which are practised as a means of regaining muscle activation and readers can refer to this work. An understanding of the nature of the weakness following a lesion of motor

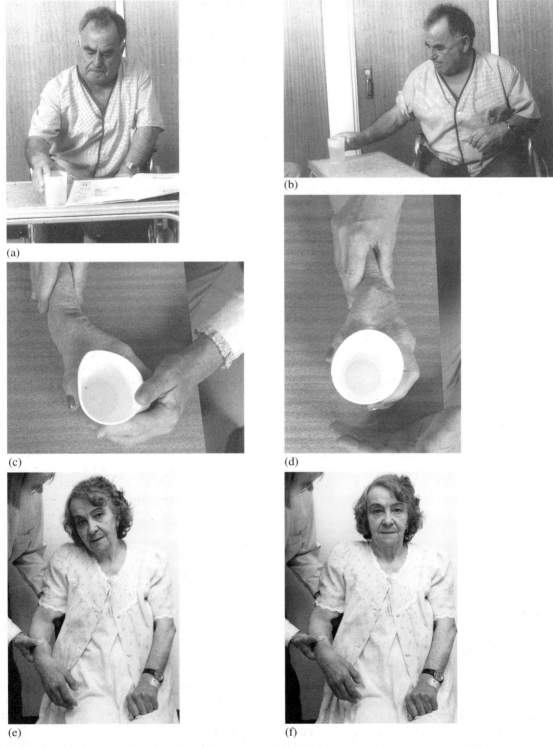

Fig. 6.15 Attempting to elicit activity in paralysed or weak muscles by practice (mental practice if physical was not possible) of critical components and training of specific actions. (*a, b*) GH external rotation and supination. Note that in (*b*) the task is made harder by a different object placement. (*c, d*) Grasping a polystyrene cup gives feedback about excessive force generation. (*e, f*) Shoulder shrugging before (*e*) and after (*f*) feedback

cortical outflow, in which muscles tend to shorten, and the pattern of movement, enables the therapist to predict which muscles in particular need to be exercised. Simple movements such as those shown in Figure 6.15 will enable the person to concentrate on activating wrist flexors and extensors, finger and thumb flexors and extensors, thumb abductors and adductors and forearm pronators and supinators. Note that the patient's objectives relate to what is to be done with the object rather than to muscle activation.

It is only relatively recently that it has been recognized that motor performance is governed to a considerable extent by objects and their 'affordances' (Gibson 1977). That is to say, objects offer possibilities for interaction. When we reach out for an object, the movement pattern reflects the object's position in relation to the body and its orientation, and what we are intending to do with it (Iberall *et al.* 1986; Rosenbaum *et al.* 1990). Objects for practice should be chosen, therefore, not only for their inherent interest and usability but also for the options they offer for hand orientation. For example, if a person has difficulty controlling the orientation of the hand and limb during reach, and reaches persistently with the shoulder internally rotated and the forearm pronated, an object can be chosen that demands a relatively externally rotated and supinated approach (Fig. 6.15*a,b*). Objects can be chosen and games played that actively encourage the action with which the person has difficulty. Objects need to be specially chosen to enable practice to take place without a struggle. Tasks should on the whole be challenging but not impossible.

Strengthening exercises

There is increasing clinical research support for repetitive practice of task-related strengthening exercises and for generalization into more functional activities. Hand grip strength, for example, is critical to many everyday tasks such as undoing a jar or lifting a saucepan and a relationship between hand grip force and a saucepan task has been reported (Turner and Ebrahim 1992).

A recent report of a randomized and controlled trial describes the effect of specific training of hand exercises (squeezing two metal bars together, rapid resisted wrist extensions performed both isotonically and isometrically) in 27 patients following stroke (Butefisch *et al.* 1995). Patients showed a significant increase in grip strength, in peak force of isometric hand extension and peak

acceleration. Most interesting, however, was the carryover to improvement of functional performance as measured on the Rivermead Motor Assessment Scale (see p. 54). That is, the biomechanical parameters improved in parallel with the functional improvement. It is also interesting that subjects did not develop increased tone and associated reactions as predicted by Bobath therapists, but instead showed (according to the Ashworth Scale; Chapter 3) a decrease in tone and a reduced tendency to elicit associated movements during the training period. The design of the study supports the investigators' view that the positive treatment effect was due to the training and not to 'spontaneous recovery'. It appears that many of the patients who showed most improvement were those who already had some muscle activity before training.

Bilateral practice

It is necessary to train bimanual actions since the two upper limbs work cooperatively in most everyday functions. For example, unscrewing a jar involves coordinating opposing forces between lid and jar. In patients with a predominantly unilateral pattern of dysfunction it is likely that training needs initially to emphasize muscle activation and task practice on the affected side. Forced use of the affected limb may also be critical to maximizing recovery of function. It is likely, however, that, even with potentially useful recovery of this limb, many individuals will not automatically acquire functionally effective bilateral hand use without practice of bilateral activities (Fig. 6.16*a*). From an early stage, they could, for example, practise getting both hands to work co-operatively to hold and manipulate an object using each hand to perform a different action (open a can, dial a telephone, Fig. 6.16*b,d*), and to work together in tasks in which the two hands do the same action either in the same direction (using a rolling pin, or rolling up a towel, Fig. 6.16*c*) or in opposite directions (using gardening shears) or in rhythmical sequential actions like arm cycling (Fig. 6.16*e*). Patients at a later stage of recovery need intensive practice of tasks which require the two limbs to time their movements to an external event (e.g., catching a ball) and which require the ability to make sensitive responses to environmental demands.

There has recently been a report that suggests that bilateral practice in which the two hands perform the same action might actually drive brain

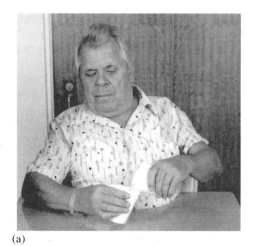
(a)

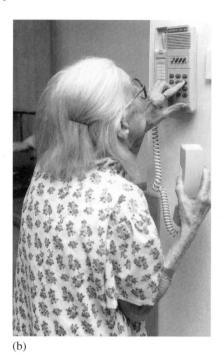
(b)

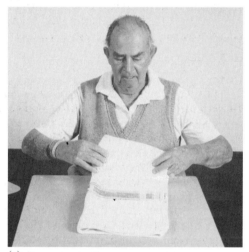
(c)

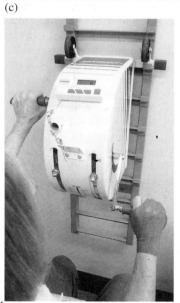
(e)

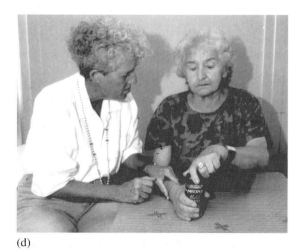
(d)

Fig. 6.16 Practice of bilateral actions gives opportunity to regain the ability to time the movement of each limb appropriately. (*a*) Pouring water from one cup to another with arms held up. (*b*) Using the telephone. (*c*) Rolling up a towel. (*d*) Unscrewing a jar. (*e*) Arm cycling

reorganization processes resulting in improved performance not only in the bimanual actions but also in unilateral actions performed by the affected limb (Mudie and Matyas 1996). There is some evidence from patient self-report that there was some transfer into other actions and patients maintained their gains over a 6-month no-training period. The authors suggest that improvement in unimanual actions by the affected limb after bilateral practice may be due to an unmasking of existing redundant connections, including uncrossed ipsilateral connections. Although unilateral activity is normally carried out via contralateral pathways, ipsilateral pathways are also theoretically capable of unimanual activation but appear under normal conditions to be inhibited (Tanji *et al.* 1988). This inhibition has been suggested to continue in hemiplegia after an acute brain lesion (Nass 1985). The positive effects reported by Mudie and Matyas support the view that the influence of the ipsilateral cortex may be stronger when its function is specifically required (Tanji *et al.* 1988).

Forced use

Limb movement may need to be forced if one limb is effectively paralysed and one is not, as in hemiplegic stroke. Taub and others (e.g., Taub 1980) have shown with both deafferented and hemiplegic monkeys that a paralysed or insensate arm was left to hang by the side when there was one effective upper limb. They referred to this behaviour as reflecting 'learned non-use', suggesting that the monkeys learned *not* to use the affected limb. However, when the intact limb was restrained and the monkey trained to use the affected limb with feedback reward, the affected limb became functional. Promising results have been reported with adults after stroke (Ostendorf and Wolf 1981; Wolf *et al.* 1989; Taub *et al.* 1993; Morris *et al.* 1997). The functional outcome for individuals with unilateral impairment is so bleak that forcing use of the affected limb while constraining the other limb becomes an obvious option. The results of the earlier Taub experiments with monkeys suggest that when therapists place the affected limb in a sling, unfortunately still a common occurence, the effect may actually be to foster the development of learned non-use of this limb, which surely is in opposition to most goals of intervention.

Guidelines for procedure can be gathered from the two major studies cited above. Taub and colleagues (1993), in their randomised controlled trial of nine patients, restrained their four subjects (a median of 4 years post-stroke) during waking hours (except during certain activities: excretory functions, activities where balance might be compromised, when sleeping) for 14 days. The unaffected limb was constrained in a resting hand splint and sling. Each weekday, patients spent 7 hours at the rehabilitation centre. They were given a variety of tasks to be carried out over 6 hours while movement of the unaffected limb was constrained. The constrained group achieved marked change, from an initially severe motor impairment to improved motor function and life-style. Furthermore, this group maintained their improvement over a 2-year period. It is important to note that, to be eligible to be included in the study, patients had to be able to extend their fingers (MCP and IP joints) at least 10° and their wrist at least 20°.

Intensity of training

The amount of time spent in physiotherapy and self-directed exercise following stroke is reported to be as little as 4 hours per week (Tinson 1989). This gives some clues as to the probable time spent in upper limb rehabilitation. One audit in an Australian rehabilitation centre (Goldie *et al.* 1992) reported 10 minutes a day. The remainder of the day is likely to involve active use of the unaffected limb and practice of a one-armed existence. Given the relative importance of hand use in daily life, it may be critical for rehabilitation staff to consider ways of increasing intensity of practice by use of relatives as training coaches, aids, forced use, access to computer-driven games.

Sensory training

In addition to motor impairments, sensory and visuospatial impairments may also affect recovery. Somatosensory impairments have been shown to benefit from specific retraining (e.g. Yekutiel and Guttman 1993). However, implicit in the concept of task-related training is the manipulation of objects with different characteristics (shapes, sizes, textures) for a variety of different purposes. It is likely that intensive task-related training provides the opportunity to practise selection of relevant somatosensory and visual information relevant to the task, in addition to a stimulus to increase attention span. Training provides the possibility of improving the person's ability to select, attend to

Feedback

As soon as the patient can activate muscles, training includes feedback regarding (1) the muscle activated (which may not be the one required); (2) the appropriateness of the force generated – such feedback can be given by the object itself (Fig. 6.15*b,c*); (3) the appropriateness of the hand path or limb configuration (Fig. 6.15*a,d*). A patient may need to pay attention to turning off an inappropriate muscle as a means of turning on its antagonist.

Electromyographic (EMG) feedback (see also p. 35) EMG feedback has been shown in several studies to assist stroke patients to regain some active function in the upper limb (Brudny *et al.* 1979; Kelly *et al.* 1979; Wolf *et al.* 1979; Balliet *et al.* 1986; Crow *et al.* 1989; Wolf *et al.* 1994). Even in apparently paralysed muscles, small voluntary muscle potentials may be present (Balliet *et al.* 1986). EMG feedback gives the patient (and therapist) information about underlying capacity for muscle activity (Fig. 6.17). Under guidance from the therapist, during task-related training with EMG attached and monitor in view, the patient can learn to turn a muscle on (or off) at will. Initially, the person may need to practise turning a particular (apparently paralysed) muscle on, learning to increase the trace on the monitor by increasing the amount the muscle contracts. A recent investigation involving specific exercise for triceps brachii (Wolf *et al.* 1994) showed that, in the group that received EMG feedback, mean EMG activity in triceps increased significantly. EMG activity also improved in the exercise-but-no-feedback group; however, this change was not significant.

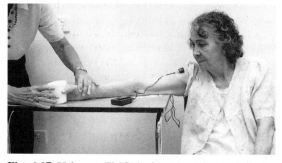

Fig. 6.17 Using an EMG device to monitor activity in deltoid muscle during attempts at reaching forward

The advantage of such a feedback system is that the patient can be encouraged to use it during the day as part of practice of particular tasks. It is likely that this aid to learning/training would enable more hours of practice than would be possible under therapist supervision. It is also likely that, for some individuals at least, practising with the monitor will be more interesting than practising alone.

Computer-generated feedback Of course, simple EMG feedback may not have as much potential to drive the person to practise as a more 'clever' device may have. For example, a recent study (Krichevets *et al.* 1995) demonstrates just how effective an interesting and interactive computer game can be. In this study, a game was set up which incorporated a lever apparatus which operated a computer game. The subject was a 13-year-old boy with Erb's palsy and virtually no active movement in the limb for which he substituted with well-practised adaptive movement patterns. The first aim was to 'break' these adaptive patterns; the second was to strengthen the main muscle groups of the limb. A special training device was made consisting of a computer and specially devised controls including counter-balancing weights. The game required accuracy from the subject in the control of spatial and temporal movement parameters. The subject's task was to move a 'sighting beam' over a submarine using a handle (see the cited article for details of apparatus). The controls were adjustable so that the movement required could be altered according to training objectives. At some point during training the boy started to activate shoulder external rotator muscles (previously inactive), and at the end of training he was able to raise the arm forward almost to shoulder height without his previous adaptive movements. The findings support the growing understanding that the most effective exercises are those in which the patient acts voluntarily, is an active participant and is motivated by the task itself and the desire to succeed.

Visual feedback Visual inputs appear critical to reaching and manipulation (e.g. Lee *et al.* 1983). A study of stroke suggests that reaching to a moving object shows better performance (smoother, faster movement with better timing) than reaching to the same object when stationary (Lee *et al.* 1984). It was suggested that recovery may be aided by exercises designed to visually drive the system. Certain other research findings suggest a dominance of vision over touch. In one study, subjects watched through a window what they thought was their own hand but was instead the experimenter's hand seen though a mirror (Rock and Harris, 1967). As a result of these findings and others, Rosenbaum (1991) suggested a training strategy for the disabled which involves the patient seeing an image of the limb with greater mobility than it actually has.

Mental practice

This may be a helpful technique for some patients, particularly when physical practice is difficult. Mental practice ('motor ideation') has been shown to affect regional cerebral blood flow (rCBF) post-stroke (Salford *et al*. 1995). This study showed a different rCBF during active arm movement compared to mental practice.

Electrical stimulation (ES)

Successful rehabilitation of upper limb function is dependent on the patient being able to regain the ability to activate muscles and to control segmental movements necessary for functional actions. It is also critical to minimize the secondary disuse changes that occur as a result of immobility. There has recently been increasing interest in the potential for new electrostimulation technologies to provide a means of stimulating muscles either to initiate or strengthen muscle activity or to reduce secondary changes in muscle.

When modern scientific scrutiny is applied to ES, it becomes clear that the effects on muscle and nerve are not at all clear, although ES has been used in physiotherapy for decades. After a review of the literature, Belanger (1991) concludes that ES appears to stimulate fast and slow motor units if the strength-training mode (high frequency/high intensity current for short periods) is used. This mode is painful and it is not known whether muscle damage can occur from inappropriate stimulation parameters or periods of use (Stokes and Cooper 1989). It appears that ES can also affect muscle fibre atrophy during immobilization, and affect muscle metabolism. The effect of ES on the re-establishing of functional motor performance is not known.

In patients following brain lesions, functional electrical stimulation (FES) – the use of multiple contraction sites to evoke a particular pattern of muscle activity – has been shown to have positive effects. These effects have been shown on recovery

of muscle function around the shoulder (Faghri *et al*. 1994) and on active wrist and finger extension (Kralj *et al*. 1993; Dimitrijevic *et al*. 1996; Pandyan *et al*. 1996; Hummelsheim *et al*. 1997). There is no evidence of generalization into improved functional activity, however, and to our knowledge there are no studies evaluating the combined effects of ES and upper limb exercise and training of actions.

ES to the hand via mesh-glove afferent ES has recently been shown to affect muscle activity after stroke. A study of 14 individuals between 8 and 69 months after stroke (Dimitrijevic *et al*. 1996) has demonstrated an increase in EMG activity in wrist extensors, increased amplitude of active wrist extension and decreased co-contraction of biceps brachii. The patients in this study all had some volitional control of wrist extension prior to the ES. ES triggered in EMG, in which ES is combined with voluntary effort, has also been reported to produce positive effects (Kraft *et al*. 1992).

It is possible that ES might prove a useful adjunct at the very least in preserving flexibility. Questions yet to be addressed include whether or not ES can enhance the effects of active exercise and training, and whether or not it has a positive effect on the condition of denervated or stiff muscle.

Orthoses

Slings or some form of orthosis are frequently recommended as a means of holding a limb in what is considered an 'optimum' position. The need for their use is very questionable and raises the issue of whether they can be a potent factor in causing learned non-use of the limb and adaptive muscle shortening. The latter is very likely, and the use of slings which hold the GH joint in internal rotation and adduction should be discontinued. The issue of shoulder supports is discussed in the Appendix to Chapter 11.

Orthoses are also recommended for stretching short muscles (or preventing muscles from shortening) (Sullivan *et al*. 1988; Ada *et al*. 1990) or for inhibiting hyperactive reflexes in individuals with dystonia or spasms following severe traumatic brain injury (TBI) (Sussman and Cusick 1979; Ada *et al*. 1990; Kitson 1991). Casting to prevent predictable muscle length changes following TBI may be effective when the individual is unconscious. *Serial casting* to stretch shortened muscles may also become necessary. Most investigations of serial casting have been of the lower limb. However, casting can also be used to stretch muscles or reduce dystonic spasms in the upper limb (Kitson 1991). (For description of casting refer to Chapter 12.)

In individuals with problems activating and controlling hand muscles, the thumb typically lies in an adducted position and web space soft tissues rapidly become short. In training, it may be helpful to support the thumb in a small orthosis so that the carpo-metacarpal joint is maintained in some abduction and opposition. The splint serves to maintain passively the extent of the grasp aperture so that, in the absence of active thumb abduction, the soft tissues between thumb metacarpal and index metacarpal do not shorten. If the splint is designed so that active abduction of the thumb, the splint may, when worn during training sessions, promote activity in the thumb muscles. A single case study (Goodman and Bazyk 1991) of a 4-year old child with cerebral palsy showed that wearing an opponens splint for 6 hours a day and all night for a 4-week period resulted in significant improvement in active range of movement and in some functional tasks. A small thumb splint can easily be made which allows hand use and which encourages thumb participation in reaching and grasping tasks during the day outside training sessions (Fig. 6.18).

Measurement

The use of a motor performance scale (e.g., Motor Assessment Scale for Stroke) enables ongoing evaluation of functional progress at regular intervals. Specific tests of aspects of hand function provide additional information. Tests of grip force, either of whole hand grip or pinch grip between thumb and index finger, may be particularly useful, since the control of grip force is a critical feature of all actions between hand and object and grip force may be a prognostic indicator of upper limb outcome (Sunderland *et al.* 1989). Relevant tests are outlined in Chapter 3.

In summary, the evidence suggests that *critical features in training of the upper limb* might be:

- Repetitive exercise/practice to activate weak/paralysed muscles
- Task-related training to improve strength and coordination
- Opportunity to practise intensively

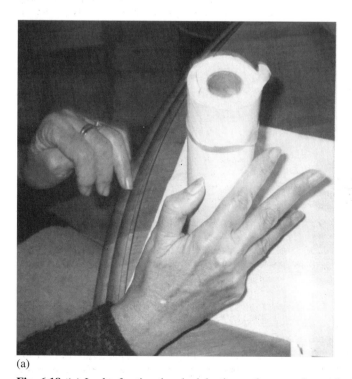
(a)

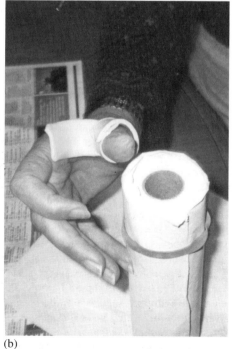
(b)

Fig. 6.18 (*a*) Lack of active thumb abduction makes grasping and releasing objects difficult. (*b*) A thumb splint holds the thumb in abduction enabling more effective practice. (Courtesy of C. Canning and C. Dean)

- Prevention of soft tissue adaptations, particularly muscle shortening, loss of extensibility and stiffness
- Prevention of painful shoulder
- Forced use of affected limb with constraint of the unaffected limb
- Avoidance of one-arm drive wheelchairs, slings and hand splints which impose immobility on the limb

Practice is likely to be enhanced by:

- Activities that provide motivation and incentive
- Activities that encourage flexibility
- Practice of concrete, interesting tasks rather than abstract actions
- Feedback

Progress is evaluated and information relevant to training is gathered by simple yet reliable and valid functional measures.

In conclusion, the major impairments affecting the upper limb following an acute brain lesion are weakness due to diminished motor outflow to muscles, diminished sensory inputs and the secondary impairments resulting from disuse and immobility. A major factor in poor recovery may be the minimal time spent in intervention and the use of outdated and apparently ineffective therapy methods. The evidence suggests, however, that there is significant scope for changes in attitude in health professionals and for new developments in motor and sensory training which could lead to a more functional outcome for a larger proportion of patients, particularly following stroke.

It seems evident, however, that some patients, even with intensive early training, regain only isolated muscle activity and cannot regain the ability to use the limb effectively. It is not known what proportion of people fall into this category (if category it is). Currently most therapy time is spent with the most impaired patients. Those with better recovery typically do not attract as much attention and tend to get discharged earlier. We would argue that, in the early stages, both groups of patients need intensive training and attention to the prevention of secondary soft tissue changes. When it is possible to predict, by testing, those individuals whose outcome for the upper limb is likely to be poor, two streams of rehabilitation can be developed. One which emphasizes preservation of soft tissue length and a simple daily programme of exercises to preserve existing muscle activity; the other emphasizing intensive task-related training, with and without therapist supervision.

If this were to happen, it may be found that the less impaired patients, who could be a larger group than yet recognized, may make a nearer to full recovery than they apparently do under most current rehabilitation regimes. Task-related training for those individuals who are approaching independence would involve training designed to address the sort of motor problems which are faced in everyday life. The use of work stations (Chapter 2), around which patients make a circuit, enables more practice time than the traditional one-to-one mode of delivery favoured by many therapists. What the severely impaired person can accomplish with exercise and training is not known and how long such training should persist is not known, yet the methods for seeking the answer to this question currently exist.

References

Ada, L., Canning, C., Kilbreath, S.L. *et al.* (1994) Task-specific training of reaching and manipulation. In *Insights into the Reach to Grasp Movement* (eds K.M.B. Bennett and U. Castiello) Elsevier, Amsterdam, pp. 239–268.

Ada, L., Canning, C. and Paratz, J. (1990) Care of the unconscious head-injured patient. In *Key Issues in Neurological Physiotherapy* (eds L. Ada and C. Canning), Butterworth Heinemann, Oxford, pp. 249–288.

Arbib, M.A., Iberall, T. and Lyons, D. (1985) Coordinated control programs for control of the hands. In *Hand Function and the Neocortex* (eds A.W. Goodwin and I. Darian-Smith), *Experimental Brain Research*, Suppl 10, Springer-Verlag, Berlin, pp. 111–129.

Balliet, R., Levy, B. and Blood, K.M.T. (1986) Upper extremity sensory feedback therapy in chronic cerebrovascular accident patients with impaired expressive aphasia and auditory comprehension. *Archives of Physical Medicine and Rehabilitation*, **67**, 304–310.

Basmajian, J.V., Gowland, C.A., Brandstater, M.E. *et al.* (1982) EMG feedback treatment of upper limb in hemiplegic stroke patients: a pilot study. *Archives of Physical Medicine and Rehabilitation*, **63**, 613–616.

Beaubaton, D. and Hay, L. (1986) Contribution of visual information to feedforward and feedback processes in rapid pointing movements. *Human Movement Science*, **5**, 19–34.

Belanger, A.Y. (1991) Neuromuscular electrostimulation in physiotherapy: a critical appraisal of controversial issues. *Physiotherapy Theory and Practice*, **7**, 83–89.

Bendz, P. (1993) The functional significance of the fifth metacarpus and hypothenar in two useful grips of the hand. *American Journal of Physical Medicine and Rehabilitation*, **72**, 210–213.

Biguer, B., Jeannerod, M. and Prablanc, C. (1982) The coordination of eye, head and hand movements during reaching at a single visual target. *Experimental Brain Research*, **46**, 301–304.

Bobath, B. (1990) *Adult Hemiplegia*, 3rd edn, Butterworth Heinemann, Oxford.

Bouisset, S. and Zattara, M. (1981) A sequence of postural movements precedes voluntary movement. *Neuroscience Letters*, **22**, 263–270.

Bourbonnais, D., Van Den-Noven, S., Carey, K.M. *et al.* (1989) Abnormal spatial patterns of elbow muscle activation in hemiparetic human subjects. *Brain*, **112**, 85–102.

Brouwer, B.J. and Ambury, P. (1994) Upper extremity weight-bearing effect on corticospinal excitability following stroke. *Archives of Physical Medicine and Rehabilitation*, **75**, 861–866.

Brudny, J., Korein, J., Grynbaum, B.B. *et al.* (1979) Helping hemiparetics to help themselves: sensory feedback therapy. *Journal of the American Medical Association*, **241**, 814–818.

Brunnstrom, S. (1970) *Movement Therapy in Hemiplegia,* Harper and Row, London.

Butefisch, C., Hummelsheim, H. and Mauritz, K-H. (1995) Repetitive training of isolated movements improves the outcome of motor rehabilitation of the centrally paretic hand. *Journal of the Neurological Sciences*, **130**, 59–68.

Carr J.H. and Shepherd R.B. (1987a) *A Motor Relearning Programme for Stroke*, Butterworth Heinemann, Oxford.

Carr J.H. and Shepherd R.B. (1987b) *Movement Science. Foundations for Physical Therapy in Rehabilitation* Aspen Publishers, Rockville, MD.

Carr, J.H. and Shepherd, R.B. (1996). 'Normal' is not the issue: it is 'effective' goal attainment that counts. *Behavioral and Brain Science*, **19**, 72–73.

Carr, J.H., Shepherd, R.B., Nordholm, L. *et al.* (1985) A motor assessment scale for stroke. *Physical Therapy,* **65**, 175–180.

Castiello, U., Bennett, K.M.B. and Paulignan, Y. (1992) Does the type of prehension influence the kinematics of reaching? *Behavioral Brain Research*, **50**, 7–15.

Castiello, U., Bennett, K.M.B. and Stelmach, G.E. (1993) The bilateral reach to grasp movement. *Behavioural Brain Research*, **56**, 43–57.

Chao, E.Y.S., An, K-N., Cooney, W.P. *et al.* (1989) *Biomechanics of the Hand*, World Scientific Publishing, Singapore.

Colebatch, J.G. and Gandevia, S.C. (1989) The distribution of muscular weakness in upper motor neuron lesions affecting the arm. *Brain*, **112**, 749–763.

Colebatch, J.G., Gandevia, S.C. and Spira, P.J. (1986) Voluntary muscle strength in hemiparesis: distribution of weakness at the elbow. *Journal of Neurology, Neurosurgery, and Psychiatry*, **49**, 1019–1024.

Colebatch, J.G., Rothwell, J.C., Day, B.L. *et al.* (1990) Cortical outflow to proximal arm muscles in man. *Brain*, **113**, 1843–1856.

Crosbie, J., Shepherd, R.B. and Squires, T.J. (1995). Postural and voluntary movement during reaching in sitting: the role of the lower limbs. *Journal of Human Movement Studies*, **28**, 103–126.

Crow, J.L., Lincoln, N.B., Nouri, F.M. *et al.* (1989) The effectiveness of EMG biofeedback in the treatment of arm function after stroke. *International Disability Studies*, **11**, 155–160.

Davies, P.M. (1985) *Steps to Follow,* Springer-Verlag, Berlin.

Davies, P.M. (1990) *Right in the Middle*, Springer-Verlag, London.

Dean, C. and Mackey, F. (1992) Motor assessment scale scores as a measure of rehabilitation outcome following stroke. *Australian Journal of Physiotherapy*, **38**, 31–35.

Dean, C. and Shepherd, R.B. (1997) Task-related training improves performance of seated reaching tasks following stroke: a randomised controlled trial. *Stroke*, **28**, 1–7.

de Souza, L.H., Hewer, R.L., Miller, S. *et al.* (1980) Assessment of arm control in hemiplegic stroke patients. 2: Comparison of arm function tests and pursuit tracking in relation to clinical recovery. *International Journal of Rehabilitation Medicine*, **2**, 10–16.

Dimitrijevic, M.M., Stokic, D.S., Wawro, A.W. *et al.* (1996) Modification of motor control of wrist extension by mesh-glove electrical afferent stimulation in stroke patients. *Archives of Physical Medicine and Rehabilitation*, **77**, 252–258.

Edwards, S. (1996) *Neurological Physiotherapy. A Problem-Solving Approach,* Churchill Livingstone, London.

Eyler, D. and Markee, J. (1954) The anatomy and function of the intrinsic musculature of the fingers. *Journal of Bone and Joint Surgery*, **36A**, 1–10.

Faghri, P.D., Rodgers, M.M., Glaser, R.M. *et al.* (1994) The effects of functional stimulation on shoulder pain in hemiplegic stroke patients. *Archives of Physical Medicine and Rehabilitation,* **75**, 73–79.

Fikes, T.G., Klatzky, R.L. and Lederman, S.J. (1994) Effects of object texture on precontact movement time in human prehension. *Journal of Motor Behavior*, **26**, 325–332.

Flanagan, J.R. and Wing, J.M. (1993) Modulation of grip force with load force during point-to-point arm movements. *Experimental Brain Research*, **95**, 131–143.

Flanagan, J.R., Ostry, D.J. and Feldman, A.G. (1993) Control of trajectory modifications in target-directed reaching. *Journal of Motor Behavior*, **25**, 140–152.

Forrest, W. and Basmajian, J. (1965) Function of human thenar and hypothenar muscles. *Journal of Bone and Joint Surgery*, **47A**, 1585–1594.

Gentile A.M. (1987) Skill acquisition: action, movement, and neuromotor processes. In *Movement Science. Foundations for Physical Therapy in Rehabilitation* (eds. J.H. Carr and R.B. Shepherd), Aspen Publications, Rockville, MD.

Gibson, J.J. (1977) The theory of affordances. In *Perceiving, Action and Knowing: Towards an Ecological Psychology* (eds R. Shaw and J. Bransford), Erlbaum, Hillsdale, NJ, pp. 67–82.

Goldie, P., Matyas, T. and Kinsella, G. (1992) Movement rehabilitation following stroke. *Research Report to the Department of Health, Housing and Community Services,* Victoria, Australia.

Goodman, G. and Bazyk, S. (1991) The effects of a short thumb opponens splint on hand function in cerebral palsy: a single-subject study. *American Journal of Occupational Therapy,* **45**, 726–731.

Gowland, C. (1982) Recovery of motor function following stroke: profile and predictors. *Physiotherapy Canada,* **34**, 77–84.

Gowland, C., deBruin, H., Basmajian, J.V. *et al.* (1992) Agonist and antagonist activity during voluntary upper-limb movement in patients with stroke. *Physical Therapy,* **72**, 624–633.

Heller, A., Wade, D.T., Wood, V.A. *et al.* (1987) Arm function after stroke: measurement and recovery over the first three months. *Journal of Neurology, Neurosurgery, and Psychiatry,* **50**, 714–719.

Hermsdorfer, J. and Mai, N. (1996) Disturbed grip-force following cerebral lesions. *Journal of Hand Therapy,* **9**, 33–40.

Hoff, B. and Arbib, M.A. (1993) Models of trajectory formation and temporal interaction of reach and grasp. *Journal of Motor Behaviour,* **25**, 175–192.

Hogan, N. and Winters, J.M. (1990) Principles underlying movement organization: upper limb. In *Multiple Muscle Systems: Biomechanics and Movement Organization* (eds J.M. Winters and S.L-Y. Woo) Springer-Verlag, New York.

Hummelsheim, H., Maier-Loth, M.L. and Eickhof, C. (1997) The functional value of electrical muscle stimulation for the rehabilitation of the hand in stroke patients. *Scandinavian Journal of Rehabilitation Medicine,* **29**, 3–10.

Iberall, T. and Lyons, D. (1984) Towards perceptual robotics. *Proceedings of IEEE International Conference on Systems, Man and Cybernetics,* Halifax, Nova Scotia, pp. 147–157.

Iberall, T., Bingham, G. and Arbib, M.A. (1986) Opposition space as a structuring concept for the analysis of skilled hand movements. *Experimental Brain Research,* **15**, pp. 158–173.

Jeannerod, M. (1981) Intersegmental coordination during reaching at natural visual objects. In *Attention and Performance* (eds. J. Long and A. Baddeley), vol. 9, Erlbaum. Hillsdale, NJ, pp. 153–168.

Jeannerod, M. (1984) The timing of natural prehension movements. *Journal of Motor Behavior,* **16**, 235–254.

Jeannerod, M. (1986) Mechanisms of visuomotor coordination: a study in normal and brain-damaged subjects. *Neuropsychologia,* **24**, 41–78.

Johansson, R.S. and Westling, G. (1984) Roles of glabrous skin receptors and sensorimotor memory in automatic control of precision grip when lifting rougher or more slippery objects. *Experimental Brain Research,* **56**, 550–564.

Johansson, R.S. and Westling, G. (1988) Programmed and triggered actions to rapid load changes during precision grip. *Experimental Brain Research,* **71**, 72–86.

Johansson, R.S. and Westling, G. (1990) Tactile afferent signals in the control of precision grip. In *Attention and Performance* (ed. M. Jeannerod) Erlbaum, Hillsdale, NJ, pp. 677–713.

Jones, R.D., Donaldson, M. and Parkin, P.J. (1989) Impairment and recovery of ipsilateral sensory-motor function following unilateral cerebral infarction. *Brain,* **112**, 112–132.

Kaminski, T.R., Bock, C. and Gentile, A.M. (1995) The coordination between trunk and arm motion during pointing movements. *Experimental Brain Research,* **106**, 457–466.

Kapandji, A.I. (1992) Clinical evaluation of the thumb's opposition. *Journal of Hand Therapy,* **5**, 102–106.

Karst, G.M. and Hasan, Z. (1990) Direction-dependent strategy for control of multi-joint arm movements. In *Multiple Muscle Systems: Biomechanics and Movement Organization* (eds J.M. Winters and S.L-Y. Woo) Springer-Verlag, New York, pp. 268–281.

Kelly, J.L., Baker, M.P. and Wolf, S.L. (1979) Procedures for EMG feedback training in involved upper extremities of hemiplegic patients. *Physical Therapy,* **59**, 1500–1507.

Kelso, J.A.S., Southard, D.L. and Goodman, D. (1979) On the coordination of 2-handed movements. *Journal of Experimental Psychology: Human Perception and Performance,* **5**, 229–238.

Kitson, A. (1991).Inhibitive castings for the upper limb: a case study. *Australian Journal of Physiotherapy,* **37**, 237–242.

Kraft, G.H., Fitts, S.S. and Hammond, M.C. (1992) Techniques to improve function of the arm and hand in chronic hemiplegia. *Archives of Physical Medicine and Rehabilitation,* **73**, 220–227.

Kralj, A., Acimovic, R. and Stanic, U. (1993) Enhancement of hemiplegic patient rehabilitation by means of functional electrical stimulation. *Prosthetics and Orthotics International,* **17**, 107–114.

Krichevets, A.N. Sirokina, E.B., Yevsevicheva, I.V. *et al.* (1995) Computer games as a means of movement rehabilitation. *Disability and Rehabilitation,* **17**, 2, 100–105.

Landsmeer, J.M.F. (1976) *Atlas of Anatomy of the Hand,* Churchill Livingstone, Edinburgh.

Lee, D.N., Lough, F. and Lough, S. (1984) Activating the perceptuo-motor system in hemiparesis. *Journal of Physiology,* **349**, 28.

Lee, W.A., Boughton, A. and Rymer, W.Z. (1987) Absence of stretch reflex gain enhancement in voluntarily activated spastic muscle. *Experimental Neurology*, **98**, 317–335.

Lemon, R.N., Bennett, K.M. and Werner, W. (1991) The cortico-motor substrate for skilled movements of the primate hand. In *Tutorials in Motor Neuroscience* (eds J. Requin and G.E. Stelmach), Kluwer, Dordrecht, pp. 477–495.

Lemon, R.N., Mantel, G.W.H. and Rea, P.A. (1990) Recording and identification of single motor units in the free to move primate hand. *Experimental Brain Research*, **81**, 95–106.

Lough, S., Wing, A.M., Fraser, C. *et al.* (1984) Measurement of recovery of function in the hemiparetic upper limb following stroke: a preliminary report. *Human Movement Science*, **3**, 247–256.

Marteniuk, R.B., Leavitt, J.L., MacKenzie, C.L. *et al.* (1990) Functional relationships between grasp and transport components in a prehension task. *Human Movement Science*, **9**, 149–176.

Marteniuk, R.B., MacKenzie, C.L. and Baba, D.M. (1984) Bimanual movement control: information processing and interaction effects. *Quarterly Journal of Experimental Psychology*, **36A**, 335–365.

Marteniuk, R.B., MacKenzie, C.L., Jeannerod, M. *et al.* (1987) Constraints on human arm movement trajectories. *Canadian Journal of Psychology*, **41**, 365–378.

Morris, D.M., Crago, J.E., DeLuca, S.C. *et al.* (1997) Constraint-induced movement therapy for motor recovery after stroke. *Neurorehabilitation*, **9**, 29–43.

Mudie, M.H. and Matyas, T.A. (1996) Upper extremity retraining following stroke: effects of bilateral practice. *Journal of Neurological Rehabilitation*, **10**, 167–184.

Muir, R.B. (1985) Small hand muscles in precision grip. In *Hand Function and the Neocortex* (eds A.W. Goodwin and I. Darian-Smith), (*Experimental Brain Research*, Suppl), **10**, Springer-Verlag, Berlin, pp. 155–174.

Muller, F. and Dichgans, J. (1994) Impairments of precision grip in two patients with acute unilateral cerebellar lesions: a simple parametric test for clinical use. *Neuropsychologia*, **32**, 265–269.

Nakayama, H., Jorgensen, H.S., Raaschou, H.O. *et al.* (1994a) Recovery of upper extremity function in stroke patients: the Copenhagen stroke study. *Archives of Physical Medicine and Rehabilitation*, **75**, 394–398.

Nakayama, H., Jorgensen, H.S., Raaschou, H.O. *et al.* (1994b) Compensation in recovery of upper extremity function after stroke: the Copenhagen stroke study. *Archives of Physical Medicine and Rehabilitation*, **75**, 852–857.

Napier, J.R. (1956) The prehensile movement of the human hand. *Journal of Bone and Joint Surgery*, **38**, 902–913.

Nass, R. (1985) Mirror movement asymmetries in congenital hemiparesis: the inhibition hypothesis revisited. *Neurology*, **35**, 1059–1062.

O'Dwyer, N., Ada, L. and Neilson, P.D. (1996) Spasticity and muscle contracture following stroke. *Brain*, **119**, 1737–1749.

Olsen, T. (1990) Arm and leg paresis as outcome predictors in stroke rehabilitation. *Stroke*, **21**, 247–251.

Ostendorf, C.G. and Wolf, S.L. (1981) Effect of forced use of the upper extremity of a hemiplegic patient on changes in function. *Physical Therapy*, **61**, 1022–1028.

Pandyan, A.D., Power, J., Futter, C. *et al.* (1996) Effects of electrical stimulation on the wrist of hemiplegic subjects. *Physiotherapy*, **82**, 184–188.

Parker, V.M., Wade, D.T. and Langton Hewer, R. (1986) Loss of arm function after stroke: measurement, frequency and recovery. *International Rehabilitation Medicine*, **8**, 69.

Putnam, C.A. (1993) Sequential motions of body segments in striking and throwing skills: descriptions and explanations. *Journal of Biomechanics*, **26**, Suppl. 1, 125–135.

Rock, I. and Harris, C.S. (1967) Vision and touch. *Scientific American*, **216**, (5), 96–104.

Rosenbaum, D.A. (1991) *Human Motor Control*, Academic Press, San Diego, CA.

Rosenbaum, D.A., Engelbrecht, S.E., Bushe, M.M. *et al.* (1993) Knowledge model for selecting and producing reaching movements. *Journal of Motor Behavior*, **25**, 217–227.

Rosenbaum, D.A., Vaughan, J., Barnes, H.J. *et al.* (1990) Constraints on action selection: overhand versus underhand grips. In *Attention and Performance* (ed. M. Jeannerod), Erlbaum, Hillsdale, NJ, pp. 321–342.

Rosenbaum, D.A., Vaughan, J., Barnes, H.J. *et al.* (1992) Time course of movement planning: selection of handgrips for object manipulation. *Journal of Experimental Psychology: Learning, Memory and Cognition*, **18**, 1058–1073.

Ryerson, S.D. (1995) Hemiplegia. In *Neurological Rehabilitation* (ed. D.A. Umphred), Mosby, St Louis, pp. 681–721.

Sahrmann, S.A. and Norton, B.J. (1977) The relationship of voluntary movement to spasticity in the upper motor neuron syndrome. *Annals of Neurology*, **2**, 460–465.

Salford, E., Ryding, E., Rosen, I. *et al.* (1995) Motor performance and motor ideation of arm movements after stroke: a SPECT rCBF study. In *Proceedings of the World Confederation of Physical Therapy Congress*, Washington, DC, p. 793.

Smith, A.M. (1981) The coactivation of antagonist muscles. *Canadian Journal of Physiology and Pharmacology*, **59**, 733–747.

Spoor, C. (1983) Balancing a force on the finger tip of a two-dimensional finger without intrinsic muscles. *Journal of Biomechanics*, **16**, 497–504.

Stokes, M. and Cooper, R. (1989) Muscle fatigue as a limiting factor in functional electrical stimulation: a review. *Physiotherapy Practice*, **5**, 83–90.

Sullivan, T., Conine, T.A., Goodman, M. *et al.* (1988) Serial casting to prevent equinus in acute traumatic head injury. *Physiotherapy Canada*, **40**, 6, 346–350.

Sunderland, A., Tinson, D., Bradley, L. *et al.* (1989) Arm function after stroke. An evaluation of grip strength as a measure of recovery and a prognostic indicator. *Journal of Neurology, Neurosurgery, and Psychiatry*, **52**, 1267–1272.

Sunderland, A., Tinson, D.J., Bradley, E.L. *et al.* (1992) Enhanced physical therapy improves recovery of arm function after stroke. A randomised controlled trial. *Journal of Neurology, Neurosurgery, and Psychiatry*, **55**, 530–535.

Sussman, M. and Cusick, B. (1979) Preliminary report: the role of short leg tone-reducing casts as an adjunct to physical therapy of patients with cerebral palsy. *John Hopkins Medical Journal*, **145**, 112–114.

Tang, A. and Rymer, W.Z. (1981) Abnormal force-EMG relations in paretic limbs of hemiparetic human subjects. *Journal of Neurology, Neurosurgery and Psychiatry*, **44**, 690–698.

Tanji, J., Okano, K. and Sato, K. (1988) Neuronal activity in cortical motor areas related to ipsilateral, contralateral and bilateral digit movement of the monkey. *Journal of Neurophysiology*, **60**, 325–343.

Taub, E. (1980) Somatosensory deafferentation in research with monkeys: implications for rehabilitation medicine. In *Behavioural Psychology and Rehabilitation Medicine* (ed. L.P. Ince) Williams and Wilkins, Baltimore, MD, pp. 371–401.

Taub, E., Miller, N.E., Novak, T.A. *et al.* (1993) A technique for improving chronic motor deficit after stroke. *Archives of Physical Medicine and Rehabilitation*, **74**, 347–354.

Tinson, D.J. (1989) How stroke patients spend their days. *International Disability Studies*, **11**, 45–49.

Trombly, C.A. (1993) Observations of improvement of reaching in five subjects with left hemiparesis. *Journal of Neurology, Neurosurgery, and Psychiatry*, **56**, 40–45.

Turner, D.P. and Ebrahim, S. (1992) Relation between handgrip strength, upper limb disability and handicap among elderly women. *Clinical Rehabilitation*, **6**, 117–123.

Twitchell, T.E. (1951) The restoration of motor function following hemiplegia in man. *Brain*, **74**, 443–480.

van Vliet, P. (1993) An investigation of the task specificity of reaching: implications for re-training. *Physiotherapy Theory and Practice*, **9**, 69–76.

Wade, D.T., Langton Hewer, R., Wood, V.A. *et al.* (1983) The hemiplegic arm after stroke: measurement and recovery. *Journal of Neurology, Neurosurgery, and Psychiatry*, **46**, 521–524.

Weir, P.L., MacKenzie, C.L., Marteniuk, R.G. *et al.* (1991a) Is object texture a constraint on human prehension? Kinematic evidence. *Journal of Motor Behaviour*, **23**, 205–210.

Weir, P.L., MacKenzie, C.L., Marteniuk, R.G. *et al.* (1991b) The effects of object weight on the kinematics of prehension. *Journal of Motor Behaviour*, **23**, 192–204.

Westling, G. and Johansson, R.S. (1984) Responses in glabrous skin mechanoreceptors during precision grip in humans. *Experimental Brain Research*, **66**, 128–140.

Wing, A.M. (1988) A comparison of the rate of pinch grip force increases and decreases in Parkinsonian bradykinesia. *Neuropsychologia*, **26**, 479–482.

Wing, A.M. and Fraser, C. (1983) The contribution of the thumb to reaching movements. *Quarterly Journal of Experimental Psychology*, **35A**, 297–309.

Wing, A.M., Lough, S., Turton, A. *et al.* (1990) Recovery of elbow function in voluntary positioning of the hand following hemiplegia due to stroke. *Journal of Neurology, Neurosurgery, and Psychiatry*, **53**, 126–134.

Wolf, S.L., Baker, M.P. and Kerry, J.L. (1979) EMG biofeedback in stroke. Effect of patient characteristics. *Archives of Physical Medicine and Rehabilitation*, **60**, 69–102.

Wolf, S.L., Catlin, P.A., Blanton, S. *et al.* (1994) Overcoming limitations in elbow movement in the presence of antagonist hyperactivity. *Physical Therapy*, **74**, 826–835.

Wolf, S.L., LeCraw, D.E., Barton, L.A. *et al.* (1989) Forced use of hemiplegic upper extremities to reverse the effect of learned nonuse among chronic stroke and head-injured patients. *Experimental Neurology*, **104**, 125–132.

Yekutiel, M. and Guttman, E. (1993) A controlled trial of the retraining of the sensory function of the hand in stroke patients. *Journal of Neurology, Neurosurgery, and Psychiatry*, **56**, 241–244.

Zajak, F.E. and Winters, J.M. (1990) Modeling musculoskeletal movement systems: joint and body-segment dynamics, musculotendinous actuation and neuromuscular control. In *Multiple Muscle Systems: Biomechanics and Movement Organization* (eds J.M. Winters and S.L-Y. Woo) Springer-Verlag, New York, pp. 121–148.

Further reading

Darian-Smith, I., Galea, M.P. and Darian-Smith, C. (1996) Manual dexterity: How does the cerebral cortex contribute? *Clinical and Experimental Pharmacology and Physiology*, **23**, 948–956.

Goodale, M.A., Milner, A.D., Jakobson, L.S. *et al.* (1990) Kinematic analysis of limb movements in neuropsychological research: subtle deficits and recovery of function. *Canadian Journal of Psychology*, **44**, 180–195.

Greene, P.H. (1982) Why is it easy to control your arms? *Journal of Motor Behavior*, **14**, 260–286.

Kelso, J.A.S., Buchanan, J.J. and Murata, T. (1994) Multifunctionality and switching in the coordination dynamics of reaching and grasping. *Human Movement Science*, **13**, 63–94.

Latash, L.P. and Latash, M.L. (1994) A new book by N.A. Bernstein: On Dexterity and its Development. *Journal of Motor Behaviour*, **26**, 56–62.

7

Balance

Introduction

The terms balance and equilibrium are often used synonymously. Balance can be considered to be the process whereby the body's equilibrium is controlled for a given purpose (Kreighbaum and Barthels 1985). Balance is also defined as the ability to control the body mass or centre of gravity (COG) relative to the base of support. Ghez (1991) describes what he calls a 'family of adjustments' which is needed in order to maintain a posture and to move. These adjustments have three goals: to support the head and body against gravity and other external forces; to maintain the centre of the body's mass (CBM) aligned and balanced over the base of support; to stabilize parts of the body while other parts of the body are moved (Ghez 1991).

The ability to balance and maintain a stable posture is integral to the execution of most movements. The functionally significant components of balance are maintenance of a posture, postural adjustments in anticipation of and during a self-initiated movement, and postural adjustments made in response to an external disturbance. Linked-segment dynamics play an important role in this control (Yang *et al.* 1990).

The adjustments we make in order to preserve equilibrium are flexible and varied due to the potential for dynamic interactions offered by the segmental linkage of which the body mass is composed. Postural adjustments are the muscle activation patterns and segmental movements that enable us to control this linkage in relation to the base of support. Movement of a body segment, whether through a self-initiated movement or an unexpected externally-imposed movement, per-turbs posture by imposing forces on adjoining and more distant segments, the destabilising forces arising from both inertia of the body segment moved and from physical contact with objects in the environment. Even the smallest movements, including taking a deep breath (Gurfinkel and Elner 1988; Bouisset and Duchene 1994), looking up or around the room, reaching for an object, need to be countered by movements of other segments.

Muscles close to the base of support, i.e., close to the fixed (supporting) segment, seem partic-ularly critical to our maintenance of a balanced body when we are moving and when we are still. In many self-initiated actions performed in both sitting and standing, activity typically begins in muscles closest to the base of support (Nashner 1977; Hirschfeld 1992; Crosbie *et al.* 1995), but this is not always the case.

In sitting on a seat, the base of support comprises the feet (on the floor) and the thighs (the amount depends on position relative to the seat and the size of the support surface); in standing, the feet form the base of support. For humans, the standing position is particularly challenging, since two-thirds of the body mass is some distance (about two-thirds of our height) above the base of support (Winter *et al.* 1990). Reducing the area of the base of support decreases the region of stability (Nashner and McCollum 1985).

Balancing the body mass while moving about is achieved by muscular activations called postural adjustments, which are known to occur before, i.e., in preparation for, a self-initiated focal limb movement (e.g., reaching out to grasp an object) as well as during the movement. Anticipatory (also called preparatory) postural adjustments occur to set up the segmental linkage in such a way that, when the hand is moved forward toward an object, for example, the body is kept steady and well balanced. In the automatic postural responses made to an unexpected destabilization, muscles are activated rapidly and in a relatively stereotyped manner. These rapid muscle activations are not, however, like reflexes, since they are appropriately scaled to achieve the goal of stability (Ghez 1991). That is to say, muscle 'responses' to stretch can adapt when necessary to ensure stability (Fig. 7.1).

Balance is constrained by the body's dynamics, including joint mobility, muscle length and strength, the physical environment, and prior experience. There is a perimeter beyond which, in standing, we cannot move the body mass without taking a step (i.e., making a new base of support) or overbalancing. The area in which we can maintain balance while moving is referred to as the 'region of reversibility' (Nashner and McCollum 1985) or 'limits of stability' (Carello *et al.* 1989). Of course, our 'perceived' limit of stability may be different if we perceive a threat to our stability brought about by visual inputs and fear or apprehension.

Balance emerges from a complex interaction of the sensory and musculoskeletal systems integrated and modified within the central nervous system (CNS) in response to changing internal and external/environmental conditions. The sensory system comprises the vestibular, visual and somatosensory systems but no one sensory system directly specifies the position of the COG (Horak *et al.* 1989). The vestibular system provides information about the position of the head in relation to gravity

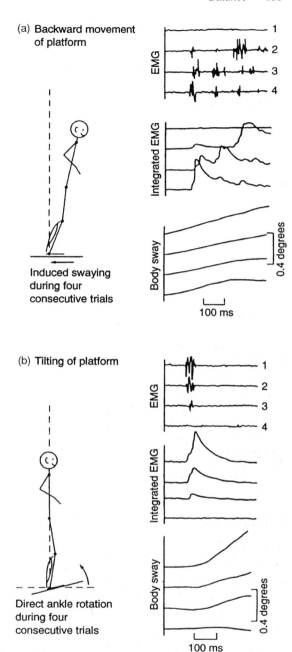

Fig. 7.1 Muscles that contract during unexpected support surface perturbation adapt according to stability needs. (*a*): Sway forward induced by unexpected backward platform movement triggers a rapid response in gastrocnemius muscle that occurs progressively earlier with repeated trials. (*b*): When the feet are unexpectedly tilted toes-up, contraction of gastrocnemius is attenuated after a few trials. In *a*, muscle activity would stabilize posture; in *b*, it has a destabilizing effect. (From Ghez 1991)

as well as to motion through linear and angular accelerations of the head. The proprioceptive system, consisting of muscle, joint and cutaneous receptors, provides information about the state of the effector apparatus, such as length and force output of muscle, our position in space and information about the environment, such as surface conditions. Proprioception provides, therefore, information about movement of the body in relation to the base of support and movement and orientation of body segments in relation to each other. Plantar cutaneous afferents have also been shown to play a marked role in balance regulation in standing (Do *et al.* 1990). The visual system has also been categorized as a proprioceptive system because it not only provides information about the environment but also about the orientation and movement of the body and thus provides exproprioceptive information (Lee and Lishman 1975).

The differing relative roles of sensory inputs is controversial, but, it is likely that they are coordinated in a task-relevant manner which is dependent on environmental circumstances. In certain types of laboratory investigations, particularly when the support surface is perturbed, able-bodied adults are said to rely primarily on somatosensory information under normal sensory conditions in which all sensory inputs are available (Nashner and Berthoz 1978). When support surface information is unreliable, for example when standing on a narrow beam, visual information increases in importance (Lishman and Lee 1973). The redundancy present within the sensory system in the maintenance of balance enables not only the verification of inputs, which may be conflicting, but also allows for compensation when one of the systems is dysfunctional (Winter *et al.* 1990).

The special role of vision

Our sensitivity to visual information appears particularly important to our skill in walking and balancing the body, since it specifies the relationship between ourselves and the properties of the environment (Owen 1985). Visual inputs tell us the position of relevant objects in the environment, our distance from them and whether they are stationary or moving. Visual information helps us judge when a moving object will reach us, or when we will land on the floor in a jump; that is to say, we can judge time-to-contact very accurately (Dietz and Noth 1978). This latter ability probably enables us to change our stride appropriately so that we correctly time when to place our foot on the kerb in

crossing the street. Time-to-contact information also helps us to walk through a crowded hall, to judge the closing doors of a lift (elevator), and to step on to an escalator.

Visual information helps us to orient ourselves vertically, although under certain conditions the information we receive may not be helpful. For example, in a dark room adults have been shown to alter their standing alignment to fit with the alignment of a luminous rod, even when it was angled away from the vertical (De Wit 1972). Another type of information comes more indirectly (i.e., not from direct visual fixation), from the optic array (see Gibson 1979). As we walk forward, for example, our surroundings move past us in an expanding optic array. In standing, visual information affects the amount we sway. Moving room experiments have shown that subjects sway inappropriately when the walls of the room move toward them or away from them. For example, in one experiment the movement of the walls away from the subjects presented similar optic array information (from peripheral vision) as would be present if they had swayed backward. Since they responded to this perceived sway (an illusion of self motion) by swaying forward, it appeared that they were rather more attuned to the visual (in this case incorrect) inputs than the proprioceptive inputs. However, the adult subjects did not fall, as did the toddlers who took part in a similar experiment (Lee and Aronson 1974). Self motion perception has been shown to be dependent on peripheral vision (e.g., Johansson 1977; Dichgans and Brandt 1978).

The sudden approach of an object or having an object (or person) close in front, provides a 'looming' effect which may evoke something like a startle response and a movement of the body backward. Therapists need to consider the effect of their standing too close in front of a patient who is having difficulty balancing. The narrower the support base and the lower the skill level of the individual, the more critical vision seems to be for balance, supporting an interaction between base of support, the availability of visual inputs and skill level (Slobounov and Newell 1994).

Given the important role of vision for our stability, we are dependent on the accuracy of the information provided by our structural environment. Owen (1985) describes some problems found with the construction of a long escalator to a subway. Lighting and wall tiling were oriented parallel to the direction of travel. Passengers had varying degrees of difficulty travelling on the escalator, with problems maintaining balance in an anteroposterior direction and even falling. At points during the trip, where there were no true horizontal or vertical references, the optic array was similar to that of a horizontal tunnel. Inputs from peripheral or central vision may have different effects on postural responses to support surface perturbations such as prevailed in the above example.

The ability to maintain a particular posture of the body (sitting, standing) and to move about in that position without falling involves:

- Generation of muscle activity to support the body mass against gravity and, therefore, to prevent collapse.
- Control of body segments in relation to each other.
- Control of body alignment in relation to the environment in which the body's COG must be maintained within the limits of stability.

The musculoskeletal components fundamental to control of balance include extensibility of soft tissue, active and passive-elastic properties of muscle. The neural components are those which control force generation and therefore strength.

Balance has been investigated under the relatively more static conditions of quiet standing, under different destabilizing physical and sensory conditions, and under natural conditions of self-initiated movement. Methods used have included monitoring the timing and sequence of muscle activation patterns using EMG; recording movement kinematics using accelerometers or cine or video motion analysis; and recording forces through the feet using a forceplate. Laboratory investigations into postural adjustments have shown that: postural adjustments are anticipatory and ongoing; they are task- and context-related; and vision provides critical 'exproprioceptive' information (Gibson 1979). Although the largest body of literature relates to balance in standing, more recently balance in sitting has also been subjected to laboratory and clinical experiments.

In daily life, there are three ways in which balance can be perturbed:

1 by an external force applied to the body itself or
2 via support surface movement and
3 by internal forces applied during a self-initiated movement.

In the first two, if perturbation is unexpected, postural adjustments occur after the perturbation in response to that perturbation. In the third, postural

adjustments precede or anticipate the perturbation as well as occurring throughout the movement. Investigations have been carried out, principally in standing, into both of these sources of perturbation.

Postural adjustments associated with self-initiated movements

In general, self-initiated actions are preceded by anticipatory or preparatory postural muscle activations and segmental movement. The probability that postural adjustment precedes a voluntary motor act was considered by Sherrington (Granit 1957), who suggested that such an adjustment would *not* be a reflex response, but that posture might be adjusted prior to an anticipated force.

Balancing in standing

The existence of postural activity prior to a movement was first established by Belenkii and colleagues (1967), who demonstrated that when subjects were asked to raise one arm as fast as possible, EMG activity of the focal muscle (anterior deltoid) and arm movement onset were preceded by activation of biceps femoris of the ipsilateral leg and contralateral sacrolumbar muscles.

Since then, other investigators have gone on to demonstrate that the anticipatory postural adjustments prior to a voluntary movement in standing appear, on the one hand, to be dependent on initial conditions, in particular on initial body posture or alignment (Lipshits *et al.* 1981; Cordo and Nashner 1982; Oddsson 1988), and, on the other hand, are specific to the forthcoming movement, the context in which it is taking place (Lee 1980; Bouisset and Zattara, 1981; Zattara and Bouisset 1986; Lee *et al.* 1987), the speed and amplitude of movement (Horak *et al.* 1984; Oddsson and Thorstensson 1987) and the amount of support provided (Cordo and Nashner 1982; Nardone and Schieppati 1988). Bouisset and Zattara (1987), by recording accelerations of limb segments, demonstrated that anticipatory muscle activity is associated with segmental movement and serves to counterbalance the inertia of forces due to movement of the arm which tends to disturb balance.

The specificity of muscle activation patterns to the intended movement has been shown in several actions (Fig. 7.2). Postural adjustments in lower limb muscles precede self-initiated pushing or pulling on a handle (Cordo and Nashner 1982). In this context, muscles are activated in a distal-to-proximal sequence, anterior lower limb muscles being activated when pushing on a handle and posterior lower limb muscles being activated when pulling on a handle. The amplitude of muscle activity also changes depending on the context. Interestingly, EMG activity in leg muscles prior to rapid, self-initiated push or pull movements of the handle was markedly decreased in amplitude if subjects were supported at the shoulder or even touched a rail with a single finger (Fig. 7.2) (Cordo and Nashner 1982). A similar result indicating the potent effect of external support was reported during heel-raising and toe-raising in standing (Nardone and Schieppati 1988).

Theoretically any muscle seems to be able to provide support. The long thumb flexor has been shown to provide postural support (Marsden *et al.* 1981). Subjects holding on to a stable rod activated their biceps brachii before their lower limb muscles when the support surface on which they were standing unexpectedly moved (Cordo and Nashner 1982). These findings are of note for clinicians since they demonstrate how conditions of support change the locus of balance. That is, support is provided by the muscles most likely to assist (Marsden *et al.* 1981).

Anticipatory leg muscle activity and movement of lower limb joints have also been recorded in *forward and backward trunk movements in standing* (Thorstensson *et al.* 1985; Crenna *et al.* 1987). The pattern and timing of head, trunk and lower limb movements appear to be dependent upon speed of movement. In addition, as one would expect, the patterns of movement differ according to whether bending takes place forward or backward.

The duration between activation of postural and focal muscles in investigations of both fast arm raising and pulling or pushing on a fixed handle have been reported to vary depending on the speed of the movement (Horak *et al.* 1984) and the degree of the expected perturbation and, therefore, the degree of postural compensation required (Bouisset and Zattara 1986). Furthermore, in very slow arm movements, there was considerable variation in the timing and sequencing of the muscles monitored and in many instances, deltoid showed the earliest measurable activity (Horak *et al.* 1984). In other words, very slow movements are not as perturbing as fast movements and, therefore, may not require anticipatory postural activation to the same extent.

There has been less investigation of *movement of the body mass in the frontal plane*. However, unpublished data indicate that, when one reaches

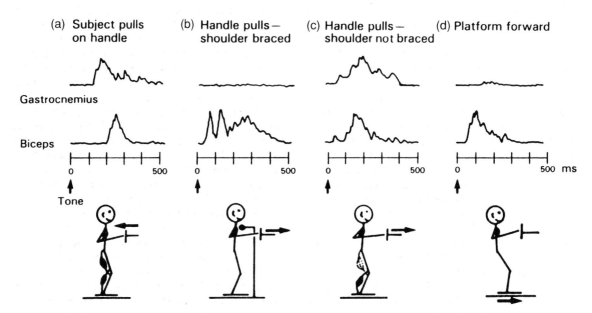

Fig. 7.2 The coordination of arm (biceps brachii) and leg (biceps femoris, gastrocnemius) muscles with different task requirements in standing – when subject is asked to pull on a handle (*a*); when the handle is unexpectedly pulled but subject is leaning against a chest support (*b*); when the handle is unexpectedly pulled with the subject free standing (*c*); and when the platform is unexpectedly moved forward (*d*). (Adapted from Nashner 1983, with permission)

out to the side in standing, the centre of pressure (COP) moves initially to the contralateral side, before moving to the side of the reaching arm. This implicates a role for the contralateral lower limb in 'pushing' the body toward the side of the reach. Studies of such actions as stepping and rapid single leg flexion, which involve shifting body mass toward the supporting leg, have similarly shown a shift of COP toward the side of the flexing leg before the shift toward the support leg (Rogers and Pai 1990, 1995). A consistent activation of hip abductor and adductor muscles has also been reported.

Postural adjustments during movements in the frontal plane occur principally at the shank–foot (invertors/evertors) and thigh–pelvis (abductors/adductors) linkages (Winter 1995). However, the hip muscles can exert far greater moments than the ankle muscles so it is considered that hip muscles probably play the greater part in balancing the upper body (Winter *et al.* 1993a).

In summary, volitional movements are associated with postural adjustments which are *anticipatory*, thus minimizing the perturbation of posture and movement, and which are *adaptable* to the conditions under which the action is carried out (Massion 1984).

Quiet stance

Although we do not often stand quite still, when we do, small movements of the body mass about the base of support occur which make up what is called postural sway. In other words, although passive elastic restoring forces are involved in these small movements, standing as still as possible is an active process, also involving changes in muscle activity (Day *et al.* 1993). The amount of sway in quiet standing varies according to a number of factors, including: environmental events which we pick up through vision, such as presence of objects moving past us (see Lee and Lishman 1975); whether or not the task requires a particularly small postural sway as in competition pistol shooting (Arutyunyan *et al.* 1969); and even how deeply we breathe (Gurfinkel and Elner 1973). The extent of postural sway increases when we close our eyes, illustrating the important role of vision in maintaining quiet stance.

Foot position and the width of base of support (Fig. 7.3) also affect the amplitude and velocity of body sway (Kirby *et al.* 1987). Sway in the frontal plane and to a lesser extent in the sagittal plane decreases when stance width is increased (Day *et al.* 1993).

Balancing in sitting

In contrast to the large number of investigations of postural muscle activity in standing subjects, there have been few investigations of postural adjustments in sitting. Nevertheless, sitting balance (measured as the ability to sit still and resist a push) has been suggested to be a good predictor of outcome following stroke (Wade *et al.* 1983; Sandin and Smith 1990).

Sitting does not present the same threat to stability as standing, due to the larger base of support. In contrast to standing, where the feet provide a small base of support, in sitting the thighs and feet make up the base of support. In sitting on the edge of a high bed, however, only the thighs are supported, which is the reason why one cannot reach as far forward or sideways in this position as in sitting on a stool or chair with feet on the support surface.

The postural adjustments made as we move about in sitting vary according to whether or not the feet are supported. If they are not, muscle activation to balance the body involves muscles linking pelvis and trunk (upper body) to the base of support (the thigh segments), i.e., muscles such as iliopsoas and gluteus maximus for movements in the sagittal plane, together with hip abductor and adductor muscles and quadratus lumborum in frontal plane movements. If the feet are on the floor, the muscles linking the upper body to the base of support include those linking shank segments to the feet, e.g., calf muscles and tibialis anterior. In both cases, trunk muscles are also active to stabilize the upper body as it moves about over the base of support.

The major functional activities carried out in sitting involve the upper limb(s). If we sit at a table with arms supported, we may need little ability to balance. However, if we are not supported by a table and we want to reach out into the workspace, we can reach much further when our feet are on the floor than when they are not (Chari and Kirby 1986). During fast reaching to a far target performed in sitting with the feet on the floor, it has been shown that the legs can play an active role as well as a supportive role as the base of support. Tibialis anterior muscles were active both before the arm started to move and during the movement, and ground reaction forces through the feet occurred in advance of arm movement (Crosbie *et al.* 1995). Tibialis anterior muscle activity, which is linked closely to the arm muscle activity just as it is to fast arm movements in standing, may

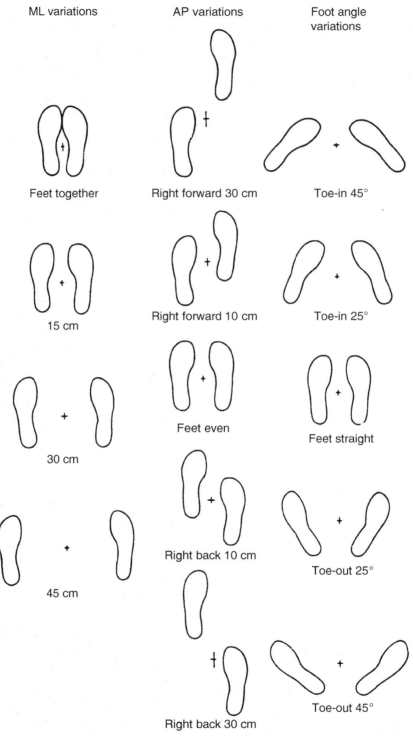

Fig. 7.3 Influence of foot position on position of centre of pressure (CP). The + sign represents the mean ± 1SD mediolateral (ML) and anteroposterior (AP) of CP positions for 10 subjects. For the AP variations of foot position, the feet were separated by 15 cm in the ML direction. (Reprinted from Kirby *et al.* (1987) The influence of foot position on standing balance. *Journal of Biomechanics*, **20**, 423–427. By permission of Elsevier Science Ltd)

provide some of the force moving the body mass forward (or diagonally sideways) toward the perimeter of the base of support. Soleus activity appears related to braking of the forward momentum and prevention of overbalancing (Fig. 7.4).

Activity of the muscles in the legs and of those which link the upper body with the thighs enable us to move our body mass about over the base of support within a certain perimeter. If we move our body mass beyond this perimeter, we overbalance

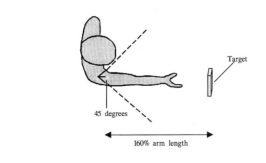

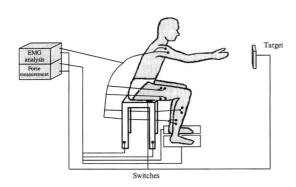

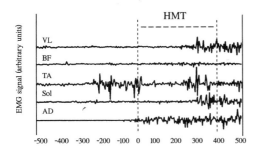

Fig. 7.4 (*top*) Laboratory set-up; (*lower*) trial from one subject showing typical EMG traces from ipsilateral vastus lateralis (VL), biceps femoris (BF), tibialis anterior (TA), soleus (S) and anterior deltoid (AD) in a forward reach

and have to make a new base of support by, for example, standing up, by moving a leg, or by falling on to our hands. A series of studies by Dean (1997) has shown that when we reach within the workspace at a comfortable speed, the legs play a less active role than in fast movement, but when we reach beyond arm's length, leg muscles are active, partly to assist in the initiation of body movement forward, partly to brake the forward movement so we do not overbalance forward. Studies confirmed that early tibialis anterior activity is associated with forward linear movement of the thighs, and therefore of body mass, and angular rotation of the shank at the ankle (Dean *et al.* 1996), and that calf muscle activity was associated with braking of forward movement and returning the body to erect sitting (Dean 1997).

Of importance to clinical practice is the fact that to reach in sitting involves not only movement of the arm but also movement of the trunk or upper body at the hips to extend the reach, together with active use of the legs to aid in balancing by making an 'active' base of support in much the same way as in standing. The distance we can reach appears to be affected by the extent of thigh support and whether one or both feet are on the floor, with the longest reach occurring with the most support (Dean 1997; Chari and Kirby 1986). Reaching sideways involves support and balance through the lower limb and is more destabilizing since the perimeter of the base of support is reached relatively early.

Postural responses to unexpected perturbations

Unexpected perturbations are typically experienced when sitting or standing on a supporting surface that moves, for example, on a train or a boat, when tripping over an obstacle or walking on a slippery surface, when pushed in a crowded street or during contact sports. Under these circumstances, postural adjustments tend to occur in response to perturbations which may be more threatening to balance, particularly if they are unexpected, than those associated with self-initiated movements. That is why we often grab hold of a stable object if we are perturbed or if we suspect we will be thrown off balance. Even under these circumstances, however, we use vision to predict the upcoming perturbation when we can and make preparatory adjustments accordingly. When we are practised at making these judgements, we may not need to hold on as the boat or vehicle moves about under us.

In laboratory settings, the response to unexpected perturbations has been examined by, for example, moving the supporting surface on which subjects stand or, alternatively, moving a handle held by subjects. Some of these investigations have also involved sensory manipulation in an attempt to identify the contribution of different sensory systems in detecting destabilization (e.g., Nashner and Berthoz 1978; Nashner *et al.* 1982).

Similar to perturbations associated with self-initiated movements, it appears that postural muscle activations in response to unexpected perturbations are specific both to the action and to the context in which that action is taking place. Muscles are activated in a distal-to-proximal sequence in response to both backward and forward platform displacements. Posterior muscles of the legs and trunk are activated to compensate for forward movement of the COG (backward displacement of the supporting surface) and anterior muscles are activated to compensate for backward displacement of the COG (Nashner and Woollacott 1979; McCollum *et al.* 1985; Nashner and McCollum 1985). It is of note that torque generated about the ankle is principally responsible for restoration of balance under these conditions (Nashner and Woollacott 1979; Nashner and McCollum 1985) reflecting the critical relationship between the fixed segment (feet) and the one directly above (the shank). Responses to unexpected perturbation have also been examined in long sitting on a movable platform (Hirschfeld 1992) and found to be as directionally specific as they are in standing (Moore *et al.* 1988).

A muscle may act as a postural muscle according to the environmental conditions prevailing at the time in responsive actions as well as in self-initiated actions. For example, in subjects who were holding on to a stable object when the support surface on which they were standing unexpectedly moved, biceps brachii functioned as a postural muscle, preventing them from losing balance (see Fig. 7.2) (Cordo and Nashner 1982).

Investigations have identified three postural synergies that are typically used in the maintenance of standing balance under different support surface conditions, which suggests that balance in the standing position is regulated and controlled by a limited number of postural synergies. The most common movement strategy in response to antero-posterior sway is the *ankle sway synergy*, in which postural adjustments are made principally at the

ankle joint and the individual sways as an inverted pendulum. In the *hip sway synergy*, postural adjustments are made principally at the hip, and, in the *suspensory synergy*, subjects flex at hip, knee and ankle to lower the COG toward the base of support (Nashner *et al.* 1979; Nashner and McCollum 1985; Horak and Nashner 1986) The hip sway synergy is considered to be used in response to large perturbations or when the supporting surface is too narrow to allow muscle activity at the ankle to exert sufficient force to restore balance (Nashner and McCollum 1985).

Such simplifying strategies may underlie the complex motor patterns that make up our daily activities. However, they may relate in the form described above only in response to unexpected perturbation. It may be more accurate to consider that the muscle activations (including postural muscle activations) that bring about balanced movement are task- and context-specific. Nevertheless, the constraints of the segmental linkage and its dynamics are major factors in the muscle activation patterns that emerge in action.

Withstanding the application of external forces

In daily life, we are often required to remain stable in standing in the presence of an external load, for example, holding a heavy object, standing in a crowd, playing a contact sport. Such forces may be applied in the sagittal or frontal plane or diagonally. It is likely that individuals with balance control impairments may have considerable difficulty coping in such a situation which requires the generation of sufficient muscle force to withstand the load and remain standing. There has, however, been relatively little investigation of this aspect of balance in either able-bodied or disabled individuals (Kobayashi and Matsui 1976; Lee *et al.* 1988; Wing *et al.* 1993).

Lee and colleagues (1988) found little difference between older (48–78 yr) and younger (20–40 yr) subjects in the maximal load they could withstand. Both groups, however, found posteriorly directed loads twice as destablizing as loads applied from the side or in an anterior direction. Interestingly, the authors found no relationship between subjects' ability to withstand a load and their scores on a clinical test which involved timed tests of standing in regular, tandem and single-leg stance, and a qualitative assessment of tilting reactions. This suggests that these tests are measuring different aspects of standing balance; the maximal load test measuring the ability to withstand loads applied externally without moving, while the clinical tests measure the ability to stand still on different sized bases of support, and assess the tilting reactions, i.e., the ability to respond to externally applied forces by moving.

Righting and equilibrium reactions

Historically, the term 'postural reflexes' has been used by physiologists to describe the mechanisms which are used to control our relationship to gravity and to enable us to maintain equilibrium in the upright position. They give us freedom to move despite our inherent instability (Martin 1967). These reflexes were categorized by Martin as antigravity mechanisms, mechanisms of postural fixation, protective, righting, locomotive, tilting reactions, and reactions to falling. These automatic responses occur when the support surface moves, when one is pushed by an external force and, in the case of the protective reactions, when one has lost balance and, in falling, makes a new base of support with the hands. It is this latter response which is responsible for so many upper limb fractures!

The early descriptions of the 'postural reflexes' were largely based on experimental evidence in animal physiology, particularly associated with brain lesion. Righting reactions (RR) were described several decades ago by Magnus and Rademaker, who observed these reactions in lesioned animals, and by Schaltenbrand and others who observed infants and children (see Magnus 1926). RR may be observed in young infants and, in exaggerated form, in mammals after decerebration experiments. RR are described as automatic reactions which produce orientation of the head in space (optical RR, labyrinthine RR, the body-on-head RR), and of the body in relation to the head and the support surface (neck-on-body RR, body-on-body RR).

Reactions that have to do with rebalancing the body when it is displaced by an external force have been termed postural fixation reactions, tilting or equilibrium reactions and parachute or protective reactions (Weisz 1938; Martin 1967). From the 1950s, Bobath was using the term postural reactions to encompass all balance-perturbing movements in response to external force (Bobath 1972; Bobath 1990). They considered postural reflex activity normally forms the necessary background for movement and functional skills (Bobath 1990).

Based on the experimental work earlier this century on lesioned animals and observational studies of human infants, righting and balance reactions were considered to make up a postural reflex mechanism, the development of which in infancy would be a critical precursor to developmental milestones and functional competence. Largely through the influence of the Bobath's work, these reactions have played a large part in the development of therapeutic activities in the last half of this century up to the present day (Bobath 1990; Davies 1990; Ryerson 1995; Edwards 1996). It is generally believed in child and adult neurological rehabilitation that part of therapy time should be spent in facilitating these righting and equilibrium (tilting) reactions (by therapist-induced perturbation or on a ball) since they form the background against which voluntary functional activity takes place (Bobath 1990). Some clinicians still consider ER and RR to be synonymous with balance (Ryerson 1995; Edwards 1996), even suggesting they precede and accompany gait (Badke and DiFabio 1985).

However, the physiological, biomechanical and psychophysical experimentation of the last few decades has resulted in increased understanding of movement and its control. In functional terms, the old dichotomy between balance and movement is less dominant as studies of functional actions are showing how difficult it is to separate postural adjustment from focal movement. Biomechanical studies are illustrating the task- and context-relatedness of postural adjustments and there is more emphasis on the examination of self-initiated movements.

The relationship of these reactions to the self-initiated movements we perform in daily life (and even the question of whether or not there is a relationship) is not clear (Hirschfeld 1992). It is likely, however, given current knowledge of the task-relatedness of postural adjustments in both self-initiated actions and in responses to unexpected perturbations, that postural reactions are very specific responses to a particular stimulus which makes an unexpected threat to stability.

Interestingly, considering the clinical emphasis on their significance, to our knowledge there has been little further investigation of these 'automatic postural reactions' since the original experiments early this century on lesioned animals, and no investigation of them in relation to functional activities. More recent experimentation on the nature and control of balance, however, has revealed the complexity of postural adjustments and balance and their dependence on task and context. Reactions to perturbations in alive, awake and active humans cannot be explained by stereotyped reactions found in lesioned animals, since a characteristic of the normal system is flexibility to task and environmental claims. That is, more recent views on how the neuromuscular system functions suggest that movement emerges in response to the demands of the task and the environment in which it is being performed (Bernstein 1967).

Nevertheless, many clinicians appear to believe that facilitating righting and tilting reactions will transfer into improved balance during self-initiated actions (Bobath 1990; Ryerson 1995). There is no evidence that this is so and it is probable that patients would regain effective balance abilities more quickly if these were trained as part of real-life situations. This view is being increasingly supported both in clinical texts (Shumway-Cook and Woollacott 1995) and by clinically-related research (Dean and Shepherd 1997).

Dynamic balance in walking

To walk straight ahead without veering to one side or increasing the base of support requires ongoing postural adjustment. The rhythm and speed of walking may mean that the actual amount of muscle activity involved in postural adjustment is minimal. If we stop mid-stride, however, it may be more difficult not to over-balance. Walking in a busy street increases the need to control balance against unexpected pushes and to control the body's path through the crowd.

Most of the literature on postural adjustments has focused on ways of keeping the body's COG safely within the supporting surface and, in particular, over the feet in upright standing. In gait, however, the COG may never pass within the area of the foot (Winter *et al.* 1990). For example, at the beginning of single support, the COG is posterior and medial to the stance heel and in double support the COG lies between the two feet. One of the problems in investigating postural adjustments in everyday activities is the difficulty in separating muscle activity into that which prevents collapse and brings about the movement, and that activity which is involved in coordinating balance. Functionally, the distinction cannot usually be made.

A recent study (Winter *et al.* 1993b) suggests that the upper body is balanced over the lower limbs during walking primarily by hip flexors and extensors in the plane of progression and hip abductor muscles in the frontal plane to counteract the imbalance of the upper body in single support. Foot placement also plays a role in balancing the body mass. Trunk muscles (e.g., erector spinae and trapezius) appear to perform a balancing function together with muscles linking the upper body with the lower limbs (e.g., gluteus maximus and lateral hamstrings).

Investigations into anticipated and unexpected perturbations during walking have demonstrated that they are context-specific and phase-dependent (Nashner 1980; Deitz *et al.* 1986; Figura *et al.* 1986; Patla 1986). When subjects are asked to pull or push on a handle during gait, the results indicate that they tend to time the push or pull to coincide with heel contact and that postural muscle activity precedes the onset of arm activity and is directionally specific (Nashner and Forssberg 1986). When Patla (1986) had subjects flex the arm rapidly at the shoulder in response to a visual cue during gait, postural activity preceded arm activity in stance phase and followed arm movement during swing. Thus, we can see how actions that are potentially destabilizing are timed to occur at an optimal time in the gait cycle to preserve stability.

Tripping, stumbling and falling

Occasionally when walking, we may trip and stumble. The source of tripping is often an uneven pavement, a misjudged step or an unseen or unexpected obstacle. Studies of stumbling due to unexpected support surface perturbation during treadmill walking and of falling forward show that context-specific adaptive bilateral muscle responses (gastrocnemius of one leg, tibialis anterior of other leg) take place to enable us to rebalance ourselves quickly (Dietz *et al.* 1984; Do *et al.* 1990). Muscle and cutaneous afferents appear to play an important role in these responses.

A trip can occur in the swing phase of walking if toe clearance is insufficient. When this occurs, knee flexors of the swinging leg and hip abductors and ankle plantarflexors of the stance leg have the shortest latencies when a trip is induced early in swing (Eng *et al.* 1994). The hip flexors respond later than these muscles and the dorsiflexor of the swinging leg, tibialis anterior, make a later and rather inconsistent response. When the trip occurs later in swing, however, the muscular response is different (Winter 1992, 1995).

Balance and ageing

In spite of a large body of literature which has attempted to characterize the effect of ageing on balance, the issue is complex and remains unclear. For example, with increasing age, there is the increased probability of the elderly individual developing specific pathologies which lead to accelerated degeneration in neural and/or musculoskeletal systems (Horak *et al.* 1989). A relatively inactive lifestyle may also result in disuse changes in the neuromuscular system, including muscle weakness and slowed response time. Horak and colleagues, in their review of postural instability in the elderly, also point out the different definitions of elderly and the relatively unselected populations typically investigated. Interestingly, when Gabell and Nayak (1984) screened a large group (1,187) of individuals of 65 years and over, they identified only 342 who were free of musculoskeletal and neural dysfunction. When the older and younger subjects in this latter group were compared on performance measures of gait, the older subjects performed as well as the younger group. The authors concluded that age-related changes in gait are due primarily to pathology.

Although postural sway has been found to increase with advancing age (e.g., Hasselkus and Shambes 1975; Hayes *et al.* 1985; Teasdale *et al.* 1991; Simoneau *et al.* 1992), there is considerable variability among subjects and this appears to be unrelated to functional ability. Furthermore, the amplitude of sway alone is not a good predictor of the likelihood of falls (Fernie *et al.* 1982). Interestingly, it has been demonstrated that aged subjects are able to decrease the amplitude of postural sway with practice (Holliday and Fernie 1979).

Disuse effects can also be common in certain groups of elderly individuals. For example, severe weakness of muscles controlling the ankle, particularly ankle dorsiflexors, was found to be present in a group of nursing home residents with a history of falls (Whipple *et al.* 1987). A combination of reduced sensation, leg muscle weakness and increased reaction time appear important factors associated with postural instability in the elderly (Lord *et al.* 1991).

The variability of sway scores in older adults may be related to inter-relationships between various musculoskeletal malalignments and impairments. In 1982, Brocklehurst and colleagues, for example, showed correlations between sway parameters and weight, scoliosis, knee angle and grip strength. Increased postural sway has also been reported in middle-aged adults with lower back dysfunction (Byl and Sinnott 1991).

One of the differences observed between younger and older subjects has been in the manner in which the body sways about the feet in standing. Where younger individuals tend to sway at the ankle when the support surface is perturbed (ankle strategy), older adults sway about the hip (hip strategy) (Manchester *et al.* 1989). The different responses in elderly subjects could reflect insufficient muscle strength to generate the necessary moment about the ankle (as shown in Whipple *et al.*'s study) or poor sensory feedback from, for example, plantar surface of the feet. Deterioration in cutaneous, visual and vestibular input has been reported in older individuals. However, it seems that it is the interaction between these systems which is critical for balance control. Older individuals (as well as the young) can shift from one sensory input to another if one input is disturbed but it appears that if two inputs are disturbed the older adults have more difficulty balancing.

In very old individuals (90–99 yr) performing self-initiated actions, it has been found that postural muscles could not be activated sufficiently far enough in advance of the focal muscle to keep from over-balancing (Mankovskii *et al.* 1980). Coactivation of muscles about a joint has also been reported under certain conditions of instability (Woollacott *et al.* 1986), but this stiffening of the limb could be an adaptation to poor timing of muscle activations and reflect a lack of skill.

Altered postural responses in elderly subjects, such as delayed onset latencies, intermittent reversal of muscle activation sequence and occasional co-contraction in lower leg muscles, have shown a tendency to improve with practice (Woollacott *et al.* 1982). In one study, although 6 of 12 subjects lost their balance on initial trials in two of the experimental conditions, all subjects but one improved on subsequent trials (Hansen *et al.* 1988). Lower limb strengthening exercises have also been shown to increase strength, improve balance and reduce falls in elderly individuals (Lord and Castell 1994; Sherrington and Lord 1997).

A major cause of balance difficulties in older adults may also be related to central and peripheral visual impairments and to visual perceptual impairments. Defective visual perception of horizontal and vertical has been implicated in falling in older adults (Tobis *et al.* 1981). Declining peripheral vision may also contribute to falls.

Movement dysfunction

Any disruption to the ability to control segmental alignment and to activate, coordinate and time muscle activity effectively and efficiently must necessarily compromise postural stability. Numerous impairments can contribute to this, including muscle weakness (Hamrin *et al.* 1982) due to poor recruitment of motor neurons, slowness of movement due to slow recruitment of motor neurons, poor timing of postural muscle activations, restriction of joint range due to adaptive soft tissue changes and loss of soft tissue extensibility, and sensory and perceptual deficits.

The control of postural adjustments is, therefore, commonly compromised in individuals with CNS dysfunction. For example, *during self-initiated movements*, individuals with Parkinson's disease have been shown to fail to generate anticipatory muscle activity in postural muscles when performing fast arm raising (Rogers *et al.* 1987). They may coactivate muscles in the lower limb, which results in stiffening the limb, rather than activate muscles in a directionally specific manner (Horak *et al.* 1988). Following stroke and head injury, muscle onset latencies may be slow which affects the ability to respond quickly to a loss of balance and to prepare for any impending disturbance to stability. Individuals with hemiplegia following stroke have been shown to demonstrate the same sequence of muscle activity in the muscles monitored (anterior deltoid, R. and L. biceps femoris, R. and L. paraspinal muscles) as that seen in normal subjects, when raising the arm with and without a weight, even though the hemiplegic subjects moved more slowly. In these individuals, there was a delay in anticipatory postural activity on the hemiplegic side which was particularly noticeable in the biceps femoris in both conditions. There are several other studies of stroke subjects performing self-initiated actions giving useful insights into the nature of impairments and of adaptations (in particular see Horak *et al.* 1984; Lee *et al.* 1988; Di Fabio and Badke 1990).

The ability to balance in standing *during a perturbation from an expected application of force* was examined in hemiplegic individuals who had to withstand the application of a maximal static load applied to the waist in the study by Lee and colleagues (1988). The patients were not able to withstand the same applied forces as either the younger or older able-bodied individuals and this was the case in both sagittal and frontal planes. This result is not surprising given that individuals after stroke have an impairment in muscle force generation (e.g., Sjostrom *et al.* 1980; Bohannon 1986), particularly with sustaining force. However, other contributing factors may be the presence of peripheral or central sensory impairments and muscle incoordination. In addition, on the clinical balance tests, the individuals with hemiplegia did not do as well as the older able-bodied subjects who, in turn, did not do as well as the younger subjects. It appears, therefore, that the clinical tests pick up impairments associated with ageing (or inactivity) and not just those associated with the brain lesion. Interestingly, the patients were no worse when force was directed toward the affected leg than to the unaffected leg.

A similar study (Wing *et al.* 1993) investigated the ability of stroke patients to withstand external forces applied mechanically to the hip in the frontal plane. As was found by Lee and colleagues, subjects were not obviously affected more by force applied to one side than to the other. However, stroke patients had more difficulty than controls in coping with the *release* of force when they had been pushed toward the affected side.

The regulation of standing balance *during unexpected perturbations* of the CBM can be compromised in a number of ways. Individuals with Parkinson's disease and with cerebellar truncal ataxia display weak or absent postural adjustments when attempting to resist displacement of a handle while standing (Traub *et al.* 1980). The appropriate synergy may be activated but the onset latency might increase. In a real-life situation, a slow response to unexpected movement of the handle one is holding for stability may result in a fall. Individuals with cerebellar dysmetria may demonstrate an excessive postural sway in standing with excessive muscle activity in response to instability which may itself cause the person to lose balance.

The ability to balance *during quiet standing* is typically examined using a forceplate to measure postural sway. Centre of pressure gives an indication of the distribution of body weight between the two feet. In individuals with hemiplegia, weight may be distributed asymmetrically, with the COP shifted towards the unaffected side (Dickstein *et al.* 1984; Sackley 1990). Higher vertical and horizontal ground reaction force magnitudes have been found in the sound leg in a group of individuals post-stroke, particularly in the anteroposterior directions, and the authors point out that this asymmetry illustrates a compensation (adaptation) for relative inactivity of the affected leg (Mizrahi *et al.* 1989). Variability of the path and amount of COP movement have also been reported (Di Fabio and Badke 1990).

The effect of immediate history and disuse changes

Disuse changes affecting many systems – cardio-vascular, musculoskeletal and neurological – may occur as a result of prolonged bed-rest or of a long period of relative inactivity in sitting, and these changes can occur in both young and older individuals (e.g., Robinson 1938; Saltin *et al.* 1968; Haines 1974; Minaire *et al.* 1974; Rayback *et al.* 1971). The resulting deficits, such as decreased VO_2 max, decreased muscle strength, decreased sensory receptiveness, all have the potential to augment balance disorders arising from impairments resulting primarily from brain lesion. Muscle weakness and secondary disuse changes in soft tissues, particularly of calf muscles, are known to affect directly the pattern of postural adjustments and therefore the ability to balance.

Many individuals who have brain lesions, partic-ularly following stroke, are elderly and may have become deconditioned prior to the lesion through an inactive lifestyle. In the period immediately follow-ing an acute lesion, a short but sometimes an extended period may have to be spent on bed-rest with the likelihood of further deconditioning. The effects will be worsened by continued inactivity and long periods spent in sitting during the rehabilita-tion period, particularly when there is little empha-sis on exercises and activities which preserve muscle length and extensibility.

In summary, the impairments underlying poor balance can include:

1 *Abnormal motor control*, with a decrease in rate and frequency of motor neuron activation and poor timing and coordination of muscle contrac-tions (i.e., loss of muscle strength and coordination).
  These problems of force and timing lead to an inability to control dynamic interactions between body segments to maintain a relatively stable posture against gravity, to respond quickly to unexpected external perturbations, to prepare for an upcoming perturbation, and to control balance during task performance.
2 *Visual, tactile, proprioceptive and vestibular impairments* which interfere with the processing of inputs from the environment and from movement itself.

Add to these impairments the secondary effects of:

3 *Adaptive behaviours*, such as stiffening the body, widening the base of support or using the arms to provide support and prevent a fall; adaptive *attitudes* such as not carrying out certain actions for fear of falling; adaptive *soft tissue changes*, which change the mechanics of movement by preventing the necessary range of joint rotations; adaptive *physiological changes*. Such adaptations prevent the person from ach-ieving flexible motor behaviour and interacting naturally with the environment.

Most adults with sensorimotor system dysfunction have problems making postural adjustments to self-initiated actions as part of a generalized motor control problem. The most commonly observed motor problems include:-

1 *Inability to generate sufficient force to support the body* (prevent collapse) in an upright posi-tion in appropriate segmental alignment.
  For example, in quiet standing a line from the COG should fall slightly in front of the lateral malleolus. Postural alignment may be affected by both mechanical and neural limitations.
2 *Inability to make effective anticipatory adjust-ments when in sitting or standing.* This may be due to delayed timing of muscular contractions and insufficient force generation which results in an inability to move about without swaying, staggering or overbalancing. Muscle weakness at the ankle, or calf muscle contracture, for example, can result in large compensatory hip and trunk movements.
3 *Difficulty with ongoing postural adjustments* due to poor timing of muscular contractions and poor grading of force output.
4 *Inability to put together in a coordinated manner the segmental rotations of which a motor act is composed.*

Since postural adjustments are a critical part of any volitional movement, the problems described above will be evident in anything the individual attempts to do, whether standing still, walking, stair climbing, standing up and sitting down or reaching for an object in sitting. It is likely that individuals may have difficulties with different aspects of preserving their equilibrium, for exam-ple, with balancing body segments while perform-ing motor actions like reaching to pick up an object or walking; with the ability to withstand externally applied forces, to brake excessive body movement;

and to move in response to an unexpected support surface perturbation.

In response to these problems, individuals with poor balance, utilize *adaptive motor behaviours* (Carr and Shepherd 1987; Shepherd 1992; Carr and Shepherd 1996). The range of mechanically possible adaptive movements has not been the subject of much investigation. However, it is likely that the adaptive behaviours listed below represent the most commonly observed (Figs. 7.5, 7.6).

Widening the base of support

This is achieved in sitting or standing by placing the legs apart. In addition, one or both legs may be externally rotated (Fig. 7.6b). The individual may walk with feet too widely spaced, or may not be able to stop without externally rotating the legs to increase the base of support still further. In standing, the individual may take a step prematurely when looking around or reaching out for an object, or may not venture to perform the full extent of a movement if it requires the CBM to move too near the edge of the perimeter of the base of support (Fig. 7.6a,c).

Using the hands for support

The individual may hold on to a stable object such as a chair or table, or clutch on to another person (Fig. 7.5a,b). This strategy, which is encouraged by the use of a support, such as a walking aid

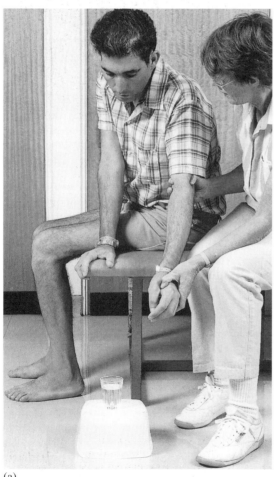

(a)

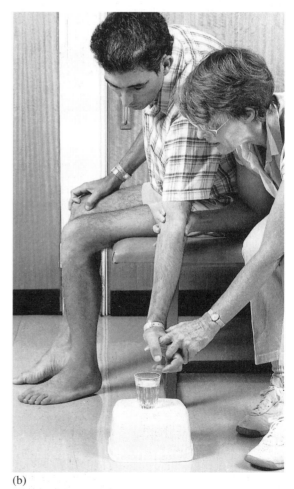

(b)

Fig. 7.5 (*a*) This man has a paretic L arm and leg, it is therefore difficult to move the body mass away from a stable position. As an adaptation, the R arm is used for support. (*b*) Assisted by the therapist, who supports his arm, he practises reaching sideways toward the glass. He is trying to use his L foot for support as this is necessary for stability when moving laterally. Note he is able to move further than in (*a*)

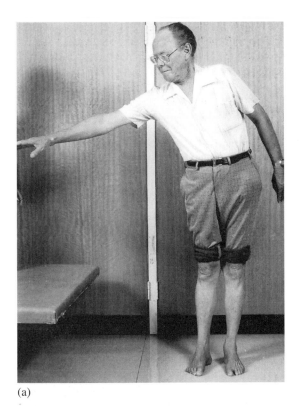

(a)

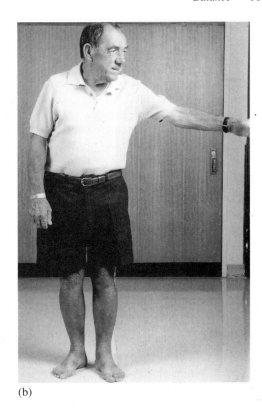

(b)

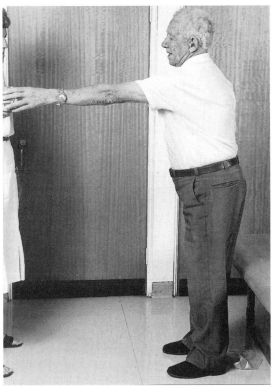

(c)

Fig. 7.6 (*a, b*) Adaptations made as a means of avoiding balancing on the weaker leg. It is possible to reach sideways by lateral movement of the spine and increasing shoulder girdle protraction. (*c*) In a forward direction, reach distance can be increased by flexion of the spine/hips and shoulder girdle protraction. However, in both directions, the distance to be reached is limited

(quadripod stick, walking frame), for standing or walking practice, has been shown to change muscle activation, kinetic and kinematic patterns.

Shifting on to the unaffected/less affected leg

This is common in standing and also affects spatial and temporal aspects of walking. It can occur in response to the fear of the weaker leg collapsing and to the relative slowness of muscle action.

Stiffening the body

This is a common adaptation in any individual who is afraid of overbalancing or who has poor control over timing and sequencing the muscles linking upper body to lower limbs and difficulty using the muscles around the ankle to correct excessive movement and to balance. Holding the body stiffly, measured as co-contraction in antagonist and agonist lower limb muscles in laboratory research, limits the excursion of movement.

The voluntary restriction of movement or stiffening of the lower limbs by antagonistic co-contraction could be a way of compensating for the inability to time muscle activity adequately. Co-contraction is typically found during learning of a motor skill when function is not optimal.

Avoiding the threat to balance

Individuals may not perform or may limit activities that threaten their balance. They align segments in ways that enable them to avoid moving the body mass too close to their limit of stability (Fig. 7.6*a,b,c*). In sitting, the individual may bend the trunk forward to reach for an object rather than sideways, since the latter involves shifting over a narrower base of support (see Fig. 7.12*a*).

In analysing motor performance and in planning appropriate intervention, it is critical to recognize the difference between primary problems affecting balance and the secondary adaptive behaviour which is the individual's way of coping with an underlying motor control impairment. Intervention should be directed toward the underlying impairment, with task-related training to improve muscle strength and control, incorporating means of preventing or avoiding adaptive behaviour as is described below. Where adaptive behaviour or soft tissue changes have already become established, it will be necessary to correct these as part of intervention. For example, it may be necessary to incorporate calf muscle stretching into the programme so that the body movement associated with reaching forward can be accomplished by dorsiflexion at the ankle. Severe soft tissue shortening may need to be corrected by serial casting (see p. 287).

Training

Assessment of balance in the clinic for practical reasons involves observational analysis. Postural adjustments are analysed initially in sitting and standing during self-initiated movements. This involves, for example, observing the individual's performance while reaching forward, sideways, down to the floor, to grasp or touch or lift up an object; while looking up at the ceiling, turning to look behind; and during walking under different conditions. As more knowledge is gained from bio-mechanical investigations of such actions and from studies of the effects of impairments on balance, so can the clinical analysis become more accurate. Some measures of balance for the purposes of evaluating change and outcome which are simple, reliable and valid, are given in Chapter 3.

The value of analysing equilibrium reactions, i.e., the ability of individuals to respond to support surface perturbations and to other external perturbations, is uncertain since these simple responses do not address the complex variety of postural impairments and adaptive motor behaviours seen in individuals with movement dysfunction. It is necessary for clinicians to understand that laboratory investigations of both self-initiated actions and responses to unexpected perturbations have repeatedly demonstrated the task- and context-specificity of postural adjustments. To continue using testing of RR and ER as the principal means of testing balance is to fly in the face of current knowledge and run the risk of wasting the patient's time on inappropriate evaluation and therapy.

For most patients, difficulties with balance can be addressed by training the types of action required in everyday life, such as standing up and sitting down, walking, stair walking, reaching to pick up objects. For example, training of standing up and sitting down (without using hands for support) is probably a most useful way to train balance for standing as well as for balance throughout the action itself (see Chapter 4).

Actions may need to be modified initially so that the postural adjustments required are relatively small, for example, reaching forward to pick up an object just beyond arm's length. The object can be moved further and further away so that the person

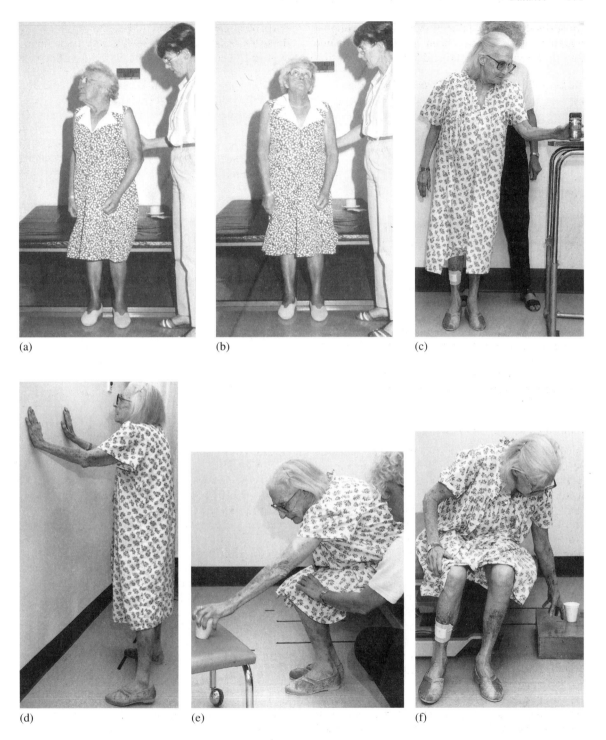

Fig. 7.7 Some methods of retraining the ability to perform simple actions in sitting and standing. They are simple because the extent of body movement is not great. (*a*) On her first attempt at standing, she practises looking around to find a target on the wall and (*b*) looking up. (*c*) Reaching sideways, attempting to move weight over L (affected) foot. (*d*) Walking sideways with some support, keeping body mass forward. (*e*, *f*) Using the L leg for support and balance

is reaching nearer to a point closest to the outside perimeter of the base of support (pushing the limits of stability). Such actions may be 'easier' for the patient because the objective of the practice is to get the object rather than to retain balance, and the goal is more concrete than abstract. Figure 7.7 shows some simple methods of retraining the ability to move the body mass about over the base of support using concrete goals. They involve quite small excursion of the body mass, as in:

● Looking up at the ceiling (anticipatory muscle activations of leg muscles ensure the CBM does not move back when the head is tilted back).
● Turning to look behind (scan the environment and pick out specified items) without moving the feet.
● Reaching forward to take an object.
● Reaching sideways.
● Reaching backwards.
● Reaching down to stool and floor.

Tasks are made progressively harder in both sitting and standing (Fig. 7.8) by such means as:

● Changing the shape of the base of support.
● Requiring increased flexion and extension of the legs.

● Increasing the object's distance from the body.
● Increasing the object's weight.
● Increasing the object's size so both hands must be used; and varying object weight.
● Changing the location of the object; moving laterally is harder than moving forward.
● Increasing speed demands.
● Requiring a quick response, as in catching a ball.
● Requiring that movement occurs in directions which are particularly hard to control for that individual.

These actions are all self-initiated and train postural adjustments, anticipatory and ongoing, as part of the actions themselves. The aim is for the person to be able to cope with the internal forces set up by the body's movement itself.

Stepping up and down exercises as described in Chapter 5 are also likely to train an individual's balance, since the movements involved present a threat to stability. In addition, such exercises help the individual regain strength and control of the lower limbs which may enable them to take more weight through the affected leg(s). Strength of muscles is a critical (although not always acknowledged) factor in preserving

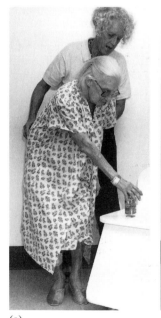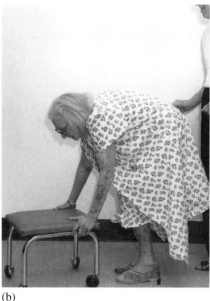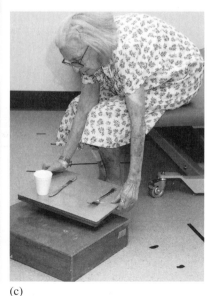

(a)   (b)   (c)

Fig. 7.8 Practice involving more difficult balancing tasks. (*a*) This reach involves hip, knee and ankle flexion and weight shift to the left. (*b*) This introduces the possibility of having to respond to the unexpected. (*c*) The task is to lift the tray without spilling water or dislodging utensils

balance. A modelling study (Kuo and Zajak 1993) suggests that the muscles which may be particularly important to strengthen are hamstrings, rectus femoris, gastrocnemius and tibialis anterior. We would add soleus, the gluteal and vasti muscles. Stepping exercises were used in a recent study (Sherrington and Lord 1997) as part of an exercise programme for elderly individuals following hip fracture. As a result of the intervention subjects had improved weight-bearing ability and reported fewer falls.

Although these exercises may need to be practised at first with some stability provided by the hands, or, preferably, by a harness, as balance (and leg muscle control) improves, the exercises can be practised without holding on, if this is possible. Balance adjustments through an affected limb can be 'forced' by including reaching movements while the individual stands with the foot of the unaffected/less affected leg on the step (see Bohannon and Larkin 1985) (see Fig. 5.19).

Sitting balance is considered a predictor of recovery from stroke (Bohannon *et al.* 1986;

Sandin and Smith 1990; Morgan 1994; Nitz and Gage 1995). It also appears highly correlated with independent locomotion at discharge (Morgan 1994; Nitz and Gage 1995). Sitting balance is not merely a matter of being able to sit still or resist external forces (as is tested in the Fugl-Meyer scale, p. 541). It infers the ability to move about in sitting and perform actions such as picking up an object from the floor. When balance is trained in sitting, therefore, emphasis is not only on the distance and direction reached but also on the need to use the lower limbs actively for balance and to extend the reach. A recent clinical study of individuals more than two years post-stroke showed that specific training designed to increase the distance that could be reached in sitting and, therefore the person's balance in sitting, showed a very positive result (Dean and Shepherd 1997). Not only could the subjects reach significantly further, and faster, but they had also regained similar muscle activation patterns and patterns of lower limb use as able-bodied subjects (Fig. 7.9). The control group did not improve.

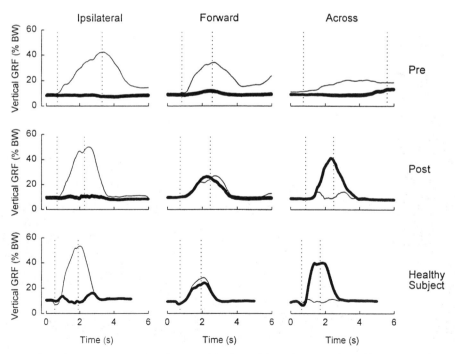

Fig. 7.9 Patterns of vertical ground reaction forces (% body weight) of one stroke subject pre- and post-training, reaching in three different directions. Heavy line: affected foot; light line: unaffected foot. Lower trace shows a healthy elderly subject reaching with the R hand for comparison. Heavy line: L foot; light line: R foot. Dotted vertical lines indicate onset and end of hand movement. (From Dean *et al.* 1997, by permission)

Other methods are used to train a person's ability to respond to external perturbations, such as:

- Standing on (and stepping on to) a moving walkway.
- Walking on a treadmill.
- Standing on a support surface which is subject to unpredictable perturbations.
- Walking in a crowded hall.
- Walking into and out of a lift (elevator).

After an acute lesion such as stroke it is unlikely that effective balance will be regained in a particular position (sitting, standing) until the individual can assume that position or is assisted to that position and can, therefore, practise. Similarly, postural adjustments are unlikely to develop as part of a specific action until that type of action is practised. It should be noted that the individual who cannot assume the upright positions of sitting and standing needs to be assisted into these positions and may, initially, need to practise reaching with some type of external constraint that controls some component of segmental alignment, for example, a soft leg splint to stop the knee from collapsing (see Fig. 5.18) or a harness to prevent a fall (see Hill *et al*. 1994) (Fig. 7.2).

Any opportunities for the person to use an external support in standing (i.e., to use the hands or be held up by the therapist) are avoided, since muscle activations are different if a part of the body other than the feet is used for providing stability. That is to say, when the therapist supports the patient, the patient's mechanism for maintaining stability changes. It has been shown in one study of a child with diplegic cerebral palsy that using a specific type of external mechanism (a body cast) for holding the segments and CBM aligned appropriately in standing was associated with markedly less co-contraction of lower limb muscles (Hirschfeld 1992). All monitored muscles were co-contracting when the child stood using a walking aid for support. When standing in a body shell, however, postural leg muscle responses to platform displacement occurred in a sequence. When he was in the body shell, the CBM projected in front of the ankle joints, that is to say with hip joints aligned over ankle joints, he was able to activate muscles more flexibly to respond to the threat to balance from the support surface perturbation. This demonstrates the importance of segmental alignment in optimizing effective postural control. It should be noted that the co-contraction

of muscles in a limb can give the impression of spasticity, although it may actually be an adaptive response to stiffen the limb and prevent collapse.

A *body harness* may be used to play a similar role. Hill and colleagues (1994) report decreased fear of falling (i.e., increased confidence) in a group of elderly individuals wearing a harness. Their results indicate that dynamic and natural movements were unhindered although they were carried out in the harness. Many of the standing exercises described in the section above could be performed in a harness (Fig. 7.10).

Movement, to be effective, must take place from an appropriate starting position, which involves body segments being appropriately aligned for the task to be performed. This is particularly critical in the early stage of training in order to avoid the habituation of adaptive movements and as a means of 'forcing' the desirable muscle activity. It is

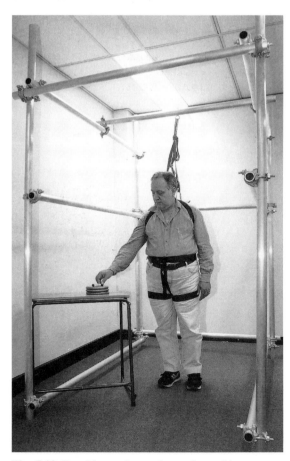

Fig. 7.10 Reaching tasks can be performed in a harness without close therapist supervision

typical, for example, for patients who have spent some time in bed to have difficulty getting their body mass sufficiently forward over the feet in standing (by movement at ankles and hips). Instead, patients tend at this stage to lean (or fall) backward, suggesting their perception of upright orientation is incorrect. Emphasis needs to be placed on the person actively moving the body forward at the ankles. The person may initially get the idea of what is required by practising walking sideways along a wall with the hands on the wall (see Fig. 7.7*d*). Objects in the environment can be used to help individuals orientate themselves. For example, a person with apparent difficulty perceiving the vertical, can be advised to line themselves up with a vertical object such as a door frame.

One way in which patients learn to adapt to poor stability is to avoid moving beyond a certain limited perimeter; i.e., the perceived limit of stability becomes very small. Concrete goals can help the person over-ride their fear of falling and the presence of the therapist close by (but not touching) can provide some emotional stability although the task may demand physical instability. Visual feedback can provide a means of training balanced movement over either a sitting or standing base of support which may provide a diversion

to overcome a reluctance to move. Computerized devices give feedback on a screen of the position of the COP as the person moves about and these make learning to move without losing stability both interesting and fun (Fig. 7.11) (Sackley and Baguley 1993).

Methods of modifying the environment to ensure the appropriate movement include outlining footprints on the floor as a way of providing information and motivation to an individual who tends to adopt a wide-based stance either in standing or while walking. Similarly, walking within a narrow track can force a narrow-based gait and provide the opportunity to practise the necessary muscle activations. Practice should always provide a challenge while still allowing the possibility of success. For example, if an individual does not have sufficient balancing ability to reach down to the floor to pick up an object in sitting or standing, the object can be placed on a box, in this way decreasing the amount of body displacement and weight shift (Fig. 7.12*a,b,c*). As the individual improves, the object can be placed progressively nearer to the floor and further away from the body mass.

Training to improve balance and the ability to move about effectively, based upon the findings of

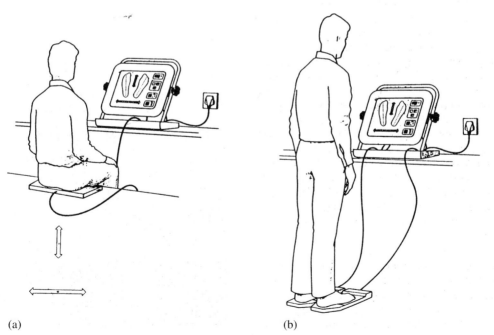

(a)   (b)

Fig. 7.11 Computerized devices such as the Balance Performance Monitor can be used to give feedback about postural sway. (Courtesy of SMS Healthcare.)

laboratory and clinical investigations, can be summarized as follows:

- Postural adjustments are task- and context-specific; they are anticipatory and ongoing in response to self-initiated movements and responsive when a change in segmental alignment is imposed from external sources.
- Adaptive motor behaviour may prevent the regaining of effective balancing in a variety of different situations.
- Vision provides exproprioceptive information and helps drive and control action.
- Modification of the environment can be used both to 'force' the desired action and to simplify the balance demands to enable active practice.
- Provision of exercises performed in standing as part of a general lower limb strengthening, stretching and coordination programme increases the time available to regain the ability to balance.

In conclusion, many laboratory investigations of postural adjustments under constrained conditions have demonstrated relatively stereotyped muscle activation patterns and motor patterns (e.g., Horak and Nashner 1986). What is clear, however, is that postural adjustments are probably stereotypical *only* under constrained and repetitive conditions. Changes in mechanical conditions engendered by different tasks in different contexts require different muscle activation and motor patterns. Furthermore, cognitive factors can also influence balance ability (Lee *et al.* 1988).

It appears that current clinical practice still emphasizes the eliciting of automatic postural reactions to an external perturbation applied by the therapist. 'Handling' and support by the therapist typically takes the place of self-initiated practice of actions such as reaching out in conditions in which the patient has to make the necessary adjustments in order to be stable. Fear on the part of the rehabilitation team that the patient is likely to fall seems to hold staff back from the intensive training that may help the patient regain the ability to balance independently. Lack of understanding of the importance of lower limb muscle strength to balance decreases the likelihood that rehabilitation will be effective in increasing balance and preventing falls, particularly in elderly individuals.

We would urge a change in attitude to balance training, with this part of rehabilitation given greater priority, and, where appropriate, the use of

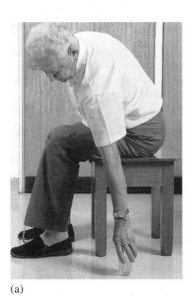 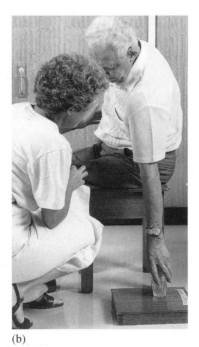 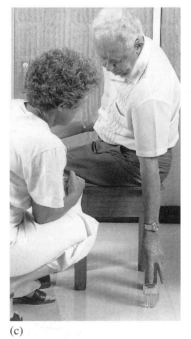

(a)   (b)   (c)

Fig. 7.12 Training reaching sideways. (*a*) He moves upper body forward and reaches back to the glass. (*b*) He can move his upper body sideways if the distance is decreased. (*c*) He practises reaching a greater distance. He will have to reach even further if he is to pick up the glass in his whole hand

a harness to allow the person to experience instability but without falling. More use could also be made of the various feedback devices available, so that the patient can practise with limited supervision and enjoy it.

References

Arutyunyan, G.A., Gurfinkel, V.S. and Mirskii, M.L. (1969) Organization of movements on execution by man of an exact postural task. *Biofizika*, **14**, 1103–1107.

Badke, M.B. and Di Fabio, R.P. (1985) Effects of postural bias during support surface displacements and rapid arm movements. *Physical Ther*apy, **65**, 1490–1495.

Belenkii, V.Y., Gurfinkel, V.S. and Paltsev, Y.I. (1967) Elements of control of voluntary movement. *Biofizika*, **12**, 135–141.

Bernstein, N. (1967) *The Coordination and Regulation of Movements*, Pergamon Press, New York.

Bobath, B. (1972) *Abnormal Postural Reflex Activity Caused by Brain Lesions*, 2nd edn, Heinemann Medical Books, London.

Bobath, B. (1990) *Adult Hemiplegia. Evaluation and Treatment*, 3rd edn, Heinemann Medical Books, Oxford.

Bohannon, R.W. (1986) Decreased isometric muscle knee flexion torque with hip extension in hemiparetic patients. *Physical Therapy*, **66**, 521–523.

Bohannon, R.W. and Larkin, P.A. (1985) Lower extremity weight-bearing under various standing conditions in independently ambulatory patients with hemiparesis. *Physical Therapy*, **65**, 1323–1325.

Bohannon, R.W., Smith, M.B. and Larkin, P.A. (1986) Relationship between independent sitting balance and side of hemiparesis. *Physical Therapy*, **66**, 944–945.

Bouisset, S. and Duchene, J-L. (1994) Is body balance more perturbed by respiration in seating than in standing posture? *Neuroreport*, **5**, 957–960.

Bouisset, S. and Zattara, M. (1981) A sequence of postural movements precedes voluntary movement. *Neuroscience Letters*, **22**, 263–270.

Bouisset, S. and Zattara, M. (1986) Chronometric analysis of the posturo-kinetic programming of voluntary movement. *Journal of Motor Behavior*, **18**, 215–223.

Bouisset, S. and Zattara, M. (1987) Biomechanical study of the programming of anticipatory postural adjustments associated with voluntary movement. *Journal of Biomechanics*, **20**, 735–742.

Brocklehurst, J.C., Robertson, D. and James-Groom, P. (1982). Skeletal deformities in the elderly and their effect on postural sway. *Journal of American Geriatrics Society*, August, 534–540.

Byl, N.N. and Sinnott, P.L. (1991) Variations in balance and body sway in middle-aged adults. *Spine*, **16**, 325–330.

Carello, C., Grosofsky, A., Reichel, F.D. (1989) Visually perceiving what is reachable. *Ecological Psychology*, **1**, 27–54.

Carr, J.H. and Shepherd, R.B. (1987) *A Motor Relearning Programme for Stroke*, 2nd edn, Butterworth Heinemann, Oxford.

Carr, J.H. and Shepherd, R.B. (1996) 'Normal' is not the issue: it is 'effective' goal attainment that counts. *Behavioural and Brain Sciences*, **19**, 72–73.

Chari, V.R. and Kirby, R.L. (1986) Lower-limb influence on sitting balance while reaching forward. *Archives of Physical Medicine and Rehabilitation*, **67**, 730–733.

Cordo, P.J. and Nashner, L.M. (1982) Properties of postural adjustments associated with rapid arm movement. *Journal of Neurophysiology*, **47**, 287–302.

Crenna, P., Frigo, C. Massion, J. *et al.* (1987) Forward and backward axial synergies in man. *Experimental Brain Research*, **65**, 538–548.

Crosbie, J., Shepherd, R.B. and Squire, T. (1995) Postural and voluntary movement during reaching in sitting: the role of the lower limbs. *Journal of Human Movement Studies,* **28**, 103–126.

Davies, P.M. (1990) *Right in the Middle*, Springer-Verlag, Berlin.

Day, B.L., Steiger, M.J., Thompson, P.D. *et al.* (1993) Effect of vision and stance width on human body motion when standing: implications for afferent control of lateral sway. *Journal of Physiology*, **46**, 479–499.

Dean, C. (1997) Stroke rehabilitation: factors affecting the performance and training of seated reaching tasks. Unpublished doctoral thesis, University of Sydney.

Dean, C.M. and Shepherd, R.B. (1997) Task-related training improves performance of seated reaching tasks following stroke: A randomised controlled trial. *Stroke*, **28**, 722–728.

Dean, C.M., Shepherd, R.B. and Adams, R. (1996) The effect of reach direction and extent of thigh support on the forces through the feet during seated reaching tasks. *Proceedings of the First Australasian Biomechanics Conference*, Sydney, Australia, p.p. 18–19.

De Wit, G. (1972) Optic versus vestibular and proprioceptive impulses measured by posturometry. *Agressologie*, **13**, 75–79.

Dichgans, J. and Brandt, T. (1978) Visual and vestibular interaction: Effects of self-motion perception and postural control. In *Handbook of Sensory Physiology*, vol. 8 (ed. R. Held, H.W. Liebowitz and H. Teuber), Springer-Verlag, Berlin.

Dickstein, R., Nissan, M. Pillar, T. *et al.* (1984) Foot–ground pressure pattern of standing hemiplegic patients: major characteristics and patterns of improvement. *Physical Therapy*, **64**, 19–23.

Dietz, V. and Noth, J. (1978) Pre-innervation and stretch responses of triceps brachii in man falling with and without visual control. *Brain Research*, **142**, 576–579.

Dietz, V., Quintern, J. and Berger, W. (1984) Corrective reactions to stumbling in man: functional significance of spinal and transcortical reflexes. *Neuroscience Letters*, **44**, 131–135.

Dietz, V., Quintern, J., Boos, G. and Berger, W. (1986) Obstruction of the swing phase during gait: phase-dependent bilateral leg muscle coordination. *Brain Research*, **384**, 166–169.

Di Fabio, R.P. and Badke, M.B. (1990) Extraneous movement associated with hemiplegic postural sway during dynamic goal-directed weight distribution. *Archives of Physical Medicine and Rehabilitation*, **71**, 365–371.

Do, M.C., Bussel, B. and Breniere, Y. (1990) Influence of plantar cutaneous afferents on early compensatory reactions to forward fall. *Experimental Brain Research*, **79**, 319–324.

Edwards, S. (1996) *Neurological Physiotherapy. A Problem-Solving Approach*, Churchill Livingstone, London.

Eng, J.J., Winter, D.A. and Patla, A.E. (1994) Neuromuscular strategies for recovery from a trip in early and late swing during human walking. *Experimental Brain Research*, **102**, 339–349.

Fernie, G.R., Gryfe, C.I., Holliday, P.J. and Llewellyn, A. (1982) The relationship of postural sway in standing to the incidence of falls in geriatric subjects. *Age and Aging*, **11**, 11–16.

Figura, F., Felici, F. and Macellari, V. (1986) Human locomotion adjustments during perturbed walking. *Human Movement Science*, **5**, 313–332.

Fitch, H.L., Tuller, B. and Turvey, M.T. (1982) The Bernstein perspective: III. Tuning of coordinative structures with special reference to perception. In *Human Motor Behaviour* (ed. J.A.S. Kelso), Lawrence Erlbaum Associates, Hillsdale, NJ, pp. 271–282.

Gabell, A. and Nayak, V.S.C. (1984) The effect of age on variability in gait. *Journal of Gerontology*, **39**, 662–666.

Ghez, C. (1991) Posture. In *Principles of Neural Science* (eds E.R. Kandel, J.H. Schwartz and T.M. Jessell), 3rd edn, Appleton and Lange, Norwalk, CT, pp. 596–608.

Gibson, J.J. (1979) *The Ecological Approach to Visual Perception*, Houghton Mifflin, Boston.

Granit, R. (1957) Systems for control of movement. In *Proceedings of the 1st International Congress of Neurological Science*, Brussels.

Gurfinkel, V.S. and Elner, A.M. (1973) On two types of static disturbances in patients with local lesions of the brain. *Agressologie*, **14D**, 65–72.

Gurfinkel, V.S. and Elner, A.M. (1988) Participation of secondary motor area of the frontal lobe in organization of postural components of voluntary movements in man. *Neurophysiology*, **20**, 7–14.

Haines, R.F. (1974) Effect of bed rest and exercise on body balance. *Journal of Applied Physiology*, **36**, 323–327.

Hamrin, E., Eklund, G., Hillgren, A.K. *et al.* (1982) Muscle strength and balance in post-stroke patients. *Upsala Journal of Medical Science*, **87**, 11–26.

Hansen, P.D., Woollacott, M.H. and Debu, B. (1988) Postural responses to changing task conditions. *Experimental Brain Research*, **73**, 627–636.

Hasselkus, B.R. and Shambes, G.M. (1975) Aging and postural sway in women. *Journal of Gerontology*, **30**, 661–667.

Hayes, K.C., Spencer, C.L., Riach, C.L., Lucy, S.D. and Kirshen, A.J. (1985) Age related changes in postural sway. In *Biomechanics IX-A*, (eds D.A. Winter, R.W. Norman, R.P. Wells *et al.*), Human Kinetic Publishers, Champaign, IL, pp. 383–387.

Hill, K.M., Harburn, K.L. Kramer, J.F. *et al.* (1994) Comparison of balance responses to an external perturbation test, with and without an overhead harness safety system. *Gait and Posture*, **2**, 27–31.

Hirschfeld, H. (1992) Postural control: Acquisition and integration during locomotion. In *Movement Disorders in Children* (eds H. Forssberg and H. Hirschfeld), Karger, Basle, pp. 199–208.

Holliday, P.J. and Fernie, G.R. (1979) Changes in the measurement of postural sway resulting from repeated testing. *Agressologie*, **20**, 225–228.

Horak, F.B., Esselman, P., Anderson, M.E. *et al.* (1984) The effects of movement velocity, mass displaced and task certainty on associated postural adjustments made by normal and hemiplegic individuals. *Journal of Neurology, Neurosurgery, and Psychiatry*, **48**, 1020–1028.

Horak, F.B. and Nashner, L.M. (1986) Central programming of postural movements: adaptation to altered support-surface configurations. *Journal of Neurophysiology*, **55**, 1369–1381.

Horak, F.B., Nashner, L.M. and Nutt, J.G. (1988) Postural instability in Parkinson's disease: motor coordination and sensory organization. *Neurology Report*, **12**, 54–55.

Horak, F.B., Shupert, C.L. and Mirka, A. (1989) Components of postural dyscontrol in the elderly: a review. *Neurobiology of Aging*, **10**, 727–738.

Johansson, G. (1977) Studies on visual perception of locomotion. *Perception*, **6**, 365–376.

Kelso, J.A.S. (1982) Coming to grips with the jargon. In *Human Motor Behaviour* (ed. J.A.S. Kelso), Lawrence Erlbaum Associates, Hillsdale, NJ, pp. 21–62.

Kirby, R.L., Price, N.A. and MacLeod, D.A. (1987) The influence of foot position on standing balance. *Journal of Biomechanics*, **20**, 423–427.

Kobayashi, K. and Matsui, H. (1976) Stability of standing posture against an external force. In *Biomechanics* vol. B (ed. P.V. Komi), University Park Press, Baltimore, MD, pp. 121–126.

Kreighbaum, E. and Barthels, K.M. (1985) *Biomechanics. A Qualitative Approach for Studying Human Movement*, 2nd edn, Macmillan, New York.

Kuo, A.D. and Zajak, F.E. (1993) A biomechanical analysis of muscle strength as a limiting factor in standing posture. *Journal of Biomechanics*, **26**, Suppl. 1, 137–150.

Latash, L.P. and Latash, M.L. (1994) A new book by N.A. Bernstein: 'On Dexterity and its Development'. *Journal of Motor Behaviour*, **26**, 56–62.

Lee, D.N. and Aronson, E. (1974) Visual proprioceptive control of standing in human infants. *Perception and Psychophysics*, **15**, 529–532.

Lee, D.N. and Lishman, J.R. (1975) Visual proprioceptive control of stance. *Journal of Human Movement Science*, **1**, 87–95.

Lee, W.A. (1980) Anticipatory control of postural and task muscles during rapid arm flexion. *Journal of Motor Behavior*, **12**, 185–196.

Lee, W.A., Buchanan, T.S. and Rogers, M.W. (1987) Effects of arm acceleration and behavioral conditions on the organization of postural adjustments during arm flexion. *Experimental Brain Research*, **66**, 257–270.

Lee, W.A., Deming, L. and Sahgal, V. (1988) Quantitative and clinical measures of static standing balance in hemiparetic and normal subjects. *Physical Therapy*, **68**, 970–976.

Lipshits, M.I., Mauritz, K. and Popov, K.E. (1981) Quantitative analysis of anticipatory postural components of a complex voluntary movement. *Fiziologiya Cheloveka*, **7**, 411–419.

Lishman, J.R. and Lee, D.N. (1973) The autonomy of visual kinaesthesis. *Perception*, **2**, 287–294.

Lord, S.R., Clark, R.D. and Webster, I.W. (1991) Postural stability and associated physiological factors in a population of aged persons. *Journal of Gerontology*, **46**, 3, M69–76.

Lord, S. and Castell, S. (1994) Physical activity program for older persons: Effect on balance, strength, neuromuscular control and reaction time. *Archives of Physical Medicine and Rehabilitation*, **78**, 208–212.

Magnus, R. (1926) Some results of studies in the physiology of posture. Part 2. *Lancet*, 18 September, pp. 585–588.

Manchester, D., Woollacott, M.H., Zederbauer-Hylton, N. and Marin, O. (1989) Visual, vestibular and somatosensory contributions to balance control in the older adult. *Journal of Gerontology*, **44**, 118–127.

Mankovskii, N., Mints, Y.A. and Lysenyuk, U.P. (1980) Regulation of the preparatory period for complex voluntary movement in old and extreme old age. *Human Physiology (Moscow)*, **6**, 46–50.

Marsden, C.D., Merton, P.A. and Morton, H.B. (1981) Human postural responses. *Brain*, **104**, 513–534.

Martin, J.P. (1967) *The Basal Ganglia and Posture*, Pitman, London.

Massion, J. (1984) Postural changes accompanying voluntary movements. Normal and pathological aspects. *Human Neurobiology*, **2**, 261–267.

McCollum, G., Horak, F.B. and Nashner, L.M. (1985) Parsimony in neural calculations for postural movements. In *Cerebellar Function* (eds J. Bloedal, J. Dichgans and W. Pratt), Springer-Verlag, Berlin.

Minaire, P., Neunier, P., Edouard, C. *et al.* (1974) Quantitative histological data on disuse osteoporosis. *Calcification Disease Research*, **17**, 57–73.

Mizrahi, J., Solzi, P., Ring, H. *et al.* (1989) Postural stability in stroke patients: vectorial expression of asymmetry, sway activity and relative sequence of reactive forces. *Medical & Biological Engineering & Computing*, **27**, 181–190.

Moore, S.P., Rushmer, D.S., Windus, S.L. *et al.* (1988) Human postural responses: responses to horizontal perturbations of stance in multiple directions. *Experimental Brain Research*, **73**, 648–658.

Morgan, P. (1994) The relationship between sitting balance and mobility outcome in stroke. *Australian Journal of Physiotherapy*, **40**, 91–95.

Nardone, A. and Schieppati, M. (1988) Postural adjustments associated with voluntary contraction of leg muscles in standing man. *Experimental Brain Research*, **69**, 469–480.

Nashner, L.M. (1977) Fixed patterns of rapid postural responses among leg muscles during stance. *Experimental Brain Research*, **30**, 13–24.

Nashner, L.M. (1980) Balance adjustments of humans perturbed while walking. *Journal of Neurophysiology*, **44**, 650–664.

Nashner, L.M. and Berthoz, A. (1978) Visual contribution to rapid motor responses during posture control. *Brain Research*, **150**, 403–407.

Nashner, L.M. and Forssberg, H. (1986) Phase-dependent organisation of postural adjustments associated with arm movements while walking. *Journal of Neurophysiology*, **55**, 1382–1394.

Nashner, L.M. and Woollacott, M. (1979) The organisation of rapid postural adjustments of standing humans: experimental and conceptual model. In *Posture and Movement* (eds R.W. Talbot and D.R. Humphrey), Raven Press, New York, pp. 243–258.

Nashner, L.M. and McCollum, G. (1985) The organisation of human postural movements: A formal basis and experimental synthesis. *Behavioral Brain Science*, **8**, 135–172.

Nashner, L.M., Black, F.O. and Wall, C. (1982) Adaptation to altered support and visual conditions during stance: Patients with vestibular deficits. *Journal of Neuroscience*, **2**, 536–544.

Nashner, L.M., Woollacott, M.H. and Tuma, G. (1979) Organization of rapid responses to postural and locomotor-like perturbations of standing man. *Experimental Brain Research*, **36**, 463–476.

Nitz, J. and Gage, A. (1995) Post stroke recovery of balanced sitting and ambulation ability. *Australian Journal of Physiotherapy*, **41**, 4, 263–267.

Oddsson, L (1988) Coordination of a simple voluntary multijoint movement with postural demands: trunk extension in standing man. *Acta Physiologica Scandinavia*, **134**, 109–118.

Oddsson, L. and Thorstensson, A. (1987) Fast voluntary trunk flexion movements in standing: motor patterns. *Acta Physiologica Scandinavia*, **129**, 93–106.

Owen, D.H. (1985) Maintaining posture and avoiding tripping. *Clinics in Geriatric Medicine*, **1**, 581–599.

Patla, A.E. (1986) Adaptation of postural response to voluntary arm raises during locomotion in humans. *Neuroscience Letters*, **68**, 334–338.

Rayback, R.S., Trimble, R.W., Lewis, O.F. *et al.* (1971) Psychobiologic effects of prolonged weightlessness 'bedrest' in young healthy volunteers. *Aerospace Medicine*, **42**, 408–415.

Robinson, S. (1938) Experimental studies of physical fitness in relation to age. *Arbeitsphysiologie*, **4**, 251–323.

Rogers, M.W. and Pai, Y-C. (1990) Dynamic transitions in stance support accompanying leg flexion movements in man. *Experimental Brain Research*, **81**, 398–402.

Rogers, M.W. and Pai, Y-C. (1995) Organization of preparatory postural responses for the initiation of lateral body motion during goal directed leg movements. *Neuroscience Letters*, **187**, 1–4.

Rogers, M.W., Kukulka, C.G. and Soderberg, G.L. (1987) Postural adjustments preceding rapid arm movements in Parkinsonian subjects. *Neuroscience Letters*, **75**, 246–251.

Ryerson, S.D. (1995) Hemiplegia. In *Neurological Rehabilitation* (ed. D.A. Umphred), Mosby, St Louis, pp. 681–721.

Sackley, C.M. (1990) The relationship between weight-bearing asymmetry after stroke, motor function and activities of daily living. *Physiotherapy Theory and Practice*, **6**, 179–185.

Sackley, C.M. and Baguley, B.I. (1993) Visual feedback after stroke with the balance performance monitor: two single-case studies. *Clinical Rehabilitation*, **7**, 189–195.

Saltin, B., Blomquist, G., Mitchell, J. *et al.* (1968) Response to exercise after bedrest and after training: A longitudinal study of adaptive changes in oxygen transport and composition. *Circulation*, **33**, Suppl. 7, 1–78.

Sandin, K.J. and Smith, B.S (1990) The measure of balance in sitting in stroke rehabilitation prognosis. *Stroke*, **21**, 82–86.

Shepherd, R.B. (1992) Adaptive motor behaviour in response to perturbations of balance. *Physiotherapy Theory and Practice*, **8**, 137–145.

Sherrington, C. and Lord, S.R. (1997) Home exercise to improve strength and walking velocity after hip fracture: A randomized controlled trial. *Archives of Physical Medicine and Rehabilitation*, **78**, 208–212.

Shumway-Cook, A. and Woollacott, M. (1995) *Motor Control. Theory and Practical Applications*, Williams & Wilkins, Baltimore, MD, pp. 221–232.

Simoneau, G.G., Leibowitz, H.W., Ulbrecht, J.S. *et al.* (1992) The effects of visual factors and head orientation on postural steadiness in women 55 to 70 years of age. *Journal of Gerontological Medicine*, **47**, M151–158.

Sjostrom, M., Fugl-Meyer, A.R., Nordin, G. *et al.* (1980) Post-stroke hemiplegia, crural muscle strength and structure. *Scandinavian Journal of Rehabilitation*, Suppl. 7, 53–61.

Slobounov, S. and Newell, K.M. (1994) Postural dynamics as a function of skill level and task constraints. *Gait & Posture*, **2**, 85–93.

Teasdale, N., Stelmach, G.E. and Breunig, A. (1991) Postural sway characteristics of the elderly under normal and altered visual and support surface conditions. *Journal of Gerontological Biological Science*, **46**, B238–244.

Thorstensson, A., Oddsson, L. and Carlson, H. (1985) Motor control of voluntary trunk movements in standing. *Acta Physiologica Scandinavia*, **125**, 309–321.

Tobis, J.S., Nayak, L. and Hoehler, F. (1981) Visual perception of verticality and horizontality among elderly fallers. *Archives of Physical Medicine and Rehabilitation*, **62**, 619–622.

Traub, M.M., Rothwell, J.C. and Marsden, C.D. (1980) Anticipatory postural reflexes in Parkinson's disease and other kinetic-rigid syndromes and in cerebellar ataxia. *Brain*, **103**, 393–412.

Tuller, B., Turvey, M.T. and Fitch, H.L. (1982) The Bernstein perspective: 11. The concept of muscle linkage or coordinative structure. In *Human Motor Behavior* (ed. J.A.S. Kelso), Lawrence Erlbaum Assoociates, Hillsdale, NJ, pp. 253–270.

Wade, D.T., Skilbeck, C.E. and Hewer, R.L. (1983) Predicting Barthel ADL score at 6 months after an acute stroke. *Archives of Physical Medicine and Rehabilitation*, **64**, 24–28.

Weisz, S. (1938) Studies in equilibrium reactions. *Journal of Nervous and Mental Disorders*, **88**, 160–162.

Whipple, R.H.,Wolfson, L.I. and Amerman, P.M. (1987) The relationship of knee-ankle weakness to falls in nursing home residents: An isokinetic study. *Journal of the American Geriatric Society*, **35**, 13–20.

Wing, A.M., Goodrich, S., Virji-Babul, N. *et al.* (1993) Balance evaluation in hemiparetic stroke patients using lateral forces applied to the hip. *Archives of Physical Medicine and Rehabilitation*, **74**, 292–299.

Winter, D.A. (1992) Foot trajectory in human gait – a precise and multifactorial motor control task. *Physical Therapy*, **72**, 45–56.

Winter, D.A. (1995) Total body kinetics: Our window into the synergies of human movement. Wartenweiler Memorial Lecture. *Proceedings of XVth Congress of ISB*, Jyvaskyla, Finland, pp. 8–9.

Winter, D.A., MacKinnon, C.D., Ruder, G.K. *et al.* (1993b) An integrated EMG/biomechanical model of upper body balance and posture during human gait. *Progress in Brain Research*, **97**, 359–367.

Winter, D.A., Patla, A.E. and Frank, J.S. (1990) Assessment of balance control in humans. *Medical Progress through Technology*, **16**, 31–51.

Winter, D.A., Prince, F., Stergiou, P. *et al.* (1993a) M/L and A/P motor responses associated with COP changes in quiet standing. *Neuroscience Research Communication*, **12**, 141–148.

Woollacott, M. H. (1993) Age-related changes in posture and movement. *Journal of Gerontology*, **48**, 56–60.

Woollacott, M., Shumway-Cook, A.T. and Nashner, L.M. (1982) Postural reflexes and aging. In *The Aging Motor System* (ed. J.A. Mortimer), Praeger, New York.

Woollacott, M.H., Shumway-Cook, A. and Nashner, L.M. (1986) Aging and postural coordination. *International Journal of Aging and Human Development*, **23**, 97–114.

Yang, J.F., Winter, D.A. and Wells, R.P. (1990) Postural dynamics in the standing human. *Biological Cybernetics*, **62**, 309–320.

Zattara, M. and Bouisset, S. (1986) Chronometric analysis of the posturo-kinetic programming of voluntary movement. *Journal of Motor Behavior*, **18**, 215–225.

Further reading

Day, B.L., Steiger, M.J., Thompson, P.D. *et al.* (1993) Effect of vision and stance width on human body motion when standing: implications for afferent control of lateral sway. *Journal of Physiology*, **469**, 479–499.

Diener, H.C., Horak, F., Stelmach, G. *et al.* (1991) Direction and amplitude precueing has no effect on automatic posture responses. *Experimental Brain Research*, **84**, 219–223.

Friedli, W.G., Hallett, M., Simon, S.R. (1984) Postural adjustments associated with rapid voluntary arm movements. 1. Electromyographic data. *Journal of Neurology, Neurosurgery, and Psychiatry*, **47**, 611–622.

Hazlegrave, C.M. (1994) What do we mean by a 'working posture'? *Ergonomics*, **37**, 781–799.

Lee, W.A. (1995) The emergence of global coordination during multijoint pulls made while standing. *Human Movement Science*, **14**, 639–663.

Massion, J. (1992) Movement, posture and equilibrium: interaction and coordination. *Progress in Neurobiology*, **38**, 35–56.

Rys, M. and Konz, S. (1994) Standing. *Ergonomics*, **37**, 677–687.

Schaeffer, L. and Bohannon, R.W. (1990) Perception of unilateral weight-bearing during unilateral and bilateral upright stance. *Perceptual and Motor Skills*, **71**, 123–128.

Part Three
Impairment and Disability Associated with Brain Lesion

8

The upper motor neuron syndrome

Introduction

It is common for both acute and chronic brain injury to involve the cortically originating motor system: the upper motor neuron, its pathways and connections. Lesions involving the cortico-fugal pathways, including the pyramidal tract, can occur at any level: in the cortex, internal capsule, brain stem or spinal cord. Such lesions may result from stroke, traumatic brain injury, multiple sclerosis, cerebral palsy or spinal cord injury.

In the neurosciences, it has been typical since Hughlings Jackson (Walshe 1961) to consider the dyscontrol characteristics associated with the upper motor neuron (UMN) syndrome as either *positive features* (abnormal behaviour) or *negative features* (impairments in muscle activation, motor control and performance) (Jackson 1958; Landau 1980; Burke 1988). This is the means of categorization used below since it has some explanatory

value for clinical practice (Carr *et al.* 1995). We have proposed another group of characteristics which we call *adaptive features*, since it appears likely that adaptive changes to neural system, muscles and soft tissues, and adaptive motor behaviours underlie some clinical signs (Fig. 8.1).

The negative and positive features appear to be relatively independent phenomena and related to the site and amount of tissue damage and spontaneous recovery processes (Landau 1980). Positive features are all exaggerations of normal phenomena or release phenomena, and include increased proprioceptive and cutaneous reflexes (spasticity). They are considered to be due to involvement of parapyramidal fibres (Shahani and Young 1980; Burke 1988), and may be related to secondary functional disturbances in surviving tissue. There is mounting evidence, however, that the negative features, the deficits in motor behaviour, including weakness, slowness of movement, loss of dexterity and fatiguability, are more disabling to the patient than the changes in muscle tone or hyperreflexia (Burke 1988; Landau 1988). Furthermore, patients themselves are usually more preoccupied with their loss of strength and dexterity, and with the stiffness associated with muscle changes, than with the manifestations of hyperreflexia.

The nature of what is called in the clinic 'spasticity' has been and remains a controversial issue. The term is typically used generically to encompass both negative and positive features: hyperreflexia, hypertonus, alteration of cutaneous reflexes and weakness (Bourbonnais and Vanden

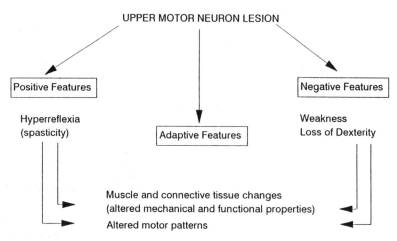

Fig. 8.1 The positive, negative and adaptive features of the upper motor neuron syndrome

Noven 1989). For example, the terms spastic hemiparesis or spastic paresis are commonly used following stroke or traumatic brain injury and in cerebral palsy. Although Hughlings Jackson considered the positive and negative features to be different in mechanism, others have assumed that the movement disability is directly related to hyperactive reflexes.

This chapter attempts to clarify the nature of the controversy, to discuss some recent research findings that are giving new, fresh insights into the nature of these clinical signs, and to make recommendations for clinical intervention based on recent research findings.

Negative features

Following a UMN lesion, there may be insufficient descending fibres converging on the final motor neuron population either to shape complex movements by graded activation of coordinating muscles or to bring motor neurons to the high frequency discharges necessary for tetanic contraction strength (Landau 1988). This insufficiency results in weakness (loss of strength of voluntary muscle action), slowness of movement and loss of dexterity and coordination. In addition, it is apparent that some disorganization of motor output at the segmental level arises which also contributes to the weakness (Tang and Rymer 1981).

When the system is in a state of shock after a lesion of acute onset, there may be a profound depression of motor function (Denny Brown 1950) in which all muscles of the affected limb(s) are involved. In this state, tendon reflexes may be decreased (hyporeflexia) or absent (areflexia). Clinically, the terms hypotonus, flaccidity, flaccid paralysis and paresis are used, interchangeably, to indicate a low state of 'tone'. Although they may be descriptive of the state of shock, the use of terms descriptive of tonus state is not particularly helpful since they are usually ill-defined (Denny Brown 1966; Eyzaguirre and Fidone 1975). It is preferable in our view to regard the absence of muscle activation as a state of paralysis or partial paralysis, since these terms are more clearly descriptive of the state of affairs.

The concept of tone itself is vague. Muscle 'tone' at rest is considered to be due exclusively to intrinsic muscle properties (Hufschmidt and Mauritz 1985). That is, normal muscle tone does not depend on neural mechanisms and any resistance to passive movement is due to mechanical factors (Burke 1988). The view that normal tone equates with a state of reflex activation of muscle at rest is no longer supportable given that there is no electrical activity in resting muscle or when a muscle is passively stretched in a relaxed subject (Fig. 8.2). Hypotonia was suggested to be an 'erroneous concept' by the authors of a study that compared relaxed normal with hypotonic limbs in a free fall test (Van der Meche and Van der Gijn 1986). They pointed out from their results that if a patient's limb feels flaccid this is the result of weakness preventing voluntary activity. Voluntary muscle activity present in most normal limbs was responsible for the resistance called 'normal tone'. They suggest that the use of the terms 'normal tone' and 'hypotonus' should be discontinued.

At rest   Voluntary contractions

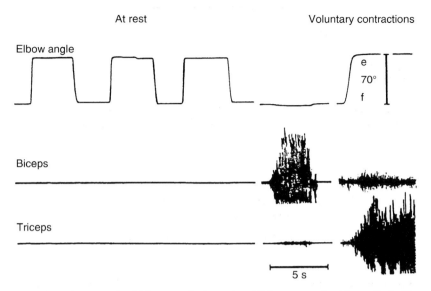

Fig. 8.2 The effects of passive stretch of biceps and triceps brachii in a normal subject. (*Left*) Abrupt stretches of 70° amplitude do not evoke any reflex activity in either muscle. (*Right*) The degree of amplification of the EMG trace when the muscles are contracted strongly by the subject (biceps in flexion; triceps in extension) is provided for comparison. (From Burke 1988, with permission)

The use of terms related to state of tone can distract the clinician from a clear understanding of the characteristics of the negative features which should usually be the focus of rehabilitative training. Such discussion of terminology is therefore not trivial, since the clinician's belief about the underlying mechanism will govern the type of therapeutic intervention. When it is understood that the patient has difficulty activating muscle, generating appropriate force and coordinating muscle forces, the clinician will use methods designed to help the patient elicit muscle activation and control movement.

Muscle weakness

The pyramidal tract is the executive pathway for volitional goal-directed movement (Phillips and Porter 1977) and any interruption to that pathway can produce considerable deficit. Interestingly, the investigation of spastic reflex activity has produced a very large body of literature, while the investigation of the mechanisms underlying muscle weakness and movement dyscontrol have been the subject of relatively less interest. However, there is general agreement that the major clinical sign is muscle weakness, or difficulty generating the necessary force for effective motor performance.

Muscle force produced is dependent upon the number and type of motor units recruited and the characteristics of both motor unit discharge and of the muscle itself. We increase muscle force by increasing the number of active motor units and increasing the firing rates of those active motor units. Firing of a motor unit results in a twitch (contraction) of the innervated muscle fibres. With an increase in firing rate, these twitches sum in order to increase and sustain force output.

Motor units are classified according to fatigue resistance and twitch tension into fast-fatiguable, fast fatigue-resistant and slow fatigue-resistant. Motor units are normally recruited in an orderly pattern, those which produce low forces being recruited first, followed by higher force-producing units as force requirements increase. Amount of force generated is matched to task demands.

After a UMN lesion, weakness is reflected in deficiencies in generating force and in sustaining force output (Bourbonnais and Vanden Noven 1989). It occurs due to loss of motor unit activation, changes in recruitment ordering and changes in firing rates. In addition, changes occur in the properties of motor units and in the morphological and mechanical properties of the muscle itself. These changes appear to be adaptations to loss of innervation, immobility and disuse.

Decreased motor unit firing rates have been reported in intrinsic hand muscles (Rosenfalck and Andreasson 1980) and in tibialis anterior (Dietz *et al*. 1986). An apparent adaptation to decreased motor neuron firing rates has been found in elbow flexor muscles of patients with hemiplegia (i.e., an abnormal force–EMG relationship) (Tang and Rymer 1981), with increased levels of EMG activity produced per unit force. Since a decrease in firing rate results in decreased tension generated by the active motor units, additional motor units would have to be recruited to counter the firing rate impairment and to enable a greater development of force. This would result in an increased sense of effort at low levels of activation, since a stronger central input would be required to generate a given level of force (Tang and Rymer 1981, p. 697). An increased sense of effort has been reported elsewhere under similar conditions (Gandevia and McCloskey 1977).

McComas and colleagues (1973) reported a 50% *decrease in functioning motor units* between the second and sixth month after stroke. They suggested that this was due to trans-synaptic changes in motor neurons following degeneration of corticospinal fibres and the tendency for surviving motor units to become slow-twitch in type. Evidence of denervation (e.g., Cruz-Martinez 1984), atrophy of some muscle fibres (especially fast-contracting fibres associated with FF and FR motor units) (Dietz *et al*. 1986), and hypertrophy of other muscle fibres (slow contracting fibres associated with slow motor units) (Edstrom 1970), have been reported.

Prolonged contraction times, particularly in fast contracting motor units, have also been reported (Young and Mayer 1982; Visser *et al*. 1985) and may be related to *changes in motor unit type*. In individuals within a month after stroke, a unique class of motor units, which are slow contracting and fatiguable and which are not present in normal muscles, have been found by Young and Mayer (1982). These authors suggested that these motor units originated from fast fatiguable units. It appears, therefore, that an increase in the proportion of functionally slow motor units may be responsible in part, along with loss or reduction in motor unit synchronization (Farmer *et al*. 1993), for the relatively slow rise to maximum tension of muscles, particularly those muscles with a high proportion of slow motor units. The fatiguability of the slow fatiguable motor units may help explain the poor endurance in sustaining muscle force output which is a common clinical observation. It is important to note that changes to muscle and motor unit may occur as a result of disuse following the brain lesion as well as of the diminished neural activation caused by the lesion.

The degree of weakness may differ for different muscle groups. Given that the pyramidal tract is the pathway for voluntary goal-directed movement, it has been suggested that interruption of this pathway produces a greater impairment in prime mover muscles (Burke 1988). For example, finger extension is usually weaker than wrist extension and both are weaker than flexion; flexor muscles of the lower limb tend to be weaker than extensors. In addition, since pyramidal innervation is denser for the distal muscles of the hand (including muscles which cross the wrist), there may be considerably more deficit in manipulation and prehension than is evident elsewhere and the greatest weakness is said to be in the intrinsic hand muscles.

Investigation of the muscles that cross the elbow has shown that the common clinical perception that the elbow extensors are weaker than the flexors is not necessarily so in individuals with hemiplegia following stroke (Sahrmann and Norton 1977; Dietz *et al*. 1981). Indeed, weakness may be more marked in flexors than in extensors (Fig. 8.3) (Colebatch *et al*. 1986).

It is commonly assumed that apparent weakness in a muscle group, such as triceps brachii, is solely due to restraint by spastic antagonists (elbow flexors). Sahrmann and Norton (1977), however, found that the primary impairment during rapid voluntary flexion and extension movements at the elbow was a limited and prolonged recruitment of the agonist muscle and delayed cessation of agonist contraction at the end of the movement. Contrary to the common belief among clinicians, they showed that the stretch reflex in the antagonist was not elicited in a way that would resist the agonist, and, therefore, that the antagonist stretch reflex was not a major contributor to the disability.

Another major cause for poor motor performance in patients with UMN syndrome is, therefore, the ineffectiveness of muscle contractions; i.e., impairments in muscle force generation and the timing of that force relative to the task at hand. Several investigations have shown a low degree of muscle (EMG) activity and abnormal muscle activation patterns in the lower limb of patients with hemiparesis during walking (Knutsson and Richards 1979). During the swing phase of gait, a low degree of EMG activity in triceps surae has

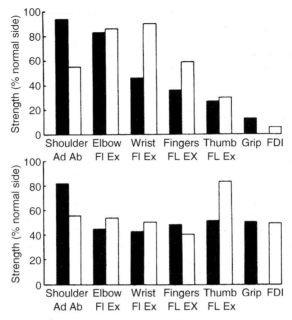

Fig. 8.3 Distribution of muscle weakness in two subjects with hemiparesis. Note that the subject shown in the top bar chart (infarct of corona radiata) shows greater distal than proximal muscle weakness; the subject in the lower chart (distal occlusion of basilar artery) shows a similar degree of involvement in all muscles tested. (From Colebatch and Gandevia, by permission)

been observed with abnormally high levels of activity in tibialis anterior (Dietz *et al.* 1981). In this example, it was evident that resistance to dorsiflexion was provided by changes in mechanical muscle fibres in the calf muscles rather than hyperactivity in calf muscle stretch receptors.

Adaptive changes in muscle such as increased stiffness of antagonists may be a major factor providing resistance to agonist contraction in some patients (Dietz *et al.* 1981). It seems likely that clinicians mistake these muscle changes for spasticity. This issue is discussed in some detail later in the chapter.

Another limitation to force generation has been assumed to come from abnormal patterns of muscle activation, including inappropriate and ungraded *co-contraction of agonist/antagonist muscles* (McLellan 1977; McLellan *et al.* 1985). Knutsson and Martensson (1980) suggested that 'antagonistic restraint' may be due to co-contraction caused by misdirected descending motor command signals, as well as facilitation of phasic stretch reflexes during voluntary effort. Co-contraction has been demonstrated in stroke patients walking (Knutsson and Richards 1979; Conrad *et al.* 1985), and in other movements (Knutsson and Martensson 1980; Berardelli *et al.* 1985). How-

ever, co-contraction of agonist and antagonist is a normal phenomenon. Furthermore, the presence of an unnecessary degree of co-contraction of antagonist muscles and of altered agonist–antagonist relationships is a similar phenomenon to that found in unskilled people as they attempt a new task. In patients, co-contraction may reflect the excessive muscle activity associated with lack of 'skill' in putting together task-related muscle activation (motor) patterns in the presence of inadequate recruitment of, for example, an agonist muscle. It is likely that patients adapt to poor strength and control by 'stiffening' the limb, i.e., by generating force full-on in muscles. Such a strategy may prevent limb collapse but in doing so may also restrict the flexibility of movement. Absence of the supraspinal control of Renshaw cells which normally accompanies voluntary movement may account for difficulty grading the strength of muscle contraction (Katz and Pierrot-Deseilligny 1982).

Slowness of muscle activation

Another manifestation of impairments in neural activation of motor units is slowness of movement and of initiating movement, to which weakness may contribute since the muscle forces needed to move, if they can be generated at all, are not built up quickly enough to carry out the movement at the usual speed. Slowness in walking (0.2–0.7 m/s for stroke subjects compared to 1.0–1.2 m/s for the able-bodied) has been reported (Giuliani 1990), and slowness in standing up from a seat (Ada and Westwood 1992).

It has been shown that, after stroke, individuals find it difficult to generate the force needed to move at high velocities (Bohannon and Smith 1987). A report from an EMG investigation showed a prolonged contraction time leading to maximum tension and a delay from onset of EMG activity to the rise in tension during the initiation of fast movements (Tsuji and Nakamura 1987). The slowing of the rate of voluntary muscle contraction is thought to be due to loss of inputs from fast large pyramidal tract neurons to motor neurons (see Burke 1988 for review). In fast alternating movements, slowness of movement appears to be associated with reduction of motor unit synchronization (Farmer *et al*. 1993). Knutsson and Martensson (1980) reported deficient capacity to accelerate motion up to a pre-set speed for slow as well as fast movements. However, they found that the capacity to develop force in fast movement was more impaired than in slow movements.

Loss of dexterity

The term dexterity has been used to describe the ability to 'fractionate' movement, to make independent movements, particularly for fine manipulation (Burke 1988). Dexterity has also been described as adroitness or skill in using the body (O'Dwyer *et al*. 1996), which infers the fine coordination of muscle activations that typifies the actions we confidently perform in our daily lives and in which we are skilled. Bernstein (1991; cited in Latash and Latash 1994) defined dexterity as the ability to solve any motor task rationally, precisely, quickly and deftly (p. 57). He suggested that dexterity, rather than being present in the motor act itself, is only present in its interaction with the changing environment. Dexterity depends on a sustained and rapid transfer of sensorimotor information between cerebral cortex and spinal cord motor neurons (Darian-Smith *et al*. 1996).

The extent to which loss of dexterity and muscle weakness are separate but related phenomena, i.e., whether or not loss of dexterity is due to weakness, is not clear. Relationships between strength of quadriceps muscles and walking speed, and

between strength of elbow flexors and the action of moving the hand to the mouth, have been reported (Bohannon *et al*. 1991; Bohannon 1992). A relationship has also been reported between grip strength and functional hand movements (Sunderland *et al*. 1989; Butefisch *et al*. 1995).

The relationship between strength (ability to generate sufficient muscle force) and dexterity (coordination of muscle activation) is unclear at the physiological level. In a functional sense, however, it is likely that they are linked, since the ability to generate force in a particular action requires the ability to generate force in synergic muscles including antagonists and muscles that stabilize the limb. Controlling synergic muscle linkages probably underlies dexterity. It is interesting that increasing muscle strength has been shown to be related to improved standing balance (Bohannon 1987, 1988).

The relationship between strength and dexterity may be more relevant (and therefore easier to show) in certain tasks. For example, a recent study used a laboratory tracking task designed to measure dexterity (of elbow flexion and extension) within the strength capabilities of subjects between 2 weeks and 24 months after stroke and a group of age-matched control subjects (Ada *et al*. 1996). Performance on the tracking task deteriorated at the faster speed in all subjects, with a more pronounced decrement for the stroke subjects, who also tended to move faster than was required to follow the targets. No statistical relationship was found between strength and dexterity in this task which required minimal muscle force generation but did require the ability to brake the forearm movement and to change direction (i.e., shift muscle activity). It is possible that the relationship between dexterity and strength may be to some extent task-related.

In summary, the negative clinical signs of weakness, slowness of movement and loss of dexterity are due to the lack of descending inputs on spinal motor neurons and impairments in coordination of motor unit activation. Inability to generate and time muscle forces are major reasons for functional disability, together with the adaptive changes that occur in soft tissues as a result of denervation, immobility and disuse.

Since clinicians have assumed that weakness of muscle is due to spastic constraint exerted by antagonists (Bobath 1978, 1990), and the dominant physiotherapy approach prioritizes the normalization of muscle tone, in particular, the inhibition of spasticity (Davies 1985; Bobath 1990; Ryerson

1995; Edwards 1996). Increased understanding of the complexity of physiological and adaptive mechanisms, however, suggests that these views can no longer be supported.

Positive features

The positive features of the UMN syndrome are the result of abnormal proprioceptive and cutaneous reflexes (Burke 1988), that is to say, reflex hyperexcitability. The characteristic clinical signs of exaggerated proprioceptive reflexes are the clasp-knife phenomenon (a velocity-dependent build-up of reflex resistance), exaggerated tendon jerk (a synchronized reflex response generated by abrupt mechanical disturbance) and clonus (a sustained reflex response set in train by tendon percussion). Exaggerated cutaneous reflexes produce a flexor withdrawal reflex, extensor and flexor spasms, which are manifestations of a severely damaged spinal cord, and a Babinski (extensor plantar) response (toe extension evoked by a stimulus provided to the plantar surface of the foot). The positive features appear to be of extrapyramidal rather than pyramidal origin but the underlying pathophysiological mechanisms remain somewhat obscure.

Spasticity has occupied a substantial amount of the neuroscience and rehabilitation literature for decades. It is the feature that most occupies the minds of clinicians whether they be from the therapy or the medical professions. However, as pointed out by Landau (1980), there is a major problem inherent in the word itself since it is commonly used clinically to signify many different features associated with brain lesions. These range from loss of strength to increased tendon jerks, and include the resistance offered to passive movement of a limb (also called hypertonus), and abnormal patterns of movement and posture. It is a fact that, for many clinicians, the term spasticity is commonly used in the clinic in a generic sense, and can cover all the phenomena seen following a UMN lesion.

This disparity in meaning has not made for ease of communication. In addition, it is becoming clear that there are other alternative explanations for some phenomena thought to be due solely to the positive neural features. For example, what is called by clinicians spastic hypertonus and described by patients as 'stiffness', may be related to mechanical and physiological changes occurring in the muscles, which are secondary adaptations.

Abnormal patterns of movement and posture may reflect behavioural adaptations to weakness and soft tissue changes rather than pathological patterns released by the lesion.

For the purpose of clarity, we accept the relatively narrow but widely accepted neurophysiological definition of spasticity as:

> a motor disorder characterized by a velocity-dependent increase in tonic stretch reflexes ('muscle tone') with exaggerated tendon jerks resulting from hyperexcitability of the stretch reflex as one component of the upper motor neuron syndrome (Lance 1980, p. 485).

This definition implies that the abnormality underlying spasticity is an adaptation of the stretch reflex. It is assumed that hyperexcitability of the reflex may cause the increased resistance to movement that the clinician feels when handling the limb of a person who has a brain lesion. However, the definition qualifies this assumption somewhat by limiting the definition to movements of particular velocities.

The stretch reflex consists of monosynaptic and polysynaptic pathways which conduct afference from various receptors, mostly from muscle spindles, but also from Golgi tendon organs (see Gordon and Ghez 1991 for a review). The phasic component of the stretch reflex (of which the tendon jerk is the best example) responds to a rapid abrupt stretch of the muscle. On the other hand, the tonic component of the reflex responds to stretch of the muscle by slow movement, and produces a graded response. For example, the tonic stretch reflex is modulated not only by the velocity of stretch but also by the length of the muscle at which the stretch occurs (Burke *et al.* 1970, 1971; Neilson and McCaughey 1982).

It is now accepted that the stretch reflex has a role in everyday activity although the nature of that role is unclear (see Davidoff 1992 for a review). We are normally able to regulate the overall responsiveness of the tonic stretch reflex and even to some extent the phasic stretch reflex (e.g., the Jendrassik manoeuvre increases the response to the tendon tap). During a movement, the reflex can be tuned up or down so that a perturbation will result in an added amount of muscle activity or not, as the situation requires (Neilson and Lance 1978; Colebatch *et al.* 1979; Gottlieb and Agarwal 1979; Rothwell *et al.* 1980; Kanosue *et al.* 1983). In other words, the stretch reflex may serve to add stiffness to a joint independently of central drive, thereby resisting a change in position. As well as the homonymous reflex pathway, there are also heteronymous pathways so that the response to stretch is also elicited in synergic muscles of the same segment (Lloyd 1943) as well as adjacent segments (Cavallari and Katz 1989). Therefore, when holding a glass of water, the stretch reflexes may be tuned up to resist a possible perturbation. If the hand is knocked, not only the muscles of the forearm, but also the muscles of the upper arm will contract to resist tipping the glass. The presence of both tonic and phasic components of the stretch reflex is, therefore, a normal phenomenon.

Normally, during relaxation, there is no electrical response even to slow or moderate stretching of the muscle (Burke 1983). However, in the presence of spasticity, where the sensitivity of the reflex is exaggerated, the individual may be unable to control the reflex, which then responds to stretch of muscle, whether appropriate or not. How relevant this phenomenon is to the functional deficit is uncertain.

Evolution of spasticity (reflex hyperexcitability)

In humans, both cerebral and spinal spasticity appear to have a slow time course of development following the initial insult, except in cases of high brain stem lesion (e.g., after traumatic brain injury), in which there may be an immediate increase in reflex state. Following stroke, reflex hyperexcitability (hyperreflexia) may be clinically evident 4–6 weeks after the lesion. According to Chapman and Weisendanger (1982), this slow time course suggests that plastic changes in synaptic connections may contribute to the development of spasticity. They point out that one response to denervation may be the formation of new synaptic connections through axonal sprouting. Since this sprouting has the same time course for development as that of hyperreflexia, the new, functional synaptic connections may actually mediate the hyperactive reflexes. Another possible response is an increase and abnormal sensitivity of pre- or post-synaptic elements to remaining afferent input, i.e., an increased chemical sensitivity. A third possibility is that previously inactive synapses may become active.

Hyperreflexia may, therefore, be the result of adaptations made by the neural system in response to neuronal disruption. In support of this is evidence that the magnitude of the reflex EMG response to short rapid stretch (found in normal subjects as well as after stroke) varies over time.

The response found one year after stroke has been found to be significantly larger than normal (Thilmann and Fellows, 1991; Thilmann *et al.* 1991a; Katz *et al.* 1992).

Of particular interest to clinicians is the evidence that the process of reorganization of remaining circuitry as well as structural changes within the CNS may be directly influenced, both positively or negatively, by certain external events (Marshall 1990; Merzenich *et al.* 1991; Lee and van Donkelaar 1995; see Chapter 2) which could include the patient's post-lesion experiences and patterns of use (including the rehabilitation process itself).

Several studies support the view that hyperactive reflexes do not necessarily constitute a major impairment to functional movement in many patients with UMN syndrome. A low incidence of hyperreflexia has been reported in a group of 24 stroke patients within 13 months of stroke (O'Dwyer *et al.* 1996). Others have reported that when subjects are asked to decrease hyperreflexia, there is no improvement in motor function (Landau 1980; Neilson and McCaughey 1982; Thach and Montgomery 1990); others that exercises designed to increase muscle strength are associated with an increase in strength and decrease in hypertonus (Butefisch *et al.* 1995) and that increases in muscle strength and active elbow movement occurred in the presence of antagonist co-contraction (Wolf *et al.* 1994).

Two other signs taken in the clinic to infer the presence of spasticity (in its wider usage) are resistance to passive movement and abnormal patterns of posture and movement. It is now evident that there may be alternative explanations for the mechanisms underlying these clinical signs. The following section examines this issue.

Resistance to passive movement (hypertonus)

'Tone' is typically tested in the clinic by passive movement of a joint or limb, by scales such as the Ashworth Scale (Ashworth 1964) and by the pendulum test (Wartenburg 1951). The nature of these tests has in a sense contributed to the controversy which exists about the nature of spasticity. Confusion arises from the fact that these clinical tests do not distinguish between the peripheral contribution due to muscle adaptations and the neural contribution due to increased stretch reflexes (Fig. 8.4). The Ashworth Scale, which grades tone according to the amount of resistance to passive movement, is an example of a scale that

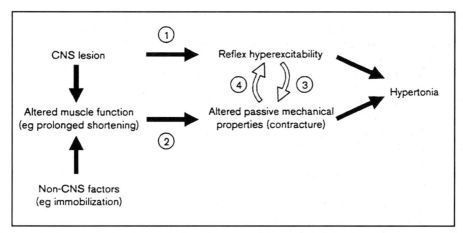

Fig. 8.4 Two mechanisms considered to underlie hypertonus (1,2). Additional mechanisms (3,4) may relate to effects flowing between reflex hyperexcitability and altered passive mechanical properties. (Reprinted from O'Dwyer and Ada 1996, with permission)

sets out to test one impairment (spasticity) but really tests another (muscle stiffness) (Bohannon and Smith 1987). Similarly, the pendulum test does not appear to differentiate between muscle length changes and hyperreflexia (Fowler *et al.* 1998).

Normal tone has traditionally been said to be a slight constant tension in muscle resulting in a modest resistance to displacement when the limbs are handled or moved passively (Ghez 1991). Therefore, the term *hypertonus* is typically used by clinicians to describe an abnormal resistance to passive movement and has traditionally been taken to reflect solely an abnormal excitability of the components of the segmental stretch reflex arc (for discussion see Powers *et al.* 1988, 1989; Thilmann *et al.* 1991b). As mentioned earlier, however, it is evident that muscle 'tone' is normally dependent on mechanical rather than neural factors. When a limb of an able-bodied person is moved passively by another individual, the response felt by the operator may vary between total relaxation (the operator takes the whole weight of the limb), some assistance (the movement is not really passive but has an active component), or some resistance (the individual contracts a muscle at an inappropriate time). If the passive movement is abrupt, it may elicit the stretch reflex, felt by the examiner as a 'catch' in the movement. However, although some resistance to passive movement may occur normally, there is no background motor unit activity in resting muscle in relaxed individuals (Burke 1988) and any resistance detected may represent a voluntary contraction by the individual. In individuals with brain lesion, resistance to passive

movement is actually determined, therefore, by several distinct components:

- physical inertia of the extremity;
- mechanical-elastic factors, particularly compliance of muscle, but also of tendon and connective tissue, and, where present,
- reflex muscle contraction (stretch reflexes) (Katz and Rymer 1989).

Since inertia of the limb does not change in the UMN syndrome, increased resistance to passive movement found on clinical examination must represent changes in the musculo-tendinous unit, i.e., contracture, and/or changes within the segmental reflex arc (Katz and Rymer 1989). Interestingly, the major positive feature patients complain of following a brain lesion is muscle stiffness, which they feel obstructs their movement. Evidence that there is a causal relationship between reflex hyperexcitability, increased resistance to passive movement and muscle contracture is lacking (O'Dwyer and Ada 1996). There is increasing evidence that mechanical and biological changes in soft tissues play a major role in resistance to both passive and active movement (Fig. 8.4).

Adaptive features: physiological, mechanical and functional changes in muscle and other soft tissue

Experimental and clinical investigations of individuals with spasticity and rigidity have confirmed that resistance to passive movement is due not only to neural mechanisms but also to changes in mechanical fibre properties of muscle and in the tendon (Dietz *et al*. 1981; Berger *et al*. 1984; Hufschmidt and Mauritz 1985; Thilmann *et al*. 1991b; Carey and Burghardt 1993), probably associated with immobility and disuse. Perry in 1980 was one of the first to point out that clinically spasticity was usually accompanied by muscle contracture. Furthermore, it is a clinical observation that the prevention of soft tissue contracture results in decreased spasticity (Perry 1980; Carr and Shepherd 1987, 1989; Ada and Canning 1990). Perry expressed the view that whether a patient's response to stretch remains just a diagnostic sign or becomes functionally obstructive is largely determined by the degree of contracture present.

In two separate studies, Dietz and colleagues (Dietz *et al*. 1981; Berger *et al*. 1982; Dietz and Berger, 1983) investigated the ankle movement of adults with stroke and children with cerebral palsy during walking. During swing phase, ankle dorsiflexion range was decreased. EMG activity showed that, although there was activity in the anterior tibial muscles, activity in plantarflexors was minimal. The authors argued that the limited dorsiflexion was due not to heightened/abnormal reflex responsiveness of the calf muscles but to changes in the mechanical properties of the muscles leading to stiffness. Following later work (Dietz *et al*., 1991), they argued that connective tissue stiffness may also contribute to the resistance. Berger and colleagues (1984) showed that, while development of force in the stance phase of walking in able-bodied subjects was coupled to EMG activity in gastrocnemius, in subjects with spasticity (hyperreflexia and Babinski sign), force was coupled to muscle length and not to gastrocnemius EMG activity. These authors proposed that hypertonus was not related to exaggerated reflexes but to changes in muscle fibres. Work carried out by others more recently makes it quite clear that altered properties in soft tissues (muscle, tendon, connective tissue) are major contributors to joint stiffness (e.g., Thilmann *et al*. 1991b).

Abnormal stiffness has been reported in subjects some time after brain lesion in the absence of reflex activity. As a result of their experimental work, Hufschmidt and Mauritz (1985) proposed that the rapid rise in resistance to movement seen on passive stretch could be explained by reference to Hill's cross-bridge theory (Hill 1968), i.e., abnormal cross-bridge connections in antagonist muscles could contribute to resistance to passive

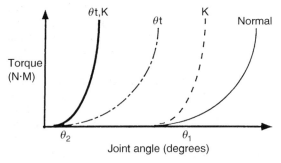

Fig. 8.5 The relationship between muscle length and tension (muscle stiffness). Normal: normal state of reflex threshold and stiffness; θt,K: represents both decreased threshold and increased stiffness; θt: decreased threshold only; K: increased stiffness. (From Rymer and Katz 1994, with permission)

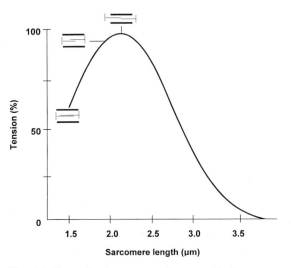

Fig. 8.6 Normally the amount of contractile force a muscle can generate depends on its length, i.e., the degree of overlap of thick and thin filaments. Around the muscle's resting length, 2.0 μm, maximum force is attained and force is progressively reduced above and below this length. No active tension develops when sarcomeres are extended to 3.6–3.7 μm because cross bridges cannot form. (Adapted from Edman, K. A. P. and Reggiani, C. (1987) The sarcomere length–tension relation determined in short muscle fibres of the frog. *Journal of Physiology*, **385**, 709–732)

movement (Figs 8.5, 8.6). These muscle changes would very likely occur in muscles which, in a relatively immobile limb, are subjected to prolonged positioning.

Changes in tendo Achilles which could underlie joint stiffness have also been described (Thilmann *et al.* 1991b). Animal experiments have shown that immobility leads to significant stiffening which is likely to be due to changes in tendon and connective tissue such as water loss and collagen deposition (Akeson *et al.* 1973).

Immobility imposed on a patient by the negative features of the UMN syndrome can result in soft tissue contracture and the resultant adaptations have an adverse effect on both the active and the passive properties of muscle (Gossman *et al.* 1982; Herbert 1988; Carey and Burghardt 1993). Evidence from animal studies shows that muscles when immobilized in their shortened position lose sarcomeres and become shorter and stiffer* (Tabary *et al.* 1972; Williams and Goldspink 1978; Witzmann *et al.* 1982).

Increased passive stiffness at the ankle joint in spastic patients has been reported even without marked clinical signs of contracture (Thilmann *et al.* 1991b). It has been proposed that muscle stiffness associated with immobility may also be due to *thixotropy*, normally a minor behaviour of muscle. A thixotropic substance is one whose stiffness and viscosity is dependent upon the past history of movement (Hagbarth *et al.*, 1985, p. 324). The term thixotropy describes tension which is almost independent of stretch velocity. Furthermore, muscle thixotropy, according to Proske and colleagues, can exert a strong influence on reflexes either by changing the size of afferent input in response to stimulus or by biasing spinal excitability levels through changes in maintained rates of afferent discharge (Proske *et al.* 1993, p. 718). Some time ago, Williams (1980) reported changes in sensitivity of spindles in immobilized muscle in animals. Spindles were activated at shorter lengths than control animals. A similar finding was reported more recently (Gioux and Petit 1993).

O'Dwyer and colleagues (1996) reported that many of the 24 post-stroke individuals they tested, habitually held their elbow in some flexion even though they did not necessarily demonstrate hyperreflexia. Changes in the properties of the muscle may lead to a new 'resting' position of the limb. Muscle spindles contribute to kinaesthetic sense and it has been suggested that the signal for limb position may be provided by the resting discharge of muscle spindles (Gregory *et al.* 1988). Position

---

* The property of muscle called stiffness is the force required to change the length of a resting muscle. (See Sinkjaer and Magnussen (1994) for discussion of passive, intrinsic and reflex-mediated stiffness in patients with hemiplegia.)

sense in a passive limb would be dependent, therefore, on the muscle's history. This may help to explain why the resting posture for, say, the upper limb, is so often with the elbow flexed when the limb is unsupported (as in standing). In sitting, if there is muscle paralysis, the arm may rest with the elbow flexed for long periods, defining, in the words of Proske and colleagues, the muscle's 'history'.

It should be noted that connective tissue in muscle also undergoes remodelling as a result of immobility and probably contributes to the increased stiffness found in shortened muscle. The soft tissue adaptations provide, therefore, a mechanical cause for the increased resistance to passive movement, in addition to forcing adaptive patterns of movement/motor behaviours.

Adaptive motor behaviour

Abnormal postures and patterns of movement may be seen following lesions involving the motor pathways. *Persistent posturing* is typically referred to in the clinic as indicative of spasticity, although there is no evidence of a relationship to hyperreflexia (see O'Dwyer *et al.* 1996). The abnormal posturing observed is more likely to reflect immobility, disuse changes to soft tissues and adaptations to the resting length of muscles. For example, it is common to see the lower limb held in flexion in individuals confined to wheelchairs (who have length-associated changes in leg muscles – short hip and knee flexors and ankle plantarflexors) and in extension in individuals who are allowed to stand and walk without specific training and exercise to improve coordination of lower limb muscles. Patients who spend the day with the shoulder joint in internal rotation and adduction, and the elbow and wrist in flexion will maintain this flexed 'resting' posture when in standing. A simple descriptive study of 10 patients 18–52 weeks following stroke showed an increase in maintained flexion of the elbow after a period spent wheeling their self-propelling chair with their unaffected hand (Cornall 1991). Abnormal posturing of a limb may, therefore, reflect the changes in resting length and increased sensitivity of spindle receptors referred to above.

Abnormal patterns of movement, rather than being a manifestation of spasticity through the 'release' of abnormal movements, may be explained as a functional adaptation to motor performance that becomes apparent when a person attempts to move in the presence of muscle paralysis and/or weakness of some muscles together with an imbalance between weaker and stronger muscle groups. When an individual following brain injury attempts a purposeful action, the movement pattern that emerges reflects the best that can be done under the circumstances, given the state of both the neural and musculoskeletal systems and the dynamic possibilities inherent in the multisegmental linkage (Shepherd and Carr 1991; Carr and Shepherd 1996). The movement pattern that emerges spontaneously can usually be interpreted by an analysis of which muscles can generate the necessary force to move a segment and which cannot.

Furthermore, movement is an effort for the patient as muscle weakness gives the perception of limb heaviness. Exaggerated force is typically generated by stronger muscles (typically in the upper limb in those with bilateral innervation such as shoulder girdle elevators and GH adductors) as the individual struggles to perform an approximation of the action required (see Fig. 6.8). In order to maintain extension of the lower limb in standing, for example, the patient may stiffen the limb by co-contracting muscles in order to prevent the limb from collapsing. Co-contraction of muscles or stiffening of a limb is often taken to reflect spasticity. It may, however, merely illustrate the adaptive capacity of the system. In addition, adaptive shortening of soft tissues will be a significant factor in the development of the abnormal movement patterns observed by clinicians, since movement is constrained by abnormally short tissues.

In some patients, although muscle activity is present, the movements which emerge are distorted. There is no reason to expect that spasticity (hyperreflexia) underlies this distortion, and the term *dystonia* (persistent posture of body part or severely distorted movement pattern) may be a more appropriate descriptor   (see Fig. 6.12) (Denny Brown 1966; Burke 1988).

Clinical intervention

While neuroscientists seek to understand the pathological mechanisms underlying the UMN lesion, the clinician needs also to identify what it is that most interferes with motor performance in order to plan appropriate rehabilitation. At the present state of knowledge, it is probably practical in a clinical sense to consider that the negative features (weakness, loss of dexterity or coordina-

tion) and the adaptive changes to muscles and other soft tissues are typically the major impairments interfering with functional motor behaviour. It appears likely that the development of disability will be less severe if soft tissue extensibility can be maintained and if rehabilitation emphasizes training the patient to control muscle activity for specific actions with task-related exercises to improve muscle force generation and synergic interrelationships. Given the nature of the changes occurring to both soft tissue and neural mechanisms, encouraging and helping the patient to be active seems a critical factor. Where the person has hemiplegia, rehabilitation must concentrate on the affected limbs being active rather than remaining immobile for long stretches of the day.

Over the past three decades, much rehabilitation practice has operated from strong beliefs both about how the system functions and the neural consequences of the lesion, many of which can no longer be supported. Many of these clinical beliefs have continued despite the publication of challenging new findings. This situation has tended to hold back not only investigations into effectiveness of various interventions, but also clinical investigations which could help elucidate the nature of recovery, adaptation and dyscontrol after brain lesions.

It has been typical for medical and therapy professions to consider spasticity as the major obstacle to improved function. As a consequence of this belief, treatment techniques in common use stress the need to 'inhibit' spasticity by drugs or toxins such as baclofen or botulinum toxin (McLellan 1977; Latash *et al.* 1989; Sutherland *et al.* 1996), or by therapist-controlled inhibition of spasticity (e.g., Bobath 1990).

It has been a long-standing clinical assumption that inhibition of spasticity will result in improved performance. There is, however, no clinical or experimental evidence to support this view (Denny Brown 1980; Landau 1980; Corston *et al.*. 1981; Neilson and McCaughey 1982; Lapierre *et al.* 1987; Bes *et al.* 1988; Landau 1988; Thach and Montgomery 1990; Richards *et al.* 1991). Suppression of hyperactive reflexes in cerebral palsy or stroke, for example, has not led to an increase in movement control (Nathan, 1969; McLellan 1977). Although people with cerebral palsy can learn to reduce hyperactive reflexes, this does not necessarily lead to improved voluntary control of movement (Neilson and McCaughey 1982). Conversely, patients have been shown to improve on a functional task despite hyperactivity in certain muscle groups (e.g., Wolf *et al.* 1989) and active exercise has been shown to decrease reflex hyper-activity (Butefisch *et al.* 1995). Consideration should be given by therapists to the possibility that efforts to inhibit muscle activity which is con-sidered to be 'spastic' may instead be inhibiting muscle activity which is needed for movement.

For some years, we (Carr and Shepherd 1987, 1989; Carr *et al.* 1995) and others (see Duncan and Badke 1987; Ada and Canning 1990; Gowland *et al.* 1992; Wolf *et al.* 1994) have argued that the major objective in rehabilitation is to train the individual to improve control over motor output during the performance of essential actions. Although training and exercise are aimed at improving motor neuron recruitment in a weak muscle, training is directed overall to the behav-ioural consequences, i.e., the motor performance deficits, of the central lesion. The behavioural consequences have the advantage of being readily identifiable with biomechanical and electromyo-graphic examination and may provide insight into the underlying pathophysiological mechanisms (Dietz 1992). The outcome of rehabilitation which is aimed at improving the performance of motor tasks can be easily tested in the clinic for effectiveness, using functional scales and bio-mechanical measures. Outcome studies so far are producing encouraging results (e.g., Visintin and Barbeau 1989; Ada and Westwood 1992; Dean and Mackey 1992; Engardt and Olsson 1992; Richards and Malouin 1992; Butefisch *et al.* 1995; Hesse *et al.* 1995; Dean and Shepherd 1997).

Such an approach makes at least one major assumption: that directing movement training toward improved performance of everyday actions (sit-to-stand, walking, reaching for an object, manipulation) provides the system with the oppor-tunity to readjust, to relearn a pattern of neuromotor activity (using what remains of the neural system) which is relevant to the individual's goal. Rather than assuming that physical treatment affects abnor-mal reflex activity or underlying tone, with an emphasis on the preparation of the patient for function by inhibiting spasticity (Bobath 1990; Mayston 1992), this more recent approach to rehabilitation is aimed directly at assisting the patient to relearn motor control and develop strength and endurance during functional motor performance. In other words, recovery (neural reor-ganization) may best be stimulated by the patient practising motor tasks under similar conditions of strength, speed and accuracy as in real life (Ada *et al.* 1996), and with similar cognitive demands.

The prevailing clinical view is that neurological rehabilitation should not only begin early but should also be active (e.g., Carr and Shepherd 1987; Richards *et al.* 1991) and it is likely that early, active and challenging rehabilitation may prevent or minimize the adaptive musculoskeletal and behavioural changes associated with the neg-ative features (see Yu *et al.* 1981). Following an acute brain lesion, some muscle activity usually becomes evident after an initial period of shock, although output is relatively uncontrolled. Lack of activity in this early period may well diminish the possibilities for return to optimal function. Fur-thermore, lack of use and prolonged immobility lead to soft tissue adaptation and 'learned non-use' (Taub 1980). Studies on neural recovery mecha-nisms in animals and humans suggest it is possible for intensive training to affect positively the recovery processes (e.g., Travis and Woolsey 1956; Taub 1980; Visintin and Barbeau 1989; Malouin *et al.* 1992; see Chapter 1). Conversely, immobility and a non-challenging environment could neg-atively affect these processes.

Immobility, which leads to contracture and increased stiffness of soft tissue, is a major consequence of a brain lesion. Patients following stroke spend long periods of inactivity, relatively motionless, in their chairs. Following severe trau-matic brain injury, immobility may be imposed by unconsciousness.

Muscle stiffness appears to reduce with active exercise of that muscle, probably due to the effects of repetitive shortening and lengthening. In addi-tion, passive stretching of muscle may introduce slack in muscle fibres allowing for freer move-ment. There is increasing interest in the probability that active exercise (and passive stretching) loos-ens thixotropic bonds in extra- and intra-fusal muscle fibres (Hagbarth *et al.* 1985). Certainly, when muscles 'feel stiff', a brief stretch for a minute or two to a muscle (or group of muscles) by the therapist or patient just before an attempt at voluntary movement often results in greater ease of movement at the joint(s) the muscle spans.

The proximo-distal and more sustained stretch-ing procedures used by Bobath therapists to 'inhibit spasticity' have been shown by Hummel-sheim and Mauritz (1993) to affect reflex hyper-excitability in muscles stretched. The authors point out, however, that there is a major drawback in the Bobath approach since voluntary active move-ments are avoided until there is maximal reduction in muscle tone. They remind the reader that hyperreflexia can also be reduced by voluntary exercise. Furthermore, a similar reduction effect was found for simple stretching in plaster cast and splint, and the effect was more long-lasting than in the case of the Bobath inhibiting procedures. The authors proposed that the effect on the muscles in both cases (therapist-induced inhibition and casting) was mechanical in nature.

Soft tissue length should be maintained, preferably by active means, but where necessary by passive means. Intervention includes the individual attempting to activate and control muscles with the limb supported. Where patients are unconscious or paralysed, however, muscle length can be maintained by a positioning programme, including the use of sandbags and inflatable splints, or by preventative casting (see Chapter 12; see also Ada *et al*. 1990). Electrical stimulation of muscles may have beneficial effects in maintaining muscle contractility where muscles are paralysed.

Where severe contractures have already occurred, a period of stretching is necessary. Manual stretching is too brief to be effective in this case (Perry 1980; Herbert 1988). Serial casting appears to be effective in maintaining and increasing calf muscle length (Booth *et al*. 1983; Barnard *et al*. 1984; Gossman *et al*. 1986; Sullivan *et al*. 1988; Moseley 1997) and may be required as a preventative measure when the patient is unconscious and incapable of comprehending instructions. The major effect of casting is on the mechanics of muscle and the objective is to stretch muscle rather than to inhibit reflex hyperactivity (Gossman *et al*. 1986). When muscles cannot be casted, prolonged passive lengthening using traction (Odeen 1981) may be necessary.

In patients who have developed severe and apparently intractable muscle hyperactivity, as can be seen in some individuals with multiple sclerosis, prolonged icing may have a positive effect (see Hummelsheim and Mauritz 1993) and botulinum toxin injections also appear to offer a means of damping down muscle activity to allow training and practice to proceed (Sutherland *et al*. 1996).

Measurement

There are many methods of measuring 'spasticity' reported in the literature, ranging from clinical scales (e.g., Ashworth 1964), tendon taps and the pendulum test (Wartenburg 1951), to neurophysiological testing requiring complex technology (for review see Katz and Rymer 1989). The Ashworth Scale and the pendulum test are not able to differentiate between hyperreflexia and a mechanical resistance to passive stretch. Resistance to passive movement can, however, be quantified by the use of dynamometers or torque motors to gauge the resistance to passive movement. In order to separate the neural component from the mechanical properties of the soft tissues, however, EMG activity in muscles has to be collected simultaneously in order to measure the neural response to stretch.

Since the major aim of neurological rehabilitation is to retrain motor function and prevent obstructive adaptations, clinical testing should involve the measurement of motor performance by functional scales such as the Motor Assessment Scale (Carr *et al*. 1985) and biomechanical measures, and measurement of muscle length using a standardized force (Ada and Herbert 1988; Moseley and Adams 1991).

Conclusion

We have set out in this chapter to describe some current and clinically relevant information about what happens following an UMN lesion. Due to the explosion of scientific findings relevant to therapeutic practice over the past 15–20 years, this information has been gleaned from a variety of sources. The major conclusions are that:

- The major primary impairments are the loss of muscle force generation and synergic muscle coordination.
- The major secondary adaptations are the structural and functional changes to muscle and there is a positive correlation between extent of muscle contracture and disability.
- The functional effects of spasticity (hyperreflexia) are unclear. However, *no* correlations have been found between:
  degree of reflex release and extent of motor disability (Landau 1988);
  hyperreflexia and hypertonia (resistance to passive stretch);
  spasticity (hyperreflexia) and weakness (O'Dwyer *et al*. 1996).

Furthermore the literature indicates that:

- Decrease in hyperreflexia does not enable a new action to be learned (Neilson and McCaughey 1982).

- Strengthening exercise is associated with a decrease in hyperreflexia (Butefisch *et al*. 1995).

Rehabilitation should thus be directed toward:

● Intensive training and practice, including task-related exercises, directed at eliciting muscle activity, controlling force generation and synergic muscle activity, strengthening muscles.
● Preserving length and extensibility (flexibility) of soft tissues.

The clinician should have a commitment to use current information in order to generate and test clinical hypotheses as a guide to the rehabilitation process. In this chapter we have attempted to illustrate how to develop logical and feasible interventions from a synthesis of the information available on the mechanisms underlying the clinical signs of the UMN syndrome.

References

Ada, L. and Canning, C. (1990) Anticipating and avoiding muscle shortening. In *Key Issues in Neurological Physiotherapy* (eds L. Ada and C. Canning), Butterworth Heinemann, Oxford, pp. 219–236.

Ada, L. and Herbert, R. (1988) Measurement of joint range of motion. *Australian Journal of Physiotherapy*, **34**, 260–262.

Ada, L. and Westwood, P. (1992) A kinematic analysis of recovery of the ability to stand up following stroke. *Australian Journal of Physiotherapy*, **38**, 135–142.

Ada, L., Canning, C. and Paratz, J. (1990) Care of the unconscious head-injured patient. In *Key Issues in Neurological Physiotherapy* (eds L. Ada and C. Canning), Butterworth Heinemann, Oxford, pp. 249–288.

Ada, L., O'Dwyer, N., Green, J. *et al.* (1996) The nature of the loss of strength and dexterity in the upper limb following stroke. *Human Movement Science*, **15**, 671–687.

Akeson, W.H., Woo, S.L.-Y., Amiel, D. *et al.* (1973) The connective tissue response to immobility: biochemical changes in periarticular connective tissue of the immobilized rabbit knee. *Clinical Orthopedics*, **93**, 356.

Ashworth, B. (1964) Preliminary trial of carisoprodol in multiple sclerosis. *Practitioner*, **192**, 540–542.

Barnard, P., Dill, H., Eldredge, P. *et al.* (1984) Reduction of hypertonicity by early casting in a comatose head-injured individual. *Physical Therapy*, **64**, 1540–1542.

Berardelli, A., Accornero, N., Hallet, M. *et al.* (1985) EMG burst duration during fast arm movements in patients with the upper motor neurone. In *Clinical Neurophysiology in Spasticity* (eds P.J. Delwaide and R.R. Young), Elsevier, Amsterdam, pp. 77–82.

Berger, W., Horstmann, G. and Dietz, V. (1984) Tension development and muscle activation in the leg during gait in spastic hemiparesis: independence of muscle hypertonia and exaggerated stretch reflexes. *Journal of Neurology, Neurosurgery, and Psychiatry*, **47**, 1029–1033.

Berger, W., Quintern, J. and Dietz, V. (1982) Pathophysiology of gait in children with cerebral palsy. *Electroencephalography and Clinical Neurophysiology*, **53**, 538–548.

Bernstein, N.A. (1991) *On Dexterity and its Development*. Physical Culture and Sports Press, Moscow (in Russian).

Bes, A., Eyssette, M., Pierrot-Desseilligny, E. *et al.* (1988) A multi-centre double-blind trial of tizanidine, a new antispastic agent, in spasticity associated with hemiplegia. *Current Medical Research Opinion*, **10**, 709–718.

Bobath, B. (1978) *Adult Hemiplegia: Evaluation and Treatment*, 2nd edn, Butterworth Heinemann, Oxford.

Bobath, B. (1990) *Adult Hemiplegia: Evaluation and Treatment*, 3rd edn, Butterworth Heinemann, Oxford.

Bohannon, R.W. (1987) The relationship between static standing capacity and lower limb static strength in hemiparetic stroke patients. *Clinical Rehabilitation*, **1**, 287–291.

Bohannon, R.W. (1988) Determinants of transfer capacity in patients with hemiparesis. *Physiotherapy Canada*, **40**, 236–239.

Bohannon, R.W. (1992) Nature, reliability and predictive value of muscle performance measures in patients with hemiparesis following stroke. *Archives of Physical Medicine and Rehabilitation*, **73**, 721–725.

Bohannon, R.W. and Smith, M.B. (1987) Interrater reliability of a modified Ashworth Scale of Muscle Spasticity. *Physical Therapy*, **67**, 206–207.

Bohannon, R.W., Warren, M.E. and Cogman, K.A. (1991) Motor variables correlated with the hand-to-mouth manoeuvre. *Archives of Physical Medicine and Rehabilitation*, **72**, 682–684.

Booth, P., Doyle, M. and Montgomery, J. (1983) Serial casting for management of spasticity in the head injured adult. *Physical Therapy*, **63**, 1960–1966.

Bourbonnais, D. and Vanden Noven, S. (1989) Weakness in patients with hemiparesis. *American Journal of Occupational Therapy*, **43**, 313–319.

Burke, D. (1983) Critical examination of the case for and against fusimotor involvement in disorders of muscle tone. In *Advances in Neurology, 39: Motor Control Mechanisms in Health and Disease* (ed. J.E. Desmedt), Raven Press, New York, pp. 133–150.

Burke, D. (1988) Spasticity as an adaptation to pyramidal tract injury. In *Advances in Neurology, 47: Functional Recovery in Neurological Disease* (ed. S.G. Waxman) Raven Press, New York, pp. 401–423.

Burke, D., Gillies, J. and Lance, J. (1970) The quadriceps stretch reflex in human spasticity. *Journal of Neurology, Neurosurgery and Psychiatry*, **33**, 216–233.

Burke, D., Gillies, J. and Lance, J. (1971) Hamstrings stretch reflex in human spasticity. *Journal of Neurology, Neurosurgery, and Psychiatry*, **34**, 464–468.

Butefisch, C., Hummelsheim, H. and Mauritz, K-H. (1995) Repetitive training of isolated movements improves the outcome of motor rehabilitation of the centrally paretic hand. *Journal of the Neurological Sciences*, **130**, 59–68.

Carey, J.R. and Burghardt, T.P. (1993) Movement dysfunction following central nervous system lesions: a problem of neurologic or muscular impairment. *Physical Therapy*, **73**, 538–547.

Carr, J.H. and Shepherd, R.B. (1987) *A Motor Relearning Programme for Stroke*, 2nd edn, Butterworth Heinemann, Oxford.

Carr, J.H. and Shepherd, R.B. (1989) A motor learning model for stroke rehabilitation. *Physiotherapy*, **75**, 372–380.

Carr, J.H. and Shepherd, R.B. (1996) 'Normal' is not the issue: it is 'effective' goal attainment that counts. *Behavioral and Brain Sciences*, **19**, 72–73.

Carr, J.H. Shepherd, R.B. and Ada, L. (1995) Spasticity: research findings and implications for intervention. *Physiotherapy*, **81**, 421–429.

Carr, J.H., Shepherd, R.B., Nordholm, L. *et al.* (1985) A motor assessment scale for stroke. *Physical Therapy*, **65**, 175–180.

Cavallari, P. and Katz, R. (1989) Pattern of projections of group 1 afferents from forearm muscles to motor neurones supplying biceps and triceps muscles in man. *Experimental Brain Research*, **78**, 465–478.

Chapman, C.E. and Wiesendanger, M. (1982) The physiological and anatomical basis of spasticity: a review. *Physiotherapy Canada*, **34**, 125–136.

Colebatch, J.G. and Gandevia, S.C. (1989) The distribution of muscular weakness in upper motor neuron lesions affecting the arm. *Brain*, **112**, 749–763.

Colebatch, J.G., Gandevia, S.C., McCloskey, D.I. *et al.* (1979) Subject instruction and long latency reflex responses to muscle stretch. *Journal of Physiology (London)*, **292**, 527–534.

Colebatch, J.G., Gandevia, S.C. and Spira, P.J. (1986) Voluntary muscle strength in hemiparesis: distribution of weakness at the elbow. *Journal of Neurology, Neurosurgery, and Psychiatry*, **49**, 1019–1024.

Conrad, B., Benecke, R. and Meick, H.M. (1985) Gait disturbances in paraspastic patients. In *Clinical Neurophysiology in Spasticity* (eds P.J. Delwaide and R.R. Young), Elsevier, Amsterdam, pp. 155–174.

Cornall, C. (1991 Self-propelling wheelchairs: The effects on spasticity in hemiplegic patients. *Physiotherapy Theory and Practice*, **7**, 13–21.

Corston, R.N., Johnson, F. and Goodwin-Austen, R.B. (1981) The assessment of drug treatment of spastic gait. *Journal of Neurology, Neurosurgery, and Psychiatry*, **44**, 1035–1039.

Cruz-Martinez, A. (1984) Electrophysiological study in hemiparetic subjects: electromyography, motor conduction and response to repetitive nerve stimulation. *Electroencephalography and Clinical Neurophysiology*, **23**, 139–148.

Darian-Smith, I., Galea, M.P. and Darian-Smith, C. (1996) Manual dexterity: How does the cerebral cortex contribute? *Clinical and Experimental Pharmacology and Physiology*, **23**, 948–956.

Davidoff, R.A. (1992) Skeletal muscle tone and the misunderstood stretch reflex. *Neurology*, **42**, 951–1009.

Davies, P.M. (1985) *Steps to Follow. A Guide to the Treatment of Adult Hemiplegia*. Springer-Verlag, Berlin.

Dean, C. and Mackey, F. (1992) Motor assessment scale scores as a measure of rehabilitation outcome following stroke. *Australian Journal of Physiotherapy*, **38**, 31–35.

Dean, C.M. and Shepherd, R.B. (1997) Task-related training improves performance of seated reaching tasks after stroke. *Stroke*, **28**, 1–7.

Denny Brown, D. (1950) Disintegration of motor function resulting from cerebral lesions. *Journal of Nervous and Mental Disorders*, **112**, 1–45.

Denny Brown, D. (1966) *The Cerebral Control of Movement*. University Press, Liverpool.

Denny Brown, D. (1980) Preface: historical aspects of the relation of spasticity to movement. In *Spasticity: Disordered Motor Control* (eds R.G. Feldman, R.R. Young and W.P. Koella) YearBook Medical Publishers, Chicago, pp. 1–15.

Dietz V. (1992) Spasticity: exaggerated reflexes or movement disorder? In *On Movement Disorders in Children* (eds H. Forssberg and H. Hirschfield), Karger, Basle pp. 225–233.

Dietz, V. and Berger, W. (1983) Normal and impaired regulation of muscle stiffness in gait: a new hypothesis about muscle hypertonia. *Experimental Neurology*, **79**, 680–687.

Dietz, V., Ketelson, U.P., Berger, W. *et al.* (1986) Motor unit involvement in spastic paresis: relationship between leg muscle activation and histochemistry. *Journal of Neurological Science*, **75**, 89–103.

Dietz, V., Quintern, J. and Berger, W. (1981) Electrophysiological studies of gait in spasticity and rigidity. Evidence that altered mechanical properties of muscle contribute to hypertonia. *Brain*, **104**, 431–449.

Dietz, V., Trippel, M. and Berger, W. (1991) Reflex activity and muscle tone during elbow movements in patients with spastic paresis. *Annals of Neurology*, **30**, 767–779.

Duncan, P.W. and Badke, M.B. (1987) Determinants of abnormal motor control. In *Stroke Rehabilitation – The Recovery of Motor Control* (eds P.W. Duncan and M.B. Badke), YearBook Medical Publishers, Chicago, pp. 135–159.

Edstrom, L. (1970) Selective changes in the sizes of red and white muscle fibers in upper motor lesions and Parkinsonism. *Journal of Neurological Sciences*, **11**, 537–550.

Edwards, S. (1996) *Neurological Physiotherapy. A Problem-Solving Approach,* Churchill Livingstone, London.

Engardt, M. and Olsson, E. (1992) Body weight-bearing while rising and sitting down in patients with stroke. *Scandinavian Journal of Rehabilitation Medicine,* **25**, 41–48.

Eyzaguirre, C. and Fidone S.J. (1975) *Physiology of the Nervous System.* YearBook Medical Publishers, Chicago.

Farmer, S.F., Swash, M., Ingram, D.A. *et al.* (1993) Changes in motor unit synchronization following central nervous lesions in man. *Journal of Physiology (London),* **463**, 83–105.

Fowler, V., Canning, C.G., Carr, J.H. *et al.* (1997) The effect of muscle length on the pendulum test. *Archives of Physical Medicine and Rehabilitation* (in press).

Gandevia, S.C. and McCloskey, D.I. (1977) Sensation of heaviness. *Brain,* **100**, 345–354.

Ghez, C. (1991) The cerebellum. In *Principles of Neural Science* (eds E.R. Kandel, J.H. Schwartz and T.M. Jessell), Appleton and Lange, Norwalk, CT, pp. 626–646.

Gioux, M. and Petit, J. (1993) Effects of immobilizing the cat peroneus longus muscle on the activity of its own spindles. *Journal of Applied Physiology,* **75**, 2629–2635.

Giuliani, C.A. (1990) Adult hemiplegic gait. In *Gait in Rehabilitation* (ed. G.L. Smidt), New York, Churchill Livingstone, pp. 253–266.

Gordon, J. and Ghez, C. (1991) Muscle receptors and spinal reflexes: the stretch reflex. In *Principles of Neuroscience* (eds R.G. Kandel, J.H. Schwartz and T.M. Jessell), 3rd edn, Appleton and Lange, Norwalk, CT, pp. 564–580.

Gossman, M.R., Rose, S.J., Sahrmann, S.A. *et al.* (1986) Length and circumference measurements in one-joint and multijoint muscles in rabbits after immobilization. *Physical Therapy,* **66**, 516–520.

Gossman, M.R., Sahrmann, S.A. and Rose, S.J. (1982) Review of length-associated changes in muscle. *Physical Therapy,* **62**, 1799–1808.

Gottlieb, G.L. and Agarwal, G.C. (1979) Response to sudden torques about the ankle in man: myotatic reflex. *Journal of Neurophysiology,* **42**, 91–106.

Gowland, C., deBruin, H., Basmajian, J.V. *et al.* (1992) Agonist and antagonist activity during voluntary upper-limb movement in patients with stroke. *Physical Therapy,* **72**, 624–633.

Gregory, J.E., Morgan, D.L. and Proske, U. (1988) After-effects in the responses of cat muscle spindles and errors in limb position sense in man. *Journal of Neurophysiology,* **59**, 1220–1230.

Hagbarth, K.-E., Hagglund, J.V., Norkin, M. *et al.* (1985) Thixotropic behaviour of human finger flexor muscles with accompanying changes in spindle and reflex responses to stretch. *Journal of Physiology,* **368**, 323–342.

Herbert, R. (1988) The passive mechanical properties of muscle and their adaptations to altered pattern of use. *Australian Journal of Physiotherapy,* **34**, 141–149.

Hesse, S., Bertelt, C., Jahnke, M.T. *et al.* (1995) Treadmill training with partial body weight support compared with physiotherapy in nonambulatory hemiparetic patients. *Stroke,* **26**, 976–981.

Hill, D.K. (1968) Tension due to interaction between the sliding filaments in resting striated muscle: the effect of stimulation. *Journal of Physiology* (London), **199**, 637–684.

Hufschmidt, A. and Mauritz, K-H. (1985) Chronic transformation of muscle in spasticity: a peripheral contribution to increased tone. *Journal of Neurology, Neurosurgery, and Psychiatry,* **48**, 676–685.

Hummelsheim, H. and Mauritz, K-H. (1993) Neurophysiological mechanisms of spasticity modification by physiotherapy. In *Spasticity: Mechanisms and Management* (eds. A.F. Thilmann *et al.*), Springer-Verlag, Berlin, pp. 426–438.

Jackson, J.H. (1958) Selected writings. In *John Hughlings Jackson* (ed. J. Taylor), Basic Books, New York.

Kanosue, K., Akazawa, K. and Fujii, K. (1983) Modulation of reflex activity of motor units in response to stretch of a human finger muscle. *Japanese Journal of Physiology,* **33**, 995–1009.

Katz, R. and Pierrot-Deseilligny, E. (1982) Recurrent inhibition of a-motor neurons in patients with upper motor neuron lesions. *Brain,* **105**, 103–124.

Katz, R.T., Rovai, G.P., Brait, C. *et al.* (1992) Objective quantification of spastic hypertonia: correlation with clinical findings. *Archives of Physical Medicine and Rehabilitation,* **73**, 339–347.

Katz, R.T. and Rymer, W.Z. (1989) Spastic hypertonia: mechanisms and measurement. *Archives of Physical Medicine and Rehabilitation,* **70**, 144–155.

Knutsson, E. and Martensson, A. (1980) Dynamic motor capacity in spastic paresis and its relation to prime mover dysfunction, spastic reflexes and antagonist coactivation. *Scandinavian Journal of Rehabilitation Medicine,* **12**, 93–106.

Knutsson, E. and Richards, C. (1979) Different types of disturbed motor control in gait of hemiparetic patients. *Brain,* **102**, 405–430.

Lance, J.W. (1980) Symposium synopsis. In *Spasticity: Disordered Motor Control* (eds R.G. Feldman, R.R. Young, and W.P. Koella), YearBook Medical Publishers, Chicago, pp. 485–494.

Landau, W.M. (1980) Spasticity: what is it? What is it not? In *Spasticity: Disordered Motor Control* (eds R.G. Feldman, R.R. Young and W.P. Koella), Year Book Medical Publishers, Chicago, pp.17–24.

Landau, W.M. (1988) Parables of palsy, pills and PT pedagogy: a spastic dialectic. *Neurology,* **38**, 1496–1499.

Lapierre, Y., Bouchard, S., Tansey, C. *et al.* (1987) Treatment of spasticity with tizanidine in multiple sclerosis. *Canadian Journal of Neurological Science,* **14**, 513–517.

Latash, L.P. and Latash, M.L. (1994) A new book by N.A. Bernstein: 'On dexterity and its Development'. *Journal of Motor Behaviour*, **26**, 56–62.

Latash, M.L., Penn, R.D., Carcos, D.M. *et al.* (1989) Short-term effects of intrathecal baclofen in spasticity. *Experimental Neurology*, **103**, 165–172.

Lee, R.G. and van Donkelaar, P. (1995) Mechanisms underlying functional recovery following stroke. *Canadian Journal of Neurological Sciences*, **22**, 257–263.

Lloyd, D.P.C. (1943) Conduction and synaptic transmission of the reflex response to stretch in spinal cats. *Journal of Neurophysiology*, **6**, 317–326.

McComas, A.J., Sica, R.E.P., Upton, A.R.M. *et al.* (1973) Functional changes in motoneurones of hemiparetic patients. *Journal of Neurology, Neurosurgery, and Psychiatry*, **36**, 183–193.

McLellan, D.L. (1977) Co-contraction and stretch reflexes in spasticity during treatment with baclofen. *Journal of Neurology, Neurosurgery and Psychiatry*, **40**, 30–38.

McLellan, D.L., Hassan, N. and Hodgson, J.A. (1985) Tracking tasks in the assessment of spasticity. In *Clinical Neurophysiology in Spasticity: Contributing to Assessment and Pathophysiology* (eds P.J. Delwaide and R.R. Young), Elsevier, Amsterdam, pp. 131–139.

Malouin, F., Potvin, M., Prevost, J. *et al.* (1992) Use of intensive task-oriented gait training program in a series of patients with acute cerebrovascular accidents. *Physical Therapy*, **72**, 781–793.

Marshall, L.F. (1990) Current head injury research. *Current Opinion in Neurology and Neurosurgery*, **3**, 4–9.

Mayston, M.J. (1992) The Bobath concept – evolution and application. In *On Movement Disorders in Children* (eds H. Forssberg and H. Hirschfield), Karger, Basle, pp. 1–6.

Merzenich, M.M., Allard, T.T. and Jenkins, W.M. (1991) Neural ontogeny of higher brain function: implications of some recent neurophysiological findings. In *Information Processing in the Somatosensory System* (eds O. Franzen and J. Westman), Macmillan Press, London.

Moseley, A.M. (1997) The effect of casting combined with stretching on passive ankle dorsiflexion in adults with traumatic head injuries. *Physical Therapy*, **77**, 240–258.

Moseley, A.M. and Adams, R. (1991) Measurement of passive ankle dorsiflexion: procedures and reliability. *Australian Journal of Physiotherapy*, **37**, 175–181.

Nathan, P.W. (1969) Treatment of spasticity with perineural injections of phenol. *Developmental Medicine and Child Neurology*, **11**, 384.

Neilson, P.D. and Lance, J. (1978) Reflex transmission characteristics during voluntary activity in normal man and patients with movement disorders. In *Cerebral Motor Control in Man: Long Loop Mechanisms: Progress in Clinical Neurophysiology* (ed. J.E. Desmedt), Karger, Basle, pp. 263–269.

Neilson, P.D. and McCaughey, J. (1982) Self-regulation of spasm and spasticity in cerebral palsy. *Journal of Neurology, Neurosurgery, and Psychiatry*, **45**, 320–330.

Odeen, I. (1981) Reduction of muscular hypertonus by long-term muscle stretch. *Scandinavian Journal of Rehabilitation Medicine*, **13**, 93–99.

O'Dwyer, N.J. and Ada, L. (1996) Reflex hyperexcitability and muscle contracture in relation to spastic hypertonia. *Current Opinion in Neurology*, **9**, 451–455.

O'Dwyer, N.J., Ada, L. and Neilson, P.D. (1996) Spasticity and muscle contracture following stroke. *Brain*, **119**, 1737–1749.

Perry, J. (1980) Rehabilitation of spasticity. In *Spasticity: Disordered Motor Control* (eds R.G. Feldman, R.R. Young and W.P. Koella), YearBook Medical Publishers, Chicago, pp. 87–100.

Phillips, C.G. and Porter, R. (1977) *Corticospinal Neurones. Their Role in Movement*. Academic Press, New York.

Powers, R.K., Campbell, D.L. and Rymer, W.Z. (1989) Stretch reflex dynamics in spastic elbow flexor muscles. *Annals of Neurology*, **25**, 32–42.

Powers, R.K., Marder-Meyer, J. and Rymer, W.Z. (1988) Quantitative relations between hypertonia and stretch reflex threshold in spastic hemiparesis. *Annals of Neurology*, **23**, 115–124.

Proske, U., Morgan, D.L. and Gregory, J.E. (1993) Thixotropy in skeletal muscle and in muscle spindles: a review. *Progress in Neurobiology*, **41**, 705–721.

Richards, C.L. and Malouin, F. (1992) Spasticity control in the therapy of cerebral palsy. In *On Movement Disorders in Children* (eds H. Forssberg and H. Hirschfield), Karger, Basle, pp. 217–224.

Richards, C.L., Malouin, F., Dumas, F. *et al.* (1991) New rehabilitation strategies for the treatment of spastic gait disorders. In *Adaptability of Human Gait* (ed. A.E. Patla), Elsevier, New York, pp. 387–411.

Rosenfalck, A. and Andreassen, S. (1980) Impaired regulation of force and firing pattern of single motor units in patients with spasticity. *Journal of Neurology, Neurosurgery, and Psychiatry*, **43**, 907–916.

Rothwell, J.C., Traub, M.M. and Marsden, C.D. (1980) Influence of voluntary intent on the human long-latency stretch reflex. *Nature*, **286**, 496–498.

Ryerson, S.D. (1995) Hemiplegia. In *Neurological Rehabilitation* (ed. D.A. Umphred), Mosby, St Louis, pp. 681–721.

Rymer, W.Z. and Katz, R.T. (1994) Mechanisms of spastic hypertonia. *Physical Medicine and Rehabilitation*, **8**, 441–454.

Sahrmann, S.A. and Norton, B.S. (1977) The relationship of voluntary movement to spasticity in the upper motor neuron syndrome. *Annals of Neurology*, **2**, 460–465.

Shahani, B.T. and Young, R.R. (1980) The flexor reflex in spasticity. In *Spasticity: Disordered Motor Control* (eds R.G. Feldman, R.R. Young and W.P. Koella),

YearBook Medical Publishers, Chicago, pp. 287–295.

Shepherd, R.B. and Carr, J.H. (1991) An emergent or dynamical systems view of movement dysfunction. *Australian Journal of Physiotherapy*, **37**, 4–5, 17.

Sinkjaer, T. and Magnussen, I. (1994) Passive, intrinsic and reflex-mediated stiffness in the ankle extensors of hemiparetic patients. *Brain*, **117**, 355–363.

Sullivan, T., Conine, T.A., Goodman, M. *et al.* (1988) Serial casting to prevent equinus in acute traumatic head injury. *Physiotherapy Canada*, **40**, 346–350.

Sunderland, A., Tinson, D., Bradley, L. *et al.* (1989) Arm function after stroke. An evaluation of grip strength as a measure of recovery and a prognostic indicator. *Journal of Neurology, Neurosurgery, and Psychiatry*, **52**, 1267–1272.

Sutherland, D.H., Kaufman, K.R., Wyatt, M.P. *et al.* (1996) Injection of botulinum A toxin into the gastrocnemius muscle of patients with cerebral palsy: a 3-dimensional motion analysis study. *Gait and Posture*, **4**, 269–279.

Tabary, J.C., Tabary, C., Tardieu, G. *et al.* (1972) Physiological and structural changes in the cat soleus muscle due to immobilization at different lengths by plaster casts. *Journal of Physiology (London)*, **224**, 231–244.

Tang, A. and Rymer, W.Z. (1981) Abnormal force-EMG relations in paretic limbs of hemiparetic human subjects. *Journal of Neurology, Neurosurgery and Psychiatry*, **44**, 690–698.

Taub, E. (1980) Somatosensory deafferentation research with monkeys: implications for rehabilitation medicine. In *Behavioral Psychology in Rehabilitation Medicine: Clinical Applications*, Williams and Wilkins, Baltimore, MD, pp. 371–401.

Thach, W.T. and Montgomery, E.B. (1990) Motor systems. In *Neurobiology of Disease* (eds A.L. Pearlman and R.C. Collins) Oxford University Press, Oxford, pp. 168–196.

Thilmann, A.F. and Fellows, S.J. (1991) The time-course of bilateral changes in the reflex excitability of relaxed triceps surae muscle in human hemiparetic spasticity. *Journal of Neurology*, **238**, 293–298.

Thilmann, A.F., Fellows, S.J. and Garms, E. (1991a) The mechanism of spastic muscle hypertonus: variation in reflex gain over time course of spasticity. *Brain*, **114**, 233–244.

Thilmann, A.F., Fellows, S.J. and Ross, H.F. (1991b) Biomechanical changes at the ankle joint after stroke. *Journal of Neurology, Neurosurgery and Psychiatry*, **54**, 134–139.

Travis, A.M. and Woolsey, C.W. (1956) Motor performance of monkeys after bilateral, partial and total cerebral decortications. *American Journal of Physical Medicine*, **35**, 273–310.

Tsuji, I. and Nakamura, R. (1987) The altered time course of tension development during the initiation of fast movement in hemiplegic patients. *Tohoku Journal of Experimental Medicine*, **151**, 137–143.

Van der Meche, F.G.A. and Van der Gijn, J. (1986) Hypotonia: An erroneous clinical concept? *Brain*, **109**, 1169–1178.

Visintin, M. and Barbeau, H. (1989) The effects of body weight support on the locomotor pattern of spastic paretic patients. *Canadian Journal of Neurological Sciences*, **16**, 315–325.

Visser, S.L., Oosterhoff, E., Hermans, H.J. *et al.* (1985) Single twitch contraction curve in patients with spastic hemiparesis in relation to EMG findings. *Electromyography and Clinical Neurophysiology*, **25**, 63–71.

Walshe, F.M.R. (1961) Contributions of John Hughlings Jackson to neurology. *Archives of Neurology*, **5**, 119–131.

Wartenberg, R. (1951) Pendulousness of the legs as a diagnostic test. *Neurology*, **1**, 18–24.

Williams, P.E. and Goldspink. G. (1978) Changes in sarcomere length and physiological properties in immobilized muscle. *Journal of Anatomy*, **127**, 459–468.

Williams, R.G. (1980) Sensitivity changes shown by spindle receptors in chronically immobilized skeletal muscle. In *Proceedings of the Physiological Society*, pp. 26P-27P.

Witzmann, F.A., Kim, D.H. and Fitts, R.H. (1982) Hindlimb immobilization: length-tension and contractile properties of skeletal muscle. *Journal of Applied Physiology*, **53**, 335–345.

Wolf, S.L., Catlin, P.A., Blanton, S. *et al.* (1994) Overcoming limitations in elbow movement in the presence of antagonist hyperactivity. *Physical Therapy*, **74**, 826–835.

Wolf, S.L., LeCraw, D.E. and Barton, L.A. (1989) Comparison of motor copy and targeted biofeedback training techniques for restitution of upper extremity function among patients with neurologic disorders. *Physical Therapy*, **69**, 719–735.

Young, J.L. and Mayer, R.F. (1982) Physiological alterations of motor units in hemiplegia. *Journal of Neurological Sciences*, **54**, 401–412.

Yu, J., Liu, C.N., Chambers, W.W. *et al.* (1981) Effects of exercise on reflexes in paraplegic monkeys. *Acta Neurobiologica Experimenta*, **41**, 271–278.

Further reading

Botte, M.J., Nickel, V.L. and Akeson, W.H. (1988) Spasticity and contracture. Physiological aspects of formation. *Clinical Orthopedics and Related Research*, **233**, 7–18.

Colebatch, J.G., Gandevia, S.C. and Spira, P.J. (1986) Voluntary muscle strength in hemiparesis: distribution of weakness at the elbow. *Journal of Neurology, Neurosurgery, and Psychiatry*, **49**, 1019–1024.

Dietz, V., Ketelsen, U.-P., Berger, W. *et al.* (1986) Motor unit involvement in spastic paresis. *Journal of the Neurological Sciences*, **75**, 89–103.

Leonard, C.T., Diedrich, P.M., Masumoto, T. *et al.* (1995) Afferent convergence from divergent sources appears to enhance the spastic patient's ability to inhibit motor neurons during an agonist contraction. *Neurology Report*, **19**, 25–27.

Moritani, T. (1993) Neuromuscular adaptations during the acquisition of muscle strength, power and motor tasks. *Journal of Biomechanics*, **26**, Suppl. 1, 95–107.

Sinkjaer, T., Toft, E., Larsen, K. *et al.* (1993) Non-reflex and reflex-mediated ankle joint stiffness in multiple sclerosis patients with spasticity. *Muscle and Nerve*, **16**, 69–76.

Taylor, D.C., Dalton, J.D., Seaber, A.V. *et al.* (1990) Viscoelastic properties of muscle-tendon units. The biomechanical effects of stretching. *American Journal of Sports Medicine*, **18**, 300–309.

Thilmann, A.F., Fellows, S.J. and Garms, E. (1990) Pathological stretch reflexes on the 'good' side of hemiparetic patients. *Journal of Neurology, Neurosurgery, and Psychiatry*, **53**, 208–214.

9

Cerebellar ataxia

In this chapter, the role of the cerebellum in relation to its possible contribution to the control of movement, the aetiology and pathology of cerebellar lesions and the clinical signs considered to reflect cerebellar dysfunction are discussed. The results of biomechanical studies of movement in patients with cerebellar lesion are examined. These descriptions are particularly helpful in planning motor training interventions since underlying mechanisms of the observable deficits are often not well understood. As Thach and colleagues (1992) point out, it is still not clear what the cerebellum does or how it does it (p. 403).

Introduction

It is clear that the cerebellum contributes to the coordination of voluntary movement. However, the way in which it contributes is not clearly understood. Control of movement is distributed throughout the central nervous system (CNS) and the cerebellum has a part to play within this distributed system. Consequently it is not always possible to associate the disordered motor control seen in individuals with lesions of the cerebellum and its connections with specific cerebellar mechanisms. Cerebellar ataxia is the descriptive term used to describe certain behaviours: the postural unsteadiness, difficulty coordinating movement and, therefore, the clumsiness experienced by individuals with cerebellar dysfunction.

The movement disorders are characterized now, as they have been since early in the century, according to the descriptive classification of Gordon Holmes (1917, 1922, 1939). In the past few years, as a result of evidence from studies in neuroscience and particularly in biomechanics, some further light has been shed on both the performance deficits associated with cerebellar lesions and the underlying impairments.

Functional role of the cerebellum

Although the cerebellum constitutes about 10% of the brain's total volume, it contains more than half the total number of neurons in the brain (Ghez 1991). The cerebellum regulates vestibular, spinal and cortical mechanisms by means of neuronal connections which are reciprocal. The cerebellum sends no pathways directly to the spinal cord but participates in at least three systems: a vestibulo-cerebellar system which modulates vestibular influences on posture and eye movements; a spino-cerebellar system which regulates muscle tone, posture and locomotion; and a cerebro-cerebellar system thought to play a role in regulating skilled movements (Gordon 1990).

The role of the cerebellum is sometimes described as enriching the quality of movement, acting as a regulatory centre for the control of motor activity and participating in the construction of synergies. Its involvement in the regulation of the intensity of movement, through its connections in the brain stem and cerebral cortex, has been accepted since the work of Rademaker (1935). Although it has generally been accepted that disorders of perception or cognition do not occur (Brooks 1986), there is some recent evidence that the cerebellum does indeed play a role in perception, cognition and language (Leiner *et al.* 1993). This may not be surprising given that movement and perception-cognition are closely related. After all, we are active participants in our environment, actively seeking out information and utilizing it to optimize the effectiveness of our goal-directed movements and to ensure that we achieve what we have set out to do.

The cerebellum may act as a comparator, comparing the motor performance occurring peripherally with motor signals from the cerebral cortex (Eyzaguirre and Fidone 1975). In this role it would compensate for errors in movement by comparing intention with performance (Ghez 1991). It has the connections to carry out this role, receiving input from the periphery and from all levels of the CNS. Inputs include internal feedback (also called corollary discharge) related to the planning and forthcoming execution of movement. That is, the cerebellum may modulate the cortical movement signal and send it back to the cortex (Flament and Hore 1986). The delayed initiation of movement found in biomechanical studies of individuals with cerebellar lesions is consistent with this hypothesis. For example, reaction time was found to be abnormally long in one study of finger movements (Inhoff *et al.* 1989). The cerebellum also receives information (external feedback) about performance from sensory receptors (visual, tactile, proprioceptive, auditory) during movement and could compare intended movement with the actual movement as it unfolds. In addition, the cerebellum projects to descending motor systems. Movements can, therefore, be corrected when they deviate from the intended course and the neural signals modified so that subsequent movements can achieve their goal.

It is generally considered that the cerebellum plays an important role in the timing and sequencing of muscle activation during movement (Eccles 1977; Gilman *et al.* 1981) and that it regulates movement and posture indirectly by adjusting the output of major descending motor systems – for example, scaling the size of the muscle contraction. The cerebellum appears to modulate spinal cord and brain stem mechanisms involved in postural control and is important for the stabilization of stance during either externally imposed perturbations or intentional actions.

Although the cerebellum contains complete motor and sensory representations of the body, lesions do not produce either paralysis or significant muscle weakness (Gordon 1990). Perceptuo-cognitive deficits have been reported, such as deficits in estimating and comparing weights held in the hand (Holmes 1917, 1939; Mai *et al.* 1989). Sasaki (1985) reported a person with hypometria on the finger-to-nose test who described an inability to visualize the target. Blood flow and metabolism studies have recently shown that mental activities related to visuo-spatial tasks or mental rehearsal of movements also involve the cerebellum (Paulin 1993). Impaired perception of time intervals and velocity of moving objects have been reported (Leiner *et al.* 1989, 1991; Schmahmann 1991). Recently Paulin (1993a) proposed that the cerebellum can be characterized as a tracking system, its role in coordinating movement arising from the need to track moving objects and the body's own movements, and to analyse the sensory consequences. It is apparent that the disruption of the normally smooth execution and coordination of movement affects the ability to carry out intentions in a manner that is appropriate to the spatial and temporal requirements of task and environment. As a result, the ability to perform tasks such as reaching out to an object, manipulating objects, walking and balancing are impaired.

Functional regions of the cerebellum

The cerebellum is a distinct and homogenous anatomic section of the brain, divided into three lobes: anterior, posterior and flocculonodular. Longitudinal furrows divide it into the midline vermis and two hemispheres. However, it is generally considered to be organized into three functional regions (Fig. 9.1), with specific inputs and outputs to and from each of these sections.

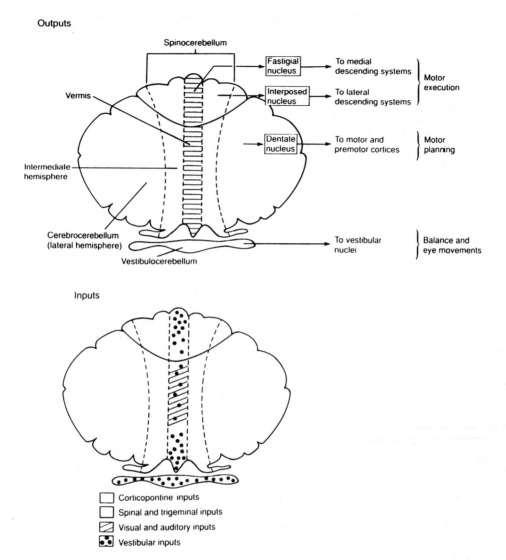

Fig. 9.1 Three functional regions of the cerebellum showing outputs (*above*) and inputs (*below*). (From Ghez 1991, by permission)

Vestibulocerebellum

The vestibulocerebellum (flocculonodular lobe) controls balance and eye movements by its output to the vestibular nuclei. This region receives inputs from the semicircular canals (signalling change in head position) and otoliths (signalling orientation of the head in relation to gravity).

Spinocerebellum

The spinocerebellum (central part of the anterior and posterior lobes, including the vermis and intermediate part of the hemispheres) has a role in controlling the ongoing execution of limb movement (Ghez 1991), including correction for error. It receives inputs from the spinal cord, and from the visual, auditory and vestibular systems. Information (feedback) from the periphery about evolving movements enables a monitoring of the operation of spinal circuits. Through its connections with the motor cortex, the spinocerebellum regulates muscle activity to compensate for variations in load encountered during movement as well as to smooth out small oscillations (Ghez 1991). In this way, the region plays a part in regulating muscle 'tone' (or stiffness), maintaining the appropriate fusimotor drive to muscle spindles.

Cerebrocerebellum

The cerebrocerebellum (lateral parts of the cerebellum) may be involved in the preparation for movement, i.e., the preparation/anticipation and initiation of movement (receiving input from the frontal association areas of the cerebral cortex), through a 'feedforward' role in modulating cortical motor outputs. Specifically, this functional region seems involved in ensuring precision in the control of the limbs, particularly during fast movement, by the precise timing of the sequence of agonist–antagonist interactions, enabling, for example, dexterity in manual tasks. A more general role in timing also appears probable, with evidence that people with lateral lesions not only suffer deficits in timing of movement but also difficulty in judging elapsed time in perceptual tasks, for example, in judging the speed of a moving visual stimulus (Ivry and Keele 1989). Recent studies suggest that the lateral cerebellar hemispheres may play a key role in the coordination of movements to a visual target (Becker *et al*. 1990). The area receives inputs from the posterior parietal lobe (Glickstein *et al*. 1985).

It appears that, although the motor pattern may be determined by higher cortical centres, details of execution are left to subcortical (notably cerebellar) control mechanisms. The cerebellum may, therefore, spare us from having to think out every movement of a limb and enable us to act automatically in this regard (Eccles 1977).

Role of the cerebellum in adaptation and motor learning

It is evident that, in its functional role in adjusting motor outputs, the cerebellum plays a major role in adapting motor performance to the requirements of the task as conditions change. It may, therefore, play a part in reorganizational and adaptive processes and in motor learning (Marr 1969; Thach *et al*. 1992; Glickstein 1992; Halsband and Freund 1993). Motor learning is thought to involve a transition from non-specific responses to highly selective associations (Brooks 1986). The cerebellum has been shown to be activated, in the absence of any motor activity, when subjects perform certain cognitive and language tasks, including mental imagery (Ryding *et al*. 1993).

Thach (1980) proposed a link between adaptation of movement to unexpected circumstances and cerebellar olivary function and suggested this as a component of motor learning (Brooks 1986). An experiment in which able-bodied subjects standing on a movable platform responded to unexpected perturbations of the support surface showed that, within a few trials, subjects had adapted their leg muscle activations to the novel conditions in order to regain their balance (see Fig. 7.1) (Nashner and Cordo 1981). This adaptation involved enhancing a muscle's response to stretch when this was useful in restoring balance, diminishing it when muscle activity would have had a disruptive effect on balance. Long-loop reflex responses can be changed, therefore, according to immediate needs; that is, they are task- and context-specific. Individuals with cerebellar lesions, however, have difficulty adapting in such a way, with response to muscle stretch being neither functional nor adaptive (Nashner and Grimm 1978).

Given that motor learning requires a transition from non-specific responses to highly selective associations (Brooks 1986), it is interesting that recent research has demonstrated that the cerebellum is involved in learning new motor routines. The function of the cerebellum and the cerebellar circuitry are modified by experience with an increase in the number of effective preferred synaptic paths (Gonshor and Melvill Jones 1976; Gilbert and Thach 1977). This modification has also been shown when cerebellar lesions follow on at some time after cerebral lesions.

To summarize, the present view is that the cerebellum is involved in:

● Initiation and control of voluntary movement
● Timing of movement/muscle action
● Moment-to-moment correction of errors
● Compensating for lesions of the cerebral cortex
● Motor learning and adaptive adjustments

Aetiology

Lesions of the cerebellum may result from developmental abnormality (e.g., hydrocephalus or hypoxia at birth), traumatic brain injury, stroke, tumour or other space-occupying lesion, infection (e.g., encephalitis), demyelinating disease (e.g., multiple sclerosis), familial or hereditary disease (e.g., Friedreich's ataxia), degenerative disease, metabolic disease (e.g., myxoedema, Wilson's disease), vascular disease (e.g., vertebro-basilar artery insufficiency) or drug and alcohol intoxications. The most common causative factor is traumatic brain injury. It is not, therefore, common to see individuals demonstrating solely the signs of cerebellar dysfunction, since such signs are usually accompanied by signs of upper motor neuron dysfunction. This may be one reason for the relative lack of studies of individuals whose dysfunction results solely from cerebellar lesion.

Clinical signs

Unilateral lesions of the cerebellum affect the ipsilateral side of the body. From knowledge of the specific afferent and efferent connections of the functional sub-divisions, dysfunction characteristics appear to reflect the different functional compartments of the cerebellum (Diener and Dichgans 1992). For example, lesions of the lateral regions are accompanied by movement incoordination related to the intent of movement and reflect problems with preparation for movement. Delays in initiating and timing movement, terminal tremor, impaired temporal coordination of multijoint movement and spatial coordination are evident. Many of the signs described by Holmes are said to reflect deficits in the lateral region, for example, dysmetria and dyssynergia.

Lesions of the vestibulocerebellum, with its connections to the vestibular system, are associated with disturbances of balance (increased postural sway with oscillations of head and trunk, staggering gait) and nystagmus. Since these disorders result from difficulty using vestibular information to coordinate movements of body and eyes, no deficits are evident when the individual is totally supported, for example, in supine.

Lesions of the central region result in problems reflecting the loss of 'updating' afferent information. Individuals find it difficult to adapt to changing circumstances. Amplitude of muscle force and timing muscle activation may, therefore, be inappropriate to the present reality as the action unfolds. Individuals with central lesions show abnormalities of balance with an absence of or diminished preparatory postural adjustments, poor timing of muscle onsets and poor recruitment of force. Actions which exemplify the impairments in force production include jumping and hopping, which may be impossible to perform, even by individuals who walk independently.

Symptoms from static lesions improve over time if the underlying disease process does not itself progress. Most individuals, however, are likely to be assisted by an exercise and training programme directed at optimizing motor performance.

The distinctive clinical signs used to categorize dysfunction, as described by Gordon Holmes, are:

- Dysmetria
- Dyssynergia
- Dysdiadochokinesia
- Rebound phenomenon
- Tremor
- Hypotonia
- Dysarthria
- Nystagmus

Recent motion analysis studies of individuals with cerebellar lesions together with an accumulation of data related to how able-bodied individuals perform everyday actions and laboratory tasks are helping to clarify the picture of the motor impairments presented so long ago by Gordon Holmes.

In clinical practice the terms used by Holmes are still commonly used. However, more biomechanical descriptors are gradually appearing in the literature. These have the advantage to the physiotherapist of providing a means by which performance can be analysed, described and measured.

Ataxia

Ataxia is the general term used to describe abnormal coordination of movements. It is demonstrated by deficits in speed, amplitude of displacement, directional accuracy and force of movement (Brown *et al.* 1990). Ataxia comprises the following movement disorders.

Dysmetria

Dysmetria (Fig 9.2*b*) is demonstrated by inaccurate amplitude of movement and misplaced force and reflects the impairment in timing of muscle force typical of cerebellar ataxia. There is excessive extent of movement or overshooting (hypermetria) (Fig. 9.3) or deficient extent of movement or undershooting (hypometria). Hypermetric movements may be more marked in small fast aimed movements and postural adjustments, while hypometria is more evident in slow movements of small amplitude (Diener and Dichgans 1992). Dysmetria is apparent at both proximal and more distal joints (Hore *et al.* 1991). The underlying

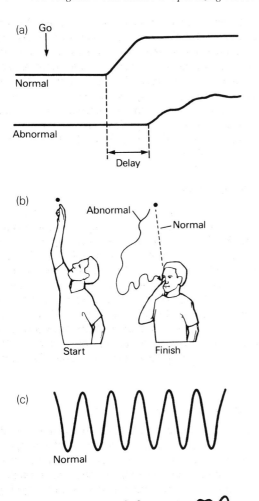

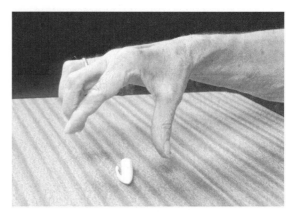

Fig. 9.3 When reaching to pick up a pen top, dysmetria is illustrated by the over-wide grasp aperture

Fig. 9.2 Typical clinical signs in cerebellar disease. (*a*) A delay in the initiation of movement. When asked to flex both elbows on signal 'Go', subject moves L arm later than R. (*b*) Moving a hand from above the head to touch the tip of the nose exhibits dysmetria, with intention tremor as the hand nears the nose. (*c*) Dysdiadochokinesia seen on the lower trace. (From Kandel *et al*. 1991, after Thach and Montgomery 1990, by permission)

impairment is thought to be in the agonist–antagonist relationship and in the duration of agonist contraction (Hallett *et al*. 1975; Brooks and Thach 1981; Becker *et al*. 1990). Lack of control is illustrated in fast movements by a picture of discontinuous velocity plots instead of the bell-shaped plots typical of controlled movement

(Brooks 1986). Fast movements are also typified by delayed onset times, hypermetria and terminal oscillations (Flament and Hore 1986). Slow movements show errors in speed and amplitude leading to decreased accuracy, with movements appearing as a series of intermittent segments performed at inappropriately high velocities (Brown *et al*. 1990).

Experimental findings have shown that although the normal triphasic (agonist/antagonist/agonist) muscle activation pattern may be present in people with cerebellar lesions during rapid or ballistic movements and also during slower movements, the first agonist burst is typically prolonged, with increased time to peak acceleration and a delayed antagonist burst (Hallett *et al*. 1991). There appears to be an inadequate scaling of acceleration duration. The disturbance in the acceleration–deceleration relationship between agonist/antagonist muscles results in lack of smoothness of movement, sometimes called a kinetic tremor.

Several studies of individuals with dysmetria point to difficulty in controlling the termination of movement (Fig. 9.4), specifically with braking or decelerating the movement. For example, when individuals with cerebellar lesions performed ballistic elbow flexion movements (Hallett *et al*. 1975), they demonstrated co-contraction of both biceps and triceps brachii which was said to result in undershooting.

It is difficult to establish in such studies how much of the dyscontrol is primary, due to the lesion itself, and how much (or what part) to the individual's adaptive strategies developed in order to move effectively despite the underlying motor

of dentate nucleus (Spidalieri *et al.* 1983; Beaubaton *et al.* 1984) have been taken to suggest that the cortico-ponto-neocerebellum loop, which has efferents to motor cortex through dentate and thalamus, is involved in movement initiation. Neurophysiological support comes from findings that neurons in cerebellar cortex and dentate nucleus change discharge frequency before cortical motor neurons (Vilis and Hore 1980; Hore and Flament 1988).

Rebound phenomenon

This phenomenon – lack of check – illustrates the dysfunction in the agonist–antagonist relationship, specifically the problem with braking of movement. It is demonstrated by asking the individual to flex the elbow isometrically against the examiner's resistance. When the resistance is suddenly released, the person is unable to stop the resultant movement, the limb overshoots and rebounds excessively. This is probably a form of hypermetria in that it illustrates the effects of a delay in the antagonistic response (Diener and Dichgans 1992).

Dysdiadochokinesia (Fig. 9.2c)

This term denotes difficulty performing rapid alternating movements. It refers to the irregular pattern of movement seen when a person performs rapid alternating movements, such as pronating and supinating the forearm or repetitive tapping. The movements are performed clumsily and slowly. As the individual persists, the errors appear to increase, with amplitude of displacement becoming greater than necessary for the action.

Tremor

Tremor is an oscillatory movement about a joint due to alternating contractions of agonists and antagonists. This tremor occurs during movement of the limb, not during rest, and is called intention, kinetic or goal-directed tremor. It is most marked at the end of the movement, for which reason it is frequently called a terminal tremor. Tremor may be greatest when visual cues are used (Sanes *et al.* 1988). This sign may also be related to difficulty controlling the deceleration phase of the movement. A postural or truncal tremor (titubation) may be present when the person is attempting to stand or sit still. Brooks (1986) describes this as a decomposition of intended postural co-contraction

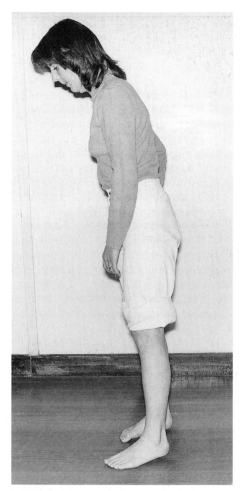

Fig. 9.4 When asked to stop walking, there may be difficulty decelerating and halting the action

control deficit. Task-dependent changes in movement strategy (Brown *et al.* 1990) used by individuals may explain the variability in some of the experimental studies.

Dysmetria has also been proposed to result from perceptuo-motor deficits. Difficulty judging velocity and predicting movement outcome (errors in the estimation of movement, either of oneself or another body) would lead to errors in action (Leiner *et al.* 1991; Paulin 1993, 1993a,b).

Delayed movement initiation (Fig. 9.2a) is demonstrated by increased reaction time (Marsden *et al.* 1977; Meyer-Lohmann *et al.* 1977; Diener *et al.* 1992). This delay has been observed in several studies to occur at all joints involved in the action and in fast and slow movements (Beppu *et al.* 1984). Results of studies of monkeys with lesions

of opposing muscles, consisting of inaccurate corrective movements of the whole body. Tremor may be the result of increases in long-latency responses (see Mauritz *et al.* 1981).

Dyssynergia

So-called 'decomposition of movement' demonstrates a lack of coordination between agonist, antagonist and other synergic muscles resulting in an absence of the normally smooth, sequential performance of various components of an action. Errors occur in the relative timing of segmental components of multijoint movements. These may be clearly seen in the heel-to-shin clinical test, in which hip and knee of the moving limb normally flex then extend in one continuous and fluid movement. The individual with cerebellar dysfunction may perform the joint components independently of each other, producing a 'decomposed' movement. There may be a failure to brace joints against forces generated by movement more distally.

Hypotonia

Hypotonia is typically defined as diminished resistance to passive movement. It is said to be manifested in some people with cerebellar lesions as an unnatural increase in joint range on passive movement, called by André-Thomas and colleagues (1960) '*passivité*' or '*extensibilite*'. The wrist, for example, can be flexed or extended beyond what would be considered its typical range. The phasic reflexes are brisk and a pendular response is evoked if the limb is unsupported. Percussion to the patella tendon is said to elicit a series of pendular oscillations.

Hypotonia could theoretically be explained by changes in tonic background activity of spinal interneurons, since cerebellar lesions lead to a decrease in phasic motor cortex neuronal discharge in some neurons (Hore and Flament 1988). It may be due to loss of the dynamic spindle response which would make the spindle less responsive to stretch. Patients seem to have difficulty increasing muscle 'stiffness'. According to some observers (e.g., Diener and Dichgans 1992), hypotonus is present only in the acute phase after a lesion. However, the mechanism remains elusive and it is not at all clear what hypotonus is or whether it is an independent entity at all. The typical method of testing, the pendular test, has been shown to be unable to differentiate between normal and cerebellar affected patients (Van der Meche and Van Gijn 1986).

The weakness complained of by some individuals may be due to a loss of the normal cerebellar reinforcement to the motor activity of the cerebral cortex. 'Weakness' may be demonstrated by a tendency for the limb to drift downwards when the individual attempts to hold the arm steady in an antigravity position. However, the production of a maximum force does not appear to be affected in cerebellar dysfunction (Mai *et al.* 1988). Rather, there may be an inability to sustain force generation which can result in the clinical sign of weakness. Difficulty maintaining a stationary antigravity posture of a limb may illustrate the difficulty an individual has in maintaining a necessary and constant force. Other examples include difficulty holding a pen to write or a knife to cut, both of which involve the sustaining of muscle force and the generation of repetitive and rapid force changes.

Dysarthria

In this disorder of speech articulation symbols of speech are normal but mechanical aspects of speech are impaired. Speech is slurred and slow with prolonged syllables (scanning speech). There may also be a lack of coordination of oral musculature and breathing.

Nystagmus

Nystagmus denotes seesaw rhythmical movements of the eyes. This is a sign of vestibular dysfunction and may be present with a lesion involving the flocculonodular lobe of the cerebellum. When seen associated with a unilateral lesion, the oscillating eye may be deflected toward the side of the lesion.

The above characteristics result in poor control when performing motor tasks, which can be summarized as: *errors of rate*, *amplitude*, *accuracy* and *force* evident during the ballistic phase of movements such as reaching and the swing phase of walking; *poor control over postural adjustments* normally interrelated with voluntary movement; *loss of fluidity of motion*, i.e., poor timing and patterning of the synergic components.

Patients attempt to accommodate their ataxia by a variety of different methods. Adaptive motor behaviours are described below. Patients may also become dependent on visual information for controlling their movements, particularly during upper limb activities (Morrice *et al*. 1990) and for balancing activities (Bronstein *et al*. 1990).

Adaptive motor behaviour

As a result perhaps of the uncertainty and unpredictability of motor performance, individuals frequently appear to restrict their actions, and hold themselves stiffly with a wide base of support (Fig. 9.5) and arms outstretched. For example, they may shorten the range through which they move, or

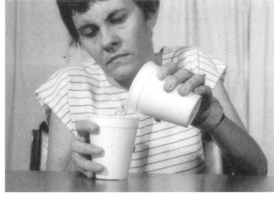

(a)

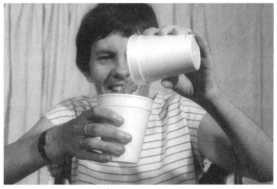

(b)

Fig. 9.6 (*a*) This task makes little demand on this person's coordination. (*b*) Practising pouring water from one cup to the other without arm support, however, increases the demands

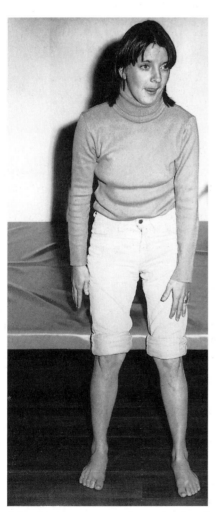

Fig. 9.5 Balancing is usually difficult, particularly where a movement (in this case standing up from sitting) requires decelerating a considerable momentum. Note the wide base of support which is also typical of poor balance

brace a segment or segments as a means of controlling dysmetria. In manipulating objects, rather than handling them at a distance from the body, the individual may confine the use of the hands to a position closer to the body or with forearms supported on a table (Fig. 9.6*a*). In reaching, a person may adapt to difficulty slowing the reach by using the support surface or object itself to brake the limb (Figs 9.7, 9.8). These behaviours decrease the number of joints (and muscles) to be controlled. In turning around, the person may take small steps instead of turning the body and pivoting on the feet. In individuals with relatively mild cerebellar signs, walking may be faster than appropriate, with large steps and a relatively wide base during double support. It is said that, at a certain level of disability, walking faster may be easier than walking slowly (Winter 1987). In this case, the ataxia and balance problems may be more clearly observed when the

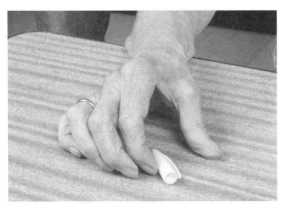

Fig. 9.7 Dysmetria is adapted for by using the table to brake hand movement when reaching to pick up the pen top (see Fig. 9.3)

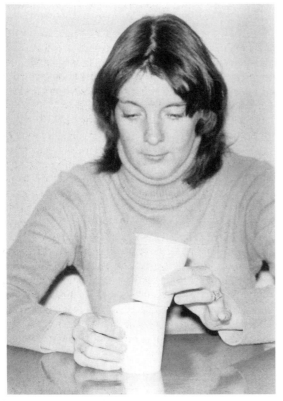

Fig. 9.8 Putting one cup into the other is difficult so she uses the cups to brake the arm movement

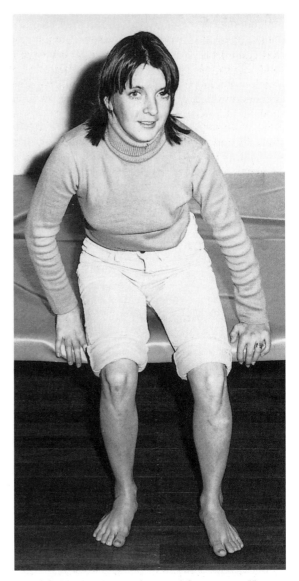

Fig. 9.9 The hands are often used for support. Here they are also used to aid in propulsion of the body mass vertically

person is asked to walk slowly. However, walking may also be slower in some individuals, particularly in those who have very poor balance. Such an individual may take small steps to help restore balance, even when attempting to stand still. The major strategy for dealing with poor balance when standing or walking is to use the upper limbs (Balliet *et al.* 1987) for support. In standing up, the hands may be used to assist at thighs-off (Fig. 9.9), perhaps adapting to a difficulty controlling the generation of extensor force required at this point in the action. Adaptive or compensatory phenomena are the person's natural response to the need to perform effective actions in the presence of incoordination.

Motor performance deficits

Much of what we know about cerebellar function has come from the study of monkeys and humans with cerebellar lesions. Since the availability of motion analysis methods, studies of biomechanical factors involved in actions performed by able-bodied individuals compared to those with cerebellar lesions are providing a clearer picture for the clinician of the nature of the movement deficits by providing information about performance which is of relevance to the clinic. Many studies have involved single joint movements and the generalizability of their results to functional motor performance may be limited. Some of the apparent conflict in the literature may arise from the different types of action being performed by the subjects. Below is a review of some more functionally relevant studies.

Postural adjustments

Postural adjustments normally precede and accompany volitional body and limb movement (e.g., Belen'kii *et al.* 1967; Bouisset and Zattara 1981; Cordo and Nashner 1982) and the muscle activation patterns which make up what are called postural adjustments appear to be specific to the task and the context in which the task is being performed (see Chapter 7). Postural adjustments (muscle activation patterns and segmental rotations), by appropriate shifts in the position of the body mass, ensure that the upcoming movement does not destabilize body equilibrium and cause either unnecessary sway or a fall. Individuals with cerebellar lesions have difficulty maintaining a stationary position (particularly in standing) and problems with balance are evident whenever they perform any actions in which the centre of body mass moves beyond a certain limited perimeter. From the few biomechanical studies available, it appears that difficulties in balancing are due in part to an inability to time and grade muscle force appropriately, related to a deficit in information related to status during ongoing movement (for example, ongoing interactions between segments in multijoint actions). In addition, subjects may have vestibular dysfunction and a derangement of peripheral retinal information processing, which have been reported from studies of eye movements (Hood and Waniewski 1984). Both these impairments can affect balance control, as does the disruption of the coordination of limb and eye movements.

Rising on tip-toes in standing

This action normally comprises an initial shift forward of the body mass. Tibialis anterior, quadriceps and biceps femoris muscles (among others) have been shown to be active prior to heel raise, tibialis anterior to rotate the shank forward (and shift the body mass forward), quadriceps and biceps to stabilize the knee prior to the generation of extensor force at the ankle by the plantarflexor (triceps surae) muscles (Diener *et al.* 1992). Timing of muscle activation and the pattern of force production is, therefore, critical to effective performance. In a recent study (Diener *et al.* 1992), 18 men and women with cerebellar (vermis) lesions were asked to rise as fast as possible on tip-toes while standing on a forceplate. Their performance was compared with that of 10 able-bodied individuals. Subjects were videotaped and EMG recordings were made of selected lower limb muscles. Two of the people with cerebellar signs were unable to perform the task. In one of these individuals, quadriceps activity built up slowly and was considerably delayed, its major burst occurring after triceps surae. Note that, whereas on average the able-bodied subjects activated the synergic quadriceps muscle some 11 ms after tibialis anterior, the subjects with cerebellar signs activated quadriceps on average 105 ms after tibialis anterior. As a result the knees flexed when the subject tried to rise on tiptoes and he had to drop back on to his heels. Among the other subjects, the deviations from normal varied. However, all of this group showed relatively delayed latencies of muscle activation. (See Holmes 1917; Hallett *et al.* 1975 for arm and hand movements.) These results clarify the nature of the deficits underlying the clinical sign of dyssynergia, with a failure of temporal coupling within synergic muscle groups that normally produces the smoothness of movement. The impairments described may underlie the difficulty commonly experienced in jumping and running.

Postural sway

In several studies, *postural sway in standing* has been found to be increased in individuals with cerebellar signs (see Mauritz *et al.* 1981; Diener *et al.* 1984; Dichgans and Diener 1987; Bronstein *et al.*, 1990), although decreased sway has been reported in patients with degenerative vermal lesions (Dichgans and Mauritz 1983). Where postural sway was increased, it seemed to be so whether eyes were open or closed. However, subjects seemed to control their unsteadiness more when they used vision (Bronstein *et al.* 1990). It should be noted that the relevance of postural sway in quiet standing as a test of balance is uncertain since postural sway seems variable even among able-bodied subjects.

A biomechanical examination of rapid arm raising performed by individuals with cerebellar lesions (Hayes 1986) showed a range of deficits in the preparatory postural adjustments. A person with pontocerebellar degeneration showed abnormal preparatory adjustments to the centre of pressure of ground reaction forces but normal postural sway. Another person with anterior lobe dysfunction and polyneuritis showed normal preparatory adjustments but grossly abnormal postural sway. Another study (Traub *et al.* 1980) involved the measurement of preparatory postural activity in triceps surae in standing subjects whose arm was subjected to perturbation. In able-bodied subjects, a slight pull by the arm to tilt the trunk forward is accompanied by a burst of EMG activity in calf muscles. The patients with ataxia had an essentially normal anticipatory reaction in muscles despite severe ataxia.

It appears that with cerebellar lesions the sequence of muscle activations can be basically preserved but is dysfunctional in terms of timing and the required fast build-up of muscle activity and therefore the proper scaling of force. For example, in the tiptoe study, delayed activation and slowed build-up of force in the quadriceps led to a failure to stabilize the knee during heel raise. Where there is too long a delay between activation of tibialis anterior and triceps surae, subjects may fall forward, illustrating the hypermetric aspect of dyscontrol. Severely disabled individuals may show no preparatory EMG activity at all and may not be able to perform the task.

Upper limb actions

There have been several studies of arm movements involving goal-directed reaching, pointing and specially designed laboratory tasks. Although many of these tasks typically involve the subjects moving as fast as possible, the results help clarify the mechanisms underlying dysfunction. Incoordination is particularly evident when individuals try to perform upper limb actions fast, although it can also be evident during slower movements. It is known that, in general, unskilled movements performed by able-bodied subjects involve a greater degree of muscle co-contraction than is evident when skill is attained. During learning to

reach for an object, a limb is normally steadied (i.e., the path/trajectory is smoothed) by means of peripheral and visual feedback. As ability improves, co-contraction of muscles is decreased. The propulsive initial burst of agonist activity is increased and the braking opposition by antagonists is reduced until optimal control is reached (Brooks 1986). Individuals with cerebellar disorders, however, in tasks which involve moving the forearm to follow a slowly moving target, show much more co-contraction of elbow muscles than able-bodied subjects (Beppu *et al.* 1984).

Even in studies of rapid single joint movements of the elbow, wrist or finger, patients with cerebellar dysfunction demonstrate an excessive extent of movement (hypermetria) at the joints being examined. One study showed that hypermetria was most marked in aimed movements with small 5 degree amplitudes (Hore *et al.* 1991). Also characteristic of fast arm movements is a picture of decreased amplitude of peak acceleration and increased amplitude of deceleration (Hore *et al.* 1991; Hallett *et al.* 1991). It seems to be typical of cerebellar disorder that acceleration of a segment is brought about by agonist muscle activation that is less vigorous and more prolonged. In addition, deceleration is associated with delay in the onset of antagonist muscle activation in slow as well as fast movements, in single joint and in multijoint movements (Hallett *et al.* 1975; Marsden *et al.* 1977; Becker *et al.* 1990; Hallett et al. 1991; Hore *et al.* 1991). Both increased duration of agonist activation and delay in antagonist activation appear to contribute to dysmetria.

In one of the few investigations of a 'natural' multijoint movement, individuals with cerebellar signs were studied as they attempted to throw a ball at a target (Becker *et al.* 1990). In performing this action, although subjects demonstrated normal sequencing of agonist arm muscles (elbow extensors, wrist flexors and hand opening), onset of antagonist biceps activation was premature. Subjects had difficulty consistently reproducing the same hand direction in a succession of movements and were, therefore, less accurate than able-bodied subjects.

Clinical assessment, measurement and evaluation

Clinical neurological tests

A series of tests are used which seem to reflect the underlying incoordination of movement. These tests were originally designed to test the major clinical signs according to Holmes. They remain useful in enabling the clinician to gain a descriptive picture of the movement deficits.

Finger-to-finger and finger-to-nose tests

The individual attempts to touch the index finger of the examiner with an outstretched arm. A fast response is encouraged as the examiner's arm is moved horizontally, the person attempting to follow. Alternatively, the individual attempts to touch in rapid succession the tip of his/her nose and the finger of the examiner. Any delay in movement initiation will be evident in this test, also terminal tremor and dysmetria. The test is done in standing if possible, and will therefore reveal any difficulty with postural stabilization during the arm movement. The tester usually notes characteristics such as time taken and presence or absence of dysmetria and tremor. The reliability of a scaled version of this test has recently been examined in individuals with traumatic head injury and found to be poor when applied by physiotherapists, although it has been reported that the time taken could be reliably evaluated (Swaine and Sullivan 1993). The apparent lack of reliability should not, however, detract from the test as a means of gaining a clear picture of terminal tremor.

Heel-to-shin test

In supine, the individual attempts to place the heel of one leg on to the shin of the other, near the knee, then to slide the heel down the shin towards the foot. Difficulty placing the heel illustrates the dysmetric component of dysfunction. The method of getting the heel on to the knee may illustrate the dyssynergic element, the individual flexing the hip and knee one after the other rather than flexing the limb in one synergic movement.

Rebound test

A strong isometric contraction of the elbow flexor muscles with the elbow flexed about 90 degree is resisted by the examiner, who suddenly releases the opposing force. Normally, release is followed by a small amplitude movement of the forearm, which returns to its initial position after it stops. In an individual with cerebellar dysfunction, the movement of the forearm continues unchecked and the person can hit themselves quite forcefully with the hand if not prevented by the examiner. EMG activity in biceps brachii has been shown to persist after release of the opposing force, with delayed activation of the triceps. This is in contrast to the normal silent period in biceps together with activation of triceps, both occurring approximately 50 ms after release (Terzuolo and Viviani 1973).

Test for rapid alternating movements

In order to detect the presence of dysdiadochokinesia, the individual is asked to pat on a firm surface with one hand, rapidly alternating between palm up and palm down; i.e., the forearm is rapidly supinated and pronated. The person with cerebellar dysfunction may perform the action slowly and with exaggerated supination and pronation range, seeming to have difficulty making the alternation. This phenomenon can be explained by the typical difficulty with movement initiation and by the dysmetria at the end of the movement (Diener and Dichgans 1992).

Romberg test for postural sway

This test is performed in standing. Subjects are asked to stand still with arms stretched forward at shoulder height, with eyes open then closed. Patients with cerebellar ataxia will show an increase in the observable body sway under the eyes closed condition.

There have been several attempts at developing quantified and meaningful tests. A recent study has reported four quantified tests for measuring ataxia (a modified Romberg, a quantified finger-to-nose test, tapping tests for both arms and legs), all of which were found to be reliable and correlated well with two other scales (see Notermans *et al.* 1994). The Romberg test can be quantified using a forceplate to measure the centre of foot pressure (Black *et al.* 1982).

Tests of motor performance

A functional activities evaluation is necessary to give a clear picture of the problems the individual is having with daily life. Suitable tests are described in Chapter 3. In evaluating functional performance, it is necessary to distinguish an individual's voluntary restriction of activity as an adaptation to the motor control deficits rather than as a primary cause of dysfunction. The ataxic characteristics may only be evident if the person is asked to change speed, to stop when asked, or to change direction. Since lack of consistency in movement is common following cerebellar lesions, it may be useful to record the number of repetitions performed in a consistent manner as a test of progress, or the number of successful repetitions in a given time. Two quantitative tests of hand coordination, the Spiral Test and Nail Test, have been developed and tested (Verkerk *et al.* 1990). (The Spiral Test is described in Chapter 3.)

Training

In general, the major objective of physiotherapy remains as it is for any individual with a lesion that affects the neuromuscular system; i.e., to train optimal and effective performance of any actions with which the individual is having difficulty (see Chapter 2). An organized training programme which ensures the opportunity for practice and which addresses the specific impairments interfering with controlled movement and effective goal achievement appears effective in either acute or chronic ataxia. For example, Balliet and colleagues (1987) reported positive results from a programme planned to reduce upper limb weight-bearing during walking in individuals with chronic cerebellar ataxia.

Given what we currently understand about the motor control deficits associated with cerebellar lesions, specific objectives to be achieved within the context of individual actions are:

● **To train control during performance of functional movements, specifically during actions such as standing up, sitting down, walking, reaching to point or to take an object:**
  – Using external constraints to provide some steadiness, where this is necessary to enable practice of tasks which would otherwise be too difficult or require gross compensation. This may involve providing support in sitting (Fig. 7.10) or a harness in standing (see Fig. 7.13).
  – Encouraging performance of smooth movements of various amplitudes and speeds, including stopping and starting at different points in the range, in order to provide practice of controlling agonist/antagonist muscle activity.
  – Training actions that require sustained force generation (such as holding objects while moving the arm) and actions that involve the production of a rapid initial burst of agonist activity (e.g., jumping, jogging, throwing a ball, see Figs 12.7, 12.8, 12.10).
  – Training coordination between segments at points of maximum instability.
  – Training actions which involve a varying amount and distribution of postural adjustment, both preparatory and ongoing.
  – Enabling practice of open as well as closed tasks to train predictive timing (e.g., bouncing a ball or hitting it with a bat, see Fig. 12.9).
  – Providing augmented feedback about relevant factors affecting performance.

● **To set up a practice environment which enables the person to develop more control (accuracy) during practice by varying, for example,**
  – Support conditions.
  – Timing constraints.
  – Environmental context.

As the person gains more control of a particular action, there are several ways in which the therapist can increase complexity so as to push the individual to the limits of their effective performance.

● **To increase complexity:**
  – Withdraw external control and guidance.
  – Reduce the possibilities for support through upper limbs.
  – Encourage increased amplitude of movement.
  – Add tasks which require speed alterations, changes in amplitude, direction and force.
  – Increase balance requirements.
  – Require that a complex movement (e.g., sit-to-stand, walking) is stopped immediately on request.
  – Reduce attentional demands of the action (e.g., by speaking during performance) to encourage automaticity.

Emphasis can be placed on interesting, challenging actions; for example, dart throwing, if necessary to a modified target, throwing a ball into a hoop, defending a wicket using a cricket bat (the bat can be used as an intermittent prop for balance); walking on a treadmill; throwing a ball through a basketball hoop (see Fig. 12.10). Each of these actions makes certain demands on the individual which help the re-establishing of control if there is plenty of opportunity for practice. Treadmill walking enforces a constant and therefore predictable external timing, a suspended harness reduces the need for postural adjustment and the amount of weight-bearing through the legs can be controlled without having to use the arms for support (see Chapter 4). Jumping actions (for example, jumping over a line on the floor, jumping down from a low step, see Fig. 12.8), provide the opportunity for practice of rapid generation of force (particularly in calf muscles), with associated synergic movements, and for switching between concentric and eccentric muscle action. The rehabilitation environment needs to allow for several hours of supervised and unsupervised practice each day.

Various forms of augmented feedback (see Chapter 2), in particular visual feedback, may assist the person to gain control over an action. Visual feedback about force production, for example, has been shown to assist patients with chronic cerebellar disease to maintain low isometric finger forces (Mai *et al.* 1989). The use of weights has been shown to decrease movement errors (Sanes *et al.* 1988) and a weighted belt may provide a means by which an individual can practise walking without using the hands for support. Many decades ago, Frenkel recommended exercises for individuals with sensory ataxia (associated with spinal cord disease). Several of these involved augmented visual input and feedback, with patients walking along a line drawn on the floor, walking between two parallel lines, and walking in footsteps drawn on floor (Krusen *et al.* 1971).

For patients who cannot maintain sitting or standing independently, actions can be practised with modifications. For example, sitting with arms supported on a table; walking sideways along a wall with arms outstretched and hands on the wall; standing up and sitting down with hands on a table in front; use of a harness suspended from the ceiling to enable safe practice of actions in standing, and of walking. A stick or cane can be used to provide some steadiness during walking practice for a person who cannot walk unaided (Balliet *et al.* 1987).

In conclusion, it is very likely that individuals with either acute or chronic ataxia are able to benefit from training and exercise that encourages practice which is graded to push the person to the full extent of their capacity, with repetitive practice and discouraging the use of the arms for support. There is as yet a paucity of clinical trials to demonstrate the effects of physiotherapy and indeed a noticeable lack of any documentation on therapy that addresses the specific motor control impairments and secondary adaptations.

References

André-Thomas, Chesni, Y. and Saint-Anne Dargassies, S. (1960) *The Neurological Examination of the Infant,* Heinemann, London.

Balliet, R., Harbst, K.B., Kim, D. *et al.* (1987) Retraining of functional gait through the reduction of upper extremity weight-bearing in chronic cerebellar ataxia. *International Rehabilitation Medicine*, **8**, 148–153.

Beaubaton, D., Trouche, E. and Legallet, E. (1984) Neocerebellum and motor programming: evidence from reaction-time studies in monkeys with dentate nucleus lesions. In *Preparatory States and Processes* (eds S. Kornblum and J. Requin), Erlbaum, London, pp. 303–320.

Becker, W.J., Kunesch, E., Freund, H.-J. (1990) Coordination of a multijoint movement in normal humans and patients with cerebellar dysfunction. *Canadian Journal of Neurological Science,* **17**, 264–274.

Belen'kii, V.Y., Gurfinkel, V.S., Palt'sev, Y.I. (1967) Elements of control of voluntary movements. *Biofizika*, **12**, 134–141.

Beppu, H., Suda, M. and Tanaka, R. (1984) Analysis of cerebellar motor disorders by visually guided elbow tracking movement. *Brain,* **107**, 787–809.

Black, F.O., Wall, C., Rockette, H.E. *et al.* (1982) Normal subject postural sway during the Romberg test. *American Journal of Otolaryngology*, **3**, 309–318.

Bouisset, S. and Zattara, M. (1981) A sequence of postural movements precedes voluntary movement. *Neuroscience Letters,* **22**, 263–270.

Bronstein, A.M., Hood, J.D., Gresty, M.A. *et al.* (1990) Visual control of balance in cerebellar and Parkinsonian syndrome. *Brain,* **113**, 767–779.

Brooks, V.B. (1986) *The Neural Basis of Motor Control,* Oxford University Press, Oxford.

Brooks, V.B. and Thach, W.T. (1981) Cerebellar control of posture and movement. In *Handbook of Physiology* (eds J.M. Brookhart, V.B. Mountcastle), 1, 2, II. American Physiological Society, Bethesda, MD, pp. 877–946.

Brown, S.H., Hefter, H., Mertens, M. *et al.* (1990) Disturbance in human arm movement trajectory due to mild cerebellar dysfunction. *Journal of Neurology, Neurosurgery, and Psychiatry,* **53**, 306–313.

Cordo, P.J. and Nashner, L.M. (1982) Properties of postural adjustments associated with rapid arm movement. *Journal of Neurophysiology,* **47**, 287–302.

Dichgans, J. and Diener, H.C. (1987) The use of short- and long latency reflex testing in leg muscles of neurological patients. In *Clinical Aspects of Sensory Motor Integration* (eds A. Struppler and A. Weindl) Springer, Berlin, pp. 165–175.

Dichgans, J. and Mauritz, K-H. (1983) Patterns and mechanisms of postural instability in patients with cerebellar lesions. In *Motor Control Mechanisms in Health and Disease* (ed J.E. Desmedt) Raven Press, New York.

Diener, H.C. and Dichgans, J. (1992) Review: Pathophysiology of cerebellar ataxia. *Movement Disorders*, **7**, 95–109.

Diener, H.C., Dichgans, J., Bootz, F. *et al.* (1984) Early stabilization of human posture after sudden disturbances: Influences of rate and amplitude of displacement. *Experimental Brain Research*, **56**, 126–134.

Diener, H.C., Dichgans, J., Guschlbauer, B. *et al.* (1992) The coordination of posture and voluntary movement in patients with cerebellar dysfunction. *Movement Disorders*, **7**, 14–22.

Eccles, J. (1977) Cerebellar function in the control of movement. In *Physiological Aspects of Clinical Neurology* (ed F.C. Rose) Blackwell, Oxford, pp. 157–178.

Eyzaguirre, C. and Fidone, S.J. (1975) *Physiology of the Nervous System*, Year Book Medical Publishers, Chicago.

Flament, D. and Hore, J. (1986) Movement and electromyographic disorders associated with cerebellar dysmetria. *Journal of Neurophysiology*, **55**, 1221–1233.

Ghez, C. (1991) The cerebellum. In *Principles of Neural Science* (eds E.R. Kandel, J.H. Schwartz and T.M. Jessell), Appleton and Lange, Norwalk, CT, pp. 626–646.

Gilbert, P.F.C. and Thach, W.T. (1977) Purkinje cell activity during motor learning. *Brain Research*, **128**, 309–328.

Gilman, S., Bloedel, J. and Lechtenberg, R. (1981). *Disorders of the Cerebellum*, Davis, Philadelphia.

Glickstein, M. (1992) The cerebellum and motor learning. *Current Opinion in Neurobiology*, **2**, 802–806.

Glickstein, M., May, J.G. and Mercier, B.E. (1985) Corticopontine projections in the Macaque: the distribution of labelled cortical cells after large injections of horseradish peroxidase in the pontine nuclei. *Journal of Comparative Neurology*, **235**, 343–359.

Gonshor, A. and Melvill Jones, G. (1976) Short-term adaptive changes in the human vestibulo-ocular reflex arc. *Journal of Physiology (London)*, **256**, 361–379.

Gordon, J. (1990) Disorders of motor control. In *Key Issues in Neurological Physiotherapy* (eds L. Ada and C. Canning), Butterworth Heinemann, Oxford, pp. 25–50.

Hallett, M., Berardelli, A., Matheson, J. *et al.* (1991) Physiological analysis of simple rapid movements in patients with cerebellar deficits. *Journal of Neurology, Neurosurgery, and Psychiatry*, **53**, 124–133.

Hallett, M., Shahani, B.T. and Young, R.R. (1975) EMG analysis of patients with cerebellar deficits. *Journal of Neurology, Neurosurgery, and Psychiatry*, **38**, 1163–1169.

Halsband, U. and Freund, H-J. (1993) Motor learning. *Current Opinion in Neurobiology*, **3**, 940–949.

Hayes, K.C. (1986) Postural instability in cerebellar ataxia. *Proceedings of 8th Annual Conference of IEEE*, Fort Worth, Texas.

Holmes, G. (1917) The symptoms of acute cerebellar injuries due to gunshot injuries. *Brain*, **40**, 461–535.

Holmes, G. (1922) Clinical symptoms of cerebellar disease and their interpretation. The Croonian lectures 1, 2. *Lancet*, **i**, 1177–1182, 1231–1237.

Holmes, G. (1922) Clinical symptoms of cerebellar disease and their interpretation. The Croonian lectures 3. *Lancet*, **ii**, 59–65, 111–115.

Holmes, G. (1939) The cerebellum of man. *Brain*, **62**, 1–30.

Hood, J.D. and Waniewski, E. (1984) Influence of peripheral vision upon vestibulo-ocular reflex suppression. *Journal of Neurological Sciences*, **63**, 27–44.

Hore, J. and Flament, D. (1988) Changes in motor cortex neural discharge associated with the development of cerebellar limb ataxia. *Journal of Neurophysiology*, **60**, 1285–1302.

Hore, J., Wild, B. and Diener, H.C. (1991) Cerebellar dysmetria at the elbow, wrist and fingers. *Journal of Neurophysiology*, **65**, 563–571.

Inhoff, A.W., Diener, H.C., Rafal, R.D. *et al.* (1989) The role of cerebellar structures in the execution of serial movements. *Brain*, **112**, 565–581.

Ivry, R.B. and Keele, S.W. (1989) Timing functions of the cerebellum. *Journal of Cognitive Neuroscience*, **1**, 136–152.

Krusen, F.H. *et al.* (1971) *Handbook of Physical Medicine and Rehabilitation*, 2nd. edn, W.B. Saunders, Philadelphia.

Leiner, H.C., Leiner, A.L. and Dow, R.S. (1989) Reappraising the cerebellum: what does the hindbrain contribute to the forebrain? *Behavioral Neuroscience*, **103**, 998–1008.

Leiner, H.C., Leiner, A.L. and Dow, R.S. (1991) The human cerebrocerebellar system: its computing, cognitive and language skills. *Behavioral Brain Research*, **44**, 113–128.

Leiner, H.C., Leiner, A.L. and Dow, R.S. (1993) Cognitive and language functions of the human cerebellum. *Trends in Neuroscience*, **16**, 444–447.

Mai, N., Bolsinger, P., Avarello, M. *et al.* (1988) Control of isometric finger force in patients with cerebellar disease. *Brain*, **111**, 973–998.

Mai, N., Diener, H.C. and Dichgans, J. (1989) On the role of feedback in maintaining constant grip force in patients with cerebellar disease. *Neuroscience Letters*, **99**, 340–344.

Marr, D. (1969) A theory of the cerebellar cortex. *Journal of Physiology*, **202**, 437–470.

Marsden, C.D., Merton, P.A., Morton, H.B. *et al.* (1977) Disorders of movement in cerebellar disease in man. In *Physiological Aspects of Clinical Neurology* (ed. F.C. Rose), Blackwell, Oxford, pp. 197–199.

Mauritz, K.H., Schmitt, C. and Dichgans, J. (1981) Delayed and enhanced long-latency reflexes as the possible cause of postural tremor in late cerebellar atrophy. *Brain*, **104**, 97–116.

Meyer-Lohmann, J., Hore, J. and Brooks, V.B. (1977) Cerebellar participation in generation of prompt arm movements. *Journal of Neurophysiology,* **40**, 1038–1050.

Morrice, B.-L., Becker, W.J., Hoffer, J.A. *et al.* (1990) Manual tracking performance in patients with cerebellar incoordination: effects of mechanical loading. *Canadian Journal of Neurological Science,* **17**, 275–285.

Nashner, L.M. and Cordo, P.J. (1981) Relation of automatic postural responses and reaction-time voluntary movements of human leg muscles. *Experimental Brain Research,* **43**, 395–405.

Nashner, L.M. and Grimm, R.G. (1978) Analysis of multiloop dyscontrols in standing cerebellar patients. *Progress in Clinical Neurophysiology,* **5**, 300–319.

Notermans, N.C., van Dijk, G.W., van der Graaf, Y. et al. (1994) Measuring ataxia: quantification based on the standard neurological examination. *Journal of Neurology, Neurosurgery, and Psychiatry,* **57**, 22–26.

Paulin, M.G. (1992) The role of the cerebellum in motor control and perception. *Brain, Behaviour and Evolution,* **41**, 39–50.

Paulin, M.G. (1993a) The role of the cerebellum in motor control and perception. *Brain Behavior Evolution,* **41**, 39–50.

Paulin, M.G. (1993b) A model of the role of the cerebellum in tracking and controlling movements. *Human Movement Science,* **12**, 5–16.

Rademaker, G.C.J. (1935) *Reactions Labyrinthiques et Equilibre,* Masson, Paris.

Ryding, E., Decety, J., Sjoholm, H. *et al.* (1993) *Cognitive Brain Research,* **1**, 94–99.

Sanes, J.N., LeWitt, P.A. and Mauritz, K.H. (1988) Visual and mechanical control of postural and kinetic tremor in cerebellar system disorders. *Journal of Neurology, Neurosurgery, and Psychiatry,* **51**, 934–943.

Sasaki, K. (1985) Cerebro-cerebellar interactions and organization of a fast and stable hand movement: Cerebellar participation in voluntary movement and motor learning. In *Cerebellar Functions* (eds J.R. Bloedel, J. Dichgans and W. Precht), Springer-Verlag, Berlin, pp. 70–85.

Schmahmann, J.D. (1991) An emerging concept: the cerebellar contribution to high function. *Archives of Neurology,* **48**, 1178–1187.

Spidalieri, G., Busby, L. and Lamarre, Y. (1983) Fast ballistic arm movements triggered by visual, auditory and somaesthetic stimuli in the monkey. II. Effects of unilateral dentate lesion on discharge of precentral cortical neurons and reaction time. *Journal of Neurophysiology,* **50**, 1359–1379.

Swaine, B.R. and Sullivan, S.J. (1993) Reliability of the scores for the finger-to-nose test in adults with traumatic brain injury. *Physical Therapy,* **73**, 71–79.

Terzuolo, C.A. and Viviani, P. (1973) Parameters of motion and EMG activities during some simple motor tasks in normal subjects and cerebellar patients. In *The Cerebellum, Epilepsy and Behavior* (eds J.S. Cooper, M. Riklan and R.S. Snider) Plenum Press, New York, pp. 173–215.

Thach, W.T. (1980) The cerebellum. In *Medical Physiology* (ed. V.B. Mountcastle), C.V. Mosby, St Louis, pp. 837–858.

Thach, W.T., Goodkin, H.P. and Keating, J.G. (1992) The cerebellum and the adaptive coordination of movement. *Annual Review of Neuroscience,* **15**, 403–442.

Traub, M.M., Rothwell, J.C. and Marsden, C.D. (1980) Anticipatory postural reflexes in Parkinson's disease and other akinetic-rigid syndromes and in cerebellar ataxia. *Brain,* **103**, 393–412.

Van der Meche, F.G.A. and Van Gijn, J. (1986) Hypotonia: an erroneous clinical concept? *Brain,* **109**, 1169–1178.

Vilis, T. and Hore, J. (1980) Central neural mechanisms contributing to cerebellar tremor produced by limb perturbations. *Journal of Neurophysiology,* **43**, 279–291.

Verkerk, P.H., Schouten, J.P. and Oosterhuis, H.J.G.H. (1990) Measurement of the hand coordination. *Clinical Neurology and Neurosurgery,* **92–2**, 105–109.

Winter, D.A. (1987) *Biomechanics and Motor Control of Human Gait,* University of Waterloo Press, Waterloo.

Further reading

Landau, W.M. (1989) Ataxic hindbrain thinking: the clumsy cerebellum syndrome. *Neurology,* **39**, 315–323.

Nashner, L.M., Horak, F.B. and Diener, H.C. (1987) Scaling postural response amplitudes: normals and patients with cerebellar deficits. *Neurology,* **37** (Suppl.), 281.

Stein, J.F. and Glickstein, M. (1992) Role of the cerebellum in visual guidance of movement. *Physiological Review,* **72**, 967–1017.

10

Somatosensory and perceptual–cognitive impairments

Introduction

Information from the environment and from our own body is processed, stored and accessed in the central nervous system by a complex interaction of neuronal networks. The response of cortical integration to a sensory stimulus is influenced by the recent history of sensory experience (Merzenich *et al.* 1988) and this may underlie the plasticity associated with the learning of tasks (Ebner and Armstrong-James 1990). Cortical integration of sensory information is also known to change dramatically with the individual's state of alertness. The response of the central nervous system to injury includes reorganization of sensory pathways which extends several synapses beyond the lesioned neurons.

Major somatosensory and/or perceptuo–cognitive impairments are found in many individuals with brain lesion and these impairments contribute to poor control of movement and have an impact upon the effectiveness of rehabilitation. Partial or complete loss of particular discrete sensations (tactile, proprioceptive) and disorders of the perceptual–cognitive system (neglect, inattention) may be evident on testing and reflected in the individual's behaviour.

Sensory impairment occurs most commonly following stroke and traumatic head injury, but is also associated with other brain lesions. Most commonly, impairments in discrete tactile and proprioceptive sensation occur together with motor impairments, and some patients with right hemisphere lesions develop perceptual–cognitive impairments such as unilateral neglect. A small number of patients suffer a purely sensory stroke as a result of a cerebrovascular accident, defined as a cerebrovascular syndrome in which sensory symptoms, persistent or transient, involve the face, arm and leg on one side (Fisher 1982). This type of stroke may be the result of an occlusive cerebrovascular lesion involving the thalamus, typically occurs in individuals with hypertension, and has a favourable prognosis.

Somatosensory impairment

Loss of tactile and proprioceptive sensation following brain lesion is relatively common, being reported in one study of stroke as up to 60% of patients (Feigenson *et al.* 1977). Pain and temperature sensation may also be impaired. The most common deficits, however, are in the discrimination and interpretation of information regarding movement (including perception of muscle force), texture and stereognosis (Critchley 1953; Maugiere *et al.* 1983). Somatosensory impairment may be a major cause of functional disability, particularly of the hand. Although an individual may recover the ability to activate muscles and control a limb and be able to demonstrate effective motor performance in the limited environment of the clinic, in the more natural environment of home the limb may not be used. Having poor feedback from the glass in one's hand, having the fork slip out of the hand while eating, not knowing whether or not a leg will collapse when stepping off the kerb, all contribute to lack of confidence. As a result, the individual may adapt to one-handed function or give up catching a bus or walking to the shops. As Carey (1995) points out, sensory impairments are often neglected in therapy and a review of therapy texts supports this view (e.g., Davies 1985).

Loss of discrete sensation, most typically from the limbs and face, represents a failure of sensory impulses to reach the relevant areas of the brain from the various sense organs of skin, joints, muscles, ears, eyes and mouth. That is, sensory inputs neither reach consciousness nor do they appear to play a role in the motor output. Light touch, pin prick and temperature are usually recognizable, although the qualitative element may be only crudely appreciated. Lesions of the brain stem may result in hemianaesthesia and/or hemianalgesia on the contralateral or ipsilateral side, depending on the lesion site. Subthalamic lesions may result in spontaneous pain (sometimes acute) down the opposite side of the body (see below). This thalamic syndrome results in considerable discomfort from touch stimuli to the skin and this discomfort usually causes, not surprisingly, some degree of depression in afflicted individuals.

Sensation functions in both regulatory and adaptive modes (Gordon 1987), guiding movements during their execution and correcting movements in order to improve the next attempt. The significance of the relationship between sensory and motor function in humans has been a continuing subject of interest to investigators. More recently, however, experimentation has been directed increasingly to the relationship between motor and sensory function during the performance of real-life tasks. As a consequence, there is now a substantial body of knowledge of relevance to

physiotherapists in developing strategies for testing and training sensory discrimination and motor performance in the clinic.

Patients with well-preserved sensation are generally believed by clinicians to achieve greater improvements in rehabilitation (Twitchell 1951; van Buskirk and Webster 1955) and several physiotherapy methods have been designed in the hope that improving sensory function will have a positive effect upon movement and function. Some of these methods involve generalized sensory stimulation ('sensory bombardment') (de Jersey 1979); others involve the use of rapid stretch to enhance muscle activity (PNF) or rely on the person picking up the 'sensation' of more normal movements induced automatically by the therapist's handling (Bobath therapy). It seems clear, however, given the evidence that the nervous system is selective in its use of sensory inputs, that non-specific sensory stimulation techniques are unlikely to be effective in improving either the perception of sensation or motor control and there is some evidence that this is so. Similarly, techniques of treatment utilized in the commonly used physiotherapy approaches (e.g., icing, brushing, positioning, passive or resisted movement) which are directed at decreasing or increasing tone and which emphasize automatic responses from the patient are likely to produce descending inhibition of sensory inputs from higher sensory centres to which they represent noise (Yekutiel and Guttman 1993). Hence, new approaches need to be developed and tested based on a more modern understanding of the relationship between sensory information and motor output, the capacity of the brain to adapt and to selectively 'attend' to those inputs which contain the most relevant information to the task at hand.

The more cognitively directed approach to motor training, proposed 10 years ago by the authors (Carr and Shepherd 1987a) applies also to sensory retraining. The provision of challenging and meaningful problems posed to the hand as sense organ (Yekutiel and Guttman 1993) may be solved more by the patient attending to, and concentrating on the form of sensory inputs and their relationship to the task being attempted. The impairment for the system to overcome is not related to the input as received from the (intact) peripheral system but involves the interpretation of those signals which are distorted by the effects of the brain lesion.

It is very likely that tactile and proprioceptive sensation is critical for the regaining of effective motor function, particularly in hand and arm use, and for the learning of new skills (Kusoffsky *et al.* 1982; Carr and Shepherd 1987a). However, the issue of whether or not people with sensory deficits can recover effective motor performance is not resolved. Monkeys with a deafferented limb have been shown to be capable of improving the use of the limb if they had training and if motivation was increased (Knapp *et al.* 1963; Ruch *et al.* 1938; Schwartzman 1972; Merzenich *et al.* 1983). When both limbs were deafferentated, however, the monkeys early after the lesions were able to use the limbs in activities such as feeding (Knapp *et al.* 1963). There is also the possibility that some motor tasks can be learned in the absence of somatosensory inputs, especially if vision is substituted (Rothwell *et al.* 1982). Whether or not the person will continue to use the limb following rehabilitation remains, however, to be further examined. Similarly, the issue of whether or not recovery of sensory (or motor) function changes after the early stage of recovery is not established. Wadell and colleagues (1987) showed with their study of stroke patients that the level of sensory recovery did not change after six months. However, patients were not specifically trained on sensory modalities and all patients were said by the authors to be very unilateral when performing daily activities. It may not be surprising that when a limb is rarely used, is used only for the simplest of tasks, or where limb use and the specific sensory deficits are not trained, that there is no stimulus for recovery to take place.

Joint position and movement sense

The recognition of movement, an awareness of its direction and of position in space, may be impaired. It may be possible for a person to recognize limb movement but not the position of the limb or the direction of the movement. These deficits are more obvious distally than proximally. Loss of position and movement sense may have a devastating effect on the person who may be unable to describe satisfactorily how it feels and what its effect is. Hodgins (1966) comments that, despite this difficulty, members of the health professions often assume they can objectively understand and describe what the patient subjectively cannot. This may add to the person's confusion and frustration, as Hodgins has illustrated for us with comments on his own problems following stroke. Proprioceptive inputs appear to be particularly important for balancing the body

mass and manipulative actions, i.e., movements which require a fine degree of control (Jeannerod *et al.* 1984; Sanes *et al.* 1985). Correlations between loss of proprioception, poor motor function and a low degree of independence in self-care have been reported (Smith *et al.* 1983).

Tactile impairments

Sensory functions which involve localization and discrimination of stimuli such as stereognosis, two-point discrimination and the ability to recognize bilateral simultaneous stimuli, may also be affected. These sensory functions are essential to effective use of the limbs. A correlation has been found between motor recovery in the hand and touch sensibility in a group of stroke patients (Smith *et al.* 1983).

Stereognosis is tactile identification of common objects and its absence is called astereognosis. It involves the recognition of physical properties including texture as well as the nature of the object. Normally touch and vision both provide this information. Stereognosis requires a normal threshold for touch in the palm of the hand. It is not an innate ability but grows and develops through appropriate experience and can develop to great heights of sensitivity in musicians and the visually impaired or can be almost absent in the hand of the person with congenital hemiplegia. The recognition of common objects is normally almost spontaneous in the adult.

Two-point discrimination is the ability to recognize two points when simultaneously applied with vision occluded. When the two points are at a particular distance from each other, and this depends on the part of the body touched, the two points are felt as one. The most sensitive areas are the lips, tongue, fingers and thumb.

There have been several studies of individuals with neural lesions in which the relationship between the sensory impairment and motor function has been described. A study of 21 people with hemiplegia following stroke found a high correlation between perception of joint position and the ability to produce coordinated limb synergies (Lee and Soderberg 1981). Rothwell and colleagues (1982) found that muscle power was virtually unaffected in a man with peripheral sensory neuropathy. However, he could not sustain constant levels of muscle contraction without feedback and was unable to perform certain everyday tasks such as writing with a pen and doing up and undoing buttons. Another person, with a sensory impairment associated with a cortical lesion, was described by Jeannerod and colleagues (1984) to have motor impairments which included slowed movements and difficulty performing coordinated finger movements. Again, there was difficulty sustaining a constant level of force. Cutaneous afferent inputs are critical for the control of movement of the hand. Johansson and Westling (1984) have shown that grip force varies according to the friction properties of the object being handled; that is, the more slippery the object the more force is generated by the finger flexor muscles. Several reports suggest that sensory impairments are linked to poor spontaneous use of a limb, particularly of the hand (Jeannerod *et al.* 1984; Dannenbaum and Dykes 1988).

Pain

Pain following stroke may originate centrally, when it is referred to as thalamic pain syndrome, or may be peripherally associated, for example, with joint damage and contractures. Central pain is said to occur in <2% of stroke patients and more commonly in left hemiplegia than in right. Teasell (1992) reviews the causes of pain following stroke.

Awareness of pain takes place in the thalamus and brain stem (Clifford 1984). Damage to the parietal cortex results in disturbed interpretation of peripheral sensations such as proprioception, localization and discrimination of stimuli. An individual with a parietal cortical lesion may neglect the affected limbs but complain of pain in them. The pathophysiology of central pain is unknown. Pain is often described as a burning or lacerating sensation with unpleasant tingling, pins and needles or numbness, and it is exacerbated by movement, stress, light touch and changes in the weather (Boivie *et al.* 1989).

Central pain is generally not amenable to treatment although subjects have been reported to respond positively to transcutaneous nerve stimulation (TENS) (Leijon and Boivie 1989). However, pain tends to subside.

Evaluation

In the clinic it is typical to test such discrete sensory modalities as light touch, pin prick, heat and cold, vibration, sense of passive movement and of position. These tests are described in standard medical texts (e.g., Bickerstaff and Spil-

lane 1989) and elsewhere (Dellon 1981; Winkler 1995). Methods of testing are, however, largely subjective, with reliability and validity unconfirmed (Lincoln *et al.* 1991). Agreement between testers has been shown to be poor in at least one study (Garraway *et al.* 1976). A recent report by Lincoln and colleagues (1991) also showed poor reliability among physiotherapists in tests of light touch, proprioception and two-point discrimination. Validity is a particular issue as the commonly used sensory tests were developed for testing peripheral nerve lesions, whereas in cerebral lesions emphasis needs to be on how the stimulus is perceived and interpreted rather than on conduction of specific peripheral nerves (Carey 1995).

Carey (1995) discusses in detail the assessment of somatosensory functions, stressing the importance of the use of quantified tests if they are to act as accurate guides to therapeutic intervention and provide meaningful information about outcome. More functionally oriented and standardized tests have been designed and reported (Carey *et al.* 1993; Yekutiel and Guttman 1993) and are described in Chapter 3. Nevertheless, even subjective tests give the therapist an estimate of the patient's sensory capacity.

Somatosensory evoked potentials (SEP) are used to study the afferent projections from the limbs to the cerebral cortex (Halliday and Wakefield 1963; Kusoffsky *et al.* 1982; Burke and Ganderia, 1988; Watanabe *et al.* 1989). SEP has also been suggested as contributing toward providing a prognosis for motor recovery, especially in the arm (Kusoffsky *et al.* 1982; La Joie *et al.* 1982; Pavot *et al.* 1986; Jacobs *et al.* 1988; Zeman and Yiannikas 1989). However, it has also been suggested that motor evoked potentials may be better able to predict recovery (Macdonell *et al.* 1989).

Training

Modern motor training is directed toward enabling the individual to perform critical everyday actions more effectively in the relevant environment and involves practice of the actions themselves with the action and/or environment being modified to enable practice to take place without disabling error. Where the person has a motor impairment, such as muscle paralysis, muscle weakness or poor control of muscles in the necessary synergic relationships for a particular task, exercises are practised in an attempt to address the specific functional deficit. This philosophy is based on the assumption that muscle activation is specific to the task and the environment in which it is being performed. The assumption is well founded in an increasing body of knowledge about the specificity of muscle action (see Chapter 2).

A similar assumption can also be made about sensory functions since it appears that the system is selective in the inputs utilized for function. It is likely that practice of meaningful tasks and specific exercises will also give the damaged system the opportunity to regain the ability to select and use those sensory inputs which are relevant to the action being practised. For example, practice of standing up and sitting down provides the opportunity to attend to and utilize inputs from tactile receptors in the soles of the feet and kinaesthetic input from muscle and joint receptors.

Early training of hand function enables sensory training to be incorporated into motor training. It is probably critical to encourage, early in the acute phase, simple exercises and activities using one and/or both hands as a means of 'driving' the reorganization of the brain and to prevent the phenomenon of 'learned nonuse'. Examples of exercises and activities are given in Chapter 6. Training of bimanual activities such as unscrewing the lid from a jar and using cutlery (Carr and Shepherd 1987a) enable the individual to regain the ability to attend both to the motor act itself and the information being received from tactile receptors. Training involves cueing the individual into the sensory information required for the task.

Encouraging the patient to concentrate on/pay attention to the relevant sensory cues (visual, tactile, muscle force etc), setting up an environment appropriate to the task, and providing verbal and visual feedback as reinforcers may not only affect motor performance but also the ability to make use of sensory inputs. Animal studies have shown that focusing attention increases the responsiveness of cells in the sensorimotor cortex (Hyvarinen *et al.* 1980).

Where a person has a specific sensory impairment, such as astereognosis, specific training can be provided to assist the person to regain sensitivity. Such training does not need to be modality-specific (Wynn-Parry and Salter 1975) which may result in poor generalizability, but rather require the solving of meaningful sensory-identification problems.

As Kusoffsky (1990) suggests, whether or not all patients with sensory deficits can benefit from motor training requires testing in the clinic. Similarly, it is not known whether specific sensory

training can affect recovery/adaptive processes within the brain itself. SEP responses in stroke patients have been reported as absent, asymmetrical or symmetrical (normal). Is this test a fair indicator of a person's potential for recovery as has been suggested (Kusoffsky 1990)? Is it possible that training could positively affect the SEPs? Animal experiments have shown that somatosensory cortical representations of skin surfaces are remodelled by use throughout life by intrinsic input selection processes and cortical maps have also been shown to reorganize following restricted cortical lesions following training (Jenkins and Merzenich 1987).

Several recent studies illustrate the potential for effective sensory retraining directed toward the cognitive manipulation of sensory information. A controlled trial of the training of sensory function, reported by Yekutiel and Guttman in 1993, demonstrated that somatosensory impairments could be improved even years after stroke. The authors also supported the view that systematic sensory retraining as well as motor training should be incorporated into rehabilitation. Training consisted of 45-minute sessions three times a week for six weeks and was based on the following principles:

- The nature and extent of sensory loss was explored with the patient.
  Emphasis was on sensory tasks the patient could do and each session started and ended with these.
- Tasks which interested the patient were chosen.
- Use was made of vision and the good hand to teach tactics of perception.
- Frequent rests and change of task were used to maximize concentration.

Tasks included identification of number of touches or lines, identification of numbers and letters drawn on the arm and hand; 'find your thumb' when blindfolded; discrimination of shape, weight and texture of objects or materials placed in the hand; passive drawing. Subjects were tested on location of touch, sense of elbow position, two-point discrimination and stereognosis. Only patients in the treatment group made large gains on the sensory tests. However, patients with left hemiplegia improved less than those with right hemiplegia, suggesting that these patients needed additional training directed at other problems such as neglect. Further work needs to be done to address the issue of whether or not these patients were able to use their affected hand more in functional activities.

Clinicians would be advised to introduce training such as described in detail by Yekutiel and Guttman and to add functional tests such as the Motor Assessment Scale (hand function items) to test the generalizability of training (see Chapter 3).

Carey and colleagues (1993) tested a programme of task-specific training with two groups of four subjects 5–26 weeks following stroke, using attentive exploration and quantitative feedback. The results showed that marked improvement took place in the tactile and proprioceptive discrimination tasks tested, and that this improvement was maintained in most subjects for several weeks.

Visual impairments

Vision is our major source of information about the environment and our place in it. Hence, it has been called 'exproprioceptive' (Gibson 1966). When one reaches out to pick up an object, there is a complex interaction between head, eye and hand movements. This is guided by visual information about location of the object and arm, and about the relationship between wrist, finger and hand movements just prior to and during the action of grasping the object (Mountcastle *et al*. 1975; Jeannerod 1988). Visually-selective neurons are driven by particular object properties such as shape and orientations (Taira *et al*. 1990).

Following stroke or head injury, individuals may demonstrate visual impairments which can have a negative impact upon their ability to engage actively in the rehabilitation process as well as through their daily life. Visual impairments may involve the reception of inputs to the eye itself due to retinal dysfunction or the perceptual–cognitive manipulations of those inputs. The latter are described below under visual field loss, and visual and visuospatial agnosia.

The therapist should be sure to be informed about the state of the person's visual system, given its critical role in movement control. Elderly individuals may have pre-existing visual impairments corrected by eye glasses, and it is important for acute care and rehabilitation staff to ensure the person wears their glasses during the day. Elderly individuals may have serious impairments such as cataract or macular degeneration and rehabilitation needs to take account of the problems encountered by the seriously visually impaired and provide the necessary aids to enable the person's active participation. An understanding of visual impairment enables the therapist to give consideration to environmental features such as glare and lighting during motor training. (See Efferson 1995, for a useful introduction to visual impairments.)

Visual field loss

Not uncommon after stroke affecting the right brain is the loss of half the visual field (hemianopsia). The term homonymous hemianopsia is used when there is loss of half the visual field on the same side of each eye, which means that objects are cut vertically. Individuals with visual field loss are unable to see objects which lie within a particular part of the visual field, which is that area we can see in front and to both sides while looking straight ahead (Fig. 10.1). The person may not appreciate this loss of vision and may not compensate by moving the head unless advised to do so. Some people rationalize the disability, suggesting their glasses need changing or the light is not good enough. The impairment may cause the person to bump into objects on that side, to miss utensils on the dinner tray or have difficulty reading.

Distinguishing a field loss from unilateral neglect is difficult. Testing for extinction (see below) enables this manifestation of unilateral neglect to be confirmed and in this case testing for visual field loss will be unreliable (Efferson 1995). For individuals with hemianopsia compensation training is usually considered necessary. This includes the use of margin markers to aid reading and of using eye and head movement to bring the point of desired focus into view.

Evidence suggests there may be little spontaneous recovery after the first 48 hours (Haerer 1973). However, work by Zihl and his group (Zihl and von Cramon 1985) suggests that the area of the blind field can be decreased by simple perceptual detection tasks with the effect modulated by attention.

Perceptual–cognitive impairments

The impairments described in this section are termed perceptual-cognitive to reflect the interactive links between perceptual and cognitive processes. While cognition can be considered the ability to process and interpret information, the term perception reflects the ability to process and interpret sensory information.

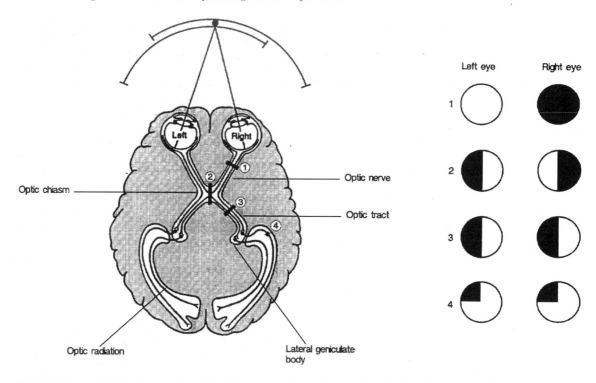

Fig.10.1 Visual field deficits produced by lesions at various points in the visual pathway. 1: Lesion of R optic nerve causes loss of vision in R eye. 2: Lesion of optic chiasm causes loss of vision in the temporal halves of both visual fields (bitemporal hemianopsia). 3: Lesion of optic tract causes complete loss of vision in opposite half of visual field (contralateral hemianopsia). 4: Lesion of optic radiation fibres causes loss of vision in upper quadrant of opposite half of visual field of both eyes. Partial lesions of visual cortex lead to partial field deficits on opposite side

Perceptual–cognitive impairments, which are more complex than the recognition of discrete sensations, may include disorders of right–left discrimination, inattention, disorders of body image, unawareness of one (usually the left) side of space. There are a number of manifestations of the latter two. Critchley in 1953 classified nine types of impairment pointing out that they are not clearly circumscribed but fuse into one another. His list included: unilateral neglect, lack of concern over the existence of hemiplegia, denial of hemiplegia with delusions (anosognosia), and loss of awareness of one body half (autotopagnosia). These are variously described as agnosias and are taken to reflect not only a failure of sensory awareness but also of cognitive awareness of the impairment.

The impairments and the associated puzzling behavioural manifestations illustrate the close links between sensory and motor processes and cognitive and perceptual processes. Their integration is critical for our existence in the environment of which we are a part. The literature on these impairments is confusing due to terminological differences which reflect the poverty of existing knowledge of underlying mechanisms and therefore difficulty with classification. In summary, perceptual–cognitive impairments are complex, little understood and sometimes demonstrated by bizarre behaviours and responses and by striking manifestations of denial.

It is understood that lesions of the *parietal lobes* lead to abnormalities of body image and perception of spatial relations. Lesions of either lobe appear to result in complex perceptual–cognitive difficulties, although it has been usual to consider that these deficits occur only after a lesion of the right (usually non-dominant) lobe. Although it appears that the more severe impairments, those which typically lead to the individual being tested, result from lesions of the right brain, it is becoming increasingly evident that lesions of the left brain are also followed by similar but less severe impairments which may only be evident on testing. Kupferman (1991) provides a useful introduction to these deficits.

Lesions of the left parietal lobe may be associated with *aphasia*, a disorder of language, and *agnosia*, an inability to perceive or know objects in the presence of normally functioning sensory pathways. Inability to recognize the form of an object by touch and therefore to recognize the object itself (*astereognosis*) may be present.

Lesions of the inferior region of the left parietal cortex give rise to a group of deficits called *Gerstmann's syndrome*, which is characterized by confusion between left and right, finger agnosia (difficulty naming fingers when they are touched), dysgraphia (difficulty writing) and dyscalculia (difficulty with mathematical calculations).

Lesions of the right parietal lobe are typically associated with a lack of appreciation of the spatial aspects of sensory input from the left side of the body and the left extrapersonal space. Affected individuals are said to suffer neglect of the left side of space. This deficit, which may be present in spite of the individual having intact somatic sensation, is typically referred to as *unilateral spatial neglect*, although a variety of other terms, such as visuospatial agnosia, are also used.

Neglect may also be evident in visual, auditory, tactile, kinaesthetic and conceptual systems. Mixed neglect is reported to differ qualitatively from unimodal neglect, in that a person with visual and auditory neglect does not behave like a person with either visual or auditory neglect (Halsband *et al.* 1985).

Deficits in the nonsyntactic processing of language may be present with inferior parietal lobe lesions, the person having trouble appreciating those aspects of a verbal message conveyed by tone, loudness and timing of words, rather than the actual sense of the words.

Apraxia

Although, following parietal lobe lesions, there may be intact comprehension and sensory and motor function, *apraxia*, a difficulty performing a willed purposeful movement or imitating movements, may be present. Geschwind (1975) defined apraxia as a disorder of learned movements not accounted for by weakness, sensory loss, incoordination, inattention or lack of comprehension. In addition, the ability to perform a task may be present when the setting is altered. Apraxia may involve any movement. It is seen to affect even lip and tongue movement. For example, a person may be unable to lick the lips when asked to do so but will be observed to do so spontaneously when eating. There have been several recent descriptions of the behaviour of individuals with apraxia which give the clinician some insight into the nature of their problems (Riddoch and Humphreys 1987; Pilgrim and Humphreys 1994).

Constructional apraxia has to do with the translation of an object from one spatial dimension to another. The defect appears to be in poor conceptualization of the spatial requirements of certain activities. The person has difficulty copying simple pictures or diagrams (Fig. 10.2). When attempting to write there may be crowding and obliquity of the words. Difficulty with arithmetic may be evident, or telling the time, sewing or constructing a model. When copying a figure, one half may be left out. The person may be unable to interpret maps or find their way about (topographagnosia).

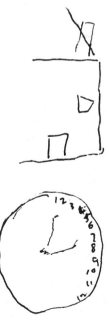

Fig. 10.2 The type of drawing made by individuals with R hemisphere parietal lobe lesion

Ideational apraxia is characterized by extreme absentmindedness and lack of purpose in various actions. For example, the person may light a match and burn the fingers instead of lighting the cigarette. It will be noticeable that the person can perform different parts of the action, i.e., pick up the matchbox, take out a match and strike it, but when asked to light a cigarette will instead do something inappropriate such as striking the cigarette on the matchbox.

Ideomotor apraxia is the inability to execute ideas or perform previously learned and skilled activities. The person may understand the purpose of the object but be unable to use it. For example, attempting to dress may involve putting the arm through the trouser leg.

Some individuals demonstrate a difficulty when attempting to walk in the early stages which may reflect apraxia. The person seems to have no idea about the movements required and may act impulsively, attempting to lift one foot without shifting weight on to the other, taking several small steps with one foot without moving the other. When helped, the person may take small steps forward with both feet while leaving the rest of the body behind. Since these individuals seem to have difficulty following instructions or responding to feedback, their behaviour may be thought to reflect intellectual deterioration rather than a lack of awareness of the appropriate movement at that time.

Three individuals with ideomotor apraxia, all with lesions that included the left parietal lobe, were investigated in a three-dimensional study of a 'slicing bread' action (Poizner *et al*. 1995). Subjects performed the action either with or without the necessary tools. Compared to healthy control subjects, the individuals with apraxia demonstrated disorganized relationships between joint movements, with deficits in phase relationships indicating impaired joint coordination. These were evident both when subjects were asked to make bread slicing movements and when they were able to use the bread and knife to perform the task. The authors suggested that their findings support the view that apraxia results from an impairment of visuo-kinaesthetic motor representations of learned movement (stored in association cortex).

Visual perceptual impairments

These may include distortion of the perception of the horizontal and vertical planes. Distorted perception of verticality has been reported in patients following stroke (Birch *et al*. 1962; DeCencio *et al*. 1970). A relationship between this visual perceptual disturbance and falling has also been reported in elderly individuals, including those who have had a stroke (Tobis *et al*. 1981).

Other problems include difficulty appreciating the three dimensional nature of objects, difficulty finding the way from place to place, discriminating numerical symbols, telling the time, visualizing a mental picture of familiar people and things, understanding the meaning of up–down, in–out, front–back.

Visual agnosia is an inability to recognize visual stimuli (faces, objects) in the presence of normally functioning vision, language and intellect (Rubens 1979). It may result from a lesion (usually bilateral) in the visual associative areas (areas 18–19).

Some individuals have difficulty with *figure-ground perception* and are unable to distinguish an object from its background. An object has to be selected from its background and isolated, this visual processing being necessary for the control of an action or to enable learning or recognition (Milner and Goodale 1993). Impairment in figure-ground perception has a particular effect on hand function and upon visual discrimination in general. A similar problem of discrimination may occur in *auditory perception* with the person unable to distinguish particular sounds from the background noise. The person may appear to be deaf or lacking in concentration.

Unilateral spatial agnosia or neglect

Individuals who do not respond to, identify or orient toward meaningful stimuli which are contralateral to the lesioned hemisphere, but whose deficit cannot be attributed to sensory or motor impairment, are said to have neglect of the body and extra-personal space contralateral to the lesion site (Ladavas *et al*. 1994). There appears to be a decreased ability to integrate visual and tactile sensory information leading to a deficit in the orientation and purposeful movement of the body in space (Brooks 1986). Although these impairments are most typically seen associated with stroke, they may also be present following traumatic brain injury or associated with a cerebral tumour. Neglect is most commonly reported following a lesion of the right hemisphere, however, it is becoming evident that some degree of visuospatial malfunction may also exist with left hemisphere lesions (Wilson *et al*. 1987).

Reported incidence of neglect varies from 29% to 85% of patients (Wilson *et al.* 1987). However, the incidence reported probably depends on tasks tested (see Schenkenberg *et al.* 1980) and in the definition of neglect. Neglect is reported to be transitory in many cases with individuals making spontaneous recovery (Wilson *et al.* 1987). However, there have been few systematic investigations and no clear consensus on evaluating neglect and it is possible that neglect persists in some individuals despite lack of obvious behavioural indications.

Severe neglect is considered to have serious effects on rehabilitation and recovery (Feigenson *et al.* 1977; Kinsella and Ford 1980; Denes *et al.* 1982; Kotila *et al.* 1986; Calvanio *et al.* 1993). Spatial disorders can involve impairments of perception, attention, memory and executive function (Calvanio *et al.* 1993). In addition, neglect is commonly accompanied by discrete sensory (tactile, proprioceptive and stereogostic) impairment, muscle weakness or paralysis, motor control deficits and visual field impairments. These latter considerably worsen the person's disability regarding one half of visual space.

In a patient with an ischaemic lesion involving right frontal lobe and basal ganglia described in a recent paper, the neglect was manifested as a 'directional hypokinesia', in which the impairment appeared to be a defective organization of arm movement toward the left side of space (Bottini *et al.* 1992). The performance of stroke subjects on reaching actions has been demonstrated by other studies. These show, with spatial and temporal kinematic analyses, that individuals with right hemisphere lesions, although demonstrating a similar pattern of movement to able-bodied controls, appeared to need more time to determine the spatial location of the target (Fisk and Goodale 1988). Goodale and colleagues (Goodale *et al.* 1990) went on to demonstrate further that hemispatial neglect can be a subtle deficit following damage to the right hemiphere, showing up only in the temporal and spatial form of movement detected on kinematic analysis. They suggest that such kinematic analyses are a valuable technique for evaluating recovery of function.

The individual with a spatial impairment may fail to dress or wash the left side of the body or shave on the left (*autotopagnosia*) or brush teeth on one side only. The left side of space appears not to be 'seen' and the patient may eat food only on one side of the plate (Fig. 10.3), start reading a sentence from the middle of the page and fail to attend to objects and people on the left side.

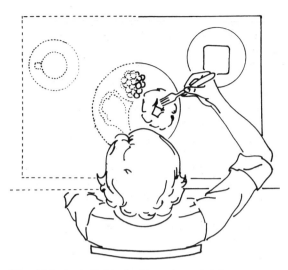

Fig. 10.3 An individual with a visuospatial impairment may only eat food on one side of the plate

Walking through a doorway, the individual may veer to one side or bump into the door frame. The person may deny the left arm or leg belongs to them, or deny the existence of hemiplegia (*anosognosia*).

The clinical signs of neglect are described both in the literature and in the clinic by different terms such as hemispatial neglect, hemispatial agnosia, hemi-inattention and hemi-neglect. The terminology in common use may be unnecessarily misleading. 'Neglect' suggests some degree of carelessness in the individual, inferring the person has a voluntary choice not to respond. Indeed it is not uncommon to hear a member of the acute care or rehabilitation staff admonishing the patient who is staring off to the right, leaning to the left, with the left arm hanging over the side of the chair with 'You're forgetting your left arm again, Mrs ——'. In a sense 'inattention' also infers that the person's behaviour is under volitional control. Perhaps the Greek word 'agnosia', which means lack of knowledge or awareness, best reflects the person's dilemma. Brain (1945) used this term since it implied a selective cognitive disorder independent of sensory and intellectual disturbance.

The variability in terminology reflects the multi-component nature of neglect and it is likely that a lack of knowledge about the underlying mechanisms is a contributing factor. It seems accepted that neglect phenomena cannot be explained in terms of a single underlying mechanism (Riddoch and Humphreys 1994). A brain lesion, even a relatively discrete one, disrupts a complete functional system, so it is difficult relating injury site to subsequent impairments.

It is, therefore, generally assumed that many different impairments are covered by the label 'neglect' (Halligan and Marshall 1992); that it is a multimodal disorder involving not only visual but also tactile and auditory awareness, complicated by weak and paralysed muscles and discrete sensory loss with denial behaviours and attitudes. Difficulties with writing, reading and drawing also come under this general heading, together with impairments of line orientation and verticality perception. It has been argued (Halligan and Marshall 1992) that the clinical symptoms regarded as making up the syndrome of neglect may have nothing more in common than the fact that there is involvement of the left side of space. Riddoch and Humphreys (1994) point out the heterogeneity of the anatomical regions implicated in neglect which has been reported in individuals following lesions to several different areas of the brain (e.g., posterior parietal lobe, frontal lobe, cingulate gyrus, thalamus, basal ganglia). However, it has been proposed that the inferior and posterior parietal cortex may be critically involved in monitoring and directing attention within the visual environment, with more anterior lesions resulting in impaired initiation and execution of movements within the contralateral side of space (Coslett *et al.* 1990).

Three main hypotheses have emerged in attempts to explain the impairment (see Ladavas *et al.* 1994):

- A *representational* hypothesis which considers the impairment to be an inability to form a whole representation of space (Bisiach and Vellar 1988);
- An *arousal* hypothesis in which the impairment is viewed as a selective loss of orienting responses to space (Heilman *et al.* 1987); and
- A *selective attention* hypothesis in which there is an imbalance in the attentional system which favours shifts to the opposite side (Kinsbourne 1987; Ladavas *et al.* 1990).

This latter hypothesis may be illustrated by the phenomenon called *extinction or tactile inattention*. Individuals with this impairment, when presented with competing stimuli applied bilaterally and simultaneously, disregard the left side stimulus in favour of the right.

Attention to the right side to the exclusion of the left seems very compelling to the affected individ-ual. Stimuli in the right field seem to provide a strong magnet, making it difficult to disengage their attention once it has been captured in the right visual field or even centrally (Posner *et al.* 1987).

Different components of attention may be affected (Ladavas et al. 1989):

- Arousal–activation mechanisms, the physiological readiness to respond to stimuli wherever they are located (Heilman and Van den Abell 1980).
- Orientation and selective attention to a space (Posner *et al.* 1987).
- Shifting attention from one target to another (Mark *et al.* 1988).
- Intention, the motor activation necessary to respond to a stimulus (Verfaelli *et al.* 1988).

For patients to be able to shift visual attention they need to be able to disengage their attention from one target, shift it to another then focus attention on this new target (Herman 1992).

Outcome for individuals with neglect may be affected by the state of the individual's brain pre-stroke. One of the sources of recovery within the lesioned brain involves the role of the intact hemisphere. Levine and colleagues (1986) reported a study which examined cerebral atrophy (ventricle size and sulcal width) in 29 individuals with right hemisphere stroke. Atrophy was not related to the stroke lesion but it pre-dated stroke. Atrophy was, however, related to neglect and to delayed recovery at 10–20 weeks among moderate to severely affected patients. These findings, according to the authors, are consistent with a significant role for the left hemisphere in determining recovery from left neglect. Recovery and trainability of everyday actions are also likely to be affected and this has been reported by Calvanio and colleagues (1993). Figure 10.4 (*top*) shows that all patients started out at one week post-stroke at a similar level but varied widely by seven weeks. The lower part shows the major source of this variability. The seven individuals had large right hemisphere lesions but the results show that the degree of recovery is inversely related to the amount of pre-stroke cortical atrophy.

Lack of awareness of impairment and denial

Responses to impairment may result in the person objecting to a reminder, acting as if an object is not present, and acknowledging its presence but still behaving as though it does not exist (Diller and Weinberg 1993).

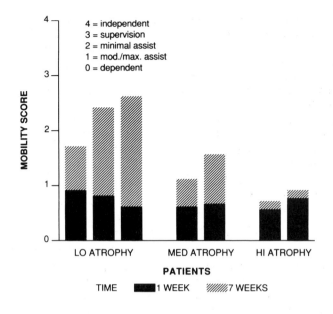

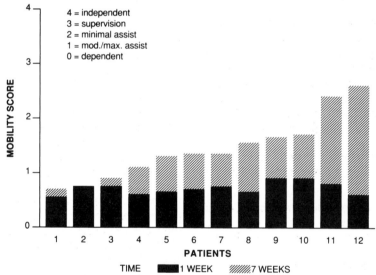

Fig. 10.4 (*top*) Variation in recovery of mobility in 12 patients with R hemisphere stroke. All were severely impaired 1 week after admission to rehabilitation; at 7 weeks, they showed varied degrees of recovery. Mobility measures were performance on getting in and out of wheelchair, wheelchair driving, ambulation and stair climbing. (*lower*) Variation in mobility of 7 of the above patients as a function of low, medium and high cortical atrophy by CT scan. (From Calvanio *et al.* (1993) by permission)

Denial of impairment is one response seen following brain lesion. Reasons for denial may range from a desire to avoid unpleasant problems or maintain positive self-regard to a lack of awareness associated with unilateral neglect. In the latter situation, understanding denial can help the therapist work out solutions to impairments with the patient.

Diller and Weinberg (1993, p. 167) categorize patients' responses into four levels:

I   Active resistance when confronted with a visuo-perceptual problem.
II Indifferent passive resistance.
III Initial resistance accompanied by perplexity on confrontation.

IV   Awareness and acceptance of the problem on a gross level but failure to come to grips with the specific ways in which the problems are played out.

They give examples of the types of behaviour commonly demonstrated in each group and indications of means by which rehabilitation can attempt to deal with the denial. Basically the task for remediation they suggest is to facilitate the patient's discovery of their own impairment when they cannot achieve this on their own.

Some physiotherapists use the term *'pusher syndrome'* in an attempt to explain the behaviour of individuals who demonstrate ipsilateral pushing, i.e., those who lean toward the hemiplegic side and resist any attempt at passive correction of posture that would move weight toward or across the midline of the body toward the non-affected side (Davies 1985; Ashburn 1995).

There has been little investigation of this phenomenon. A recent Danish study (Pedersen *et al.* 1996) sought to investigate the incidence of ipsilateral pushing, establish whether or not there is such a syndrome, and determine the effect of pushing on functional recovery. The incidence was found to be 10% of the 327 subjects studied. However, the diagnosis of 'pusher' was provided by therapist observation and not by any standardized or reliable measure. All patients with unilateral pushing had the more severe strokes. Interestingly, they were no more likely to suffer neglect or anosognosia than the non-pushers, were distributed evenly between left- and right-sided lesions, and, although they spent longer in rehabilitation, their functional outcome was not affected by ipsilateral pushing.

The authors proposed that there was, therefore, no support for the so-called 'pusher syndrome', in the sense of a syndrome encompassing both physical and neuropsychological symptoms. Pedersen and colleagues found an increased involvement of crus posterior of the internal capsule, suggesting damage to sensory pathways, but there was no special association with parietal lobe involvement.

There is some anecdotal evidence that individuals with this problem have an impairment in judging the vertical (verticality perception). It often appears that patients have experienced a change in their perception of the midline of their body, which can explain the anxiety and even fear expressed if they are moved by the therapist into a more symmetrical sitting position. A recent study

(Karnath *et al.* 1991) found evidence that the midline of the trunk and/or head serves as a plane for dividing space into a right and left sector. The trunk midline serves as a physical anchor for the calculation of internal egocentric coordinates for representing the position of the body relative to external objects.

It is our experience that the tendency to push usually disappears after a short period of balance training (see Chapter 7), as patients regain their ability to move about in sitting and standing. In our view, it is possible that the techniques used in Bobath therapy, which involve the patient being moved about by the physiotherapist, may reinforce the abnormal behaviour and cause it to persist for longer. If an individual's midline of body has shifted to one side, being moved over by the therapist to the opposite side would be perceived as a large excursion away from the egocentric midline. Affected patients are clearly distressed when attempts are made to move them to the unaffected side and appear to cope much better when trained to move actively toward that side, with visual cueing and appropriate rewards and feedback provided. It is sometimes helpful to point out that they are being misled about the nature of vertical and to encourage them to look at objects they 'know' to be vertical (i.e., the leg of a bed, a door frame); i.e., to intellectualize the 'idea' of vertical and to try to align themselves with known vertically oriented objects.

Evaluation

Evaluation is typically carried out by a neuropsychologist. However, careful observation of the person's behaviour may reveal many aspects of the impairment and provide explanations of poor performance in general motor training in addition to useful clues for the neuropsychologist and therapist regarding specific points to be addressed in rehabilitation.

Neuropsychological asessment of visuospatial neglect includes various simple perceptual motor tasks involving, for example, line crossing (Albert 1973), cancellation tasks (Diller and Weinberg 1977) and drawing and copying tasks. Other tests include drawing from memory, copying complex figures, performing visual matching tasks.

Wilson and colleagues (1987) argue that such tests are not relevant to the problems encountered in everyday life. Just as tests of motor performance in everyday actions such as reaching, walking and standing up give an indication of what must be achieved in movement rehabilitation, so, Wilson and colleagues argue, behavioural tests of a selection of everyday skills provide the grounding for specific rehabilitation strategies, despite the absence of clearly defined underlying mechanisms.

The Rivermead Behavioural Inattention Test (see Chapter 3) was developed to provide such information (Stone *et al.* 1987, 1991; Wilson *et al.* 1987, 1988). It consists of items such as dialling a telephone, reading a menu, copying an address and following a map. It has been shown to be a valid and reliable test.

The verticality test is a simple subjective test which can be carried out by the therapist to indicate whether or not a person perceives the vertical correctly. It involves holding an object such as a ruler, stick or pencil in front of the person at different orientations including the vertical and asking the person to say which orientation is vertical. Alternatively, the individual being tested is asked to match a ruler to the orientation of the examiner's ruler (Efferson 1995).

The auditory perception test involves for example, snapping the fingers by the person's ear. It is another simple test to enable the therapist to gain some indication of hearing capacity.

Individuals who disregard one stimulus over another if applied bilaterally and simultaneously are said to demonstrate what is called *tactile inattention or extinction*. This disability causes the person to be unaware of stimulation on the affected side when this stimulus has to compete with a stimulus to the sound side. The ability to recognize both stimuli requires normal tactile localization, i.e., the person has to be able to localize one spot when it is touched. Therefore, tactile localization needs to be tested before the test for tactile inattention.

Training

Treatment regimes for perceptual–cognitive impairments are difficult to develop due to the lack of a clear understanding of the underlying mechanisms. Nevertheless, it seems likely that specific training to improve a person's active performance on functionally relevant and concrete tasks, with emphasis on the individual paying attention to and orienting to the relevant objects and their position in space, would result in improvement on these tasks. Given the importance of the visual system in our interactions with the external world, emphasis on vision is a critical part of motor training, particularly early after brain lesion. The individual is encouraged to look around, to scan the environment, to talk about what can be seen; to look at what they are doing; to look at the therapist during a demonstration; to link vision and tactile inputs in deciding on the best way to hold a glass.

Soderbach and colleagues (1992) demonstrated that use of video feedback assisted patients with neglect to perceive and interpret, and partially to overcome, their neglect behaviour.

Specific attention training, in which voluntary orienting of attention, was used, has been shown to be effective in reducing visual neglect and visual extinction (Ladavas *et al.* 1994). The rehabilitation procedure was aimed at training individuals to overcome their bias to the right by directing their attention to stimuli shown in the left visual field.

Lennon (1994) found in her study of one subject that some problems resolved spontaneously immediately the person returned home. Difficulty negotiating an obstacle course showed improvement with cueing by the therapist but no generalization to other settings (at home, outside). However, the person's spouse was able to use cueing to help the person negotiate other environments leading to fewer collisions and falls. Tactile cueing (stroking) with weight-bearing and repetitive motor practice using Bobath therapy (as described in Davies 1985) did not produce any improvement in either motor neglect or spatial awareness.

Emphasis in Bobath therapy is on the therapist moving the patient, with responsive movements made by the patient, with less emphasis on the patient actively moving about themselves. The probability that movement initiated by the therapist might not be the optimal method of helping the person overcome the impairment is supported by several investigations. In a study involving a visual target search in which targets had to be manually identified, there was significantly less neglect when the left (affected) hand was used compared to the right (unaffected) (Joanette *et al.* 1986). Results of another study of one individual (Robertson and North 1993) suggest that self-initiated and intentional movements of the affected limb may reduce visual neglect by moving the limb about in the neglected part of extrapersonal space. Their results showed that passive movement of the left hand did not reduce neglect of that hand. Active movement, however, reduced neglect but not extinction, supporting the generally held view that different mechanisms subserve sensory extinction from those underlying neglect. A later report (Robertson and North 1994), replicating this result with two other subjects, suggests that improvements seen in neglect may disappear during bilateral active hand use. This suggests that bilateral tasks need to be trained (see Chapter 6).

Overall, rehabilitation aims to address specific deficits by increasing the person's awareness of the nature of their problem and by training them to reorient their attention as particular situations require. Training takes place as part of the practice of motor tasks, such as walking, standing up and sitting down, reaching for and manipulating objects, in sitting and standing. However, specific training may also need to be provided to address highly task-related perceptual–cognitive impairments. Such training is typically carried out by a neuropsychologist or occupational therapist with reinforcement provided during motor training sessions with the physiotherapist.

From the studies available to date, some **general principles** can be outlined for use by the physiotherapist during the **training of motor tasks**. These principles are taught to friends and relatives as well as to the affected individual as a means of reinforcement during visits and at home.

- Increase the person's awareness and understanding of the inattention and suggest strategies for overcoming the problem. Knowing that they are not mad or senile is very reassuring for the individual.
- Emphasize the need (and advantages) of visual scanning using interesting items as targets, introducing games to the training (How many objects can you see on that wall?). Rather than asking the person to turn to the left all the time, suggest he/she searches for a particular object instead.
- Increase the complexity of the tasks – assembling objects scattered on the table.
- Encourage the person to deal with what seems odd and to use head and eye movement to locate apparently missing objects.
- Use markers to help the person anchor their vision – explain the reason for this. In reading, encourage the person not to start reading a line until the eye has scanned to the marker on the left of the page.
- Teach the person to slow down if they are being impulsive.
- If inattention reappears during training, give the person time and assistance in becoming reoriented before going on.
- Both therapist and relatives should avoid using words with negative connotations and be sure

not to nag. For example, it may be better to say 'see if you can find' a particular object rather than 'turn to the left'.
- Fatigue and performance decrements during training can be ameliorated by feedback (Fleet and Heilman 1986).

One implication from research in the area of unilateral attentional disorders is that training should involve specific cues found in everyday life (Robertson 1994). Cueing the patient to attend to the affected side has been shown to improve neglect (Posner *et al.* 1982). Conversely, neglect is exacerbated by presenting stimuli on both sides simultaneously (Riddoch and Humphreys 1994).

Due to the observed problems with transference of training effects from one task to another (Gouvier 1987; Wagenaar and Beek 1992) and the failure of positive results to persist after training ceases (Gordon *et al.* 1985), it seems clear that at this stage of our knowledge training to enable the individual to regain control over the affected limbs during the practice of everyday and meaningful tasks may be the preferable means of improving neglect. Lennon (1994) also suggests that training strategies should be incorporated that are specific and relevant to the tasks that individuals are likely to encounter in everyday life. With the general concept of specific and meaningful training, auditory feedback (Robertson and Cashman 1991) may also be effective in enabling individuals with attentional deficits to achieve more effective motor function. Computerized scanning and attentional training programmes have not been found to be successful at generalizing into other more real-life tasks or to be maintained once training has ceased (Robertson *et al.* 1990).

In the *acute phase*, the manifestations of perceptual–cognitive impairments may be very pronounced, and early efforts to increase the person's awareness and understanding of the deficits may be critical to their general wellbeing and confidence. It is also important to help the person avoid the confusion they experience and the depression that may result from a feeling that they are mentally incompetent. Although it is said that the more profound impairments typically improve spontaneously (Wade *et al.* 1988), while more subtle manifestations may persist (Heilman *et al.* 1985), early intervention may make a great deal of difference to how both patient and those who are in contact with the patient (relatives, therapists, physicians) view the situation. One training strategy which may be effective is to help the person use intellectual knowledge both as a substitute for their lack of direct information and as a means of regaining direct knowledge. Items 1 and 3 below illustrate the use of this strategy.

Some examples of early training include:

1 **Where awareness of verticality is impaired:**
   - Explain with a rod that the eyes and brain are providing incorrect information/playing tricks and suggest the person focuses on an object known to be upright (such as the legs of the bed) and try to 'see' them as upright.

2 **Where the person falls or leans (or 'pushes') toward the affected side in sitting:**
   - A small cushion placed under the left buttock may be sufficient to enable the person to sit upright.
   - Repetitive exercises such as reaching down to pick up a desirable object from the floor in front, with the object gradually being placed more and more toward the right may help the person learn to orient toward the right. The tasks should be varied, interesting and sufficiently difficult to provide a challenge.

3 **Where the person neglects food to the left of the plate:**
   - The person is encouraged to find the food on the left by using touch – exploring the plate with the fork or with fingers (see Lawson 1962). When food is located on the left, the person is encouraged to identify what that food is and to concentrate on picking it up with the fork and eating it.

4 **Where a person has difficulty paying attention to the left during training:**
   - Keep the right space free of competing stimuli; suggest the person does not talk while trying to pay attention; forewarn of a coming change in activity.
   - Start with the person attending centrally, or even to the right, i.e., start where the person can cope, then try to move their attention toward the left.
   - Use eye contact as a magnet to draw the person's attention to the left. Reward eye contact on the left with a smile.

If neglect is seen principally as a lateralized attentional deficit, rehabilitation needs to emphasize the training of attentional processes. Training of attention is a critical part of motor training which sets out to enable the individual to regain effective performance. It has been suggested that tasks which make demands on the right hemisphere may boost the depleted attentional resources of that hemisphere causing increased arousal and consequently decreased neglect of the left side (Riddoch and Humphreys 1994).

In conclusion, despite the fact that somatosensory loss is relatively common following brain lesion, and stroke in particular, it remains a somewhat neglected problem (Carey 1995). The same can probably be said about visual and perceptual–cognitive impairments. Such impairments cause considerable difficulty for the individual through their impact on activities which require information about the environment. Recently developed rehabilitation methods directed at training specific functional actions depend on learning by the patient for their success (e.g., Carr and Shepherd 1987a,b). Such methods are likely to assist the person with somatosensory, visual and perceptual–cognitive impairments since they involve active participation of the individual, use of the environment to facilitate interaction, an emphasis on the need to pay attention to the task, and the practice of concrete tasks. However, it seems likely, and there is some supporting evidence, that specific retraining of sensory awareness, with emphasis on paying attention to relevant sensory inputs is necessary for some individuals. In addition, some individuals who have severe cognitive deficits will need additional training of, for example, such cognitive processes as memory and attention.

References

Albert, M.L. (1973) A simple test of neglect. *Neurology*, **23**, 658–664.

Ashburn, A. (1995) Behavioural deficits associated with the 'pusher' syndrome. *Proceedings of World Congress of Physiotherapists*, Washington, DC, p. 819.

Bickerstaff, E.R. and Spillane, J.A. (1989) *Neurological Examination in Clinical Practice*, 5th edn, Blackwell Scientific, London.

Birch, H.G., Belmont, I., Reilly, T. *et al.* (1962) Somesthetic infuences on perception of visual verticality in hemiplegia. *Archives of Physical Medicine and Rehabilitation*, **43**, 556–560.

Bisiach, E. and Vellar, G. (1988) Hemineglect in humans. In *Handbook of Neuropsychology* (eds F. Bollar and J. Grafman), Elsevier, Amsterdam, pp. 195–222.

Boivie, J., Leijon, G. and Johansson, I. (1989) Central post-stroke pain: a study of the mechanisms through analysis of the sensory abnormalities. *Pain*, **37**, 173.

Bottini, G., Sterzi, R. and Vallar, G. (1992) Directional hypokinesia in spatial hemineglect: a case study. *Journal of Neurology, Neurosurgery, and Psychiatry*, **55**, 562–565.

Brain, W.R. (1945) Speech and handedness. *Lancet*, **2**, 837–842.

Brooks, V.B. (1986) *The Neural Basis of Motor Control*, Oxford University Press, New York.

Burke, D. and Gandevia, S.C. (1988) Interfering cutaneous stimulation and the muscle afferent contribution to cortical potentials. *Encephalography and Clinical Neurophysiology*, **70**, 118–125.

Calvanio, R., Levine, D. and Petrone, P. (1993) Elements of cognitive rehabilitation after right hemisphere stroke. *Behavioral Neurology*, **11**, 25–57.

Carey, L.M. (1995) Somatosensory loss after stroke. *Critical Reviews in Physical and Rehabilitation Medicine*, **7**, 51–91.

Carey, L.M., Matyas, T.A. and Oke, L.E. (1993) Sensory loss in stroke patients: effective training of tactile and proprioceptive discrimination. *Archives of Physical Medicine and Rehabilitation*, **74**, 602–611.

Carr, J.H. and Shepherd, R.B.(1987a) *A Motor Relearning Programme for Stroke*, 2nd edn, Butterworth Heinemann, Oxford.

Carr, J.H. and Shepherd, R.B. (1987b) A motor learning model for rehabilitation. In *Movement Science. Foundations for Physical Therapy in Rehabilitation* (eds J.H. Carr and R.B. Shepherd) Butterworth Heinemann, Oxford.

Clifford, D.B. (1984) The somatosensory system and pain. In *Neurological Pathophysiology* (eds A.L. Pearlman and R.C. Collins), 3rd edn, Oxford University Press, New York, p. 74.

Coslett, H.B., Bowers, D., Fitzpatrick, E. *et al.* (1990) Directional hypokinesia and hemispatial inattention in neglect. *Brain*, **113**, 475–486.

Critchley, M. (1953) *The Parietal Lobes*, Hafner, New York.

Dannenbaum, R.M. and Dykes, R.W. (1988) Sensory loss in the hand after sensory stroke: therapeutic rationale. *Archives of Physical Medicine and Rehabilitation*, **69**, 833–839.

Davies, P.M. (1985) *Steps to Follow: A Guide to the Treatment of Adult Hemiplegia*, Springer-Verlag, Berlin.

DeCencio, D.V., Leshner, M. and Voron, D. (1970) Verticality perception and ambulation in hemiplegia. *Archives of Physical Medicine and Rehabilitation*, **51**, 105–110.

Denes, G., Semenza, C., Stoppa, E. *et al.* (1982) Unilateral spatial neglect and recovery from hemiplegia. A follow-up study. *Brain*, **105**, 543–552.

de Jersey, M. (1979) Report on a sensory programme for patients with sensory deficits. *Australian Journal of Physiotherapy*, **25**, 165.

Dellon, A.L. (1981) *Evaluation of Sensibility and Re-education of Sensation in the Hand*, Williams and Wilkins, Baltimore, MD.

Diller, L. and Weinberg, J. (1977) Hemi-inattention and rehabilitation. The evolution of a rational treatment program. In *Advances in Neurology*, 18 (eds E.A. Weinstein and R.P. Friedland), Raven Press, New York.

Diller, L. and Weinberg, J.(1993) Response styles in perceptual retraining. In *Advances in Stroke Rehabilitation* (ed. W.A. Gordon), Andover Medical Publishers, Boston, pp. 162–182.

Ebner, F.F. and Armstrong-James, M.A. (1990) Intracortical processes regulating the integration of sensory information. In *Progress in Brain Research* (eds P. Coleman, G. Higgins and C. Phelps), Elsevier Science Publishers, Amsterdam, pp. 129–141.

Efferson, L. (1995) Disorders of vision and visual perceptual dysfunction. In *Neurological Rehabilitation* (ed D.A. Umphred), 3rd edn, Mosby, St Louis, pp. 769–801.

Feigenson, J.S., McCarthy, M.L., Greenberg, S.D. *et al.* (1977) Factors influencing outcome and length of stay in a stroke rehabilitation unit. Part 2. Comparison of 318 screened and 248 unscreened patients. *Stroke*, **8**, 657–662.

Fisher, C.M. (1982) Pure sensory stroke and allied conditions. *Stroke*, **13**, 434–447.

Fisk, J.D. and Goodale, M.A. (1988) The effects of unilateral brain damage on visually guided reaching: hemispheric differences in the nature of the deficit. *Experimental Brain Research*, **72**, 425–435.

Fleet, W.S. and Heilman, K.M. (1986) The fatigue effect in unilateral neglect. *Neurology*, **36** (Supplement 1), 258.

Garraway, W.M., Akhtar, A.J., Gore, S.M. (1976) Observer variation in the clinical assessment of stroke. *Age and Ageing*, **5**, 233.

Geschwind, N. (1975) The apraxias: neural mechanisms of disorders of learned movement. *American Scientist*, **63**, 188–195.

Gibson, J.J. (1966) *The Senses Considered as Perceptual Systems*, Houghton Mifflin, Boston.

Goodale, M.A., Milner, A.D., Jakobson, L.S. *et al.* (1990) Kinematic analysis of limb movements in neuropsychological research: subtle deficits and recovery of function. *Canadian Journal of Psychology*, 44, 180–195.

Gordon, W.A., Hibbard, M.R., Egelco, S. *et al.* (1985) Perceptual remediation in patients with right brain damage: a comprehensive program. *Archives of Physical Medicine and Rehabilitation*, **66**, 353–359.

Gordon, J.(1987) Assumptions underlying physical therapy intervention: theoretical and historical perspectives. In *Movement Science. Foundations for Physical Therapy in Rehabilitation* (eds J.H. Carr and R.B. Shepherd), Butterworth Heinemann, Oxford.

Gouvier, W.D. (1987) Assessment and treatment of cognitive deficits in brain-damaged individuals. *Behavior Modification* **11**, 312–328.

Halliday, A.M. and Wakefield, G.S. (1963) Cerebral evoked potentials in patients with dissociated sensory loss. *Journal of Neurology, Neurosurgery, and Psychiatry*, **26**, 211–219.

Halligan, P.W. and Marshall, J.C. (1992) Left visuospatial neglect: a meaningless entity? *Cortex*, **28**, 525–535.

Halsband, U., Gruhn, S. and Ettlinger, G. (1985) Unilateral spatial neglect and defective performance in one half of space. *International Journal of Neuroscience*, **28**, 173–195.

Heilman, K.M. and van den Abell, T. (1980) The right hemisphere dominance for attention: the mechanism underlying hemispheric asymmetries of inattention (neglect). *Neurology* **30**, 327–330.

Heilman, K.M., Bowers, D., Coslett, H.B. *et al.* (1985) Directional hypokinesia: prolonged reaction times for leftward movements in patients with right hemisphere lesions and neglect. *Neurology*, **35**, 855–859.

Heilman, K.M., Bowers, D., Valenstein, E. *et al.* (1987) Hemispace and hemispatial neglect. In *Neurophysiological and Neuropsychological Aspects of Spatial Neglect* (ed. M. Jeannerod), Elsevier, Amsterdam, pp. 115–150.

Herman, E.W.M. (1992) Spatial neglect: new issues and their implications for occupational therapy practice. *American Journal of Occupational Therapy*, **46**, 207–216.

Hodgins, E. (1966) Listen: the patient. *New England Journal of Medicine*, **274**, 657–661.

Hyvarinen, J., Poranen, A. and Jokinen, Y. (1980) Influence of attentive behavior on neuronal responses to vibration in primary somatosensory cortex of the monkey. *Journal of Neurophysiology*, **43**, 870–883.

Jacobs, H., Vanderstaeten, G., Van Laere, M. *et al.* (1988) SEPs and central somatosensory conduction time in hemiplegics. *Electromyography and Clinical Neurophysiology*, **28**, 355–360.

Jeannerod, M. (1988) *Neural and Behavioural Organization of Goal-Directed Movements*, Oxford University Press, Oxford.

Jeannerod, M., Michel, F. and Prablanc, C. (1984) The control of hand movements in a case of hemianaethesia following a parietal lesion. *Brain*, **107**, 899–920.

Jenkins, W.M. and Merzenich, M.M. (1987) Reorganization of neocortical representations after brain injury: a neurophysiological model of the bases of recovery from stroke. In *Progress in Brain Research, 71* (eds F.J. Seil, E. Herbert and B.M. Carlson), Elsevier Science, New York, pp. 249–266.

Joanette, Y., Brouchon, M., Gauthier, L. *et al.* (1986) Pointing with left versus right hand in left visual field neglect. *Neuropsychologia*, **24**, 391–396.

Johansson, R.S. and Westling, G. (1984) Roles of glabrous skin receptors and sensorimotor memory in automatic control of precision grip when lifting rougher or more slippery objects. *Experimental Brain Research*, **56**, 550–564.

Karnath, H.O., Schenkel, P. and Fischer, B. (1991) Trunk orientation as the determining factor of the 'contralateral' deficit in the neglect syndrome and as the physical anchor of the internal representation of body orientation in space. *Brain*, **114**, 1997–2014.

Kinsbourne, M. (1987) Mechanisms of unilateral neglect. In *Neurophysiological and Neuropsychological Aspects of Spatial Neglect*, (ed. M. Jeannerod),

Elsevier, Amsterdam, pp. 69–86.

Kinsella, G. and Ford, B. (1980) Acute recovery patterns in stroke patients. Neuropsychological factors. *Medical Journal of Australia*, **2**, 663–666.

Knapp, H.D., Taub, F. and Berman, A.J. (1963) Movements in monkeys with deafferented forelimbs. *Experimental Neurology*, **7**, 305–315.

Kotila, M., Niemi, M-L. and Laaksonen, R. (1986) Four-year prognosis of stroke patients with visuospatial inattention. *Scandinavian Journal of Rehabilitation Medicine*, **18**, 177–179.

Kupferman, I. (1991) Localization of higher cognitive and affective functions: The association cortices. In *Principles of Neural Science* (eds E.R. Kandel, J.H. Schwartz and T.M. Jessell), 3rd edn, Appleton & Lange, Norwalk, CT, pp. 823–838.

Kusoffsky, A. (1990) *Sensory Function and Recovery after Stroke*, Karolinska Institute, Stockholm.

Kusoffsky, A., Wadell, I. and Nilsson, B.Y. (1982) The relationship between sensory impairment and motor recovery in patients with hemiplegia. *Scandinavian Journal of Rehabilitation Medicine*, **14**, 27–32.

Ladavas, E., Del Pesce, M. and Provinciali, L. (1989) Unilateral attention deficits and hemispheric asymmetries in the control of visual attention. *Neuropsychologia*, **27**, 353–366.

Ladavas, E., Menghini, G. and Umilta, C. (1994) On the rehabilitation of hemispatial neglect. In *Cognitive Neuropsychology and Cognitive Rehabilitation* (eds M.J. Riddoch and G.W. Humphreys), Erlbaum, London, pp. 151–172.

Ladavas, E., Petronio, A. and Umilta, C. (1990) The deployment of visual attention in the intact field of hemineglect patients. *Cortex*, **26**, 307–317.

La Joie, W.J., Reddy, N.M. and Melvin, J.L. (1982) Somatosensory evoked potentials: their predictive value in right hemiplegia. *Archives of Physical Medicine and Rehabilitation*, **63**, 223–226.

Lawson, I.R. (1962) Visual-spatial neglect in lesions of the right cerebral hemisphere. *Neurology*, **12**, 23–33.

Lee, K.C. and Soderberg, G.L. (1981) Relationship between perception of joint position sense and limb synergies in patients with hemiplegia. *Physical Therapy*, **10**, 1433–1437.

Leijon, G. and Boivie, J. (1989) Central post-stroke pain – the effect of high and low frequency TENS. *Pain*, **38**, 187.

Lennon, S. (1994) Task specific effects in the rehabilitation of unilateral neglect. In *Cognitive Neuropsychology and Cognitive Rehabilitation* (eds M.J. Riddoch and G.W. Humphreys), Erlbaum, London, pp. 187–203.

Levine, D.N., Warach, J.D., Benowitz, L. *et al.* (1986) Left spatial neglect: Effects of lesion size and premorbid brain atrophy on severity and recovery following right cerebral infarction. *Neurology*, **36**, 362.

Lincoln, N.B., Crow, J.L., Jackson, J.M. *et al.* (1991) The unreliability of sensory assessments. *Clinical Rehabilitation*, **5**, 273–282.

Macdonell, R.A.L., Donnan, G.A. and Bladin, P.F. (1989) A comparison of somatosensory evoked and motor evoked potentials in stroke. *Annals of Neurology*, **25**, 147.

Mark, V.W., Kooistra, C.A. and Heilman, K.M. (1988) Hemispatial neglect affected by non-neglected stimuli. *Neurology*, **38**, 1207–1211.

Mason, C. and Kandel, E.R. (1991) Central visual pathways. In *Principles of Neural Science* (eds E.R. Kandel, J.H. Schwartz and T.M. Jessell), Appleton and Lange, Norwalk, CT, pp. 420–438.

Maugiere, F., Desmedt, J.E. and Courjon, J. (1983) Astereognosis and dissociated loss of frontal or parietal components of somatosensory evoked potentials in hemispheric lesions. *Brain*, **106**, 548.

Merzenich, M.M., Kaas, J.H., Wall, J. *et al.* (1983) Topographic reorganization of somatosensory cortical areas 3b and 1 in adult monkeys following restricted deafferentation. *Neuroscience*, **8**, 33.

Merzenich, M.M., Recanzone, G., Jenkins, W.M. *et al.* (1988) Cortical representational plasticity. In *Neurobiology of the Neocortex* (eds P. Rakic and W. Singer), Wiley, New York, pp. 41–67.

Milner, A.D. and Goodale, M.A. (1993) Visual pathways to perception and action. *Progress in Brain Research*, **95**, 317–337.

Mountcastle, V.B., Lynch, J.C., Georgopoulos, A. *et al.* (1975) Posterior parietal association cortex of the monkey: command functions for operations with extrapersonal space. *Journal of Neurophysiology*, **38**, 871–908.

Pavot, A.P., Ignacio, D.R., Kuntavanish, A. *et al.* (1986) The prognostic value of somatosensory evoked potentials in cerebrovascular accidents. *Electromyography and Clinical Neurophysiology*, **26**, 333–340.

Pedersen, P.M., Wandel, A., Jorgensen, H.S. *et al.* (1996) Ipsilateral pushing in stroke: incidence, relation to neuropsychological symptoms, and impact on rehabilitation. The Copenhagen Stroke Study. *Archives of Physical Medicine and Rehabilitation*, **77**, 25–28.

Pilgrim, E. and Humphreys, G.W. (1994) Rehabilitation of a case of ideomotor apraxia. In *Cognitive Neuropsychology and Cognitive Rehabilitation* (eds M.J. Riddoch and G.W. Humphreys), Erlbaum, London, pp. 271–286.

Poizner, H., Clark, M.A., Merians, A.S. *et al.* (1995) Joint coordination deficits in limb apraxia. *Brain*, **118**, 227–242.

Posner, M.I., Cohen, Y., and Rafal, R.D. (1982) Neural systems control of spatial orienting. *Philosophical Transactions of the Royal Society of London,* **B298**, 187–198.

Posner M.I., Walker, J.A., Friedrich, F.A. *et al.* (1987) How do the parietal lobes direct covert attention? *Neuropsychologia*, **25**, 135–145.

Riddoch, M.J. and Humphreys, G.W. (1987) Perceptual and action systems in unilateral visual neglect. In *Neurophysiological and Neuropsychological Aspects of Spatial Neglect* (ed. M. Jeannerod), Elsevier, Amsterdam.

Riddoch, M.J. and Humphreys, G.W. (1994) Towards an understanding of neglect. In *Cognitive Neuropsychology and Cognitive Rehabilitation* (eds M.J. Riddoch and G.W. Humphreys), Erlbaum, London, pp. 125–149.

Robertson, I.H. (1994) The rehabilitation of attentional and hemi-attentional disorders. In *Cognitive Neuropsychology and Cognitive Rehabilitation* (eds M.J. Riddoch and G.W. Humphreys), Erlbaum, London, pp. 173–186.

Robertson I. and Cashman, E. (1991) Auditory feedback for walking difficulties in a case of unilateral neglect: a pilot study. *Neuropsychological Rehabilitation*, **1**, 175–183.

Robertson, I.H. and North, N, (1993) Active and passive activation of left limbs: Influence on visual and sensory neglect. *Neuropsychologia*, **31**, 293–300.

Robertson, I.H. and North, N.T. (1994) One hand is better than two: motor extinction of left hand advantage in unilateral neglect. *Neuropsychologia*, **32**, 1–11.

Robertson, I.H., Gray, J.M., Pentland, B. *et al.* (1990) Microcomputer-based rehabilitation for unilateral left visual neglect: a randomised controlled trial. *Archives of Physical Medicine and Rehabilitation*, **62**, 476–483.

Rothwell, J.C., Traub, M.M., Day, B.I. *et al.* (1982) Manual motor performance in a deafferented man. *Brain*, **105**, 515–542.

Rubens, A. (1979) Agnosia. In *Clinical Neuropsychology* (eds K. Heilman and E. Valenstein), Oxford University Press, New York.

Ruch, T.C., Fulton, J.F. and German, W. (1938) Sensory discrimination in monkey, chimpanzee and man after lesions of the parietal lobe. *Archives of Neurology and Psychiatry*, **39**, 919–938.

Sanes, J.N., Mauritz, K.H., Dalakas, M.C. *et al.* (1985) Motor control in humans with large-fibre sensory neuropathy. *Human Neurobiology*, **4**, 101–114.

Schenkenberg, T., Bradford, D.C. and Ajax, E.T. (1980) Line bisection and unilateral spatial neglect in patients with neurologic impairment. *Neurology*, **30**, 509–517.

Schwartzman, R.J. (1972) Somatesthetic recovery following primary somatosensory projection cortex ablations. *Archives of Neurology*, **27**, 340.

Smith, D.L., Akhtar, A.J. and Garraway, W.M. (1983) Proprioception and spatial neglect after stroke. *Age and Ageing*, **12**, 63–69.

Soderbach, I., Bengtsson, I., Ginsburg, E. *et al.* (1992) Video feedback in occupational therapy: Its effect in patients with neglect syndrome. *Archives of Physical Medicine and Rehabilitation*, **73**, 1140–1145.

Stone, S.P., Wilson, B. and Rose, F.C. (1987) The development of a standard test battery to detect, measure and monitor visuo-spatial neglect in acute stroke. *International Journal of Rehabilitation Research*, **10**, 110.

Stone, S.P., Wilson, B., Wroot, A. *et al.* (1991) The assessment of visuo-spatial neglect after acute stroke.

Journal of Neurology, Neurosurgery, and Psychiatry, **54**, 345–350.

Taira, M., Mine, S., Georgopoulos, A.P. *et al.* (1990) Parietal cortex neurons of the monkey related to the visual guidance of hand movement. *Experimental Brain Research,* **83**, 29–36.

Teasell, R.W. (1992) Pain following stroke. *Critical Reviews in Physical and Rehabilitation Medicine,* **3**, 205–217.

Tobis, J.S., Nayak, L. and Hoehler, F. (1981) Visual perception of verticality and horizontality among elderly fallers. *Archives of Physical Medicine and Rehabilitation,* **62**, 619–622.

Twitchell, T.E. (1951) The restoration of motor function following hemiplegia in man. *Brain,* **74**, 443–480.

van Buskirk, C. and Webster, D. (1955) Prognostic value of sensory defect in rehabilitation of hemiplegics. *Neurology,* **5**, 407–411.

Verfaelli, M., Bowers, D. and Heilman, K.M. (1988) Attentional factors in the occurrence of stimulus-response compatibility effects. *Neuropsychologia,* **26**, 435–444.

Wade, D.T., Wood, V.A. and Hewer, R.L. (1988) Recovery of cognitive function soon after stroke; a study of visual neglect, attention span and verbal recall. *Journal of Neurology, Neurosurgery and Psychiatry,* **51**, 10–13.

Wadell, I., Kusoffsky, A. and Nilsson, B.Y. (1987) A follow-up study of stroke patients 5–6 years after their brain infarct. *International Journal of Rehabilitation Research,* Supplement 5, **10**, 103–110.

Wagenaar, R.C. and Beek, W.J. (1992) Hemiplegic gait: a kinematic analysis using walking speed as an analysis. *Journal of Biomechanics,* **25**, 1007–1015.

Watanabe, Y., Shikano, M., Ohba, M. *et al.* (1989) Correlation between somatosensory evoked potentials and sensory disturbance in stroke patients. *Clinical Electroencephalography,* **20**, 156–161.

Wilson, B., Cockburn, J. and Halligan, P. (1987) Development of a behavioral test of visuospatial neglect. *Archives of Physical Medicine and Rehabili-*

tation, **68**, 98–102.

Wilson, B., Cockburn, J. and Halligan, P. (1988) *Behavioral Inattention Test.* Titchfield, Hants, Thames Valley Test Co, UK.

Winkler, P.A. (1995) Head Injury. In *Neurological Rehabilitation* (ed D.A. Umphred), 3rd edn, Mosby, St Louis.

Wynn-Parry, C.B. and Salter, M. (1975) Sensory reeducation after median nerve lesions. *The Hand,* **8**, 250–257.

Yekutiel, M. and Guttman, E. (1993) A controlled trial of the retraining of the sensory function of the hand in stroke patients. *Journal of Neurology, Neurosurgery, and Psychiatry,* **56**, 241–244.

Zeman, B.D. and Yiannikas, C. (1989) Functional prognosis in stroke: Use of somatosensory evoked potentials. *Journal of Neurology, Neurosurgery and Psychiatry,* **52**, 242.

Zihl, J. and von Cramon D. (1985) Restitution of visual function in patients with cerebral blindness. *Journal of Neurology, Neurosurgery, and Psychiatry,* **42**, 312.

Further reading

Apfeldorf, M. (1962) Perceptual and conceptual processes in a case of left-sided spatial inattention. *Perceptual and Motor Skills,* **14**, 419–423.

Goodale, M.A., Milner, A.D., Jakobson, L.S. *et al.* (1990) Kinematic analysis of limb movements in neuropsychological research: Subtle deficits and recovery of function. *Canadian Journal of Psychology,* **44**, 180–195.

Humphreys, G. and Riddoch, M.J. (1987) *To See But Not to See: A Case Study of Visual Agnosia,* Lawrence Erlbaum, Hillsdale, NJ.

Riddoch, M.J. and Humphreys, G.W. (eds) (1994) *Cognitive Neuropsychology and Cognitive Rehabilitation,* Lawrence Erlbaum, Hove, UK.

11

Stroke

Introduction

Aetiology and pathology

Stroke or cerebrovascular accident refers to neuro-logical signs and symptoms that result from disease involving blood vessels. The brain is highly susceptible to disturbance to its blood supply. Anoxia and ischaemia lasting only seconds can cause neurological signs, and within minutes, irreversible neural damage. Although the cerebro-vasculature has specific anatomical and physio-logical features that are designed to protect the brain from circulatory compromise, when these protective mechanisms fail, the result is a stroke. The terms stroke or cerebrovascular accident are used to describe neurological signs and symptoms, usually focal and acute, that result from diseases involving blood vessels.

Diseases of the blood vessels are among the most common serious neurological disorders (Brust 1991). Disorders of the cerebral circulation include any disease of the vascular system that causes ischaemia or infarction of the brain or spontaneous haemorrhage into the brain or sub-arachnoid space. Strokes are either occlusive (due to closure of a blood vessel) or haemorrhagic (due to bleeding from a vessel). Both types of stroke may occur at any age from many causes including cardiac disease, infection, trauma, neoplasm, vas-cular malformation and immunological disorders. The three most commonly recognized risk factors include hypertension, diabetes mellitus and heart disease, with hypertension the most important of these factors.

Most occlusive strokes are due to atherosclerosis and thrombosis or embolus and most haemorrhagic strokes are associated with hypertension or aneur-ysm. Haemorrhage may occur at the brain's surface (extraparenchymal), for example, from rupture of a congenital aneurysm at the circle of Willis, causing a subarachnoid haemorrhage. Alter-natively, haemorrhage may be intraparenchymal, occurring from rupture of vessels damaged by long-standing hypertension which may cause a blood clot or haematoma within the cerebral hemispheres, in the brain stem or the cerebellum. Rapid intracerebral accumulation of blood under arterial pressure may act as an expanding lesion, displacing or compressing adjacent brain tissue. Haemorrhage may result in ischaemia (insufficiency of blood supply depriving tissue of both oxygen and glucose) or infarction. The effect of an intracerebral haematoma may limit the blood supply to adjacent brain tissue. If ischaemia is temporary, there may be little or no pathological evidence of tissue damage. When ischaemia is sufficiently severe and prolonged, neurons and other cellular elements die (infarction).

The most commonly seen stroke syndrome is caused by infarction in the territory of the mid-cerebral artery with contralateral weakness, sensory loss, homonymous hemianopsia (visual field impairment) and, depending on which hemisphere is involved, either language disturbance (in general, a left hemisphere lesion) or impaired spatial perception (in general, a right hemisphere lesion). A history of abrupt loss of focal cerebral function of some kind constitutes the fundamental basis of the stroke diagnosis.

Cerebral infarction is responsible for about 80% of all first strokes, primary intracranial haemorrhage for about 10% and subarachnoid haemorrhage for about 5 %. These proportions are similar in all places where they have been reliably assessed by computerized tomography (CT) scanning (Warlow 1993).

The vulnerability of the brain to ischaemic damage makes it likely that prevention of stroke rather than improved management is the key to decreasing morbidity and mortality. Changes in lifestyle relating to diet, exercise and tobacco may make important contributions to further reduction in the incidence of stroke (Jamrozik *et al.* 1994).

Classification

Although classification of cerebrovascular disease can be complex, three practical definitions are adequate for most clinical purposes (Warlow 1993). *Transient ischaemic attack* (TIA) is an acute loss of focal cerebral or monocular function with symptoms lasting less than 24 hours which, after adequate investigation, is presumed to be due to embolus or thrombiotic vascular disease (Warlow and Morris 1982). Residual but functionally unimportant neurological signs may persist for longer. A *stroke or cerebrovascular accident* (CVA) comprises rapidly developing clinical symptoms and/or signs of focal and at times global loss of cerebral function, with symptoms lasting more than 24 hours with no apparent cause other than that of vascular origin (Hatano 1976). There is a wide range of severity, from recovery in a few days, through persistent disability to death. Since there is no qualitative difference between TIA and ischaemic stroke, the term *reversible ischaemic attack* (RIA) may be used to describe TIA, and mild ischaemic strokes associated with no persistent neurological disability. *Arteriosclerotic dementia* is deterioration in previously normal intellect and/or memory due to repeated episodes of cerebral ischaemic infarction or haemorrhage.

Incidence

After coronary heart disease and cancer, stroke is the third most common cause of death in western countries and is the most important single cause of severe disability in people living in their own homes. Interestingly, the annual incidence rate for first ever stroke per 1000 head of population varies little between countries where it has been measured systematically (e.g., Europe, United States of America, Japan and Australasia). In Australia, the rate according to the age group has been reported as 2.9 (55–64), 5.8 (65–74) and 9.6 (75–84) per 1000 head of population (Ward *et al.* 1988). Mortality appears to vary between countries. It is not clear whether this is due to racial, environmental or social factors.

It is clear that about 25% of strokes occur below the age of 65 and about 50% below the age of 75. Although there are considerable methodological problems in comparing incidence, stroke mortality rises rapidly with age (Bonita and Beaglehole 1992), with age-standardized death rates attributed to stroke varying considerably between (Bonita *et al.*, 1990) and within countries (Franks *et al.* 1991). In Australia, for example, the age-standardized stroke mortality rate was reported in 1990 as 60 for men and 45 for women per 100,000 (Bonita *et al.* 1990). Prevalence is extremely difficult to measure since some patients die early after onset and many of the survivors are not disabled. A typical estimate of prevalence is about 5/1000 but this depends on many factors including population age structure (Wade, Langton Hewer *et al.* 1985).

Blood supply to the brain

Efficient blood flow to the central nervous system delivers oxygen, glucose and other nutrients and removes carbon dioxide, lactic acid and other meta-

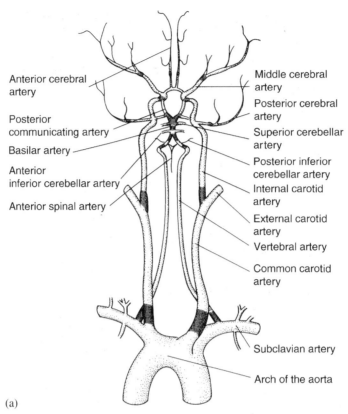

Anterior cerebral
artery

Posterior
communicating artery

Basilar artery

Anterior
inferior cerebellar artery

Anterior spinal artery

Middle cerebral
artery

Posterior cerebral
artery

Superior cerebellar
artery

Posterior inferior
cerebellar artery

Internal carotid
artery

External carotid
artery

Vertebral artery

Common carotid
artery

Subclavian artery

Arch of the aorta

(a)

Fig. 11.1 (*a*) The blood vessels of the brain. Dark areas indicate common sites of atherosclerosis and occlusion. (From Kandel, E.R., Schwartz, J.H. and Jessell, T.M. (eds) (1991) *Principles of Neural Science*, 3rd edn. p. 1042. Appleton and Lange, Norwalk, CT, by permission)

bolic products. At rest, the brain, which is only 2% of total body weight, receives 15% of the cardiac output of blood and consumes about 25% of the total inspired oxygen. The brain receives this rich supply of blood through four major arteries, two vertebral arteries and two internal carotid arteries (Fig. 11.1*a*) which anastomose at the base of the brain to form the circle of Willis. The protective importance of the circle of Willis is illustrated by the fact that minor deviations from the classic structure are common. The four major arteries branch intracranially to form the main arterial branches of the brain (Fig. 11.1*b*). Extensive anastomatic connections between blood vessels can protect the brain when part of its vascular supply is blocked.

Acute stroke

Survival after stroke

About 20% of first-ever stroke patients die within a month, the prognosis being much better for

cerebral infarction than for intracerebral haemorrhage (about 10% vs 50% dead) (Bamford *et al.* 1990). Mortality in the first few days is almost always due to the brain lesion itself, intracerebral haemorrhage or large cerebral infarcts with associated oedema causing brain shift and herniation or direct disruption of vital brain stem centres by the lesion. Sudden death only occurs as a consequence of intracranial haemorrhage (Bamford *et al.* 1990). Deaths after the first week are more likely to be due to indirect consequences of the brain lesion (e.g., bronchopneumonia and pulmonary embolism) or concurrent cardiac disease.

After the first month, the risk of death declines (about 6% per annum) but it is still about twice that in the general population because stroke patients are particularly likely to die of a further stroke and even more likely to die of the consequences of ischaemic disease (Dennis *et al.* 1993). The best single predictor of early death after stroke is an impaired level of consciouness within the first 24 hours.

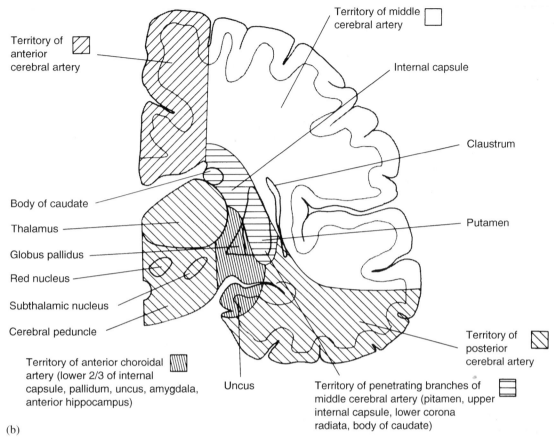

Fig. 11.1 (*b*) Cerebral arterial areas. (From Kandell, E.R., Schwartz, J.H. and Jessell, T.M. (eds) (1991) *Principles of Neural Science*, 3rd edn. p. 1042. Appleton and Lange, Norwalk, CT, by permission)

Admission to hospital

All stroke patients deserve hospital admission for diagnosis since management and prognosis vary with the exact diagnosis (Levine 1987). However, rates of admission to hospital vary widely, presumably reflecting the resources available to the general practitioner, local or national guidelines, the proximity and suitability of a hospital with an available bed which is prepared to take stroke patients, expectations of the patient, and family, and cost (Warlow 1993).

Undoubtedly, it is impossible to care for some patients at home for a number of reasons, including the severity of stroke, whether or not the person lives alone, whether or not a spouse or close relative is able to assist. Clearly, well-organized care from professionals who are familiar with and have a particular interest in stroke leads to better outcome than haphazard care. This may explain why the prog-

nosis for patients admitted to specialized *stroke units* seems to be better than those admitted to general medical units (Indredavik *et al.* 1991). One reason may be that the stroke patient does not have to compete for attention with patients who are ostensibly more ill. A review of randomized controlled trials published between 1962 and 1993, in which management of stroke patients in a specialized unit was compared with that in general medical wards, concluded that management of stroke patients in a stroke unit is associated with a sustained reduction in mortality (Langhorne *et al.* 1993) and may have some impact on functional outcome (Ottenbacher and Jannell 1993).

General medical management of all strokes

Although specific medical management may differ depending on the type of lesion, the overall aims are:

1 to make the correct diagnosis;
2 to establish the reason for stroke and the underlying cause, particularly if treatable;
3 to attempt to reduce early mortality and later disability by maintenance of vital functions, treatment of systemic complications, recognition and treatment of any cause of neurological deterioration;
4 to initiate secondary prevention in patients who might benefit;
5 to treat any coincidental disorders, for example, cardiac failure, and angina;
6 to rehabilitate patients surviving the first few days (Warlow 1993).

Ideally, most stroke patients should have a CT scan (Donnan 1992). Particular indications for early CT scan in acute patients include uncertain diagnosis, atypical progression, exclusion of intracerebral haemorrhage (CT scan will identify cerebral haemorrhage acutely), and in a young patient (Warlow 1993). The CT scan is typically normal shortly after onset of stroke and, if the lesion is less than about 0.5 cm in diameter or in the posterior fossa, the scan may remain normal. With larger infarcts a low density area begins to appear, due to increasing brain water content, within a few hours. Magnetic resonance imaging (MRI) is more sensitive but less specific than CT, so that although many more lesions are shown, it can be difficult to decide which is relevant to current symptoms. Positron emission tomography (PET) and single photon emission tomography (SPET) are interesting research tools but as yet are of little clinical relevance (Warlow 1993).

Specific medical and surgical treatment

Despite numerous suggested treatments for acute ischaemic stroke, there is still no routine treatment which, given early, increases the numbers of independent survivors (Sandercock and Willems 1992). Other than the occasional need to relieve hydrocephalus, there is no specific treatment for primary intracerebral haemorrhage apart from removing the haematoma. However, this is controversial because the natural history is so variable. Specific treatment of subarachnoid haemorrhage involves surgery to clip a ruptured aneurysm or remove a ruptured malformation if technically feasible. Carotid reconstructive surgery is sometimes recommended for patients with well-defined carotid disease, with normal or near normal

neurological status, and who are good surgical risks (Levine 1987).

When a stroke causes more than mild disability, good *nursing* in the initial acute stage is vital to ensure that the patient is comfortable, well hydrated, fed and toileted, is monitored reliably, turned regularly and suitably positioned, that the airway is kept clear and swallowing is safe. Pneumonia is the most common serious medical complication following stroke. Factors that contribute to the development of pneumonia include bed rest, immobility, hypoventilation and aspiration. A patient's ability to protect the airway is frequently impaired temporarily following stroke for one or more of the following reasons: depressed level of consciousness; diminished gag reflex; and an impaired swallowing mechanism. Nutrition and hydration can be compromised by altered consciousness, dysphagia, reduced mobility or depression. Provision of adequate fluids, care of the skin and avoidance of urinary retention and bowel impaction are all important nursing procedures.

Physiotherapy for the unconscious patient

Brain tissue needs adequate oxygenation to function and the respiratory system relies on drive from the brain to control ventilation. Brain function is affected by cerebral blood flow which is compromised by cerebrovascular disease and can be altered in the presence of oedema following stroke. Physiotherapy is required to prevent retention and pooling of secretions, atelectasis and bronchopneumonia, and may include the following interventions.

Respiratory function

● Regular and frequent turning.
● Techniques of percussion and vibration to the chest, and rib springing. Postural drainage if indicated or if the patient is unconscious for a prolonged period, and if necessary some form of intubation and mechanical suction.

Musculoskeletal integrity

● *Range of motion exercises.* It is generally routine to move the patient's limbs through a range of motion each day with the aims of improving circulation, and preventing stiffness. Whether or not these intended aims are accomplished is unknown. However, passive movements may add to the person's comfort. When passively moving the glenohumeral joint particular care should be taken to avoid damage to the soft tissues and impingement at the glenohumeral joint which is likely to occur when passively moving the arm into abduction without external rotation.

- *Positioning* to maintain at-risk muscles and soft tissue in a lengthened position and to prevent muscle shortening and increased stiffness (e.g., at-risk muscles in the upper limb include internal rotators and adductors of the shoulder and long finger and thumb flexors, at-risk muscles in the lower limb include the plantarflexors, hip and knee flexors).
- *Active exercises* and *task-related training* should be instituted as soon as the person is conscious.

Early active exercise (in sitting and standing) started as soon as the patient becomes conscious, reduces the likelihood of medical complications associated with bed rest, for example, pneumonia and deep vein thrombosis which are common after stroke.

Prognosis

Immediately after stroke it is difficult to predict the extent of eventual recovery. After about two weeks post-stroke, good prognostic signs include urinary continence, young age, mild stroke, rapid improvement, good perceptual abilities and no cognitive disorders. However, even with the use of mathematical models, it is impossible to predict outcome with sufficient accuracy to influence management (Warlow 1993) since there are patients who improve unexpectedly and others who do poorly despite having a good predicted prognosis (Bonita and Beaglehole 1988; Barer and Mitchell 1989; Lincoln *et al*. 1990; Jørgenson *et al*. 1995). Overall, it would appear from a review of outcome studies in the United States of America, Great Britain and Sweden that the most powerful predictors of functional recovery and eventual discharge home among survivors are the initial functional disability and the patient's age, although age may be a 'stand in' for other medical, psychological and psychiatric factors, none of which is strong enough to emerge alone (Alexander 1994). Other important predictors of poor outcome appear to be poor premorbid functioning and incontinence (Cifu and Stewart 1996).

The great majority of patients who survive the first month after a stroke will improve, many returning to pre-stroke levels of function. Approximately 50–60% of stroke survivors become functionally independent, with little difference between those whose stroke was due to cerebral infarction, primary intracerebral haemorrhage or subarachnoid haemorrhage. Overall, about 90% of stroke survivors go home (Legh-Smith *et al*. 1986). In the recently completed Copenhagen study, for example, 81% of those who survived their stroke went home (Jørgensen *et al*. 1995). However, the functional outcome of stroke rehabilitation does not necessarily predict placement after discharge. Some families take home individuals who require considerable care.

Recovery stage

In general, active rehabilitation can commence, if there is no progression of neurological deficits and provided the patient is medically stable, within 48 hours (Feigenson, 1979; Hayes and Carroll 1986). Primary goals of early rehabilitation are to prevent secondary emotional, intellectual and physical deterioration and to prepare the patient and relatives for the challenges ahead. Morale may be raised by making sure that a patient succeeds in early attempts to move and communicate. A comparison of two groups of patients, one which began rehabilitation within 3 days after acute hospital admission and another which commenced rehabilitation after 4–15 days, indicated that the early intervention group was discharged earlier, was more likely to walk independently and to go home (e.g., Hayes and Carroll 1986). In a comprehensive review of the literature on outcome following stroke, delay in onset of rehabilitation correlated with poor outcome in a number of studies (Cifu and Stewart 1996). Rehabilitation early after stroke has also been suggested to improve long-term social and economic costs (Dombovy *et al*. 1986).

The traditional view of neurological rehabilitation is that it reduces impairment and minimizes disability. Intensive rehabilitation is expensive and there are, in most countries, limited and diminishing resources. In attempts to address the role of rehabilitation in reducing disability and improving quality of life, there is an ongoing debate in the literature on major issues such as: Is rehabilitation for stroke effective? Where should rehabilitation take place? When should it start? and, Who are most likely to benefit from intensive rehabilitation? Studies on these issues tend to be inconclusive. There are several major methodological problems in evaluating outcome studies which include:

- The variety of measurement tools used including functional measures.
- Different practices between the centres studied (e.g., when rehabilitation commences and length of stay).
- Assessment of physical performance unrelated to function.
- Most importantly, the failure of authors to describe or define accurately the interventions used.

Another important question is: What type of movement rehabilitation is most effective at improving functional outcome? It is argued in this book that newer, more scientifically based and active task-related training of motor performance and fitness, and a deeper understanding of the need to prevent deleterious musculoskeletal changes may result in a better outcome than the commonly used approaches. This is particularly so given that there is only equivocal support for the effectiveness of these approaches (e.g., Bobath/NDT, Brunnstrom). What patients **do** following stroke, the **use** to which they put their affected limbs, and their **experiences**, appear to affect brain reorganization (Chapter 1). It is becoming clear that the amount and type of physical and mental activity, and the attitude and motivation of the patient, will impact upon brain reorganization post-stroke.

The sensorimotor, cognitive, psychological and behavioural impairments that may be seen in patients following stroke vary from patient to patient. Some of the most typical are discussed below.

Sensorimotor impairments

The site and size of the cerebrovascular lesion and the amount of collateral blood flow initially determine the degree of motor deficit which may range from slight incoordination to complete paralysis of the upper and lower limbs and face. Paralysis and/or weakness on one side of the body is referred to as hemiplegia or hemiparesis. The coexistence of sensory deficits adds to the overall motor deficits, the two systems being so closely interrelated.

Lesions of the cortical motor areas and their projections cause characteristic symptoms. Hughlings Jackson first recognized and described two types of abnormal function: the negative signs which reflect the loss of particular functions controlled by the damaged system, for example, impaired innervation of spinal motor neurons and,

as a result, impaired muscle activation and weakness; and the positive signs, for example, hyperreflexia (spasticity), that may emerge after the lesion. Over the past 20 years, it has been increasingly recognized that the major functional deficits following stroke are largely due to the negative features (e.g., Landau 1974, 1988; Burke 1988) (see Chapter 8 for review). Motor deficits may also resemble parkinsonian bradykinesia or cerebellar ataxia. Secondary musculoskeletal complications of soft tissue contracture as well as shoulder pain (see Appendix) are common sequelae of stroke.

The effects of muscle weakness on function can be summarized as difficulty in:

- Eliciting and sustaining muscle activity.
- Generating and timing force.
- Generating and controlling synergistic muscle activity.
- Supporting, propelling and balancing the body mass over the feet.
- Lack of dexterity (defined as lack of skill).

These impairments are initially the result of deficits in descending innervation of spinal motor neurons. They may be augmented as time passes by secondary neural and soft tissue changes due to disuse.

Motor and sensory loss have the greatest effect in the hand since more proximal limb and trunk muscles tend to have greater representation in both hemispheres (Brust 1991). For example, paraspinal muscles are hardly ever weak in unilateral cerebral lesions. Similarly, the facial muscles of the forehead and the muscles of the pharynx and jaw are represented in both hemispheres and are usually spared. Tongue weakness is variable.

Sensory loss tends to involve discriminative and proprioceptive modalities more than affective modalities. Pain, touch and temperature sensitivity may be impaired, or seem changed, but are usually not lost unless the lesion is peripheral to the thalamus when they may be associated with anaesthesia. Joint position sense may be severely impaired, there may be loss of two-point discrimination and stereognosis, and failure to recognize a touch stimulus if another is simultaneously delivered to the intact side of the body (called tactile extinction) (see Chapter 10).

In the initial stage following stroke, the system is in a state of cerebral shock, but as a result of reparative processes such as reduction of cerebral oedema, absorption of damaged tissue and improved local vascular flow, the patient starts to improve and there is evidence of returning muscle activity, although output is relatively uncontrolled. This reflects the return to function of undamaged neural tissue (see Chapter 1) and is known as the period of spontaneous recovery.

Adaptive motor behaviour

When an individual following stroke attempts to move or perform a purposeful action, the movement pattern that emerges reflects the individual's 'best' attempts given the state of the system (Shepherd and Carr 1991). In a sense, the action is performed in the most biomechanically advantageous manner given the effects of the lesion, the dynamic possibilities inherent in the musculoskeletal linkage and the environment in which the action is performed. Such adaptive movements seem to illustrate the ability of the lesioned system to put an action together spontaneously out of what remains of the various subsystems (neural, musculoskeletal). Added to the primary problem of muscle weakness arising from the lesion, the patient is forced to be inactive. This enforced immobility leads to secondary adaptation of soft tissue, particularly muscle, those tissues which are held in a shortened position becoming shorter and stiffer, and to declining physical fitness.

Adaptive movements emerging secondary to the impairment represent both the initial attempts of the individual to move, using muscles that can be most easily activated, as well as the restraining effects of adaptive length-associated changes in muscles and other soft tissue. That is, the way in which the patient attempts to achieve a goal reflects the degree and distribution of muscle weakness and loss of soft tissue extensibility which impose mechanical restraints on movement.

Some muscles are weak or paralysed due to diminished neural activation. Movement is, therefore, difficult for the patient, exaggerated force typically being generated by stronger and more easily activated muscles as the individual struggles to perform an approximation of the action required to carry out a task (see Fig. 6.8). It is very likely that these attempts at movement, together with adaptive shortening of soft tissue, may be significant factors in the development of the abnormal 'spastic' patterns observed, described and inhibited by Bobath clinicians.

Functional motor training

The patient should be considered an active participant in a rehabilitation process designed to optimize performance of functional actions. Given that biomechanical information is now available about many everyday actions, the analysis and training of actions, such as standing up and sitting down, walking, reaching and manipulation, are based on models of these actions built out of normative data.

Training methods take account of movement biomechanics, muscle characteristics, environmental context, and of pathology and the nature of impairments. We have suggested that the methods used in training should be similar to those already shown to be effective in promoting motor learning and in increasing motor skill, muscle strength and endurance in healthy subjects. The techniques used for encouraging learning include goal identification, instruction, auditory and visual feedback, manual guidance and practice.

Details of common problems of movement following brain lesions, with specific analysis and training are given in Chapters 2 and 4–7. General principles of training following stroke include:

- Anticipate and prevent soft tissue contracture, preferably by active means but if necessary by passive means. Muscles and muscle groups most at risk of shortening include ankle plantarflexors (particularly soleus), hip flexors and adductors, internal rotators and adductors of the shoulder joint, elbow flexors, forearm pronators, wrist and finger and thumb flexors.
- Elicit muscle activity utilizing kinesiological principles such as elimination of gravity, eccentric concentric/isometric contraction, and such techniques as electromyographic (EMG) feedback and functional electrical stimulation (FES). Critical muscles (those which are essential to major functions) to concentrate on are hip/knee/ankle extensors for support in standing, shoulder girdle elevators, shoulder flexors/abductors and external rotators for reaching, wrist and finger extensors, thumb abductors and rotator for grasp and release.
- Train motor control using concrete goals. For example, train the person to activate muscles synergistically, to activate muscles at a particular length, to sustain a muscle contraction under certain load conditions, to generate and utilize momentum, to increase speed of movement, all for a particular goal, such as standing up, walking, reaching.
- Increase muscle strength by increasing repetitions and load relevant to specific actions, for example, hip/knee/ankle extensors for standing up and sitting down, stair climbing and descent.

- Modify the action or environment to achieve a particular outcome when the person can only perform with significant and maladaptive and ineffective movements.
- Mobilize 'stiff' joints, for example, wrist, shoulder and thoracic spine, using peripheral joint or spinal mobilization methods.
- Train endurance and cardiovascular responses by, for example, increasing number of repetitions, distance walked.

Active training of critical actions should commence as soon as vital signs are stable. The patient should be dressed in clothes suitable for exercising, including suitable shoes. A typical physiotherapy session should include practice of actively controlling the sitting and standing positions, moving actively within these positions, with practice of tasks which are typically performed in both sitting and standing (particularly reaching beyond arm's length), standing up and sitting down, walking and manipulation.

Turning on to the intact side and sitting up over the side of the bed are critical to the re-establishment of independence. However, for individuals who cannot perform these without assistance or gross adaptation, it is important to help them into the sitting position (Fig. 11.2a–c). In this way, training to re-establish swallowing, communication, visual scanning of the environment, attentional capacity and the ability to balance and move can start early.

Bed mobility exercises may be a waste of time in the early stages, time being better spent practising activities in sitting and standing. Emphasis on rolling over is probably also misplaced since it takes time away from training in upright positions.

Individuals following stroke do not need to learn how to '*transfer*' the body mass from one surface to another, as does a person following spinal cord injury. Rather, they need to practise standing up and sitting down from one chair or surface to another with both feet on the ground. Nurses also need to understand this and know the critical features of standing up and sitting down in order to be able to assist appropriately.

The problem with the term 'transfers', which is commonly used in rehabilitation, is two-fold. For the patient, the term has no meaning, certainly not in relation to standing up which it does not resemble. For the staff, it tends to have a special meaning, again not necessarily related to active standing up. With increasing understanding of the need to train tasks, the term 'transfers' is not relevant to stroke patients who are attempting to relearn the action of standing up and sitting down. A critical factor enabling the person to attempt, with assistance, to stand up is the provision of a higher than normal seat (or bed) (Fig. 11.3).

There is a persistent belief in physiotherapy that strengthening exercises are not necessary following stroke, which is surprising given the fact that diminished or absent neural innervation of muscle is a major primary impairment and that muscle weakness also occurs secondarily due to disuse resulting from imposed immobility. Interestingly, *strength training* studies in healthy subjects indicate that a number of neural adaptations occur in the process of getting stronger in terms of the ability to:

- Recruit more motor units.
- Increase the frequency of motor unit discharge or both.
- Increase the synchronization of motor unit activity (e.g., Hakkinen and Komi 1983; Rutherford and Jones 1986; Rutherford, 1988).

That is, strength training is in large part a matter of neural adaption. Since impairment of motor unit activity is a major problem after stroke, it seems reasonable to assume that muscle strengthening would be beneficial.

Inaba and colleagues (1973) demonstrated that stroke patients who performed exercises to increase strength were more independent at one month than patients who received either functional training and stretching, or additional active exercises. More recently, Nugent and colleagues (1994) investigated the relationship between the number of repetitions of a weight-bearing exercise to strengthen the lower limb extensors (Carr and Shepherd 1990), and performance on the walking item of the Motor Assessment Scale (Carr *et al.* 1985). Subjects did stepping exercises with the affected foot on a small step (5–12 cm range) raising and lowering their body mass by extending or flexing the affected hip, knee and ankle (see Fig. 5.22). A maximum of 60 repetitions of the exercise was done each day. For patients who were able to stand on their affected limb and step forward with the intact limb at the start of training, a relationship was found between the number of repetitions subjects performed and improved outcome on the MAS score. This finding suggests not only that the more these subjects exercised the better they did

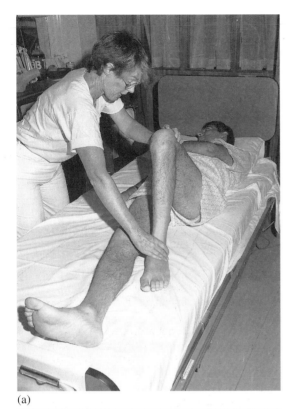

(a)

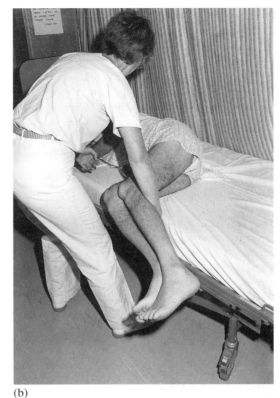

(b)

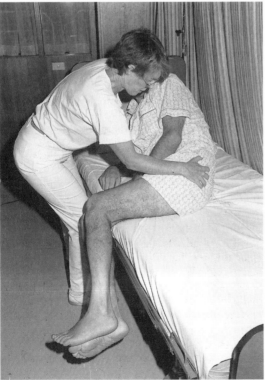

(c)

Fig. 11.2 Sitting up over the side of the bed. (*a*) He is able to push through his L foot (affected side) to turn on to his R side if the therapist (or nurse) stabilizes the foot and leg. (*b*) He gets the idea of sitting up over the side of the bed from his intact R side. Therapist assists by lowering the legs. (*c*) He flexes his head sideways while the therapist assists him into sitting, one hand on the top of his pelvis and the other hand under his R shoulder. Once sitting, training of dynamic sitting balance commences with his feet on the floor

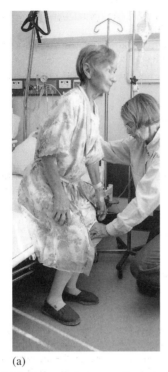

(a)

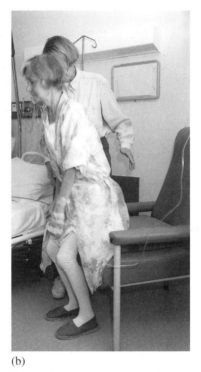

(b)

Fig. 11.3 Both bed and chair are adjusted to a suitable height to enable practice of STS and SIT with (*a*) manual guidance to stabilize the foot and (*b*) stand-by assistance

but also that the stepping exercise enabled patients to achieve the aim of improving walking. For patients who could not stand and step forward at initial assessment, there was no relationship between the number of repetitions and walking outcome. However, these patients achieved independent walking of at least 3 m by the end of training.

It is important that specific therapy aims are directly related to improving functional performance as in the above study. That is, specific lower limb strength training exercise needs to be accompanied by training and practice of walking. There can, however, be a disparity between the achievement of stated physiotherapy aims and improvement in functional performance. For example, the stated aims of physiotherapy in a study designed to investigate the outcome of a 4 week comprehensive programme to improve walking in mildly affected stroke patients (Hesse *et al.* 1994b), were to improve weight acceptance and push-off as described by Davies (1985). Following treatment a change in ground reaction forces indicated better weight acceptance and push-off through both legs. Functional performance, however, did not

improve. Functional performance was measured in the following ways:

1 10 m walk on level ground at maximum velocity;
2 walking endurance (self-adopted speed, limit of 600 m); and
3 stair climbing (self-adopted speed with or without handrail, limit 90 stairs).

Notably, the patients were already able to walk 20 m independently and without aids when they commenced physiotherapy. The physiotherapy these patients received did not enable them to improve functional performance, suggesting that the physiotherapy aims and methods were not appropriate. The authors also reported that patients were discouraged from walking as it was believed this might encourage spasticity. It is therefore likely that physiotherapy was geared to too low a level for these individuals.

Below are some examples of scientifically based interventions in which changes in performance have been observed and measured. These studies illustrate the effectiveness of *task-related training* of everyday actions.

Walking

Richards, Malouin and colleagues (Malouin *et al.* 1992; Richards *et al.* 1993) have demonstrated that stroke patients can tolerate both early and active gait training following stroke. The training consisted of loading the affected limb, resisted exercises on an isokinetic device and walking on a treadmill with supportive harness. Richards and colleagues (1993) reported a significant difference in walking velocity in the experimental group at the end of 5 weeks' training compared with walking velocity in two control groups, one conventional physiotherapy group, and another that emphasized early and intensive conventional therapy but did not focus on walking. Conventional physiotherapy was reported to be based on Bobath and Brunnstrom approaches.

Treadmill walking with suspension harness

This is increasingly being suggested for rehabilitation of walking and shown to be associated with positive outcomes (e.g., Waagfjord *et al.* 1990, Malouin *et al.*, 1992, Richards *et al.* 1993, Hesse, Jahnke *et al.* 1994; Hesse *et al.* 1995). The evidence to date suggests this is an effective way to augment gait training.

Hesse and colleagues (1994a) examined the effects of treadmill walking on nine patients who could not walk at all or required the assistance of at least one person. These patients had already received regular physiotherapy rehabilitation (Bobath/NDT) for at least 3 weeks without marked improvement in their walking ability. Patients started treadmill walking for 15 minutes per session and within 5 days they had increased this time to 30 minutes. After 25 treadmill training sessions, endurance and walking velocity had increased as had cadence and stride length. It is notable that conventional (Bobath) physiotherapy emphasized 'preparation' in supine and practice of 'components' of walking. Practice of walking itself was not encouraged in order to avoid 'stereotyped mass synergies'. These synergies were claimed by the physiotherapists to occur in the absence of sufficient trunk and lower limb control. It is obvious that the treadmill provided the opportunity for the patients to practise the complete walking cycle.

There may be several major benefits in the use of a treadmill with or without supportive harness to augment walking training:

- It allows walking practice without danger or fear of falling.
- Inter- and intra-limb timing parameters can be practised before the patient has sufficient muscle strength to support body weight fully.
- It eliminates the need to use adaptive movements, e.g., using the upper limbs for support and balance to compensate for lower limb muscle weakness.
- Speed of the treadmill can be increased, thereby forcing the patient to walk faster.
- It forces stepping, probably through stretch facilitation of hip flexors and calf muscles at the end of stance phase and the fact that taking a step is 'forced' by the moving belt.
- It loads the affected lower limb and enables the patient to practise the complete walking cycle.
- Patients can practise on their own or with minimal supervision.
- If performed long enough, treadmill walking has the potential to increase endurance.

Initially the physiotherapist (or an aide) may need to help to move the affected leg forward in order to give the patient the idea of the movement.

Other studies have shown positive effects of task-related training: on sit-to-stand (e.g., Ada and Westwood, 1992; Ada *et al.* 1993; Engardt *et al.* 1993) and on balancing and reaching in sitting (e.g., Dean and Shepherd 1997). These are discussed in Chapters 4 and 7.

Forced-use

Following both deafferentation and surgical interruption of the pyramidal tract in monkeys, Taub (1980) suggested that muscle weakness and paralysis led to secondary behavioural adaptation, which he called *learned non-use*. That is, the animal's attention was diverted toward the intact contralateral limb and it learned not to use the affected limb. However, when the intact limb was restrained and the affected limb was specifically trained with feedback reward, the affected upper limb became functional.

Three papers (Wolf *et al.* 1989; Taub *et al.* 1993; Morris *et al.* 1997) provide convincing evidence for forced-use of the affected upper limb in humans following stroke. In these studies, forced-use involved restricting the intact upper limb and training the affected limb. Subjects in these studies had their stroke at least one year prior to commencing the forced-use and training regime. Taub and colleagues followed up their subjects over a two year period and found that the subjects in the forced-use group had maintained their gains. For the control group, who participated in procedures designed to focus attention on the affected upper limb, only one measure showed some moderate improvement and this was lost during the follow-up period.

Exercise capacity

It is well known that there is a strong relationship between disuse/inactivity and accelerated ageing. Reduction in levels of physical activity as a consequence of stroke leads to a deterioration in both exercise capacity and physical condition. Added to this, many individuals following stroke are elderly and the seventh decade appears a critical age for accelerated decline in function (Cunningham *et al.* 1982) so some individuals may be deconditioned before their stroke. Regular exercise in the healthy elderly has been shown to have beneficial effects on cardiovascular fitness (Morey *et al.* 1989), skeletal muscle strength (Flatarone *et al.* 1990; Lord and Castell 1994), flexibility and general well-being (Lampman 1987). Similar improvements in elderly individuals with other disease have also been demonstrated (Morey, *et al.* 1989). It is evident that increased muscle strength and flexibility are due to improved neural recruitment patterns as well as to muscle hypertrophy (Fiatarone *et al.* 1990). Exercise training to enhance exercise capacity should be initiated early in the rehabilitation process and continue after discharge.

Clinical studies indicate that stroke patients at least one year after stroke are able to improve motor performance with training (e.g, Wade *et al.* 1992, Taub *et al.* 1993, Dean and Shepherd 1997). Tangeman and colleagues (1990) suggest that one reason may be that patients, once they get home, see how their disability affects their daily lives and are, therefore, keen to improve their performance. Individuals in this study commented that the stress of the acute phase prevented them from participating fully during initial rehabilitation.

There is also a suggestion of a continuing decline in mobility in stroke patients over time, after rehabilitation is concluded (Wade et al. 1992). This may be due to the effects of inactivity and poor self-image on motivation and reflect the need for access to exercise classes for disabled and/or elderly individuals following rehabilitation.

Although individuals following stroke are known to have low endurance to exercise (King

et al. 1989), there is little documentation of the need for and the role of aerobic exercise training to maximize functional performance. Potempa and colleagues (1995) report the results of a randomized control trial of stroke subjects: one group had passive range of motion exercises for 30 minutes for 10 weeks and the other group exercised on an adapted cycle ergometer for 30 minutes, three times per week for 10 weeks. Baseline aerobic capacity of subjects was less than similarly aged able-bodied but hypertensive subjects. At the end of the study only the exercise group showed significant improvement in maximum O_2 consumption, workload and exercise time. This group also showed significantly lower systolic blood pressure. Improvement in aerobic capacity was also correlated with improved function on the Fugl-Meyer Index. More recently Potempa and colleagues (1996) have reviewed the advantages and disadvantages of exercise modalities and make some recommendations in relation to maximizing physical performance in stroke patients.

Some years ago, Brinkman and Hoskins (1979) reported the benefits of an exercise programme which consisted of stationary bicycling for individuals following discharge from stroke rehabilitation. The results indicated improved physical fitness in most subjects, inasmuch as the heart rate response to a constant load was lower at the end of the 12 week programme. On completion of the study, subjects reported increased self-esteem and several subjects reported change in various aspects of their general behaviour. For example, one person commenced gardening and another could once again comb her hair. It seems reasonable to assume that the increased self-esteem and feeling of well-being engendered by the exercise programme gave these individuals the confidence and drive to improve their performance in other activities.

The results of these two studies highlight the benefits of aerobic exercise training to improve both the physical and mental well-being of individuals following stroke. Figure 11.4 illustrates a MOTOmed Pico Leg Trainer, which can be used to increase strength and endurance, and is easily adapted to different environments.

Aids

Provision of aids should be carefully considered and aids not substituted for exercises and training directed toward increasing muscle strength and control.

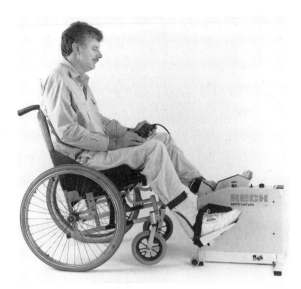

Fig. 11.4 Exercising on a MOTOmed Pico Leg Trainer. (Courtesy of Reck, Reckstrasse 1–3, D-88422 Betzenweiller, Germany)

Orthoses   The value of orthoses following stroke is a matter of some debate. Some form of splinting may be necessary to lengthen shortened soft tissue. Serial casting, designed to lengthen soft tissues progressively, is necessary if adaptive changes have not been prevented.

For orthoses designed to improve functional performance or allow practice of an action, there should be a congruence between the goals of training and the rationale behind the design of the orthosis. Ankle-foot orthoses (both rigid and hinged) have typically been suggested to compensate for the effects of impairments on walking, in particular inadequate dorsiflexion in swing and mediolateral subtalar instability during stance (e.g., Montgomery 1987; Ryerson 1995). However, the use of such an orthosis may force adaptive behaviour on the individual by interfering with the ankle plantarflexion which occurs at the beginning of stance for foot flat and at the end of stance for heel- and push-off. Such adaptive behaviour may be inconsistent with the aim of walking training. Conversely, there is some evidence that in some individuals walking with an orthosis is more energy-efficient, although this is not conclusive. Ankle supports typically used in sport may be effective in helping stabilize an ankle by preventing excessive inversion of the foot.

Orthoses can be designed to optimize muscle activity at a particular length. For example, a splint or strapping to hold the thumb abducted at the carpometacarpal joint may facilitate practice of grasp and release. Strapping can be used to alter the direction of a muscle's pull or prevent adaptive movements at the glenohumeral joint. Strapping at the back of the knee (see Fig. 5.20*b*) may prevent knee hyperextension in stance caused by rotation backward of the shank at the ankle, due to muscle weakness or decreased extensibility of the soleus.

One-arm drive wheelchairs   Although propelling a wheelchair with the intact arm and leg may promote early independence, it is likely to focus attention on the intact side. The use of a wheelchair in this way is inconsistent with the aim of directing the person's attention to the affected side and driving the reorganization of the lesioned central nervous system to enable optimal recovery of function in affected limbs. If early independence in mobility is desirable for a person unable to walk independently, some form of motorized transporter is preferable.

Walking aids   Aids such as parallel bars, walking frame, quadripod (four-point cane) and another person's arm are frequently advocated for individuals with poor balance and support through the lower limbs during standing and walking. However, these aids all rely on weight-bearing through one or both upper limbs and the patient may learn to depend on the arms for balancing. This is counter to the aim of training the person to balance the body mass over the feet using lower limb muscles. It is very likely, with current rehabilitation practices, that a person may spend considerably longer walking with a frame or quadripod or propelling a wheelchair than in practising balance and walking under the guidance/coaching of the physiotherapist.

Walking aids may actually prevent the person taking advantage of physiotherapy training since, from a biomechanical perspective, they impose mechanical restrictions on walking by affecting, for example, speed and movement pattern. A *quadripod stick* shifts the centre of pressure (distribution of total forces applied by the human body to its supporting surface) toward the intact side and therefore encourages weight-bearing through the intact lower limb. Walking with a *walking frame* has been found to increase heart rate by 22% (Hamzeh et al. 1988), substantially change hip and knee motion, particularly restricting hip motion, and decrease the speed of walking (Crosbie 1993). Although all walking aids impose some mechanical constraint, a simple *walking stick* interferes less with balance and walking and provides some assistance.

Language, cognitive and affective impairments

Modern cognitive psychology and brain science have led us to appreciate that all mental processes consist of perceiving, thinking, learning and remembering, and even the simplest task requires the coordination of several regions of the brain (Kandel 1991a). Impairments following stroke can be categorized as disorders of language that also interfere with cognitive function (dysphasia/aphasia); disorders of perception–cognition (i.e., of perception, orientation, memory, executive functioning); depression, and other emotional and behavioural disturbances. All these impairments affect the individual's mental state and have the potential to affect significantly the individual's ability to participate in and benefit from rehabilitation. Perceptual–cognitive impairments, such as unilateral neglect or agnosia, are described in Chapter 10.

Aphasia

The aphasias (usually dysphasia, since there is rarely a total loss of language) are disturbances of language caused by an insult to specific regions of the brain (usually regions of the left cerebral cortex), with lesions in different parts of the cortex causing selective disturbances. The damage to the brain may also affect other cognitive and intellectual skills. Since language is distinguished from other kinds of human communication by its creativity, form, content and use, and since, in both its written and spoken forms, it represents social and interactive activities (Mayeux and Kandel 1991), loss or impairment have a profound effect on the individual.

The aphasias are distinct from disorders of speech which result from weakness and incoordination of the muscles controlling the vocal apparatus, which are classified as: dysarthria, a disturbance of articulation; and dysphonia, a disturbance in vocalization.

There is no universally accepted classification for the aphasias. However, several types can be distinguished (Mayeux and Kandel 1991). Wernicke's aphasia is characterized by a deficit in comprehension and severe difficulty in reading and writing. In Broca's aphasia, comprehension is usually preserved but language expression is affected. This latter may range from almost complete loss of language expression to a slowed, deliberate speech utilizing only key words and simple grammatical structure. Comprehension of both spoken and written language is less disturbed than in Wernicke's aphasia. Other types of aphasia include: anomic aphasia, a difficulty finding the correct words, and global aphasia, an inability to speak or comprehend language, read or write, repeat or name objects.

The stroke patient with aphasia suddenly finds he/she is unable to understand spoken language, read, speak or write and to communicate the simplest needs. These deficits isolate the individual and may, not surprisingly, lead to anger and frustration as attempts to communicate fail. Early diagnosis of language impairment by a speech pathologist is essential to identify the patient's specific problems so that the family and rehabilitation team can understand the nature and extent of the communication deficits and the best ways of communicating with the individual.

Individuals with language impairment usually experience some degree of spontaneous improvement (Wade *et al.* 1986). However, persisting problems may have profound and pervading consequences for the individual's quality of life and employment opportunities, and lead to a feeling of social isolation. Automatic speech, or the ability to count or recite something familiar that does not require thought mechanisms, may return more quickly than other forms of expressive language.

Intervention varies with the type and severity of aphasia. Below are some suggestions to assist physiotherapists to communicate with aphasic patients before they have the benefit of an assessment and plan of management by the speech pathologist:

- Do not exclude the individual from the conversation, or answer for him/her.
- Keep sentences short and simple without too much information.
- Provide time for the person to respond and to switch from one topic to another.
- Phrase questions so that they can be answered with yes/no or some other form of response where there is expressive aphasia.
- Use gestures, situational cues, visual prompts, facial expression to enhance communication/comprehension.
- Engage in eye contact since eye contact facilitates communication and more positive attitudes (Mehrabian 1969).

- Be honest in establishing communication and a relationship with the individual. For example, if the therapist does not understand a response it is better to say so and ask the individual to try again. Prompts such as 'Is it about your appointment time?' may help. Try some diverting behaviour if the individual becomes very frustrated.
- Discourage perseveration on words and phrases as it interferes with real communication.

Cognitive function

Although many patients eventually return to full mental capacity following stroke, it is certain that not enough time and thought are spent on retraining intellectual function. For example, Kinsella and Ford (1980) found that although stroke patients made physical gains during rehabilitation, there was little or no improvement in mental functioning. The authors commented that the reason may have been the lack of any specific mental stimulation. Although they point out that this result could be attributed to the insensitivity of the tests or the size of the group, it is also probable that, where there are cognitive problems, improvement will not occur without specific training and an intellectually stimulating environment.

There is an ongoing debate concerning the effectiveness of cognitive retraining. Some of the debate centres on criticism of the methodology used in reported studies (e.g., Robertson 1993), while some focuses on the role of cognitive impairment as a predictor of long-term outcome. Meanwhile the physiotherapist and other clinicians have to deal daily with patients with perceptual–cognitive impairments (Chapter 10).

It should be noted that neuropsychological cognitive tests may demonstrate a variety of impairments in elderly stroke patients, not all of which would have a marked effect on everyday life. Some impairments may have been present before stroke with no apparent effect upon ability to function in their own environment.

It is likely that individuals may have coped quite well with everyday levels of stress despite certain cognitive impairments. Clearly, however, some patients with impairments in mental functioning following stroke are unable to cope with the demands placed on them by their sensory–motor and/or language impairments and the stress imposed by the unfamiliar environment in which they find themselves. These people require evaluation and training for their specific impairments in order to assist them to participate actively in the rehabilitation process and return to functional activities. One deficit for which specific training may be required is memory.

Individuals with *memory impairments* require a neuropsychological assessment to identify deficits and strengths and weaknesses, combined with direct assessment of specific problems by, for example, observation (Wilson 1995). Wilson (1989) lists eight points to encourage individuals with memory problems to encode, store and recall information:

- Simplify information.
- Reduce the amount of information given at any one time.
- Ensure there is minimal distraction.
- Make sure information is understood, for example, ask the person to repeat the information in his or her own words.
- Encourage the person to link or associate information with material already known.
- Encourage the person to ask questions.
- Use the 'little and often' rule (Baddeley, 1992).
- Make sure learning occurs in different contexts to promote generalization.

Physiotherapists should utilize these points to help memory-impaired individuals during motor training.

Other strategies include rearranging the environment, for example, having rooms clearly labelled, direction markers on the floor, so that the individual has to rely less on memory. Use of external aids such as notebooks, diaries and microcassettes should also be encouraged. These are strategies we all use; however, memory-impaired people may need encouragement to use them, concerned that they may become 'dependent' on them. Wilson (1995) reports how a woman who could not find her way around a rehabilitation centre dictated the directions on to a microcassette which she listened to when she needed to find a particular department.

The use of internal mnemonic strategies is well documented. However, many memory-impaired individuals may not have the necessary concentration to use these strategies. Wilson (1991) reported that when patients used techniques to improve their memory they mostly relied on written lists, calendars or wall charts rather than internal strategies.

Dementia

Dementia is a serious and progressive decline in mental function, in memory, and in acquired intellectual skills (Goldman and Côté 1991). About 15% of all cases of dementia are caused by stroke (sometimes repeated small infarcts) and some individuals may have been demented prior to stroke.

Normal ageing is associated with characteristic changes in the brain and behaviour that vary widely among individuals but in most cases do not seriously compromise the quality of life. Although dementia is age-related, it is not an inevitable consequence of ageing and the majority of individuals age without substantial loss of intellect. The neurobiological processes of age-related mental changes are poorly understood (Goldman and Côté 1991).

Depression

Depression is a common sequela of stroke. Prevalence is difficult to determine and has been reported to vary with the diagnostic criteria used (Hibbard *et al.* 1993). There is some evidence that it is more common in lesions of the left hemisphere than the right (e.g., Robinson and Szetela 1981).

The major criteria reflecting depression in the wider community include disturbed sleep (usually insomnia but sometimes over-sleeping), loss of energy, difficulty concentrating, feelings of worthlessness, weight loss or gain, restlessness or slowing down of thought and actions, and suicidal thoughts (Kandel 1991b). When these criteria are applied to patients with stroke, however, they may reflect the effects of hospitalization and disenchantment with the rehabilitation process rather than be manifestations of altered mood (Hibbard *et al.* 1993).

Depression may not only affect participation in rehabilitation and long-term outcome but may also compound cognitive dysfunction (Bolla-Wilson *et al.* 1989). There is some evidence that depression and learned helplessness share parallel symptoms (Peterson *et al.*, 1993). Learned helplessness is a phenomenon first observed in laboratory animals by Seligman (1975), which he described as maladaptive passivity. A rehabilitation setting in which the individual is not given any responsibility may facilitate this passivity. It should be noted that depression is commonly said to be misdiagnosed as dementia in the elderly (Brocklehurst 1985).

Depression needs to be carefully assessed, taking into account the presence of aphasia, denial of illness and mental status. The patient's family may be able to help in identifying changes from pre-stroke behaviour as well as areas of dissatisfaction with rehabilitation.

One of the first steps in evaluation is to ensure that depressive symptoms are not due to medica-tion (e.g., sedatives, hypnotics) or environmental factors (e.g., interruption of sleep habits or perceived lack of opportunity for training and activity in rehabilitation). Effective medical treatment depends on accurate diagnosis and may include a trial of antidepressant drugs, psychiatric intervention or counselling. Mild symptoms usually respond to greater encouragement from staff and family and to active participation and observable success in motor retraining.

Other emotional and behavioural disturbances

Anxiety, outbursts of uncontrolled behaviour and hostility can also occur following stroke but are much less common than depression (AHCPR 1995). Apathy and 'undue cheerfulness' have also been described, particularly in individuals with right hemisphere stroke (Price 1990).

A stroke takes place suddenly and often without warning. The fear associated with loss of independence may be overwhelming. Alterations in self-image and self-worth are common and these affect adversely the individual's motivation and ability to participate fully in active rehabilitation. Concerns about possible dependency and how this may affect the individual's social and economic situation may cause a great deal of stress.

Positive attitudes towards the individual by all members of staff are critical to help him/her cope. Having the patient dress as soon as possible in day clothes, encouraging both men and women to take an interest in their appearance, all help to improve an individual's self-image and have a positive affect on all those with whom he/she comes in contact.

Educational programmes for patients and families include lectures and group discussions on the pathophysiology of stroke, the meaning of symptoms, the adaptability of the brain, the physical and emotional affects of stroke, ways of communicating, coping strategies, planning for discharge, and community participation in rehabilitation. Some of the benefits from such programmes are decreased anxiety, more effective family involvement in the rehabilitation process and increased maintenance of rehabilitation gains after discharge.

If a patient appears unmotivated, the cause should be investigated. A person's behaviour is to some extent a consequence of the limitations imposed by the damage to the brain, which results in difficulty in moving to achieve a goal and in perceptual and thinking processes, slowness in registering and retaining recent information, inability to give proper language expression to what is perceived, along with emotional turmoil. A lack of understanding of a patient's behaviour and of ways of remediating the problems may result in the individual being incorrectly labelled as unmotivated and this may result in failure to take the necessary action. Poor motivation and mood 2 weeks after stroke have been reported to be highly correlated with failure to benefit much from rehabilitation and with a poor outcome a year later (Henley *et al.* 1985). This result raises the question of whether or not there is sufficient psychological help and attention to suitability of the environment for patients after stroke.

Dysphagia

Dysphagia, or difficulty swallowing, is a common problem following stroke and may lead to aspiration of saliva, food or liquids. The prevalence is hard to determine. However, likelihood of dysphagia increases for those patients with bilateral hemisphere or brain stem strokes (Schmidt *et al.* 1994).

Medical complications associated with dysphagia include aspiration pneumonia, dehydration and malnutrition. Early detection and treatment is important in preventing both aspiration and dehydration from inadequate oral intake. Primary difficulties are incoordination of the oral and pharyngeal phases of swallowing and delayed or absent triggering of the swallow reflex, or both. Problems with the oral phase of swallowing are relatively easily identified while observing the patient's facial alignment and expression and attempts at eating and drinking. Problems include dribbling from the mouth, difficulty controlling the bolus and closing the jaw, a tendency to attempt to swallow incompletely chewed food, collection of food between the gums and cheek and choking and coughing when swallowing. The frequency of dysfunction in the pharyngeal phase of swallowing is probably underestimated by observation (Schmidt *et al.* 1994). Videofluoroscopy using a modified barium swallow may be used to evaluate the pharyngeal phase of swallowing and the mechanism of aspiration in patients whose problem persists beyond the early stage of recovery. Those with severe dysphagia who do not respond to training may require nasogastric tube feeding.

Specific training to improve swallowing (Carr and Shepherd 1987) should be commenced as soon as dysphagia is identified. The re-establishment of effective swallowing may be aided by the person sitting up at a table at meal time, and having food he/she enjoys. Meals should be carefully super-vised until the person has become competent in preparing and swallowing the bolus. The large majority of people respond quickly and well to specific training.

Incontinence

Urinary incontinence is common but usually transient following stroke. Clearly, some of the problems are related to motor and sensory impairments, difficulty communicating (which interferes with making the need known to others), enforced immobility, as well as to cognitive deficits and inability to recognize the need to void. There is, however, some evidence of neurological deficits leading to either retention or overflow or both (e.g., Gelber *et al.* 1993). Gelber and colleagues summarize the major mechanisms for post-stroke incontinence as: disruption of the neuromicturition pathways resulting in bladder hyporeflexia and urgency incontinence; incontinence associated with cognitive and language deficits, with normal bladder function; and bladder hyporeflexia and overflow incontinence associated with concurrent neuropathy or medication. Urodynamic studies are useful in diagnosing the cause of incontinence.

Detrusor hyperreflexia (associated with a functional reduction in bladder capacity) was the most common cystometric finding in a group of stroke patients with urinary problems (Khan *et al.* 1990). The authors suggest that this finding may reflect a high prevalence of involuntary contractions in elderly people in general. These individuals may have been continent prior to stroke but the combination of impaired mobility and involuntary contractions of the detrusor may lead to urinary incontinence.

Early assumption of the standing position and early ambulation usually helps the individual overcome incontinence. If it does not, a bladder training programme may be instituted.

A bladder training programme involves timed voiding. Use of a commode or toilet should be encouraged rather than a bed pan or bottle. Men should stand to void. Fluid balance (intake/output), frequency and timing of voiding are documented to assess the individual's voiding pattern prior to starting bladder training. The physiotherapist needs to communicate with the nursing staff about the programme in order to reinforce voiding cues, ensure access to toilet facilities and avoid embarrassing accidents during treatment which add to the individual's loss of self-esteem and interfere with time spent in active rehabilitation. Any individual in whom urinary incontinence cannot be overcome with a bladder training programme should be referred to a urologist for evaluation to identify treatable medical conditions such as an enlarged prostate. It is at least possible that persistent incontinence is secondary to poor cognitive function (Wade, Langton Hewer, *et al.* 1985).

Alteration in bowel function, either diarrhoea or constipation, may be associated with immobility. Constipation is by far the more common and is assessed and treated by attention to pre- and post-stroke bowel habits, diet and activity.

The role of the family in stroke rehabilitation

The effects of stroke and stroke rehabilitation are mostly described in terms of functional gains. The consequences of stroke on everyday life of the patient and family are typically inadequately described and poorly understood. Patients are seldom asked to evaluate their experiences during rehabilitation although there are several insightful publications written by individuals who have survived a stroke and rehabilitation (e.g. Griffiths 1970; Brodal 1973; Hewson 1988, 1996).

Major challenges for the individual after a stroke are coming to terms with the losses associated with disability or handicap, coping with a changed identity as a disabled person and with the way this affects self-image and social relationships. The process of adjustment may take considerable time and go through several phases (Lewinter and Mikkelsen 1995).

There is some evidence that family interactions can affect eventual outcome either positively or negatively (Evans *et al.* 1987). This probably depends on the strength of the relationship prior to stroke. The most important rationale for involving the family in stroke rehabilitation is their role in reinforcing positive patient behaviours and assisting the patient to exercise and practise. Evans and colleagues (1992) caution, however, that expecting families to assist with treatment when they are not coping well themselves can be counter-productive.

The majority of individuals who survive a stroke return to live at home and the alteration in family lifestyle can be considerable. In a review of the literature, Evans and colleagues (1992), identify the need for family education, advocacy and supportive counselling to foster cooperation and social support after stroke. There are several clinical studies which indicate that the level of functioning at discharge from rehabilitation decreases after that discharge (e.g., Andrews and

Stewart 1979; Wade *et al.* 1992). Both inadequate family education and preparation for the patient's return home may be one reason for these findings. Another may be a lack of emphasis on the need for continuing exercise and training after discharge.

Sexual concerns are rarely addressed by the patient, spouse or professional team, yet sexual dysfunction has been found to be common after stroke (Monga *et al.* 1986) and a source of disharmony in a relationship. In a semi-structured interview in which individuals were asked to report on their experiences in rehabilitation, those interviewed expressed a need for more sexual counselling (Lewinter and Mikkelsen 1995). One subject reported that sexual concerns were a taboo subject and that some staff members 'fled' when it was introduced, highlighting the need for sexual issues to be addressed during rehabilitation. Many post-stroke sexual problems are related to emotional causes such as fear, dependency in self-care, anxiety and changes in body image.

Return to the community

In a follow-up study 5–6 years after stroke in Sweden, patients who experienced a good quality of life were all married, lived at home, participated in active leisure activities and were continuing to train/exercise on their own (Wadell *et al.* 1987). A community-based stroke group can play an important role; for example, the Stroke Recovery Association of Australia is a social and self-help organization for stroke persons and their families. Weekly group meetings organized by members at different locations offer a rewarding experience for people who have had a stroke, providing emotional and social support and assisting in the transition back into the community (Sutherland and Baker 1979; Dyson 1984).

In conclusion, there is evidence overall that physiotherapy in a general sense improves outcome in rehabilitation following stroke. The extent of recovery is likely in large part to reflect a person's experiences and the activities in which he/she participates. There is a growing body of evidence which suggests that the adult nervous system is capable of reorganizing after damage and that environmental factors, including the amount of activity (i.e., use), affect the extent of and actually drive neural reorganization (Chapter 1). It is doubtful, however, that much current clinical rehabilitation (including physiotherapy) actually takes these factors into account. The authors agree with Ernst (1990) who suggests that many widely used physiotherapy approaches lack scientific background. Although recent evidence of the effectiveness of specific active training and muscle strengthening is promising, it is doubtful that current physiotherapy approaches are providing optimal training at the present time. It is very likely that an increased understanding of human movement and of task-related intensive training in a stimulating and challenging environment will begin to give a clearer picture of the potential for brain reorganization and recovery after an acute brain lesion.

References

Ada, L. and Westwood, P. (1992) A kinematic analysis of recovery of the ability to stand up following stroke. *Australian Journal of Physiotherapy*, **38**, 135–142.

Ada, L., O'Dwyer, N. and Nailson, P.D. (1993) Improvement in kinematic characteristics and coordination following stroke quantified by linear systems analysis. *Human Movement Science*, **12**, 137–153.

AHCPR (1995) *Clinical Practice Guidelines, 16, Poststroke Rehabilitation*. US Department of Health and Human Services, Rockville, MD.

Alexander, M.P. (1994) Stroke rehabilitation outcome. A potential use of predictive variables to establish levels of care. *Stroke*, **25**, 128–134.

Andrews, K. and Stewart, J. (1979) Stroke recovery: he can but does he? *Rheumatology and Rehabilitation*, **18**, 43–48.

Baddeley, A.D. (1992) Memory theory and memory therapy. In *Clinical Management of Memory Problems* (ed. B.A. Wilson and N. Moffat) 2nd ed, Chapman and Hall, London, pp. 1–31.

Bamford, J., Dennis, M. and Sandercock, P. *et al.* (1990) The frequency, causes and timing of death within 30 days of a first stroke: the Oxfordshire Community Stroke Project. *Journal Neurology, Neurosurgery and Psychiatry*, **53**, 824–829.

Barer, D.H. and Mitchell, J.R.A. (1989) Predicting the outcome of acute stroke: Do mulitvariate models help? *Quarterly Journal of Medicine*, **74**, 27–39.

Bolla-Wilson, K., Robinson, R.G., Starkstein, S.E. *et al.* (1989) Lateralization of dementia of depression in stroke patients. *American Journal of Psychiatry*, **146**, 627–634.

Bonita, R. and Beaglehole, R. (1988) Recovery of motor function after stroke. *Stroke*, **19**, 1497–1500.

Bonita, R. and Beaglehole, R. (1992) Stroke mortality. In *Population Based Studies of Stroke* (ed. J.P. Whisnant), International Medical Review Series, Butterworth Heinemann, Oxford, pp. 1–30.

Bonita, R., Stewart, A. and Beaglehole, R. (1990) International trends in stroke mortality 1970–85. *Stroke*, **21**, 989–992.

Brinkman, J.R. and Hoskins, T.A. (1979) Physical conditioning and altered self-concept in rehabilitated patients. *Physical Therapy*, **59**, 859–865.

Brocklehurst, J.C. (1985) *Textbook of Geriatric Medicine and Gerontology*, 2nd edn. Churchill Livingstone, London.

Brodal, A. (1973) Self-observation and neuroanatomical considerations after a stroke. *Brain*, **96**, 675–694.

Brust, J.C.M. (1991) Cerebral circulation: stroke. In *Principles of Neural Science* (ed. E.R. Kandell, J.H. Schwartz and T.M. Jessell), 3rd edn. Appleton and Lange, Norwalk, CT, pp. 1041–1049.

Burke, D. (1988) Spasticity as an adaptation to pyramidal tract injury. In *Advances in Neurology, 47: Functional Recovery in Neurological Disease* (ed. S.G. Waxman), Raven Press, New York, pp. 401–423.

Carr, J.H. and Shepherd, R.B. (1987) *A Motor Relearning Programme for Stroke*, 2nd edn. Butterworth-Heinemann, Oxford, pp. 73–83.

Carr, J.H., Shepherd, R.B., Nordholm, L. *et al.* (1985) Investigation of a new motor assessment scale for stroke. *Physical Therapy*, **65**, 175–180.

Carr, J.H. and Shepherd, R.B. (1990) A motor learning model for rehabilitation of the movement disabled. In *Key Issues in Neurological Physiotherapy* (ed. L. Ada and C. Canning), Butterworth-Heinemann, Oxford, pp. 1–24.

Cifu, D.X. and Stewart, D.G. (1996) A comprehensive, annotated reference guide to outcome after stroke. *Critical Reviews in Physical and Rehabilitation Medicine*, **8**, 39–86.

Crosbie, J. (1993) Kinematics of walking frame ambulation. *Clinical Biomechanics*, **8**, 31–36.

Cunningham, D.A., Rechniter, D. A., Pearce, M.E. *et al.* (1982) Determinants of self-selected walking pace across ages 19 to 66. *Journal of Gerontology*, **37**, 560–564.

Davies, P.M. (1985) *Steps to Follow*. Springer-Verlag, New York.

Dean, C. and Shepherd, R.B. (1997) Task-related training improves performance of seated reaching tasks after stroke. *Stroke*, **28**, 722–728.

Dennis, M., Burn, J., Sandercock, P. *et al.* (1993) Longterm survival after first ever stroke: the Oxfordshire Community Stroke Project. *Stroke*, **24**, 796–800.

Dombovy, M.L., Sandok, B.A. and Basford, J.R. (1986) Rehabilitation for stroke: a review. *Stroke*, **17**, 363–369.

Donnan, G.A. (1992) Investigations of patients with stroke and transient ischaemic attacks. *Lancet*, **339**, 473–477.

Dyson, J. (1984) A voluntary stroke club. *Physiotherapy*, **40**, 79.

Engardt, M., Ribbe, T. and Olsson, E. (1993) Vertical ground reaction force feedback to enhance stroke patients' symmetrical body-weight distribution while rising/sitting down. *Scandinavian Journal of Rehabilitation Medicine*, **25**, 41–48.

Ernst, E. (1990) A review of stroke rehabilitation and physiotherapy. *Stroke*, **21**, 1081–1085.

Evans, R.L., Bishop, D.S., Matlock, A.L. *et al.* (1987) Family interaction and treatment adherence after stroke. *Archives of Physical Medicine and Rehabilitation*, **68**, 513–517.

Evans, R.L., Hendricks, R.D., Haselkorn, J.K. *et al.* (1992) The family's role in stroke rehabilitation. A review of the literature. *American Journal of Physical Medicine and Rehabilitation*, **71**, 135–139.

Feigenson, J.S. (1979) Stroke rehabilitation: effectiveness, benefits, and cost. Some practical considerations. *Stroke*, **10**, 1–4.

Fiatarone, M.A., Marks, E.C., Ryan, N.D. *et al.* (1990) High-intensity strength training in nonagenarians. *Journal of the American Medical Association*, **263**, 3029–3034.

Franks, P.J., Adamson, C., Bulpitt, P.F. *et al.* (1991) Stroke death and unemployment in London. *Journal of Epidemiology and Community Health*, **45**, 16–18.

Gelber, D.A., Good, D.C., Laven, L.J. *et al.* (1993) Causes of urinary incontinence after acute stroke. *Stroke*, **24**, 378–382.

Goldman, J. and Côté, L. (1991) Aging of the brain: dementia of the Alzheimer's type. In *Principles of Neural Science* (eds E.R. Kandell, J.H. Schwartz and T.M. Jessell), Appleton and Lange, Norwalk, CT, pp. 974–983.

Griffiths, V. (1970) *A Stroke in the Family*. Pitman, London.

Hakkinen, K. and Komi, P.V. (1983) Electromyographic changes during strength training and detraining. *Medicine and Science in Sports and Exercise*, **15**, 455–460.

Hamzeh, M.A., Bowker, P. and Sayegh, A. (1988) The energy costs of ambulation using two types of walking frame. *Clinical Rehabilitation*, **2**, 119–123.

Hatano, S. (1976) Experience from a multicentre stroke register: a preliminary report. *Bulletin of the WHO*, **54**, 541.

Hayes, S.H. and Carroll, S.R. (1986) Early intervention care in the acute stroke patient. *Archives of Physical Medicine and Rehabilitation*, **67**, 319–321.

Henley, S., Petit, S., Todd-Pokropek, A. *et al.* (1985) Who goes home? Predictive factors in stroke recovery. *Journal of Neurology, Neurosurgery and Psychiatry*, **48**, 1–6.

Hesse, S., Bertelt, C., Jahnke, M.T. *et al.* (1995) Treadmill training with partial body weight support compared with physiotherapy in nonambulatory hemiparetic patients. *Stroke*, **26**, 976–981.

Hesse, S., Bertelt, C., Schaffrin, A. *et al.* (1994a) Restoration of gait in nonambulatory hemiparetic patients by treadmill training with partial body-weight. *Archives of Physical Medicine Rehabilitation*, **75**, 1083–1097.

Hesse, S.A., Jahnke, M.T., Bertelt, C.M. *et al.* (1994b) Gait outcome in ambulatory hemiparetic patients after

a 4-week comprehensive rehabilitation program and prognostic factors. *Stroke*, **25**, 1999–2004.

Hewson, L. (1988) *Stroke: a Family Affair*. Collins Dove, Blackburn, Victoria, Australia.

Hewson, L. (1996) *The Stroke Jigsaw: Lorna's Story*. An Integrated Resource Package, The University of Newcastle, Newcastle, Australia.

Hibbard, M.R., Gordon, W.A., Stein, P.N. *et al.* (1993) A multimodal approach to the diagnosis of post-stroke depression. In *Advances in Stroke Rehabilitation* (ed. W.A. Gordon), Andover Medical Publishers, Boston, pp. 185–214.

Inaba, M.K., Edberg, E., Montgomery, J. *et al.* (1973) Effectiveness of functional training, active exercise and resistive exercises for patients with hemiplegia. *Physical Therapy*, **53**, 28–35.

Indredavik, B., Bakke, F., Solberg, R. *et al.* (1991) Benefit of a stroke unit: a randomised control trial. *Stroke*, **22**, 1026–1030.

Jamrozik, K., Broadhurst, R.J., Anderson, C.S. *et al.* (1994) The role of lifestyle factors in the etiology of stroke. A population-based case-control study in Perth, Western Australia. *Stroke*, **25**, 51–59.

Jørgensen, H.S., Nakayama, H., Raaschou, H.O. *et al.* (1995) Outcome and time course of recovery in stroke. Part 1: outcome. The Copenhagen stroke study. *Archives of Physical Medicine Rehabilitation*, **76**, 399–405.

Kandel, E.R. (1991a) Brain and behavior. In *Principles of Neural Science* (ed. E.R. Kandell, J.H. Schwartz and T.M. Jessell), Appleton and Lange, Norwalk, CT, pp. 5–17.

Kandel, E.R. (1991b) Disorders of mood: depression, mania, and anxiety disorders. In *Principles of Neural Science* (eds E.R. Kandel, J.H. Schwartz and T.M. Jessell), Appleton and Lange, Norwalk, CT, pp. 869–883.

Khan, Z., Starer, P., Yang, W.C. *et al.* (1990) Analysis of voiding disorders in patients with cerebrovascular accidents. *Urology*, **35**, 265–270.

King, J.L., Guarracini, M., Lenihan, L. *et al.* (1989) Adaptive exercise testing for patients with hemiparesis. *Journal of Cardiopulmonary Rehabilitation*, **9**, 237–242.

Kinsella, G. and Ford, B. (1980) Acute recovery pattern in stroke patient. *Medical Journal of Australia*, 13 December, pp. 653–666.

Lampman, R. (1987) Evaluating and prescribing exercise for elderly patients. *Geriatrics*, **8**, 63–65.

Landau, W.M. (1974) Spasticity: the fable of the neurological demon and the emperor's new therapy. *Archives of Neurology*, **31**, 217–219.

Landau, W.M. (1988) Parables of palsy, pills and PT pedagogy: A spastic dialectic. *Neurology*, **38**, 1496–1499.

Langhorne, P., Williams, B.O., Gilchrist, W. *et al.* (1993) Do stroke units save lives? *Lancet*, **342**, 395–398.

Legh-Smith, J., Wade, D.T. and Langton-Hewer, R. (1986) Services for stroke patients one year after stroke. *Journal Epidemiological Community Health,* **40**, 161-165.

Levine, R.L. (1987) Diagnostic, medical, and surgical aspects of stroke management. In *Stroke Rehabilitation The Recovery of Motor Control* (eds P.W. Duncan and M.B. Badke), Year Book Medical Publishers, Chicago, pp. 1–47.

Lewinter, M. and Mikkelsen, S. (1995) Patients' experience of rehabilitation after stroke. *Disability and Rehabilitation,* **17**, 3–9.

Lincoln, N.B., Jackson, J.M., Edmans, J.A. *et al.* (1990) The accuracy of predictiions about progress of patients on a stroke unit. *Journal of Neurology, Neurosurgery and Psychiatry,* **53**, 972-975.

Lord, S. and Castell, S. (1994) Effect of exercise on balance, strength and reaction time in older people. *Australian Journal of Physiotherapy,* **40**, 83–88.

Malouin, F., Potvin, M., Prevost, J. *et al.* (1992) Use of an intensive task-oriented gait training program in a series of patients with acute cerebrovascular accidents. *Physical Therapy,* **72**, 781–789.

Mayeux, R. and Kandel, E.R. (1991) Disorders of language: the aphasias. In *Principles of Neural Science* (eds E.R. Kandel, J.H. Schwartz and T.M. Jessell), Appleton and Lange, Norwalk, CT, pp. 834–851.

Mehrabian, A. (1969) Significance of posture and position in the communication of attitude and status relationships. *Psychology Bulletin,* **71**, 359–372.

Monga, T.N., Lawson, J.S., Inglis, J. (1986) Sexual adjustment in stroke patients. *Archives of Physical Medicine and Rehabilitation,* **67**, 19–22.

Montgomery, J. (1987) Assessment and treatment of locomotor deficits in stroke. In *Stroke Rehabilitation: The Recovery of Motor Control* (eds P.W. Duncan and M.B. Badke), YearBook Medical Publishers, Chicago, pp. 223–259.

Morey, M.C., Cowper, P.A., Feussner, J.R. *et al.* (1989) Evaluation of a supervised exercise program in a geriatric population. *Journal of the American Geriatric Society,* **37**, 348–354.

Morris, D.M., Crago, J.E. and De Luca, S.C. *et al.* (1997) Constraint-induced movement therapy for motor recovery after stroke. *Neurorehabilitation,* **9**, 29–43.

Nugent, J.A., Schurr, K.A. and Adams, R.D. (1994) A dose-response relationship between amount of weight bearing exercise and walking outcome following cerebrovascular accident. *Archives Physical Medicine Rehabilitation,* **75**, 399–402.

Ottenbacher, K.J. and Jannell, S. (1993) The results of clinical trials in stroke rehabilitation research. *Archives of Neurology,* **50**, 37–44.

Peterson, C., Maier, S.F. and Seligman, M.E.P. (1993) *Learned Helplessness A Theory of Personal Control.* Oxford University Press, Oxford.

Potempa, K., Braun, L.T., Tinknell, T. *et al.* (1996) Benefits of aerobic exercise after stroke. *Sports Medicine,* **21**, 337–416.

Potempa, K., Lopez, M., Braun, L.T. *et al.* (1995) Physiological outcomes of aerobic exercise training in hemiparetic stroke patients. *Stroke,* **26**, 101–105.

Price, T.R. (1990) Affective disorders after stroke. *Stroke,* **21** (Suppl 11)**,** 12–13.

Richards, C.L., Malouin, F., Wood-Dauphinee, S. *et al.* (1993) Task-specific physical therapy for optimization of gait recovery in acute stroke patients. *Archives of Physical Medicine and Rehabilitation,* **74**, 612–620.

Robertson, I.H. (1993) Cognitive rehabilitation in neurologic disease. *Current Opinion in Neurology,* **6**, 756–760.

Robinson, R.G. and Szetela, B. (1981) Mood changes following left hemipheric brain injury. *Annals of Neurology,* **9**, 447–453.

Rutherford, O.M. (1988) Muscular coordination and strength training implications for injury rehabilitation. *Sports Medicine,* **5**, 196–202.

Rutherford, O.M. and Jones, D.A. (1986) The role of learning and coordination in strength training. *European Journal of Applied Physiology,* **55**, 100–105.

Ryerson, S.D. (1995) Hemiplegia. In *Neurological Rehabilitation* (ed. D.A. Umphred) Mosby, New York, pp. 681–721.

Sandercock, P. and Willems, H. (1992) Medical treatment of acute ischaemic stroke. *Lancet,* **339**, 537-539.

Schmidt, J., Holas, M., Halvorson, M.S. *et al.* (1994) Videofluoroscopic evidence of aspiration predicts pneumonia and death but not dehydration following stroke. *Dysphagia,* **9**, 7–11.

Seligman, M. (1975) *Helplessness on Depression, Development and Death.* San Francisco, W.H. Freeman.

Shepherd, R.B. and Carr, J.H. (1991) An emergent or dynamical systems view of movement dysfunction. *Australian Journal of Physiotherapy,* **37**, 4–5,17.

Sutherland, J. and Baker, G.H.B. (1979) Group support for relatives of stroke patients. *Occupational Therapy,* September, pp. 216–217.

Tangeman, P.T., Banaitis, D.A., and Williams, A.K. (1990) Rehabilitation of chronic stroke patients: changes in functional performance. *Archives of Physical Medicine and Rehabilitation,* **71**, 876–880.

Taub, E. (1980) Somatosensory deafferentation research with monkeys. In *Behavioral Psychology and Rehabilitation Medicine* (ed. L. Ince), Williams and Wilkins, Baltimore, MD, pp. 371–401.

Taub, E., Miller, N.E., Novack, T.A. *et al.*, (1993) Technique to improve chronic motor deficit after stroke. *Archives of Physical Medicine and Rehabilitation,* **74**, 347–354.

Waagfjord, J., Levangle, P.K. and Certo, C.M.E. (1990) Effects of treadmill training on gait in a hemiparetic patient. *Physical Therapy,* **70**, 549–558.

Wade, D.T., Collen, F.M., Robb, G.F. *et al.* (1992) Physiotherapy intervention late after stroke and mobility. *British Medical Journal*, **304**, 609–613.

Wade, D.T., Langton Hewer, R., David, R.M. *et al.* (1986) Aphasia after stroke: natural history and associated deficits. *Journal of Neurology, Neurosurgery and Psychiatry*, **49**, 11–16.

Wade, D.T., Langton Hewer, R., Skillbeck C.E. *et al.* (1985) *Stroke, a Critical Approach to Diagnosis, Treatment and Management.* Chapman and Hall, London.

Wade, D.T., Wood, V.A. and Langton Hewer, R. (1985) Recovery after stroke – the first 3 months. *Journal of Neurology, Neurosurgery and Psychiatry*, **48**, 7–13.

Wadell, I., Kusoffsky, A. and Nilsson, B.Y. (1987) A follow-up study of stroke patients 5–6 years after their brain infarct. *International Journal of Rehabilitation Research*, **10**, 103–110.

Ward, G., Jamrozik, K. and Stewart-Wynne, E. (1988) Incidence and outcome of cerebrovascular disease in Perth, Western Australia. *Stroke*, **19**, 1501-1506.

Warlow, C. P. (1993) Disorders of cerebral circulation. In *Brain's Disorders of the Nervous System* (ed. J Walton), Oxford University Press, Oxford, pp. 197–268.

Warlow, C. P. and Morris, P.J. (1982) Introduction. In *Transient Ischaemic Attacks* (eds C.P. Marlow and P.J. Morris), Marcel Dekker, New York.

Wilson, B. A. (1989) *Memory Problems After Head Injury.* National Head Injuries Association, Nottingham.

Wilson, B.A. (1991) Long-term prognosis of patients with severe memory disorders. *Neuropyschological Rehabilitation*, **1**, 117–134.

Wilson, B. A. (1995) Management and remediation in brain-injured adults. In *Handbook of Memory Disorders* (eds A.D. Baddeley, B.A. Wilson and F. N. Watts) John Wiley, Chichester, pp. 451–479.

Wolf, S.L., Lecraw, D.E., Barton, L.A. *et al.* (1989) Forced use of hemiparetic upper extremities to reverse the effect of learned nonuse among chronic stroke and head-injured patients. *Experimental Neurology*, **104**, 125–132.

Further reading

Ada, L. and Canning, C. (eds) (190) *Key Issues in Neurological Physiotherapy.* Butterworth-Heinemann, Oxford.

Carr, J.H. and Shepherd, R.B. (1987) *The Motor Relearning Programme for Stroke*, 2nd edn. Butterworth-Heinemann, Oxford.

Carr, J.H. and Shepherd, R.B. (1987) *Movement Science Foundations for Physical Therapy in Rehabilitation.* Butterworth-Heinemann, Oxford.

Kapur, N. (1995) Memory aids in the rehabilitation of memory disordered patients. In *Handbook of Memory Disorders* (eds A.D. Baddeley, B.A. Wilson and F. N. Watts), John Wiley, Chichester, pp. 533–556.

Appendix
The shoulder in stroke

Secondary musculoskeletal complications, resulting in glenohumeral subluxation stiffness and shoulder pain are common sequelae of neurological impairment, particularly following stroke (Bohannon *et al.* 1986; Roy *et al.* 1994). Figures of up to 84% of patients with shoulder pain have been cited (Najenson *et al.* 1971; van Ouwenaller *et al.* 1986; Roy *et al.* 1994) and pain and stiffness around the shoulder have been reported to occur as early as two weeks after stroke (Brocklehurst *et al.* 1978). However, in the clinic a diagnosis of 'hemiplegic shoulder pain' may be given with little attempt to provide an accurate diagnosis of the causes of the pain and where an individual without a stroke would usually receive a specialized examination, this may not occur following stroke.

Considerable space is occupied in the literature on issues related to the painful shoulder, yet shoulder pain remains ubiquitous and seems accepted as a 'natural' and largely unpreventable entity (for exception see Roy *et al.* 1994). For the person with the pain, movement of the arm becomes increasingly difficult, sleep is interfered with and life, including much of rehabilitation, becomes an effort (Savage and Robertson 1982). The person who has pain on movement remains immobile; if there is pain at rest, the person may withdraw from collaborating in rehabilitation (Braun *et al.* 1971).

Shoulder pain is recognized as a substantial cause of poor recovery of upper limb function following stroke (Cailliet 1980; Griffin and Reddin 1981) and recently, pain on movement has been reported to be a predictor of outcome (Roy *et al.* 1995). This relationship to poor recovery is to be expected given the fact that a significant degree of pain will cause an inhibition of muscle action at the shoulder (Bechtol 1980). Pain may be localized to the shoulder or may radiate down the arm. Localized tenderness over supraspinatus or biceps brachii may be present. Pain may be present at rest or only on passive or attempted active movement.

Why does pain occur?

Examination of the sequelae of brain lesion affecting the sensorimotor systems implicates some probable causative mechanisms. Decreased descending inputs to spinal motor neurons lead to muscle paralysis and weakness. This leads in turn to immobility of the limb or, where there are some muscles with intact innervation, to muscle imbalance (Bohannon and Smith 1987), with active, stronger muscles moving the limb segments in what become preferred directions.

Muscle paralysis and the effect of gravity and non-use can lead to a downward displacement of the humeral head. This may or may not be associated with pain. Indeed the relationship between pain and glenohumeral (GH) subluxation is not really understood and remains controversial (Bohannon *et al.* 1986; Bohannon 1988; Van Langenberghe and Hogan 1988; Joynt 1992; Roy *et al.* 1995).

Muscle paralysis, weakness and disuse

It is typically observed that it is individuals with severe muscle paralysis who develop shoulder pain and stiffness (Najenson *et al.* 1971; Jensen 1980; Brandstater and Basmajian 1987; Roy 1988) and an association between pain and reduced shoulder shrug has been reported (Wanklyn *et al.* 1996). One study of 30 individuals following stroke has reported a significant correlation between shoulder pain and strength of shoulder external rotator and abductor muscles (Bohannon 1988) and it was suggested that muscle weakness may lead to pain because the weak muscles were not able to move the joint to prevent adhesive capsulitis.

The relative immobility of the limb caused by paralysis or extreme weakness results in adaptive changes in the soft tissues around the shoulder which are synonymous with disuse. That is to say, muscle paralysis and weakness result in immobilization and disuse as effectively as any splint.

Adaptive structural changes

The structural changes that occur within the musculoskeletal system as a result of muscle weakness, immobilization and disuse are well known and include *muscular, capsular and ligamentous length changes* (structures either shortening or lengthening), *changes in muscle stiffness*, and *degenerative changes in joint structure and bone*. Bohannon and colleagues (Bohannon *et al.* 1986) found that a painful shoulder in individuals who have had a stroke was not only related to weakness but also was significantly correlated with diminished range of external rotation of the GH joint, in addition to weakness of GH abduction, external rotation and 'stiffness'. Soft tissues become shorter and stiffer due to the same factors as pertain during any form of immobilization (see Chapter 8).

These adaptations to muscle and joint capsule effectively impose their own restrictions on joint movement (whether passive or active). The tissues that shorten are those which are held short because of the preferred or imposed resting position of the limb. Individuals who spend a large part of the day in sitting with the affected arm by the side and hand in lap, for example, will develop adaptive shortening of the GH adductors and internal rotators, as well as of elbow flexors, forearm pronators, wrist and finger flexors, and thumb adductors (see Fig. 6.9). Severely limited external rotation is very common after stroke (see Bohannon *et al.* 1986), and this is not surprising given the extreme internal rotation in which the shoulder typically rests for large parts of the day and night. It should be noted also that loss of external rotation is also typically associated with capsulitis in the non-stroke population. Where loss of external rotation occurs rapidly despite preventative positioning and active exercise into external rotation, capsulitis should be suspected. Another diagnostic sign of capsulitis is a report of pain at night.

Disuse in the non-stroke population is known to cause abnormalities in shoulder structures, such as subacromial bursitis, and biceps and supraspinatus tendinitis. These conditions are associated with pain. Muscle contracture and reduced range of motion have been shown to be associated with joint changes typical of adhesive capsulitis (Bruckner and Nye 1981; Rizk *et al.* 1984). Even young adults have been shown to develop abnormalities of shoulder structures due to disuse; for example, increased calcium deposits have been found in supraspinatus of typists compared to file clerks who move their arms more freely (Bechtol 1980).

Decreased painless range of elevation has been reported to occur with increasing age (Saario 1963). This may be because relatively few of our daily activities require full elevation of the arm. Alternatively, it may reflect an increase in thoracic kyphosis and/or stiffness. Older adults have an increased chance of having abnormalities of capsule, bursae and humeral head, such as humeral head arthritis (Peat 1986). Degenerative changes in periarticular soft tissues occurring with increasing age include: thickening and shredding of biceps brachii tendon; calcific deposits in rotator cuff tendons; thinning and fraying of supraspinatus muscle (De Palma 1983). Hakuno and colleagues (1984) in a study of 77 people with hemiplegia, reported that the incidence of capsular tears did not differ between affected and unaffected side, however, there were more adhesive changes in the affected shoulder. Whether or not these findings are related to decreased use of the limb or to previous injury is not known but both are possibilities. The point is, however, that older adults may have degenerative changes in the shoulder prior to the stroke, suggesting that particular care should be taken with the shoulder as soon as a person is admitted to acute care following stroke.

Trauma to the unprotected arm

This has been implicated in the cause of shoulder pain (Cailliet 1980; Jensen 1980). Certainly capsulitis is known to follow on from even relatively minor trauma in the non-stroke population. Following stroke, when the limb is moved passively by its own weight or by the individual or another person, the altered mechanics of the joint caused in part by the limitations on movement imposed by the altered length of tissue, together with thoracic stiffness, can subject bone and soft tissue to stresses which can cause pain or eventually lead to pain.

Soft tissues in the vicinity of the joint may be traumatized by various events occurring to the paralysed and defenceless shoulder, causing or aggravating pre-existing adhesive capsulitis, biceps or supraspinatus tendinitis or subacromial bursitis. A recent study (Wanklyn *et al.* 1996) investigated factors associated with shoulder pain. The authors reported that lifting the patient by pulling on the arm was a rather common occurrence, even when staff had been advised not to. Interestingly, those patients who needed help with 'transfers', i.e., getting in and out of bed and standing up, were most likely to suffer shoulder pain, which implicates pulling on the arm as a causative factor.

Passive range of motion exercises, including overhead pulley exercises, have been implicated in injury or activation of previously symptomatic abnormalities of the paralysed shoulder (Cailliet 1980; Griffin 1986; Kumar *et al.* 1990). The probability of damage is likely to increase if paralysis persists. Adaptive shortening of scapula muscles, for example, rhomboids and trapezius, could prevent the scapula from rotating and protracting when the arm is passively moved into elevation and this could result in small tears to scapulo-humeral muscles. This is magnified by contracture of muscles linking scapula to humerus. Impingement of soft tissues may occur if the head of humerus is compressed against the scapula when the shoulder is passively flexed or abducted without the accompanying GH rotation, for example, external rotation during abduction (Hawkins and Murnaghan 1984) (Fig. 11.5).

Spasticity has been suggested as a cause of pain in the shoulder through 'spastic' contracture of scapula retractors and GH joint adductors, and abnormal movement patterns (Bobath 1990; Ryerson 1995). The assumption is that the muscles hold the limb immobilized because they are spastic. This assumption has misled therapists into believing that inhibition of spasticity will overcome the stiffness and pain. In addition, some therapists generally believe that muscle weakness is not a major problem following a neural lesion. Perhaps as a result of such beliefs, rehabilitation personnel do not place emphasis on developing methods of prevention, diagnosis and intervention which might prevent the painful stiff shoulder in many patients and lead to rational methods of treatment should a painful condition occur. It is notable that recent textbooks which contain chapters referring to stroke do not mention degenerative or traumatic GH joint impairments (e.g., Ryerson 1995; Edwards 1996), their prevention or treatment.

In summary, although there may be other specific causes of a painful stiff shoulder for a particular individual, it is evident that there are some strong contenders for principal contributors:

- Immobility and prolonged posturing with arm by the side associated with muscle weakness or paralysis.
- Pre- and post-stroke degenerative conditions.
- Adapted stiff contracted soft tissues.
- Compounding effects of injury to the shoulder post-stroke.

These factors are amenable to intervention; some could actually be prevented (Griffin 1986; Shep-

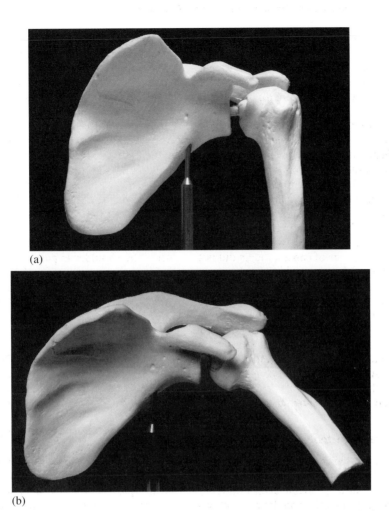

(a)

(b)

Fig. 11.5 (*a*) Scapular–humeral anatomical relationships: External rotation of the humerus during abduction (*b*) ensures that the greater tuberosity of the humerus rotates out of the way of the acromion process

herd and Carr 1998). A recent study of shoulder pain in 67 individuals following stroke found that the amount of shoulder pain was related most to loss of motion. Amount of pain was unrelated to subluxation, spasticity, strength or sensation (Joynt 1992).

Reflex sympathetic dystrophy (RSD), also called shoulder–hand syndrome, is characterized by pain, stiffness, swelling and discoloration of the involved limb. Reports citing frequency of RSD are variable and it has been reported in up to 39% of individuals following stroke (Brandstater and Basmajian 1987; Roy *et al.* 1994). Its cause is unknown but immobility and GH joint inflammation appear to contribute.

It has been suggested that *brachial plexus lesions* can occur following stroke (Kaplan *et al.* 1977). Such a lesion would compound the problem

of muscle paralysis. However, the difficulties inherent in distinguishing plexus lesion from the effects of the cortical lesion, make an accurate diagnosis problematic (Kingery *et al.* 1987).

Glenohumeral joint malalignment and subluxation

GH joint malalignment and subluxation are reported to occur in patients with little or no voluntary movement after stroke (Grossen-Sils and Schenkman 1985; Van Langenberghe and Hogan 1988). Malalignment appears to occur early in the flaccid limb due to severe paralysis of the muscles around the GH joint, which is common in many individuals immediately after stroke (Poulin de Courval *et al.*

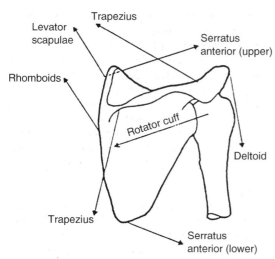

Fig. 11.6 Muscles of the shoulder girdle and major forces acting on the shoulder girdle. (From Peat 1986, after Dvir and Berme 1978, by permission)

1990), to the effects of gravity (weight of the limb) and of limb position (Fig. 11.6). As a result of muscle paralysis or extreme weakness, support and protection of the GH joint are dependent upon joint capsule, ligaments and non-active muscles. The combination of a dependent resting position and paralysis or severe weakness of muscles linking the humerus to the scapula or spine (such as supraspinatus; Basmajian and Bazant 1959) causes stretching and lengthening of soft tissues around the GH joint in the absence of preventative methods. Early lengthening of the joint capsule has been shown by arthrography (Miglietta *et al.* 1959).

The mechanism of subluxation is generally considered to include the downward rotation of the scapula caused by the weight of the limb, which positions the glenoid fossa more vertically (Cailliet 1991). However, downward rotation of the scapula may not be a significant feature (Arsenault *et al.* 1991) and, in a recent report, no evidence of a relationship between scapula and humeral orientation and GH subluxation was found (Culham *et al.* 1995). Culham and colleagues pointed out that there was, therefore, no evidence that 'low tone' in scapular muscles contributes to downward rotation of scapula as has been suggested (Davies 1985; Ryerson and Levit 1991).

Subluxation has been proposed as a contributing factor in the development of shoulder pain (Chaco and Wolf 1971; Najenson *et al.* 1971; Griffin and Reddin 1981; van Ouwenaller *et al.* 1986; Roy *et al.* 1995). The mechanism suggested is one of traction on rotator cuff and superior joint capsule, the resulting stretch causing pain. However, there has been no explanation of why this should cause pain, and there is no direct evidence linking subluxation with pain. One cause of pain on movement could be the pinching of the lengthened capsule, caught between joint surfaces during movement in certain parts of range. This appears evident in some patients as a sharp pain which can be relieved by gentle distraction of the joint during assisted movement of the limb.

Although subluxation has been implicated in shoulder pain, several studies report patients with subluxation who have no pain, even when subluxation was moderate to severe (Smith *et al.* 1982; Arsenault *et al.* 1991). Subluxation has also been reported to be associated with an increased incidence of RSD (Tepperman *et al.* 1984; Roy et al. 1994). Whatever the relationship of subluxation to pain, attempts should be made to prevent or minimize it, since stretched capsule and muscles about the GH joint are likely to impact on the regaining of control of the limb.

Prevention of secondary musculoskeletal changes, damage to the shoulder complex, subluxation and pain

Prevention depends on anticipation, i.e., on an awareness of the susceptibility of older people to shoulder injury (AHCPR 1995) and of the probable causative mechanisms following stroke. The literature is replete with studies of the incidence of painful shoulder after stroke and the sequelae. Prevention is, however, rarely mentioned.

Anticipation involves the therapist and patient knowing in advance which muscles and other soft tissues are at risk of shortening and which therapy and general handling methods have the potential to damage the unprotected shoulder. There needs also to be an awareness of the benefits associated with active exercise to elicit and strengthen muscle activity and gain optimal control of the limb. We know for certain that the problem occurs in a large proportion of patients; we understand a great deal about the causative mechanisms. The next step is to investigate methods of prevention.

A protocol for prevention of shoulder joint stress, trauma and pain

Such a protocol can describe best practice to be carried out by all staff from the time the individual

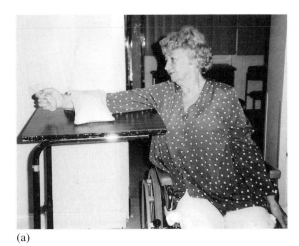

(a)

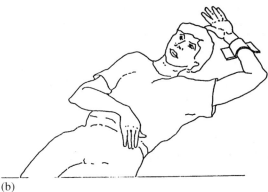

(b)

Fig. 11.7 Examples of positions for preserving length in shoulder muscles. (*a*) Sitting at a table, (*b*) lying down. A sandbag can be used to keep the arm in position. In (*a*) and (*b*), the patient exercises to improve grip strength (particularly of 4th and 5th fingers which are weak) and full finger extension (*b*, Courtesy of C. Dean)

is admitted to the acute care facility. The protocol is tested for effectiveness by monitoring the presence of pain, GH joint range of motion and functional use of the limb. A preventative protocol can involve:

- **Positioning procedures**
  To prevent changes in soft tissue length, particularly of GH adductor and internal rotator muscles. Specified periods of time are spent stretching these muscles (Fig. 11.7).
- **Avoidance of certain handling methods**
  To protect the GH joint, avoid lifting or pulling by the arm, and passive range of motion exercises performed by staff with limited knowledge of the shoulder region. A stick-on logo or strapping used to support the arm may

be effective in drawing attention to the shoulder and act as a warning to staff (Fig. 11.8).
- **Supporting the arm in sitting**
  To prevent limb weight from stretching soft tissues around the GH joint. The limb is supported in flexion on a table, and for specified periods of the day in abduction and external rotation. When the patient is not exercising, the arm must not rest in GH internal rotation but in mid-rotation. In standing or when practising walking, strapping may provide sufficient support for the limb.
- **Exercise**
  To regain active muscle contraction, increase strength and control of muscles of the shoulder region. A specified period of time is spent exercising the upper limb, both supervised by the therapist, and unsupervised but monitored.

The US Department of Health and Human Services (AHCPR 1995), in their clinical practice guideline, advocate supporting the limb on a table attached to the wheelchair; using a sheet (the Australian lift, Fig. 11.9, can also be used) to lift the patient up in bed rather than the arms; including external rotation of the GH joint in exercises that take the arm beyond 90° flexion or abduction. AHCPR cautions against self-ranging exercises through flexion or overhead pulleys and points out that supports and slings are controversial due to potential complications from immobilization.

Below are some suggestions for early motor training which, given the relationship between muscle weakness, muscle shortening and pain, are a critical part of the prevention protocol. These are discussed in more detail in Chapter 6.

- Exercises to elicit muscle activity with the muscle at different lengths. When muscle activation is present, exercises to train controlled movement of the shoulder (Fig. 11.10): for example, in the supine position, with the hand on the head, attempting to adduct horizontally (see Fig. 6.13), with the arm in elevation, attempting to raise the arm from the bed (Fig. 11.10).

Note: These exercises are motivating for the patient as innervation to the pectoral muscles is often either intact or recovers early. It may be possible to perform a lengthening (eccentric) contraction when a shortening (concentric) contraction cannot be elicited. The therapist and patient have to search for signs of muscle action together. Muscle activity is frequently present under the right conditions, even in an apparently flaccid limb.

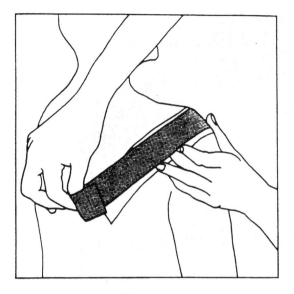

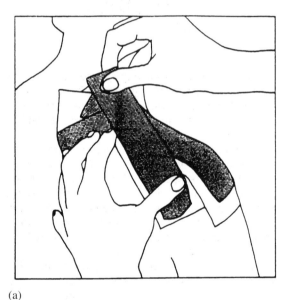

(a)

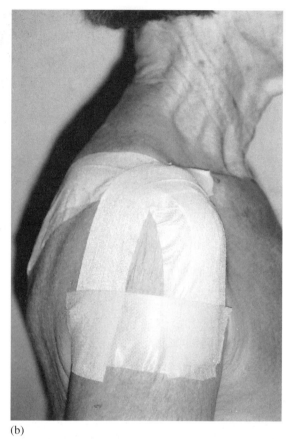

(b)

Fig. 11.8 Strapping to provide some support for the upper limb. (Courtesy of J. McConnell)

- Verbal feedback by the therapist, who monitors muscle activation by palpation and by EMG feedback (see Fig. 6.17).
- Exercises are progressed as soon as muscles are active to enable the individual to activate a number of muscles synergistically to achieve a goal.
- Shoulder shrugging exercises can be practised by the patient several times a day and may be important for overcoming the 'dragging' effect of a heavy immobile limb (see Fig. 6.15e,f).

The patient may feel a sudden pain in the shoulder in a certain part of GH joint range, particularly in supine with the arm around 90°. This may be due to impingement of the humeral head against soft tissues at the joint surface and can usually be overcome by the therapist applying a small amount of traction, enough to distract the humeral head from impact with the scapula while the person practises, say, touching the head, as a means of exercising elbow extensor muscles. This distraction is a temporary measure enabling exercise to

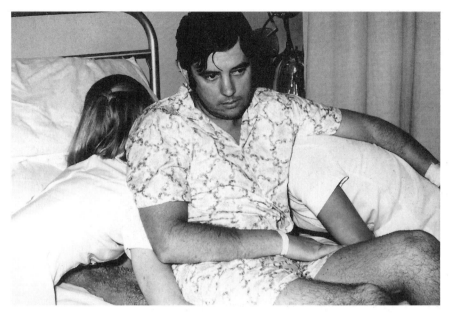

Fig. 11.9 The 'Australian' lift enables staff to move a person in bed without pulling on the paretic arm

continue. The person practises moving the limb through small arcs, avoiding but getting close to the painful arc at first then moving throughout range as soon as possible. The resultant increase in strength and control of muscles around the joint through active exercise often resolves the problem of pain.

Note that supine, the arm at 90° is a position suitable for eliciting and training muscle activity around the shoulder in a person with severe muscle weakness since the muscle force required to move is not as great as with the arm at the side. However, training is also carried out in sitting with the arm supported on a table (see Fig. 11.10) and this is where it can start in the person with more muscle strength.

Electrical stimulation of paralysed muscles around the shoulder has been shown to decrease existing subluxation (Baker and Parker 1986). Recently, Faghri and colleagues (1994) tested the effects of functional electrical stimulation (FES) of posterior deltoid and supraspinatus muscles with 26 individuals early after stroke. They found a significant decrease in subluxation (on radiography), and a significant increase in arm function, EMG activity of shoulder muscles and range of motion compared to the control group. The experimental group received FES to posterior deltoid and supraspinatus 6 hours a day for 6 weeks.

It is likely that electrical stimulation and support of the limb on a table are most critical early after stroke to prevent stretching of the capsule and ligaments, since many patients with early motor training recover at least sufficient muscle power to maintain the GH joint in normal alignment (Anderson 1985).

A variety of *slings and supports* have been suggested to prevent and correct GH joint subluxation. Slings, supports and other aids can be categorized as: *total support* (triangular sling, hemi-sling, wheelchair arm trough or table); *partial support* (Hook hemi-harness, Royal South Sydney harness, other cuff slings); and *axillary support* (Bobath shoulder roll).

Most aids are designed principally to take the weight of the arm either totally or partially (Chaco and Wolf 1971). Many have been shown to be ineffective either in preventing subluxation or in correcting it once it has occurred. Several are contraindicated because of their probable effect in producing disuse adaptations (triangular sling, various forms of hemi-sling), malalignment of the humeral head laterally (Bobath roll) and the phenomenon of learned non-use.

In a radiographic analysis, the authors examined the effects in the sitting position of five different slings (triangular sling, hemi-sling, the Hook hemi-harness, the Bobath roll and support of the arm on a pillow in sitting) on one patient with a subluxed shoulder. We found that resting the arm on a pillow was the only method that made any difference to the

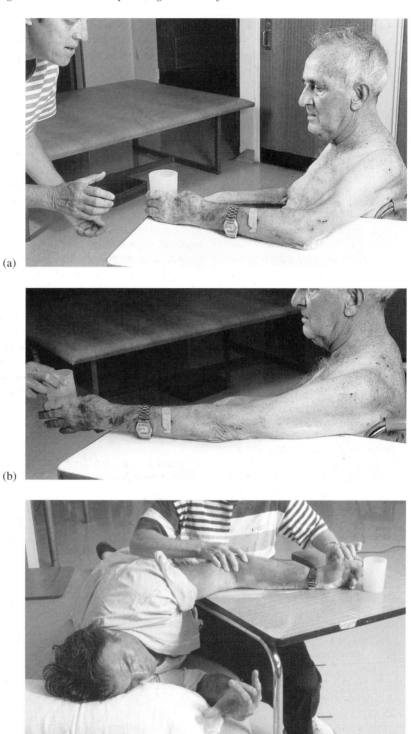

Fig. 11.10 (*a*) Attempting to reach forward to pass the glass of water. (*b*) He has sufficient muscle activity to reach forward if his arm is supported on the table. (*c*) Another position in which to elicit muscle activity around the shoulder (same person as in Fig. 6.8)

subluxation (Carr and Shepherd 1987a). Other radiographic studies of various slings show that several of them can correct to some extent an existing subluxation (Moodie *et al.* 1986; Williams et al. 1988; Brook *et al.* 1991; Zorowitz *et al.* 1995). However, the considerable disadvantages of most of these slings appear to outweigh the advantages.

Those which involve axillary support (e.g., Bobath roll) have been shown to produce unwanted malalignment, specifically horizontal displacement of the humeral head in the glenoid fossa (Zorowitz *et al.* 1995). Slings which hold the arm in an adducted, internally rotated position (e.g., triangular sling, hemi-slings), although they may be effective in reducing the extent of subluxation, have serious disadvantages. We have already seen that immobilization of the arm is likely to cause degenerative changes (and probably pain) in the shoulder joint, particularly but not only in elderly individuals, as well as atrophy of the muscles of that arm (Bruton 1985). An internally rotated and adducted shoulder position, if maintained for a length of time, will result in soft tissue contracture (at the elbow as well as shoulder) and pain. It is also likely that such support will augment the tendency, already well known (Taub *et al.* 1993), for the individual to ignore the affected limb and develop learned non-use, since it is tucked away out of sight. Similar criticisms can be levelled at the varieties of hemi-sling which have been developed. It should be noted that none of these studies investigated either the long term effects of the devices nor their effect in preventing subluxation.

Support of the limb on a table while the person is in a wheelchair appears an effective means of reducing subluxation (Moodie *et al.* 1986; Boyd and Garland 1986; Williams *et al.* 1988). This simple method is likely also to be effective in preventing subluxation although this has not been tested. Table support has the added advantage of allowing the individual to practise hand and arm activities or, in the absence of voluntary movement, the hand can at least be seen and movements practised mentally. Prevention of shortening of GH internal rotator muscles appears to be critical and measures need to be instituted very early to ensure that the GH joint rests in mid-rotation when the subject is not exercising and not in internal rotation. Arm troughs on the wheelchair can be used to support the GH joint in mid GH rotation.

Strapping with hypoallergenic tape can be applied as in Figure 11.8 to provide some support for the GH joint and to control humeral head position with upward and backward pressure. The tape needs to be checked regularly and additional pieces of strapping applied as necessary. In one study of a different type of strapping (Ancliffe 1992), it was reported that it was noted by staff that the presence of the strapping had the effect of drawing their attention to the need to protect the shoulder from injury.

In summary, the protocol outlined above involves spending periods of the day with the limb supported in different ways on a table, including a wheelchair arm trough, in order to stretch at-risk muscles. It is designed to avoid a dependent upper limb, prevent shortening of at-risk muscles such as internal rotators and adductors; to train muscle activity around the shoulder and to ensure practice is regular and frequent throughout the day. The use of strapping to the shoulder to provide some support and to correct humeral alignment in standing and walking is worth investigation, a sling may be useful when the person is being showered during the acute stage, and a logo on the shoulder during the day may warn staff not to pull on the arm. EMG feedback (providing information for therapist as well as the patient) and electrical stimulation to muscles around the shoulder can be used as part of the protocol.

Evaluation and treatment of the already painful shoulder

Evaluation

For the purpose of diagnosis and intervention, evaluation is carried out by specialized staff such as orthopaedist, radiologist and manipulative physiotherapist.

Pain   Keeping records of shoulder pain is critical for ensuring quality of care while the patient is in hospital or the rehabilitation unit and to monitor efforts made to prevent pain. It is necessary, therefore, to use some method of quantification, and several methods exist, including the McGill Pain Questionnaire (Melzack 1975; Arsenault *et al.* 1991).

Range of motion   A simple standardized measure of extent of horizontal abduction and external rotation is shown in Fig. 11.12 (Ada and Canning, 1990). This is useful for monitoring changes in this critical part of range and as a guide to intervention. It is important to measure the extent of external

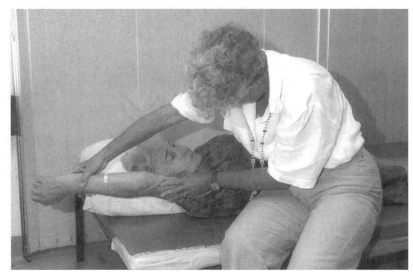

Fig. 11.11 Attempting to raise the arm from the pillow. Therapist ensures arm does not move too far into elevation, and that, as the person activates shoulder adductor muscles, the arm is moved in a path close to the head

rotation and a gravity goniometer has been reported to have test-retest reliability (Andrews and Bohannon 1989).

GH joint subluxation Typical methods of evaluation used in the clinic include: palpating the suprahumeral space and comparing it to the other side or measuring the space using calipers. These methods are usually considered to lack precision, and recently a reliable and valid method of measuring subluxation radiographically has been reported (Boyd *et al.* 1993; Hall *et al.* 1995). However, a study which compared the results of several clinical (palpation and anthropometric measures) and two-dimensional radiographic measures against a three-dimensional measure (Prevost *et al.* 1987), concluded that all the methods tested had an acceptable level of accuracy for clinical studies directed at shoulder subluxation.

Treatment

It is not surprising that secondary musculoskeletal complications have been found to be associated with poor functional outcome. What is surprising is the lack of theoretical or data-based discussion in the copious literature on painful shoulder and subluxation following stroke on the significance of:

● adaptive changes, such as soft tissue shortening and stiffness,

● weakness of muscles surrounding the shoulder and
● pre-existing and post-stroke inflammatory or degenerative GH joint changes

in the production of pain. Individuals who develop shoulder pain but who have not had a stroke typically receive a diagnosis and intervention from professionals skilled in the area of musculoskeletal mechanics and orthopaedics. If a person has had a stroke, however, they may not obtain this specialized assistance.

An accurate diagnosis enables a more rational attempt at therapy. When a diagnosis of inflammatory disorder such as capsulitis or tendinitis is made, local medical treatment for pain typically involves injection of anti-inflammatory and analgesic substances to break the pain cycle and enable active movement. Injection of 1% lidocaine in the subacromial area gave moderate or marked relief to half a group of patients who received it, suggesting, according to the authors, that the subacromial area is a pain-producing location in a number of people (Joynt 1992).

Local treatment for the painful shoulder was described nearly two decades ago as including intra-articular injections of a local anaesthetic or steroid agent (Cailliet 1980). Range of motion exercises and ultrasound were found to be ineffective in relieving pain in a randomized trial reported in 1972 (Inaba and Piorkowski 1972). Current methods of local treatment applied in non-stroke

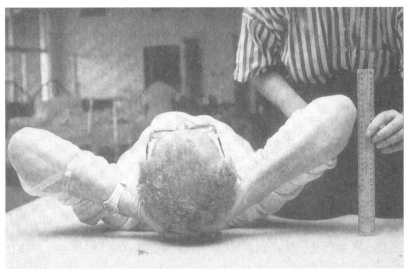

Fig. 11.12 A simple method of measuring horizontal abduction and external rotation using a ruler. (From Ada and Canning 1990, by permission)

patients include passive joint mobilising exercises, transcutaneous electrical stimulation (TENS) (Leandri *et al.* 1990) and active exercise. (See Corrigan and Maitland 1994 for details of various methodologies.)

Active exercise consists of gently coaxing active movement. The principle is to train active movement within the pain-free range available, encouraging the patient to extend the range of movement, with a caution to stop before the onset of pain. Patients with entrenched pain may need help coping with this (for example, using methods such as TENS) in order to enable an exercise and stretching programme to be commenced.

Following stroke, where active movement is difficult due to muscle paralysis or weakness, exercises such as those shown in Figures 11.10 and 11.11 will usually enable the person to gain some movement of the GH joint, although this may not be significant enough to allow the effective performance of daily actions. Some muscles involved as prime movers in GH movement (GH adductors, including pectoralis major and latissimus dorsi) and shoulder girdle elevators can usually be activated early after stroke. Exercises can be done after a local injection is given, or passive joint mobilization, if pain relief is necessary.

Passive joint mobilization (e.g., gentle accessory glides) may be effective in mobilising the joint if pain and stiffness persist (Corrigan and Maitland 1994). Movements that exacerbate pain must be

avoided and passive mobilizing is followed by active exercise. Some elderly patients may have a degree of flexion deformity of the thoracic spine and/or thoracic spine stiffness. When exercises are done in supine lying, care should be taken not to exercise the limb in an excessive degree of GH flexion (see Fig. 11.10), which may occur if the thoracic spine position is not taken into account. In addition, it is likely that many elderly individuals have a pre-stroke adaptive limitation of GH flexion since most daily activities do not require motion at extremes of flexion. Mobilizing the thoracic spine may be useful in individuals with GH pain where thoracic range of movement is limited.

Where *reflex sympathetic dystrophy* is considered to be a major cause of pain, treatment methods include high dose anti-inflammatory agents, steroid therapy, pain medications, sympathetic nerve blocks, heat, compression and exercise to increase range of movement (AHCPR 1995) and task-related exercises to train control of muscles in functional activities. Given the perceived relationship between inactivity and RSD, exercise of the limb in the early stages after stroke is particularly important (Chu *et al.* 1981). Positioning of the limb in different segmental alignments between exercise sessions is critical to ensure soft tissue length changes do not occur, as they rapidly will do if the limb is persistently maintained in one position. The patient will need a great deal of encouragement because of the pain which will tend to discourage active movement. Chu and colleagues (1981) reported that most of the patients they encountered were pain-free within a few days on a regime of steroids, oedema reduction, positioning and exercise, with oedema subsiding in a week.

In conclusion, certain information related to mechanisms of shoulder pain after stroke needs to be collected in order to utilize and test more rational and effective methods of intervention. Such information would include: identifying the factors predisposing most commonly to pain on a particular clinical unit; evaluating the effect of preventative protocols on incidence of pain and/or subluxation; examining the effects of more modern methods of intervention for pain, such as peripheral joint mobilizations, injected analgesic or anti-inflammatory drugs and exercise.

Nevertheless, a great deal is already known about potential factors causing shoulder-related pain:

- **Pre-stroke factors** such as: the degeneration present in the shoulders of some individuals.
- **Post-stroke factors** such as: the effects of immobility, prolonged GH positioning in adduction and internal rotation; disuse resulting from paralysis and severe weakness of soft tissue peri-joint structures (capsule, ligaments and muscles); the compounding effects of stress and trauma to the joint from forced passive movement and excessive traction.

Given that a painful shoulder will lead in many individuals, according to Cailliet (1980), to disuse atrophy, disability, depression, drugs and dependence, intensive effort should be made in both the acute and rehabilitation stages to prevent the cycle of immobility, soft tissue shortening and traumatic injury to joint structures and shoulder pain, using information we already have available. As can be seen from the discussion above, prevention requires anticipation. Most interest is typically generated, however, both in clinical practice and in the literature, in the problem of already existing pain, stiffness and subluxation. It appears that little attempt is made to work systematically to prevent the preventable sequelae of stroke. Given the predisposition of the elderly shoulder to painful musculoskeletal conditions, particular emphasis on prevention should be given to this group of individuals very early after stroke. Methods of positioning and active exercise as a means of preventing disuse adaptation (particularly muscle and capsular contracture) and of increasing active

control of the limb are in little evidence despite the emphasis placed on such procedures in several texts (Carr and Shepherd 1987a,b; Ada and Canning 1990; Ada *et al.* 1994).

If a painful shoulder develops, accurate diagnosis is possible using radiographic and other methods widely available to the non-stroke population, as are treatment methods for adhesive capsulitis, biceps and supraspinatus tendinitis should they occur. The individual following stroke who develops a painful shoulder should have access to the same medical and therapeutic interventions as does the general population.

Finally, it remains to be proved, first, whether or not shoulder pain and subluxation are preventable in many individuals post-stroke, and second, that preventing (or treating) shoulder pain improves outcome following stroke. Answering these questions should be a priority in stroke rehabilitation.

References

Ada, L. and Canning, C. (1990) *Key Issues in Neurological Physiotherapy*, Butterworth-Heinemann, Oxford.

Ada, L., Canning, C.G., Carr, J.H. *et al.* (1994) Task-specific training of reaching and manipulation. In *Insights into the Reach to Grasp Movement* (eds K.M.B. Bennett and U. Castiello), Elsevier, Amsterdam, pp. 239–268.

AHCPR (1995) *Clinical Practice Guideline 16: Post-Stroke Rehabilitation*, US Department of Health and Human Services, Rockville, MD.

Ancliffe, J. (1992) Strapping the shoulder in patients following a cerebrovascular accident (CVA): a pilot study. *Australian Journal of Physiotherapy*, **38**,(1), 37–41.

Anderson, L.T. (1985) Shoulder pain in hemiplegia. *American Journal of Occupational Therapy*, **39**, 11–19.

Andrews, A.W. and Bohannon, R.W. (1989) Decreased shoulder range of motion on paretic side after stroke. *Physical Therapy*, **69**, 768–772.

Arsenault, A.B., Bilodeau, M., Dutil, E. *et al.* (1991) Clinical significance of the V-shaped space in the subluxed shoulder of hemiplegics. *Stroke*, **22**, 867–871.

Baker, L.L. and Parker, K. (1986) Neuromuscular electrical stimulation of the muscles surrounding the shoulder. *Physical Therapy*, **66**, 1930–1937.

Basmajian, J.V. and Bazant, F.J. (1959) Factors preventing downward dislocation of the adducted shoulder joint. *Journal of Bone and Joint Surgery*, **41A**, 1182–1186.

Bechtol, C.O. (1980) Biomechanics of the shoulder. *Clinical Orthopaedics and Related Research*, **146**, 37–41.

Bobath, K. (1972) Letter to the editor. *Physical Therapy,* **52**, 444–445.

Bobath, B. (1990) *Adult Hemiplegia: Evaluation and Treatment, 3rd edn,* Heinemann, London.

Bohannon, R.W. (1988) Relationship between shoulder pain and selected variables in patients with hemiplegia. *Clinical Rehabilitation,* **2**, 111–117.

Bohannon, R.W., Larkin, P.A., Smith, M.B. *et al.* (1986) Shoulder pain in hemiplegia: statistical relationship with five variables. *Archives of Physical Medicine and Rehabilitation,* **67**, 514–516.

Bohannon, R.W. and Smith, M.B. (1987) Assessment of strength deficits in eight paretic upper extremity muscle groups of stroke patients with hemiplegia. *Physical Therapy,* **67**, 522–525.

Boyd, E. and Garland, A. (1986) Shoulder supports with stroke patients: A Canadian survey. *Canadian Journal of Occupational Therapy,* **53**, 61–68.

Boyd, E.A., Goudreau, L., Eng, P. *et al.* (1993) A radiological measure of shoulder subluxation in hemiplegia: its reliability and validity. *Archives of Physical Medicine and Rehabilitation,* **74**, 188–193.

Brandstater, M.E. and Basmajian, J.V. (eds) (1987) *Stroke Rehabilitation,* Williams and Wilkins, Baltimore.

Braun, R.M., West, F., Mooney, V. *et al.* (1971) Surgical treatment of painful shoulder contracture in stroke patient. *Journal of Bone and Joint Surgery,* **53**, 1307–1312.

Brocklehurst J.G., Andrews, K., Richards, B. *et al.* (1978) How much physical therapy for patients with stroke. *British Medical Journal,* **1**, 1307–1310.

Brook, M.M., de Lateur, J., Diana-Rigby, C. *et al.* (1991) Shoulder subluxation in hemiplegia: effects of three different supports. *Archives of Physical Medicine and Rehabilitation,* **72**, 582–586.

Bruckner, F.E. and Nye, C.J.S. (1981) A prospective study of adhesive capsulitis of the shoulder ('frozen shoulder') in a high risk population. *Quarterly Journal of Medicine,* **198**, 191–204.

Bruton, J.D. (1985) Shoulder pain in stroke patients with hemiplegia or hemiparesis following a cerebrovascular accident. *Physiotherapy,* **71**, 1, 2–4.

Cailliet, R. (1980) *The Shoulder in Hemiplegia,* F.A. Davis, Philadelphia.

Cailliet, R. (1991) *Shoulder Pain,* F.A. Davis, Philadelphia.

Carr, J.H. and Shepherd, R.B. (1987a) *A Motor Relearning Programme for Stroke,* 2nd edn, Butterworth Heinemann, Oxford.

Carr, J.H. and Shepherd, R.B. (1987b) In *Movement Science. Foundations for Physical Therapy in Rehabilitation* (ed J.H. Carr and R.B. Shepherd) Aspen, Rockville, MD.

Chaco, J. and Wolf, E. (1971) Subluxation of the glenohumeral joint in hemiplegia. *American Journal of Physical Medicine,* **50**,139–143.

Chu, D.S., Petrillo, C., Davis, S.W. *et al.* (1981) Shoulder–hand syndrome: importance of early diagnosis and treatment. *Journal of the American Geriatrics Society,* **29**, 58–60.

Corrigan, B. and Maitland, G.D. (1994) *Musculoskeletal and Sports Injuries,* Butterworth-Heinemann, Oxford.

Culham, E.G., Noce, R.R. and Bagg, S.D. (1995) Shoulder complex position and glenohumeral subluxation in hemiplegia. *Archives of Physical Medicine and Rehabilitation,* **76**, 857–864.

Davies, P.M. (1985) *Steps to Follow. A Guide to the Treatment of Adult Hemiplegia,* Springer-Verlag, Berlin.

De Palma, A.F. (1983) *Surgery of the Shoulder,* 3rd edn, JB Lippincott, Philadelphia.

Edwards, S. (1996) *Neurological Physiotherapy. A Problem-Solving Approach,* Churchill Livingstone, London.

Faghri, P.D., Rodgers, M.M., Glaser, R.M. *et al.* (1994) The effects of functional electrical stimulation on shoulder subluxation, arm function recovery, and shoulder pain in hemiplegic stroke patients. *Archives of Physical Medicine and Rehabilitation,* **75**, 73–79.

Griffin, J.W. (1986) Hemiplegic shoulder pain. *Physical Therapy,* **66**, 12, 1884–1893.

Griffin, J. and Reddin, G. (1981) Shoulder pain in patients with hemiplega. *Physical Therapy,* **61**, 1041.

Grossen-Sils, J. and Schenkman, M. (1985) Analysis of shoulder pain, range of motion, and subluxation in patients with hemiplegia. *Physical Therapy,* **65**, 182.

Hakuno, A., Sashika, H., Ohkawa, T. *et al.* (1984) Arthrographic findings in hemiplegic shoulders. *Archives of Physical Medicine and Rehabilitation,* **65**, 706–711.

Hall, J., Dudgeon, B. and Guthrie, M. (1995) Validity of clinical measures of shoulder subluxation in adults with poststroke hemiplegia. *American Journal of Occupational Therapy,* **49**, 526–533.

Hawkins, R.J. and Murnaghan, J.P. (1984) The shoulder. In *Adult Orthopaedics* vol. 2 (eds R.L. Cruess and W.R. Rennee), Churchill Livingstone, New York.

Inaba, M.K. and Piorkowski, M. (1972) Ultrasound in treatment of the painful shoulder in patients with hemiplegia. *Physical Therapy,* **52**, 737–741.

Jensen, E.M. (1980) The hemiplegic shoulder. *Scandinavian Journal of Rehabilitation Medicine,* **12** (Suppl.), 113–119.

Joynt, R.L. (1992) The source of shoulder pain in hemiplegia. *Archives of Physical Medicine and Rehabilitation,* **73**, 409–413.

Kaplan, P.E., Meredith, J., Taft, G. *et al.* (1977) Stroke and brachial plexus injury: a difficult problem. *Archives of Physical Medicine and Rehabilitation,* **58**, 415–418.

Kingery, W.S., Date, E.S. and Bocobo, C.R. (1987) The absence of brachial plexus injury in stroke. *American Journal of Physical Medicine and Rehabilitation,* **72**, 127–134.

Kumar, R., Matter, E.J., Mehta, A.J. *et al.* (1990) Shoulder pain in hemiplegia. The role of exercise. *American Journal of Physical Medicine and Rehabilitation,* **69**, 205–208.

Leandri, M., Parodi, C.I., Corrieri, N. *et al.* (1990) Comparison of TENS treatments in hemiplegic shoulder pain. *Scandinavian Journal of Rehabilitation Medicine*, **22**, 69–72.

Melzack, R. (1975) The McGill pain questionaire: major properties and scoring methods. *Pain*, **1**, 277.

Miglietta, O., Lewitan, A. and Rogoff, J.B. (1959) Subluxation of the shoulder in hemiplegic patients. *New York State Journal of Medicine*, **59**, 457–460.

Moodie, N.B., Brisbin, J. and Morgan, A.M.G. (1986) Subluxation of the glenohumeral joint in hemiplegia: evaluation of supportive devices. *Physiotherapy Canada*, **38**, 151–157.

Najenson, T., Yacubovich, E. and Pikielini, S. (1971) Rotator cuff injury in shoulder joints of hemiplegic patients. *Scandinavian Journal of Rehabilitation Medicine*, **3**, 131.

Peat, M. (1986) Functional anatomy of the shoulder complex. *Physical Therapy*, **66**, (12), 1855–1865.

Poulin de Courval, L., Barsauskas, A., Berenbaum, B. *et al.* (1990) Painful shoulder in the hemiplegic and unilateral neglect. *Archives of Physical Medicine and Rehabilitation*, **71**, 673–676.

Prevost, R., Arsenault, A.B., Dutil, E. *et al.* (1987) Shoulder subluxation in hemiplegia: a radiologic correlational study. *Archives of Physical Medicine and Rehabilitation*, **68**, 782–785.

Reading, A.E. and Newton, J.R. (1978) A card sort method of pain assessment. *Journal of Psychosomatic Research*, **22**, 503.

Rizk, T.E., Christopher, R.P., Pinals, R.S. *et al.* (1984) Arthrographic studies in painful hemiplegic shoulders. *Archives of Physical Medicine and Rehabilitation*, **65**, 254–256.

Roy, C.W. (1988) Shoulder pain in hemiplegia: a literature review. *Clinical Rehabilitation*, **2**, 35–44.

Roy, C.W., Sands, M.R. and Hill, L.D. (1994) Shoulder pain in acutely admitted hemiplegics. *Clinical Rehabilitation*, **8**, 334–340.

Roy, C.W., Sands, M.R., Hill, L.D. *et al.* (1995) The effect of shoulder pain on outcome of acute hemiplegia. *Clinical Rehabilitation*, **9**, 21–27.

Ryerson, S.D. (1995) Hemiplegia. In *Neurological Rehabilitation* (ed. D.A. Umphred), 3rd edn, Mosby, St Louis, pp. 681–721.

Ryerson, S. and Levit, K. (1991) The shoulder in hemiplegia. In *Physical Therapy of the Shoulder* (ed R. Donatelli), Churchill Livingstone, New York, pp. 117–145.

Saario, L. (1963) The range of motion of the shoulder joint at various ages. *Acta Orthopaedica Scandinavia*, **33**, 366.

Savage, R. and Robertson, L. (1982) The relationship between adult hemiplegic shoulder pain and depression. *Physiotherapy Canada*, **34**, (2), 86–90.

Shepherd, R.B. and Carr, J.H. (1998) The shoulder following stroke: preserving musculoskeletal integrity. *Topics in Stroke Rehabilitation*, **4**, 35–53.

Smith, R.G., Cruikshank, J.G., Dunbar, S. *et al.* (1982) Malalignment of the shoulder following stroke. *British Medical Journal*, **284**, 1224.

Taub, E., Miller, N.E., Novak, T.A. *et al.* (1993) A technique for improving chronic motor deficit after stroke. *Archives of Physical Medicine and Rehabilitation*, **74**, 347–354.

Tepperman, P.S., Greyson, N.D., Hilbert, L. *et al.* (1984) Reflex sympathetic dystrophy. *Archives of Physical Medicine and Rehabilitation*, **65**, 442–447.

Van Langenberghe, H.V.K. and Hogan, B.M. (1988) Degree of pain and grade of subluxation in the painful hemiplegic shoulder. *Scandinavian Journal of Rehabilitation Medicine*, **20**, 161–166.

van Ouwenaller, C., Laplace, P.M., and Chantraine, A. (1986) Painful shoulder in hemiplegia. *Archives of Physical Medicine and Rehabilitation*, **67**, 23–26.

Wanklyn, P., Forster, A. and Young, J. (1996) Hemiplegic shoulder pain (HSP): natural history and investigation of associated features. *Disability and Rehabilitation*, **18**, 497–501.

Williams, J.M. (1982) Use of electromyographic feedback for pain reduction in the spastic hemiplegic shoulder: a pilot study. *Physiotherapy Canada*, **34**, 327.

Williams, R., Taffs, L. and Minuk, T. (1988) Evaluation of two support methods for the subluxated shoulder of hemiplegic patients. *Physical Therapy*, **68**, (8), 1209–1214.

Zorowitz, R.D., Idank, D., Ikai, T. *et al.* (1995) Shoulder subluxation after stroke: a comparison of four supports. *Archives of Physical Medicine and Rehabilitation*, **76**, 763–771.

Further reading

Crawford, H.J. and Jull, G.A. (1993) The influence of thoracic posture and movement on range of arm elevation. *Physiotherapy Theory and Practice*, **9**, 143–148.

Dvir, Z. and Berme, N. (1978) The shoulder complex in elevation of the arm: a mechanism approach. *Journal of Biomechanics*, **11**, 219–225.

Kronberg, M., Nemeth, G. and Brostrom, L-A. (1990) Muscle activity and coordination in the normal shoulder. *Clinical Orthopaedics and Related Research*, **257**, 76–85.

Roy, C.W. (1988) Shoulder pain hemiplegia: a literature review. *Clinical Rehabilitation*, **2**, 35–44.

12

Traumatic brain injury

Introduction

Trauma is the commonest cause of death under the age of 35 years in most developed countries and head injury is the commonest cause of accidental death. Head injury or traumatic brain injury (TBI) are terms used to describe a physical injury to the brain, by an external mechanical force or projectile, that results in loss of consciousness, post-traumatic amnesia and neurological deficits. Precise measures of prevalence and mortality within various populations are difficult to assess. TBI is most commonly the result of road accidents, industrial and sporting accidents, attempted suicides and interpersonal violence. The sequelae can have a devastating effect on the individual's lifestyle and future aspirations, creating general health and social problems, causing disruption for family members and marital strain, affecting role-relationships and fostering economic hardship (McKinlay *et al.*, 1981).

The beginning of the systematic study of the effects of TBI can be traced to World War II. In this early work, much was learned about the deficits following penetrating injuries to the brain in servicemen with gunshot wounds. The majority of TBI individuals seen in hospitals these days are classified as closed TBI, i.e., the skull is not actually penetrated.

The type of trauma sustained in road accidents (e.g., blunt impact or acceleration–deceleration) usually results in diffuse brain damage with a variety of physical, cognitive and behavioural problems. As the younger age groups tend to be over-represented and because life expectancy is often near normal (Jennett and Teasdale 1981), the role of rehabilitation is critical in order to maximize quality of life by reducing disability and handicap.

Following a period of unconsciousness, the majority of individuals are left with a combination of physical and cognitive impairments which vary as a consequence of the severity of the lesion, the nature of brain damage and medical complications. Changes in behaviour, mood and personality after TBI have been documented and are considered by many clinicians to be among the most difficult problems to manage effectively. Behaviour problems range from minor irritability and passivity to disinhibited and psychotic behaviour. Cognitive, behavioural and personality changes are far more frequently associated with long-term functional disability and family stress than are physical handicaps (McKinlay *et al.* 1981; Brooks *et al.* 1986).

Epidemiology

It has been suggested that TBI is one of the five most prevalent neurological conditions affecting the central nervous system (CNS), together with cerebrovascular disease, epilepsy, Parkinson's disease and migraine (Wade and Langton Hewer 1987). Prevalence estimates and incidence reports vary depending on such factors as whether or not all grades of severity and all who are hospitalized are included. Incidence also varies depending on location, since urban areas account for a higher incidence than country areas (Frankowski 1985). Some countries, e.g. the UK, Japan and Sweden, have half as many fatal TBIs as the USA (Jennett, 1989, 1990). The incidence of TBI in Australia is approximately 180–200 per 100,000 per year, per head of population. Five to ten per cent of these are classified as severe.

In the UK, it has been estimated that each year a million patients are admitted to Accident and Emergency (A&E) departments. Of these, 5000 die and 1500 are left with permanent brain damage each year (Jennett 1986). However, although the annual attendance rate at A&E departments of individuals with TBI is high, less than a quarter of these tend to be admitted to hospital.

In all studies, males outnumber females by at least 2:1, and the injuries in which males are involved tend to be more severe. Several risk factors have been suggested as predisposing individuals to the likelihood of sustaining a TBI. The most common factor cited is alcohol intake before the injury (Levin *et al.* 1982) and about half of all injuries are transport related. Compulsory use of helmets for both motor bike riders and cyclists has helped to reduce the severity of injuries that occur (Sosin *et al.* 1990; Wasserman and Buccini 1990).

The pattern and severity of injury as well as the resulting outcome are extremely variable and are dependent in part on the criteria used for classification. The overall mortality from TBI amongst those seen in A&E is relatively small since most of these individuals have minor TBI. Mortality for severe TBI patients in coma from the time of impact, however, is high. Approximately 33–50% of these individuals die (Jennett and Teasdale 1981; Hans *et al.* 1989) and 15–20% survive with persistent and severe disability (Murray *et al.* 1993). Of those who survive, outcome is typically defined by global categories listed on the Glasgow Outcome Scale (GOS) as: death; persistent vegetative state; severe disability; moderate disability; good recovery (Jennett and Teasdale 1981). Even those who

achieve a good recovery on the GOS may have significant psychological impairment that interferes with a return to premorbid levels of function (Whyte and Rosenthal 1993). The economic and social impact is enormous. Estimates of return to work vary considerably depending on the selection criteria for the vocation being studied (Ben-Yishay *et al.* 1987).

Those patients who suffer a loss of consciousness of less than 6 hours and post-traumatic amnesia (PTA) of less than 24 hours, encompass the vast majority of TBI individuals. Only a small percentage of these individuals are likely to have persistent problems. In injuries commonly referred to as mild, the individual may not suffer any loss of consciousness, although there may be a period of brief altered consciousness, and the individual returns to normal activities after several days without any problems. In other 'mild' injuries, a post-concussional syndrome consisting of headaches, vertigo, fatiguability, dizziness, or impairment of memory may persist for months or even years (e.g., Gronwall and Wrightson 1975; Rimel *et al.* 1981). Impairment of information processing, attention and reaction time may continue for up to 3 months and can be cumulative in individuals with repeated minor head injury (MacFlynn *et al.* 1984). Both animal studies (Povlishock *et al.* 1983) and magnetic resonance imaging scans of humans (Levin *et al.* 1987) have shown that axonal injury can occur even with relatively minor injury.

Pathophysiology

TBI may occur as a result of a direct blow to the head, or the head may be injured indirectly from an impact to other parts of the body. Direct injury may be blunt or penetrating. Blunt or acceleration–deceleration injuries commonly result in multiple injuries of the body as well as widespread brain damage. The impact to the head may cause scalp injuries, deformation of the skull with or without fractures, or depressed fractures which may lacerate and perforate the dura mater and brain.

Mechanism of brain damage

The mechanisms that produce brain damage in trauma are varied and complex and include both intracranial and extracranial factors (Table 12.1). Intracranial mechanisms of brain damage are typically divided into *primary damage*, in which

Table 12.1 Classification of mechanisms of brain damage following trauma. Reprinted from Mendelow, A.D. (1993a) by permission

Extracranial mechanisms
  Hypoxia
  Hypotension
Intracranial mechanisms
  Primary brain damage
    diffuse axonal injury
    lacerations
    contusions
  Secondary brain damage
    haemorrhage
      extradural
      intradural
    brain swelling
      venous congestion
      oedema: vasogenic
        cytotoxic
        interstitial
    infection
      meningitis
      abscess

contusions or axonal disruption. Acceleration–deceleration and rotational forces that commonly result from motor vehicle accidents produce diffuse axonal injury. Such lesions may be microscopic or they may combine into focal macroscopic lesions with a predilection for the midbrain, pons, corpus callosum and white matter of the cerebral hemispheres (Blumbergs *et al.* 1989). Diffuse axonal injury is primarily responsible for the initial loss of consciousness. Although the actual mechanism of axonal injury is not clear, it includes microscopic haemorrhage in white matter (Mendelow and Teasdale 1983).

Cerebral contusion or cortical bruising occurs principally at the crests of the gyri and expands to variable depths depending on the severity of the injury. Contusions occur primarily on the undersurface of the frontal lobes and at the temporal tips, regardless of the site of impact (Mendelow and Teasdale 1983). In contrast to diffuse axonal damage, contusions may result from relatively low-velocity impact such as in blows to the head and falls. They may also cause multiple small intracerebral haemorrhages and occasionally more extensive bleeding. Cerebral contusions are not directly responsible for loss of consciousness but are risk factors for development of seizures, and may produce focal cognitive and sensorimotor deficits (Mendelow and Teasdale 1983).

Another form of primary brain damage is laceration following penetration of the brain by a projectile or skull fragment. Associated with these, there is often a surrounding zone of damage caused by release of kinetic energy (Mendelow 1993a).

the effects are largely immediate, and delayed or *secondary damage* that occurs some time after the injury. Both affect the eventual morbidity and mortality of the individual. In general, primary brain damage produces an immediate effect on level of consciousness while secondary brain damage produces a late deterioration in the level of consciousness and development of focal signs. Hypoxic and ischaemic brain damage can be minimized by effective and early resuscitation. It is chiefly in the treatment of secondary brain damage, which is potentially preventable or treatable, that medical and surgical intervention has advanced over the past decade or so.

The injuries associated with extracranial mechanisms are many and may include fractures to the extremities, spine (with or without spinal cord damage) and pelvis, damage to the rib cage and underlying organs, rupture of abdominal viscera, and facial injuries. These insults and the associated haemorrhage are often responsible for ischaemic brain damage largely as a result of hypoxia and hypotension.

Primary brain damage

In its mildest form primary brain damage manifests as concussion, which is a state of unconsciousness due to a form of diffuse axonal injury of a minor nature (Oppenheimer 1968). On impact, some brain tissue is irreparably damaged by grey matter

Secondary brain damage

The primary injury may set in motion a series of processes that result in more severe and widespread brain damage. The three main causes of secondary brain damage are haemorrhage, brain swelling and infection. Other causes of secondary brain damage include systemic factors such as blood loss and hypotension, pulmonary injury and cardiac or respiratory arrest.

Intracranial *haemorrhage* may occur as a result of laceration. It may develop within the brain itself or on its surface. Haemorrhages are referred to as subarachnoid, subdural, extradural or intracerbral, according to their location. Secondary haemorrhage may occur due to displacement of the brain which may result from raised intracranial pressure due to oedema, or from a space-occupying lesion such as a haematoma.

Venous congestion, an increase in cerebral blood volume, may cause *brain swelling*, but later *brain oedema* (swelling of brain cells), which takes longer to develop, may be more common. Brain oedema may depress metabolic activity of intact neurons and cause ischaemia in intact neural structures and thus functional impairment. If these processes remain unresolved, they may contribute to further damage of relatively spared neural structures.

Infection of the brain, which may cause further damage, may occur from open fractures, cerebrospinal fluid rhinorrhoea or iatrogenically from ICP monitoring (Mendelow and Teasdale, 1983).

Any factor that leads to increased intracranial pressure (ICP) can decrease cerebral perfusion pressure and cause ischaemic damage. For example, expanding haematomas or acute hydrocephalus lead to dramatic pressure changes (Mendelow and Teasdale 1983). Vasogenic oedema through disruption of the blood-brain barrier can occur in tissue near areas of contusion (Tornheim *et al.* 1984). Increase in cerebral blood volume and, therefore, ICP, may be caused by hypoxia, hypercapnia or venous obstruction. Once increased, ICP compromises perfusion, and further cytotoxic oedema creates a self-perpetuating cycle (Mendelow and Teasdale 1983). Intractable increases in ICP can lead to diffuse ischaemic injury, focal vascular occlusion and herniation of brain tissue.

Measures of severity and outcome

Initial coma is universal in individuals with severe brain injury and up to a half of patients in coma for longer than 6 hours die without ever regaining consciousness. About 10% remain unresponsive one month after injury with the remainder emerging from coma and gradually improving in function (Braakman *et al.* 1988). Depth and duration of coma and length of PTA are considered to be indices of severity of TBI and predictors of outcome, with longer periods of coma and PTA typically being associated with poorer outcomes.

The Glasgow Coma Scale (GCS) (Teasdale and Jennett 1974) is the most widely used measure of the severity of the injury and has provided clinicians with a relatively precise definition of coma (Chapter 3). The GCS was designed to provide a system of monitoring the comatose patient that is consistent when used by different observers, and the results of which are easily accessible to different members of the team. It consists of three features which are independently

observed: eye opening; motor response and verbal monitoring. Change in the degree of impairment of consciousness is typically the best indicator of both improvement in overall function of the brain and development of intracranial complications, some of which require immediate intervention to prevent secondary brain damage.

A comatose state is operationally defined as a GCS of 8 or less for a period of 6 hours or longer (Teasdale and Jennett 1974). Coma is defined as: not opening the eyes; not obeying commands; and not uttering understandable words. Individuals who remain unresponsive for more than a few weeks can evolve into a vegetative state which is characterized by the presence of spontaneous sleep-wake cycles but absence of cortical activity judged behaviourly (Jennett and Plum, 1972). The patient appears to be 'awake but not aware'.

The GCS taken in the first few days following injury is highly predictive of outcome at 6 months as measured by the Glasgow Outcome Scale (GOS) (Jennett and Teasdale 1981) with a score of less than 8 usually predictive of poor outcome. The addition to the scale of the assessment of several brain stem reflexes (Born *et al.* 1985) and multimodal evoked potentials (Rappaport 1986) have both been reported to improve the prognostic value of the GCS.

Prediction of severity by means of the GCS depends on the evaluation of both depth and duration of altered consciousness. Coma duration alone is a poor predictor of outcome for many patients with brief periods of coma (Gronwall 1989) but is said to be a good predictor for more serious injuries. The commonly accepted criteria for classifying severity of trauma (Bond 1986) are:

Mild: GCS 13–15, ≤20 minutes coma duration
Moderate: GCS 9–12, no longer than 6 hours coma duration
Severe: GCS ≤8, >6 hours coma duration

The distinction between mild, moderate and severe TBI, however, is often arbitrary and many descriptive outcome studies combine subjects with these different levels of severity.

Duration of PTA, which has typically been used to measure severity of injury (Bond 1990), correlates well with GCS rating. PTA was first used by Russell (1932) as an indication of the severity of a head injury in terms of duration of loss of full consciousness. PTA is now characterized by the inability to lay down memories reliably from one day to the next as assessed subjectively. The assessment of PTA is likely to be unreliable in A&E when other considerations such as immediate medical attention are uppermost. PTA can also be difficult to determine when confounded by alcohol abuse or when it is brief (McMillan 1990). In spite of these drawbacks, duration of PTA is highly correlated with ultimate outcome, with PTA greater than 14 days associated with a greater likelihood of persisting deficits (Jennett and Teasdale 1981).

Shores and colleagues (1986) developed and tested a simple, easy to administer clinical scale, the Westmead PTA Scale (Chapter 3), for measuring PTA. The scale takes approximately 3 minutes to administer and has been successfully administered with only a minimum of training. A follow-up study (Shores 1989) suggests that duration of PTA, as measured on the Westmead scale, can be used as an objective measure for predicting neuropsychological (verbal learning, non-verbal problem-solving) outcome of blunt head injury. Interestingly, when patients recovered from PTA, as operationally defined by the scale, marked changes in behaviour and increased participation in therapy were noted.

The GOS (Chapter 3), consisting of five categories ranging from good recovery to death (Jennett and Bond 1975), has been shown to have a high degree of interrater reliability in large international multicentre studies (Jennett and Teasdale 1981). In spite of its reported limitations, (for example, the global categories do not provide a real indication of functional abilities), the GOS continues to be used widely to describe outcome. In attempts to address the perceived shortcomings, several other instruments have been developed, such as the Disability Rating Scale (Rappaport *et al.* 1982).

In general, it is reported that the majority of recovery takes place within the first 6 months following injury. Many factors may affect the recovery process including pre-injury medical and psychological factors, age, gender and demographic variables such as marital status and socioeconomic status (MacNiven 1994). In a study of 102 individuals admitted to hospital following TBI, 56% had blood alcohol levels of ≥ 0.10 (Sparedo and Gill 1989). The authors reported that these individuals were hospitalized for longer, remained agitated for longer and had a lower cognitive status on discharge than the remaining subjects. Dresser and colleagues (1973) and others have reported that the degree of emotional stability and pre-injury mental endowment have a considerable effect on future employment probability. Delayed medical complications may include epilepsy, meningitis, chronic subdural haematoma and post-traumatic hydrocephalus (Mendelow 1993a).

Management of acute traumatic brain injury

TBI presents a considerable problem of management. Preservation of life and prevention of secondary brain damage are the first priorities in the emergency treatment of the brain-injured and multi-injured individual, involving the expertise of a wide range of health professionals. Skilled and forward-looking management in the immediate stage can prevent many subsequent disabilities, a fact which must not be overlooked in the urgent concern to save life (Hitchcock 1971). Increased availability of computerized tomography scans and magnetic resonance imaging have meant that haematoma and other acute complications associated with TBI can be detected before they cause neurological deterioration.

There is no typical clinical picture following TBI. Nevertheless, the first priorities on admission to hospital are resuscitation, assessment of the airways and prevention of inhalation. TBI patients are preferably nursed in a neurosurgical or specialized brain-injury intensive care unit and there is some evidence to suggest that the provision of these facilities improves outcome (Mendelow 1993a) Initial management may include neurosurgical intervention designed to evacuate haematoma, reduce brain oedema and treat hydrocephalus. Monitoring of vital signs and coma are routinely performed and in most instances intracranial pressure is also monitored. Observation of progression of the clinical picture from the moment of injury is critical to management. Any patient whose level of consciousness deteriorates should be considered to have a haematoma (Mendelow 1993a) and requires immediate investigation.

Respiratory function

The management of the brain-injured individual varies depending on the severity of the problems. The management of respiratory function of the comatose brain-injured patient is complex. It requires an understanding of the relationship between pulmonary, cardiovascular and neurological function, and of the mechanical and physiological effects of respiratory techniques, since inappropriate intervention can exacerbate the problems of hypoxia and hypercapnia. Establishment of an adequate airway is paramount since it ensures adequate oxygenation, protection of the airway from inhalation (e.g., of vomitus) and reduction in ICP.

Control of breathing is normally a complex interaction of a number of mechanisms. Brain tissue requires adequate oxygenation in order to function and the respiratory system relies on drive from the brain to control ventilation. In the brain-injured patient, lung function may be compromised by damage to the respiratory centres of the brain, or associated injuries such as rib fractures, as well as pre-existing lung disease. Similarly, brain function may be compromised by damage to tissue or blood vessels, altered cerebral blood flow, oedema, changes in arterial blood pressure, or respiratory failure (Ellis 1990).

The space inside the cranium is occupied by the brain and its coverings, blood vessels, together with blood and cerebrospinal fluid. The sum of these three volumes is normally constant, so that an increase in any one occurs at the expense of the others. Since the skull is rigid the space available is finite and an increase in intracranial mass associated with haemotoma or oedema, for example, causes an increase in ICP. As ICP rises, cerebral blood flow falls. The relationship between ICP and cerebral blood flow can be described by the following equation:

cerebral perfusion pressure = mean arterial blood pressure – intracranial pressure (e.g., Rowland *et al.* 1991).

If cerebral perfusion pressure reaches a critical low, ischaemia results.

As ICP rises, there is increasing depression of consciousness, increase in systemic arterial blood pressure, bradycardia, and irregular breathing. With a further increase in ICP, there is deep coma, a progressive fall in systemic arterial blood pressure, the pupils are fixed and dilated and at this stage a fall in cerebral perfusion pressure which deprives the brain of oxygen (Plum and Posner 1980). This in turn increases cerebral oedema and the cycle continues (Mendelow 1993b). Progressive expansion of the mass within the cranium may cause brain shift from where pressure is rising to a compartment where it is lower. This may eventually lead to herniation of brain tissue because of the limited confines of the skull. For example, a mass above the tentorium may push the brain stem and part of the cerebral hemisphere down through the tentorial hiatus, causing compression, ischaemia and oedema of the midbrain and resulting in ischaemia and further oedema of the hemispheres.

Patients who have adequate arterial blood gases, a GCS score of greater than 8, no respiratory dysfunction or signs of deterioration, are usually not ventilated but their inspired oxygen concentration is increased since the oxygen requirements of the damaged brain are greater than those of the undamaged brain (Frost 1985).

It is generally agreed that mechanical ventilation is beneficial in the acute phase following TBI in patients whose PaO_2 is less than 60 mmHg and $PaCO_2$ is greater than 45 mmHg (e.g., Frost 1985,1987; Jennett 1985). With signs of deterioration or a GCS score of less than 8, patients may also be paralysed and sedated. Ventilation and the associated paralysis and sedation decrease cerebral blood volume and prevent potentially noxious stimuli and inadequate respiration from causing further brain damage. Paralysis and sedation are usually discontinued after 3 days, and, when patients are able to maintain adequate blood gases, they are extubated. If prolonged mechanical ventilation is required, a tracheostomy may be necessary.

The major aims of physiotherapy intervention as part of the team involved in prevention of secondary brain damage are to:

● improve respiratory function and
● prevent respiratory failure and secondary brain damage

by ensuring adequate ventilation and clearing of excessive secretions. The major respiratory problems amenable to intervention are hypoventilation, impaired mucociliary clearance, hyperventilation and ventilation/perfusion mismatch (Ada *et al.* 1990). The reader is referred to a discussion on the effects of specific techniques on pulmonary, cardiovascular and neurological status (Ellis and Rader 1990) and examples of clinical reasoning exemplified in several case studies (Ada *et al.* 1990).

General nursing/medical care includes maintenance of fluid and electrolyte balance and nutrition, eye and skin care, regular turning, monitoring of vital signs, ICP and level of consciousness (GCS). Impaired consciousness and coma may lead to complications and eventually to preventable disability if steps are not taken to prevent them. For example, the eyes may need to be taped closed and lubricated periodically to prevent corneal damage from abrasion or dryness.

Of primary importance in the management of TBI individuals is the rapid recognition of deterioration. Monitoring of ICP is thought to affect outcome since it enables early recognition of intracranial hypertension (e.g., Frost 1987) and prevention of secondary brain damage (Shapiro 1975; Frost 1985). It is critical that ICP is monitored during any physiotherapy intervention and, should it begin to rise, intervention should be modified accordingly. Postural drainage typically needs to be modified since the head-dependent position is contraindicated where there is a risk of increasing ICP.

The other major goal of physiotherapy during the acute phase when the patient is comatose and therefore immobilized, is the prevention of muscle and soft tissue contracture in order to maintain musculoskeletal integrity.

Musculoskeletal integrity

Impaired motor control following from the brain lesion, associated with paralysis, muscle weakness, spasticity, ataxia or a combination of these, along with coma, effectively immobilize the individual following TBI, who is then vulnerable to the musculoskeletal and cardiovascular adaptations associated with bed rest, reduced physical activity and disuse. Soft tissue changes and reduced cardiovascular fitness are likely to impede rehabilitation by interfering with active and intense training designed to improve motor performance.

Immobilization of skeletal muscle is known to induce both muscle atrophy and impairment of contraction. Muscle tissue responds selectively and differentially to the demands placed on it, altering its structure (length, volume, cross-sectional area) in response to changes in the operating conditions (Tabary *et al.* 1976,1981). Muscle force production and levels of physical activity have an important relationship with other components of the musculoskeletal system such as tendons, ligaments and bones. Deprivation of mechanical stresses normally imposed on the skeleton by the musculature can result in demineralization of the skeleton (McLellan 1993). Furthermore, loading of bones and joints is important in order to preserve bone mass and density and to maintain healthy articular cartilage (Akeson *et al.* 1980).

Soft tissue contractures are reported to be common following TBI (e.g., Yarkony *et al.* 1987).

Muscles at particular risk of shortening due to the effects of position (and immobilization) include hip and knee flexors, ankle plantarflexors and invertors, shoulder adductors and internal rotators, elbow flexors, forearm pronators, wrist and finger flexors, thumb flexors and adductors or any other muscle held persistently at a short length. Animal studies have shown that when muscle is subjected to imposed and maintained change in length, it undergoes anatomical, biochemical and physiological changes that are neither obvious nor readily considered (Gossman *et al.* 1982). These length-associated changes can be induced by many factors including immobilization, muscle imbalance, postural malalignment or, as is typical, a combination of these. Furthermore, these changes start to occur within a few hours of immobilization and can have a profound effect on motor performance.

A typical animal model used in studying the effect of imposed changes of length on muscle involves immobilizing a joint (for review see Goldspink and Williams 1990). When immobilized in a shortened position, muscle loses sarcomeres while muscle immobilized in a lengthened position adds sarcomeres. Loss of sarcomeres results in the remaining sarcomeres being pulled out to a length which affects the ability of the muscle to generate tension, maximum tension being developed at the immobilized length (Tabary *et al.* 1972; Williams and Goldspink 1973; Williams 1990). Connective tissue in muscle immobilized in a shortened position also loses its extensibility, with the result that there is increased resistance to passive stretch, i.e., muscles becomes shorter and stiffer. In functional terms, an increase in stiffness of muscle has an adverse effect on motor function since it will take an increased amount of force to lengthen the muscle actively during movement. It is thought that connective tissue remodelling is associated with lack of movement, both in terms of lack of stretch applied and reduced muscle activity, whereas the stimulus for muscle fibre adaptation results from the imposed length. Range of joint motion is reduced, therefore, both by the shortening of muscle fibres and by loss of muscle compliance (increased stiffness). In addition to impaired muscle compliance, ligament, joint capsule and tendon also lose extensibility following immobilization (Akeson *et al.* 1980).

Electrically induced constant contraction of the muscle when it is held at a shortened length appears to exaggerate the rate and quantity of sarcomere loss (Tabary *et al.* 1981). Spasticity and dystonic posturing following severe TBI may, therefore, lead to more rapid development of contracture.

Muscle weakness and atrophy are well known adaptations associated with disuse. Interestingly the effect of disuse in non-trained healthy subjects has been found to be most obvious in highly active antigravity muscles, such as triceps surae (White *et al.* 1984), particularly the slow-twitch soleus and quadriceps. For example, atrophy of quadriceps has been detected as early as 3 days after immobilization (Lindboe and Platou 1984). The decrease in muscle strength, found when a muscle is immobilized in the shortened position, appears to be greater than that attributable to decrease in size alone.

The major aim in preserving musculoskeletal integrity in the comatose and paralysed individual is to prevent or minimize adaptive changes in soft tissue, in particular to prevent muscle shortening and increased stiffness by:

- Maintaining at-risk muscles and soft tissues in a lengthened position for periods of the day.
- Loading bone and cartilage.
- Moving limbs to aid maintenance of flexibility of joints, soft tissues and muscles.

The comatose patient is *positioned* in side lying or semi-prone. A pillow placed between the slightly flexed legs prevents them from adducting. The upper limb may be positioned on a pillow with the shoulder girdle protracted and the elbow extended. Inflatable plastic blow-up splints may be useful in maintaining position. The supine position should be avoided if possible where this position stimulates dystonic posturing or reflex hyperactivity.

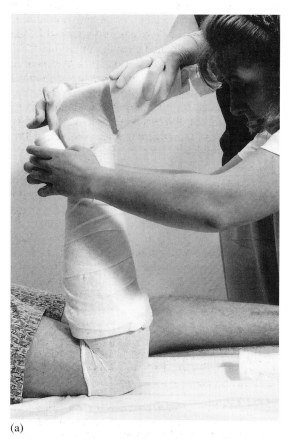

(a)

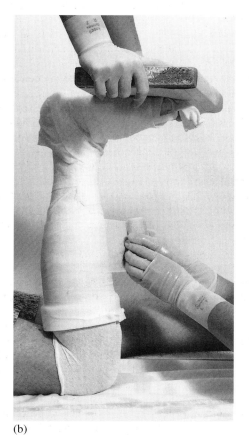

(b)

Fig. 12.1 Application of cast. (*a*) Application of stockinette and padding over bony prominences prior to casting. (*b*) Soleus muscle is stretched into maximum obtainable dorsiflexion using a board placed on the plantar surface of the foot while the cast is applied. Note that with the knee in flexion gastrocnemius muscle is not lengthened over both joints. (From Moseley, A. (1997) The effect of casting combined with stretching on passive ankle dorsiflexion in adults with traumatic head injuries. *Physical Therapy*, **77**, 240–259, by permission)

The terms decerebrate and decorticate are sometimes used to describe the posturing of human patients with brain lesions. Decerebrate and decorticate posturing have been demonstrated experimentally in animals. Following ablation procedures at a certain level of ablation, the animal demonstrates a decerebrate posture in which all four limbs are held in extension. At a higher level of ablation, the animal demonstrates a decorticate posture in which the forelimbs show an increase in flexion and lower limbs an increase in extension.

Although recommended in most rehabilitation texts, it is unclear whether or not *passive range of motion (PROM) exercises* have any effect on preventing development of contracture and how often or how many repetitions would be required. From results of animal experiments, it is doubtful whether PROM exercises have any effect on preventing contracture development in the immobile TBI individual unless muscles at risk of shortening are stretched for at least 30 minutes every day (Williams 1990). PROM exercises may also have deleterious effects on soft tissue. A possible relationship between trauma produced by passive movements and periarticular heterotopic ossification was reported many years ago (Silver 1969). Passive ranging performed too vigorously or in too large a range can cause micro tears in muscle. Such tears cause bleeding into the muscle which leads to ossification, or myositis ossificans, a form of heterotopic ossification, and further loss of mobility. Early signs of myositis include decreased range of movement, increased pain and swelling. The most common sites are around the elbow, shoulder and hip (Horn and Garland 1993).

Since spasticity is velocity-dependent (see Chapter 8), PROM exercises performed too quickly may cause an increase in hyperreflexia. Conversely, in the presence of muscle weakness and paralysis, PROM exercises performed at the end of range may overstretch and damage periarticular connective tissue. This is especially likely in joints that rely on the braking activity of muscles for protection at end of range, such as the glenohumeral joint (Ada *et al.* 1990).

If passive exercises are the only way of moving joints in the comatose patient, they should probably be performed slowly, with care taken at the end of range not to cause abnormal stress. In this case, passive movements of the limbs also provide an opportunity to make some contact with the individual, the therapist (or relative) describing the movements being performed.

The use of *serial casting* has been found to be effective in both preventing (Sullivan *et al.* 1988) and correcting calf muscle contracture (Booth *et al.* 1983; Moseley 1997). Applying casts with muscle in a lengthened or neutral position stretches the connective tissue elements and may provide a stimulus for the muscle to add sarcomeres to the muscle fibre as reported in animal studies (Tabary *et al.* 1972). Sullivan and colleagues (1988) comment that casting has been more successful when patients at risk of developing calf muscle contracture are immediately placed in casts rather than waiting for contracture to occur. Other joints may also require serial casting either to prevent or correct muscle contracture.

The critical features in applying casts are described by Sullivan and colleagues (1988) and Ada and colleagues (1990). Casts are applied with minimum padding in order to prevent movement and ensure a sustained stretch (Fig. 12.1*a*). When casting a two-joint muscle, a lengthened position is more easily achieved if the cast is applied while the muscle is not lengthened over the other joint (Fig 12.1*b*). Monitoring of circulation is initiated as soon as casts are applied and they need to be changed regularly to examine the condition of the skin. Another reason for changing casts regularly is to measure joint range to ensure that muscle shortening is in fact being prevented/corrected (Fig. 12.2). The therapist applying the cast needs to be technically

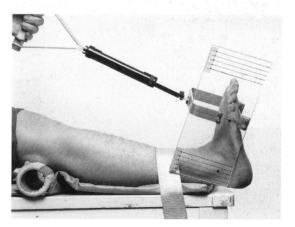

Fig. 12.2 A torque-controlled measurement procedure. A known torque is applied to produce passive ankle dorsiflexion in a standardized testing position. Ankle angle is measured using skin surface markers and photography. (From Moseley, A. (1997) The effect of casting combined with stretching on passive ankle dorsiflexion in adults with traumatic head injuries. *Physical Therapy*, **77**, 240–259, by permission)

skilled in order to prevent complications. Muscle relaxants and sedating drugs may be necessary to achieve a lengthened position in the awake individual. These drugs, however, tend to depress brain function and should be avoided if possible.

As soon as vital signs are stable, in particular blood pressure and ICP, *periods of sitting* (Fig. 12.3) and *standing*, if necessary with external constraints, are instituted. The standing position loads bones, and applies stretch to soft tissue predisposed to developing contracture, e.g., lower limb flexors. Patients can be placed in the upright standing position on a *tilt table* (Fig. 12.4). This procedure does not produce dynamically distributed compression forces through the bones as would occur in the natural process of standing up. However, if patients need to be stood up slowly to control blood pressure changes, a tilt table is essential. Furthermore, using a tilt table may be the

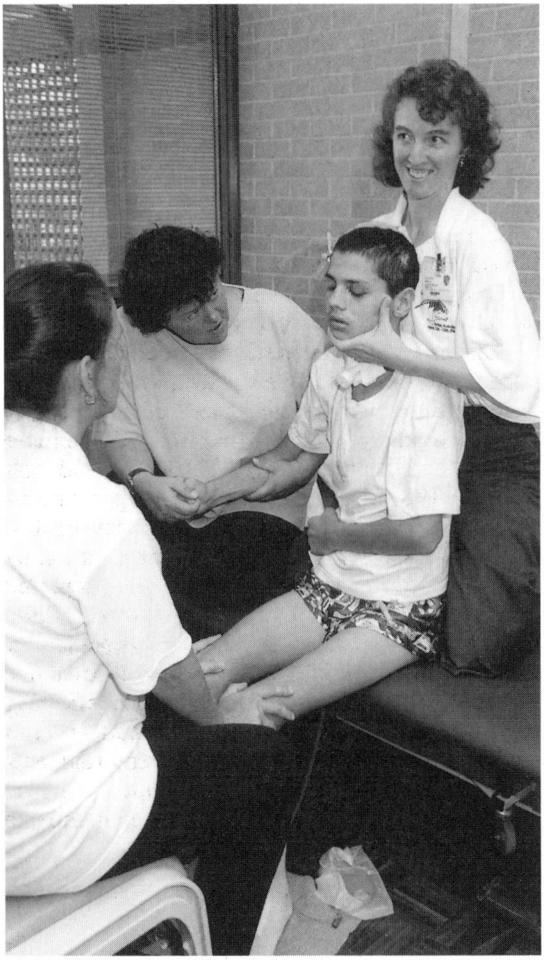

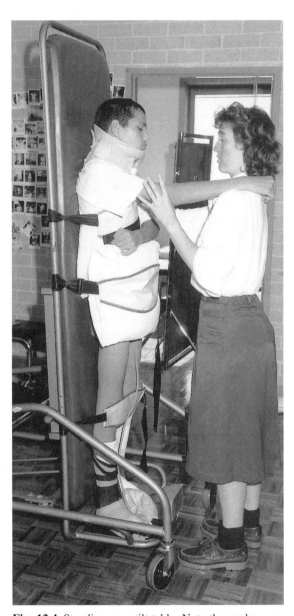

Fig. 12.4 Standing on a tilt table. Note the wedge under the L foot. A high table placed in front of a tilt table enables participation in cognitive, reaching and manipulative activities while adjusting to the vertical position

Fig. 12.3 This young man requires external constraint to sit with the head and trunk erect and feet stabilized on the floor. A mirror enables the training therapist to get some feedback about sitting alignment and the boy's engagement with his environment. His mother is encouraging him and another therapist holds his feet on the floor

only way to get a person into standing and to stay there for a sufficiently long period to stretch soft tissue at risk of shortening.

Since the upright position is vital for the proper functioning of many organs, other possible benefits of having the patient stand for periods during the day may include:

● Stimulation of internal functions such as bowel movements and bladder emptying.
● Improved ventilation (the abdominal contents move down giving more space for lung expansion, redistributing air flow to basal lobes, and changing perfusion/ventilation ratio).
● Decreased ICP as cerebral venous return is increased provided autoregulation is intact.

Since the upright position can result in large drops in cerebral blood flow if autoregulation is compromised, blood pressure and ICP should be monitored during initial attempts to stand the patient.

Maintaining functional muscle length is critical to the re-establishing of active self-initiated functional movement. For motor training to be effective, muscles must be of functional length not only so that movement of the necessary amplitude can be performed but also so that the muscles can generate tension over the necessary range of movement. Note that it is only by lengthening the muscle that the range over which the muscle can actively generate tension can be increased. Casting may be imperative if exercise and training are not sufficient to lengthen muscle actively.

The environment of the comatose patient

Coma is a state of unconsciousness in which there is neither arousal nor awareness. Eyes remain closed and there is an absence of sleep/wake cycles. The definition implies that there is no motor response to command and no speech. Coma exists in the early period after injury and usually lasts no longer than 3–4 weeks. The vegetative state describes a condition in which the patient demonstrates no signs of cognition but may return to wakefulness with the eyes open in response to verbal stimuli. Although sleep/wake cycles, normal blood pressure and normal respiration are present, the patient is unable to engage in verbal interaction or produce organized, discrete motor responses (Garner and Valadka 1994).

As a result, there is a need to organize the environment around the comatose TBI individual. If environmental effects are not considered, the unconscious person is not only deprived of normal sensory input but many of the necessary observations may produce stimulating and painful sensory input throughout 24 hours each day (e.g., turning, tracheal stimulation, attention to hygiene, feeding). The physiotherapist's contribution needs to take account of the timing of interventions.

Family involvement, education and counselling are important considerations. Both family and team members need to understand the importance of speaking to the patient, of the need to consider the patient's feelings during conversation around the bed, of the need to preserve a sense of dignity by ensuring that he or she is appropriately covered, and of providing specific input which encourages some active response from the patient. The family can provide important information about the patient's favourite name, interests, likes and dislikes.

Coma stimulation or coma arousal programmes

Such programmes, with the goals of improving arousal and responsiveness, have been developed but remain controversial (Ellis and Rader 1990; Wood 1991). The rationale for these programmes has arisen from the need to avoid the known negative effects of sensory deprivation and to change the environment systematically in an attempt to prompt the patient to respond in a more specific and appropriate way. Briccolo and colleagues (1980) have described prolonged unconsciousness as a 'race against time'. In view of this, a number of attempts to reduce coma duration by means of sensory stimulation have been reported (e.g., Pierce *et al.* 1990; Mitchell *et al.* 1990; Freeman 1987). However, results are somewhat equivocal. More evidence is required to establish the usefulness of such a procedure in affecting outcome. Wood (1991) argues that habituation to environmental stimuli occurs when environments do not control certain sensory input such as overexposure to radio and television constantly in the background.

Recovery from coma

Recovery manifests itself with periods of opening of the eyes. This is evidence that the mechanisms concerned with wakefulness are recovering. The next phase is the utterance of words in individuals who are not going to remain vegetative and are not aphasic. Initially these utterances are random and occasional and the patient may start to carry out instructions. Some individuals demonstrate a period of noisy, disinhibited behaviour: cursing, attempting to get out of bed and displaying aggressive behaviour to anyone who is nearby.

The individual is usually amnesic in this period of disturbed behaviour (Jennett and Teasdale 1981). During the period of PTA there is severe anterograde memory disorder (amnesia for events occurring after the precipitating trauma) in association with other problems such as disorientation and restlessness. There may be poor participation in motor training and other aspects of rehabilitation due to confusion, agitation or inappropriate behaviour. The individual may have difficulty in initiating appropriate behaviours or may demonstrate impulsivity.

The intensity and duration of this stage of recovery varies considerably. It is unclear whether or not these behaviours reflect damage to different areas of the brain, are associated with pretraumatic personality traits of the individual, or are related to the environment or some combination of these. Factors such as a full bladder or pain from associated injuries about which the patient is unable to communicate appropriately may add to the person's frustration.

This phase can be difficult for both relatives and staff to deal with but it is important that the patient's natural recovery is not impeded by heavy sedation. Families require reassurance since, having ceased to fear for the survival of the individual, they may now be very concerned about the future.

Investigations suggest that the end of PTA is a crucial stage in the recovery process and that it is associated with the restoration of other mental skills. The individual may demonstrate changes in personality which are only obvious to those who knew him/her prior to the injury. This stage is often complicated by the individual's apathy rather than by overactivity and this requires a different approach by therapists in order to utilize appropriate behavioural and environmental strategies to facilitate active participation in training. The establishment of daily testing on the Westmead PTA Scale (Shores *et al.* 1986) has been found useful by all members of the rehabilitation team by alerting them to the existence of a specific mental state which interferes with rehabilitation. While in a state of PTA, 'carryover' of training from one session to the next may be limited.

Patients who demonstrate erratic and irrelevant behaviour may be subject to outbursts of violence and impulsivity. Families need early counselling to

be able to cope with altered behaviour, to be prepared for difficulties likely to occur, and be given some short-term objectives as well as some hint of the ultimate degree of recovery that is expected.

The re-establishment of swallowing, unassisted breathing, effective coughing and communication through facial expression, gesture and language is essential if the patient is to resume more normal function. At the stage when the patient is emerging from coma, the establishment of an unambiguous and easy to produce yes/no response is critical to re-establishing some form of communication. Options to augment communication include eye contact, facial expression, gesture and communication boards – with letters (Fig. 12.5), symbols or pictures.

Once patients can breathe unaided for several minutes they are disconnected from the ventilator for short periods. Tension and anxiety, which may precipitate respiratory distress, are to be avoided. Periods of unassisted breathing are increased in duration and frequency. Articulation, phonation and eating are dependent upon control of breathing. Patients who have both a nasogastric and tracheostomy tube need training to improve coordination of these functions once the tubes are removed. Sitting with erect trunk and head are critical pre-requisites for swallowing, improved lung expansion and coughing as well as fostering orientation, eye contact and communication. If the individual cannot sit unsupported or hold the head

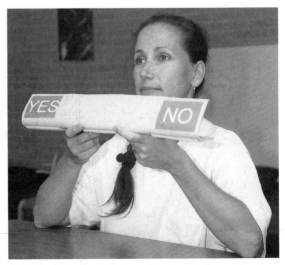

Fig. 12.5 Critical to communication is the need to establish a Yes/No response

upright some form of external restraint may be necessary (Fig. 12.6).

The reticular formation (neurons in the brain stem extending through the medulla, pons and midbrain) is considered to mediate aspects of arousal (Kelly and Dodd 1991). It is likely, therefore, that the erect position facilitates arousal by providing a change in the orientation of the head and neck. Standing is also critical for proper functioning of many organs, including regaining control over continence.

In summary, aims in the acute phase of management of the TBI individual are to:

- Monitor the patient's level of coma and vital signs.
- Improve respiratory function.
- Preserve musculoskeletal integrity.
- Facilitate arousal and active engagement.

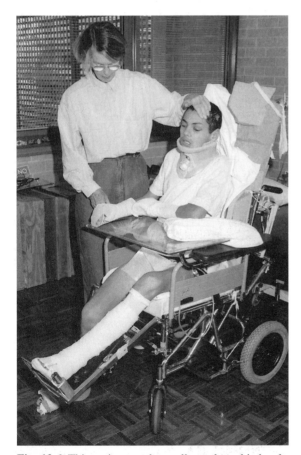

Fig. 12.6 This patient needs a collar to keep his head upright. In this way, visual information is not distorted when he opens his eyes. He is wearing orthoses and casts to stretch long finger flexors and calf muscles

Rehabilitation: an overall view

Rehabilitation of the TBI individual requires the provision of comprehensive interdisciplinary rehabilitation services including physiotherapist, occupational therapist, orthotist, social worker, psychologist, neuropsychologist and vocational rehabilitation counsellor. Rehabilitation should begin in the acute surgical/intensive care unit and continue in a rehabilitation centre or the person may visit the rehabilitation centre from home or transitional living centre, an arrangement which helps the person bridge the gap between hospital-based facilities and re-entry into the community. At periodic intervals, the patient and family need assistance in coming to terms with the person's changing physical, mental and social capabilities. Rehabilitation of the severely brain-damaged individual may continue for many years and some patients will require long-term care.

The issue of predicting outcome, time course and degree of recovery is complex and may be affected by many factors. The study of outcome from rehabilitation of TBI has been hampered by the lack of agreement upon methods for monitoring the process of recovery, or the degree of recovery finally reached, as well as the diversity of populations studied. However, multicentre studies over the past few decades make it possible to provide rough guidelines based on probability statistics for predicting outcome in individual patients.

TBI is by nature a diffuse and multifocal insult. For this reason there is great variability in sensorimotor, cognitive, behavioural and personality impairments depending on many factors including the pattern, extent and severity of the damage. The therapist is faced with understanding the complex interaction of the many physical, cognitive and behavioural deficits.

Cognitive and memory deficits and personality changes

It has long been realized that it is the cognitive and memory deficits and the personality changes that have the most profound consequences in terms of rehabilitation and social reintegration. Jennett and Teasdale (1981) describe the effect of these deficits on the family and the individual. As these authors point out, suffering a TBI, even brief concussion, is a significant experience for anyone. The severely injured person wakes up after days or sometimes weeks unable to recall anything that occurred in that time. Unbeknown to the individual, relatives have been fearing for his or her life but are now concerned about mental status. Insight into the situation and implications for the future, however, may take weeks to develop. It is often only when the TBI individual goes home that the extent of the effects of the injury on the person and the family are fully realized.

One of the mental capacities that TBI individuals have most difficulty with is the ability to adapt to and to cope with new and different stresses. Some individuals become depressed, some deny their disability, others may be so euphoric that they do not appreciate their plight. Some may become so distressed by their condition that they react with anger and frustration, placing blame on therapists, doctors and relatives for their situation. The relatives may also react with frustration, depression or denial. Another factor thought to influence the psychological reaction to severe TBI is pretraumatic psychosocial status of the individual and family.

The so-called *frontal pattern of behaviour* (Walsh 1985) falls somewhere between behavioural and cognitive deficits. It is increasingly understood that disorganized behaviour seen after frontal lobe damage underlies deficits in many cognitive functions (Lezak 1995). Behavioural problems associated with prefrontal damage include decreased productivity or lost initiative, difficulty making mental or behavioural shifts in attention, or in making changes in movement. Problems modulating ongoing behaviour may show up as impulsivity and disinhibition. The patient may also be incapable of planning or of sustaining goal-directed behaviour. Whatever the nature of symptoms, many individuals with frontal lobe disorders seem to have poor judgement and poor adaptability to new situations and are unable to achieve rewarding personal relationships or steady and successful employment (Newcombe 1993).

A wide variety of *cognitive* deficits has been reported, including disorders of learning and memory, complex information processing (including speed and planning), and disorders of perception and communication (Prigatano 1986; Brooks 1990). The reader is referred to Further Reading on these complex topics.

Memory complaints, ranging from trivial forgetfulness to profound, permanent amnesia (in which cognitive abilities may be intact except for delayed memory), are frequently made by patients and their relatives. The exact nature of memory

disturbances (encoding, storage and retrieval of information) are difficult to unravel, and the influence of other factors such as low motivation, poor morale and depression should not be underestimated. Comparatively little is known about the long-term prognosis of memory disorders following TBI with confusing reports in the literature (Wilson 1995). There is, however, evidence that patients and their relatives can be helped to cope with the everyday difficulties they are likely to experience. In a follow-up study of 59 brain-damaged patients, 29 of whom had sustained a TBI, only one third had improved since the end of rehabilitation although many subjects had improved during rehabilitation. Wilson (1991) suggests that an encouraging finding was that most subjects were using more aids, strategies and techniques to compensate for their difficulties compared with the number they had been using at the end of rehabilitation. In Wilson's view, these results are less bleak than would have been anticipated several years earlier (Wilson 1995).

Sarno's detailed studies (1980, 1984) have shown that *impaired communication* is a common consequence of TBI. It is unclear, however, whether such disorders should be called language deficits or deficits in complex processing and lack of attention (Brooks 1990). For example, confabulation, tangential speech and perseveration may be due to attentional disturbances. Except in the case of focal left hemisphere damage, language dysfunction following TBI differs considerably from the aphasias seen following stroke. Adequate speech is often present but language may be ineffective. Whereas individuals with aphasia often communicate better than they talk, TBI patients frequently talk better than they communicate (Milton and Wertz 1986). Strategies for optimizing language and communication are described in several texts (Adamovich 1990; Ylvisaker and Urbanczyk 1994). These strategies should be reinforced across all disciplines so that consistent language demands occur in all environments.

In the period of recovery characterized by confusion and generally inappropriate behaviour, communication management is similar to overall behaviour management and includes tolerance for slow and cumbersome speech, use of orientational and pertinent cues, strategies to focus attention (addressing the individual by name, waiting for eye contact, and use of prompts), and positive interaction with the individual. Other ways of encouraging communication summarized by Ylvisaker and Urbanczyk (1994) include:

- Simplifying language in both form and content.
- Modifying the environment so that communication is likely to be successful.
- Using natural contextual cues.
- Communicating respect for the individual.
- Redirecting agitated or perseverant behaviour.

Three aspects of behaviour are typically described when analysing the nature of change in *personality*. *Drive* is usually reduced and the apathy that results is often described as laziness or simply slowness. This lack of drive interferes with successful and active participation in rehabilitation. Combined with a lack of drive there may be *affective* changes toward euphoria which may lead individuals to claim that they are better than they really are. This may lead to a passive acceptance of their condition. Emotional lability, inexplicable bouts of crying or, less often, inappropriate or exaggerated laughing may also be present. Deficits in *social restraint and judgement* may be characterized by tactless and hurtful behaviour toward others. The individual may be subject to outbursts of rage that are out of character and an inability to control individual feelings of dislike and frustration. In turn, these changes are associated with marital and family breakdown, social isolation and unemployment (Zencius *et al.* 1990).

Cognitive and personality deficits can produce overtly inappropriate sexual advances toward uninterested individuals. Rehabilitation staff members and relatives are often discomforted by these behaviours and have difficulty in coping effectively with them.

Management and remediation of memory disorders

A neuropsychological assessment as described by Howieson and Lezak (1995) provides a picture of the patient's cognitive strengths and weaknesses. An assessment and observation of everyday problems is also necessary to supplement the information gathered from more formal neuropsychological testing and to classify the problems to be tackled (Wilson 1995). General guidelines for helping people with memory problems and their families are outlined on page 257. Other strategies include adaptation of the environment (e.g., colour coding), the use of external aids, and internal strategies such as mnemonics and rehearsal techniques (Wilson 1995).

Behaviour management

Socially unacceptable or socially deviant actions present serious management problems for the rehabilitation team and family. These actions may be so severe that they preclude the individual from rehabilitation. Furthermore, if these disorders persist, they are considerable barriers to acceptance back into the community (Eames *et al.* 1990). There is evidence from both group (Eames and Wood 1985) and single case studies (Hegel 1988; Zencius 1990) that behavioural management can be effective in improving behaviour which in turn tends to increased cooperation with therapists, for example, and in carrying out essential living skills.

Behaviour modification in a structured environment is based on positive reinforcement (tokens, privileges, interest, attention and praise) of all appropriate behaviour and the strict avoidance of such reinforcement of inappropriate and socially unacceptable behaviours (Eames and Wood 1985; Wood 1987a). It is important to note that a token economy structure has been shown to enable rehabilitation to proceed despite behavioural disorders that had previously made it impossible (Eames and Wood 1985).

The goals of treatment are summarized as (Eames *et al.* 1990):

- Reward all instances of appropriate behaviour.
- Withhold rewards that are currently maintaining maladaptive behaviour.
- Withhold all sources of positive reinforcement for a brief period after each instance of maladaptive behaviour (time-out from positive reinforcement).
- Apply a predeclared penalty following the maladaptive behaviour.
- Apply an aversive consequence following extremely severe or resistant maladaptive behaviour.

Time-out procedures are based on the assumption that many behaviours are reinforced (and therefore develop and are maintained) by the attention they receive from staff, peers and family. As a consequence, the individual receives some reward for inappropriate/maladaptive behaviour. Some form of time-out, therefore, has a punishing effect. For a detailed description of behaviour modification techniques see Wood (1987a,b) and Eames and colleagues (1990).

In severely affected individuals, closed units which enable consistency of approach and reduce inappropriate input from relatives, have been found to be particularly effective (Eames and Wood 1985). In these severe cases, treatment may take at least 3–6 months or longer, with a period of 15–18 months likely to be optimal. The results of a follow-up study show a high percentage of these individuals achieved lasting improvements in behaviour and in personal and social independence (Eames and Wood 1985).

Task-related training

Due to the diffuse nature of TBI, primary sensori-motor impairments are variable and complex and may include weakness, rigidity, reflex hyper-activity, cerebellar ataxia, tremor, dyskinesia, sensory loss (impairments in basic sensation or of perceptual processing) and commonly a combina-tion of these. Added to these neurological impair-ments, some individuals may have other associated physical injuries, including fractures, spinal cord injury and frequently cranial nerve injury (Table 12.2). Many individuals also enter rehabilitation with secondary musculoskeletal, respiratory, cardi-ovascular and metabolic sequelae, and in some instances a combination of all of these, which interferes with performance of everyday activities and skills. Furthermore, low aerobic capacity and increased fatiguability may limit the individual's ability to participate in motor training. The major objective of physiotherapy is to train optimal and effective performance of any action which the individual cannot perform or can only perform with difficulty.

The physiotherapist needs an understanding of the pathophysiology of the primary sensorimotor

impairments (see Chapters 8–10) and the adapta-tions or compensations that emerge as the patient attempts to perform everyday actions. The major role of the physiotherapist is to train the individual to perform more effectively those everyday actions, such as walking, sit-to-stand, reaching and manipulation, which are difficult. Motor training in these actions is described in Chapters 2 and 4–7. Some other important details of physiotherapy intervention particularly relevant to rehabilitation of the individual with TBI, however, are discussed below.

Physiotherapy *evaluation* of the TBI individual involves observation and analysis of sensorimotor impairments and the gathering of information about the individual's communication, cognitive, behavoural deficits and any other relevant informa-tion, such as deficits or loss of one of the special senses, hearing, taste or vision (e.g., presence of double-vision, blurred vision). All of these deficits affect the individual's ability to participate actively in motor training. Early assessment may be complicated because the patient is dysphasic, may have a short attention span, inappropriate or antisocial behaviours and impaired short-term memory. The physiotherapist needs to consider physical, cognitive and social demands of the task in order to clarify where task breakdown occurs. In other words, problems in functional performance may be due not only to primary sensorimotor impairments but also to distraction from perform-ing the task because of irritability, short-term memory loss, short attention span, apathy or lack of motivation.

It is the authors' opinion that the focus of *measurement* should be on real world functional performance, i.e., performance of everyday actions as measured on a functional scale, e.g., the MAS (Carr *et al.* 1985) or the Rivermead Motor Assessment (Lincoln & Leadbitter 1979). Some special-purpose tests, e.g., sensory tests (Chapter 10), walking and running velocity (Chapter 3), motor fitness tests (Rossi and Sullivan 1996) are also used to establish the major reason for impaired motor performance and/or to get a baseline meas-ure. When muscle contracture is present, measure-ment of joint range using standardized procedures (Ada and Herbert, 1988) is necessary in order to monitor effectiveness of intervention aimed at reducing stiffness and increasing muscle extensi-bility. Measurement of muscle strength may be helpful. However, measurement of isolated mus-cles does not indicate how that muscle works in a multijoint movement (e.g., the ability to sustain a

Table 12.2   Cranial nerves most commonly affected in TBI

Cranial nerve	Deficits
I	Anosmia (loss of sense of smell)
III IV V	Diplopia (double vision)
VII	Facial paralysis
VIII	Hearing loss Tinnitus Vertigo (spatial disorientation characterized by a feeling of turning or having objects rotate about oneself – disturbance in balance)

contraction, to time a contraction within a synergy to achieve a specific goal).

Some critical factors in motor training for the TBI individual are to:

- Direct the individual's attention to the critical biomechanical features of the action.
- Modify the task to achieve success.
- Organize the environment to force use and participation.
- Practise routines using the same verbal cues.
- Provide concrete goals (rather than abstract ones).
- Decrease prompts as performance improves.
- Monitor performance throughout the day.
- Provide reinforcers.
- Establish goals for each session.
- Give feedback that is concrete and accurate.
- Graph progress for the individual.
- Provide pictorial (and/or written) instructions.
- Evaluate effects of training.

Physiotherapy should be biased toward functional performance of concrete tasks (Figs 12.7, 12.8), with enjoyable activities (Figs 12.9, 12.10) and exercise (Fig. 12.11).

To keep the patient focused on practising tasks, the physiotherapist needs to be inventive and creative to ensure that the activities practised in therapy are perceived as relevant to the individual's needs. It is only in a more natural and challenging environment, e.g. walking in a busy corridor, entering and exiting a lift, crossing a busy street, rather than the artificial setting of the therapy centre that the individual may gain insight into his or her deficits and the need to train and practise.

Some TBI individuals simply fail to act without extensive cuing and imposed structure. Since the cognitive and behavioural deficits tend to predominate after TBI, a highly structured, consistent and reinforcing environment is required to ensure active participation in training as well as sufficient time-on-task to improve performance. Steps in structuring environmental settings to change behaviour during therapy sessions include systematic observation and assessment, and the provision of a comprehensive continuum of structure throughout the rehabilitation centre with reinforcement by all staff and relatives. Less restrictive options can be instituted as improvement occurs.

For example:

- Observe patient's behaviour in different settings and with different people.

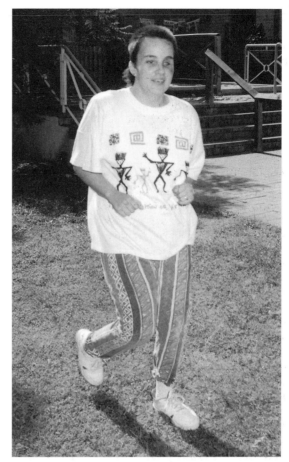

Fig. 12.7 This woman has cerebellar signs. Jogging involves rapid bursts of muscle activity in a cyclical fashion. Stopping and starting in response to a command or as part of a game are also practised

- Analyse environmental variables that affect the patient's behaviour either positively or negatively.
- Remove variables that trigger or reinforce unwanted/maladaptive behaviours and replace them with variables that reinforce desired behaviours.
- Evaluate effects of environmental modification.
- Progress and modify intervention to facilitate further improvement.

Examples of successful treatment programmes using this type of structure can be found in Lincoln (1978,1981). The use of behavioural techniques to teach dressing and washing skills after severe brain injury are described by Giles and Clark-Wilson (1988).

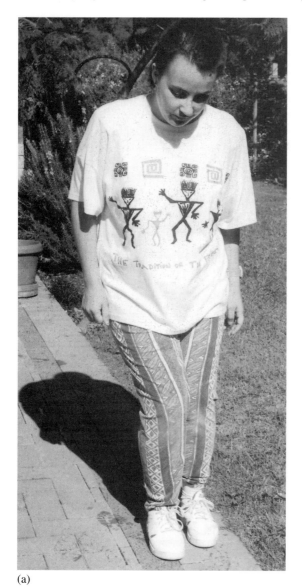

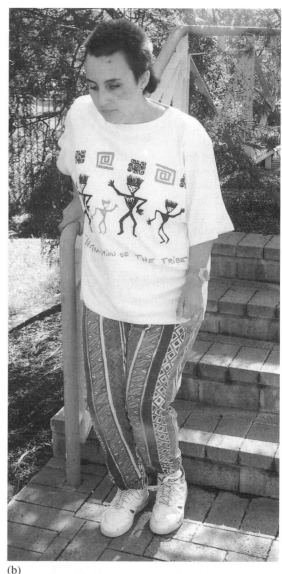

(a)   (b)

Fig. 12.8 Jumping (*a*) from side-to-side keeping the feet together and (*b*) jumping off a step. Both these actions involve the production of a rapid initial burst of agonist extensor activity to propel the body upward from the flexion counter-movement without a pause between the two

Swallowing dysfunction (dysphagia)

Obstacles to eating include both cognitive (difficulty following instructions, difficulty concentrating, poor motivation) and oromotor deficits (Winstein 1983). Analysis of swallowing dysfunction includes an evaluation of reflexive and voluntary components of function and training is instituted to improve control (see Carr and Shepherd 1987 for details). Orofacial deficits may include inability to swallow, inadequate lip and jaw close, an aversion to certain textures in the mouth, inability to chew, and abnormal reflex activity such as a hyperactive bite reflex, and a hypo- or hyperactive gag reflex. Facial asymmetry may also be present as a result of impaired motor control or damage to the facial nerve.

Patients who have frequent coughing fits and episodes of clinical aspiration may benefit from videofluoroscopy to aid evaluation of the

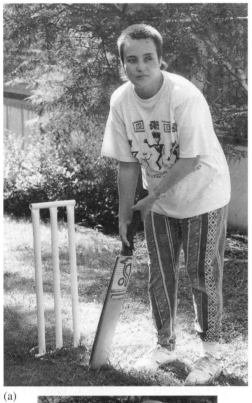

(a)

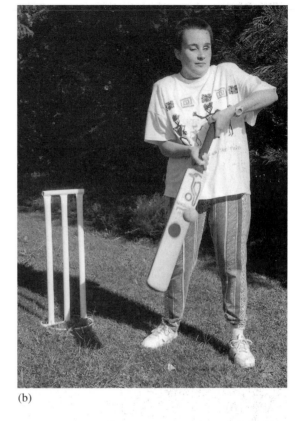

(b)

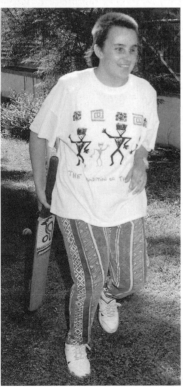

(c)

Fig. 12.9 Playing cricket enables her to improve balance and coordination along with eye–hand coordination and predictive time-to-contact from a relatively stable position (*a*) with the bat on the ground, (*b*) raising the bat to hit the ball and (*c*) running between wickets carrying the bat

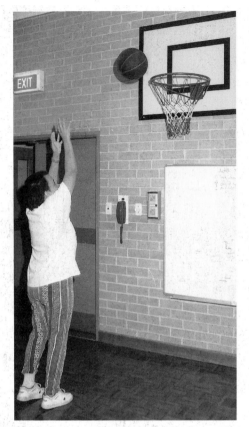

Fig. 12.10 Goal throwing. Note that she has not been able to generate a sufficiently rapid and powerful burst of muscle activity to propel her on to her toes. Heel-raising exercises (see Fig. 5.23) may increase strength and control in calf muscles

pharyngeal phase of swallowing. Swallowing disorders are best treated through an experienced member of the team (physiotherapist, occupational therapist or speech pathologist) assuming responsibility for evaluation and treatment, with all team members, particularly those present at meal times, following recommended procedures and precautions. The prognosis for functional recovery with training is very good (Winstein 1983).

Bladder and bowel incontinence

Obstacles to bladder and bowel continence likewise include both neurogenic and cognitive deficits. Slowed mobility, poor communication and impaired initiation also contribute to incontinence. Neurogenic bladder dysfunction is assessed by noting the frequency and volume of individual voids and measuring the post-void residual. A bladder training programme can then be instituted (see p. 259 for more detail).

Cardiovascular deconditioning

Not only are many patients very deconditioned at the start of active rehabilitation, but also after discharge from rehabilitation, TBI individuals have been found to have reduced cardiovascular fitness, as measured by VO_2 peak, compared with their able-bodied counterparts (Becker *et al.* 1978; Hunter *et al.* 1990; Jankowski and Sullivan 1990).

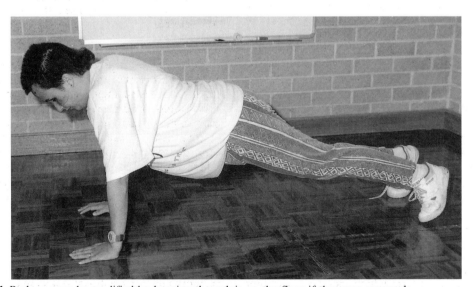

Fig. 12.11 Push-ups can be modified by keeping the pelvis on the floor if the arms are weak

Sullivan and colleagues (1990) recommend that all patients engage in physical activity for at least half the working day in challenging activities throughout rehabilitation (e.g., long jump, weight lifting, 1 km walks or jogs, cross country walks; competitive activities either against oneself or others). It is interesting to note that Sullivan and colleagues describe the atmosphere in group sessions designed to increase flexibility, strength and coordination as being akin to that found in a health club.

Benefits of a physical conditioning programme include:

- Increased cardiovascular fitness and prevention of cardiovascular disease.
- Decreased resistance to physical fatigue.
- Enhanced ability to participate in other aspects of the rehabilitation programme.
- Improved self-confidence by accomplishing targets of behaviour.
- Establishing general healthy behaviour.
- Assisting in gaining normal sleep patterns.
(Sullivan *et al.* 1990).

A self-report of a final year medical student (Moran 1972) who survived a severe (21 days PTA) head injury in the final year of his medical degree tells how he increased his mental and physical abilities by running (1 mile) and doing push-ups. Subsequently, Moran (1976) reported six case studies in which vigorous exercise played a major role not only in combating depression, emotional lability, regression and fatigue but also in developing self-confidence and initiative.

Physical conditioning programmes have resulted in improvements in oxidative capacity as measured by maximum oxygen consumption. A group of individuals who underwent circuit training (stationary cycling, rope skipping, jogging and stair climbing) demonstrated significant improvement in aerobic capacity (Jankowski and Sullivan 1990). Given that exercise intensity was relatively low because these individuals were incapable of exercising at the established intensity, the authors suggest the result may have been due to the rather prolonged interval training. Hunter and colleagues (1990) also found a significant increase in VO_{2max} following a similar physical conditioning programme (using treadmill, mechanical stairs and bicycle ergometer).

An attempt has been made to establish reliability in a battery of motor performance and fitness tests in children and adolescents (age range 8–17) (Rossi and Sullivan 1996). The components tested were based on criteria which included flexibility,

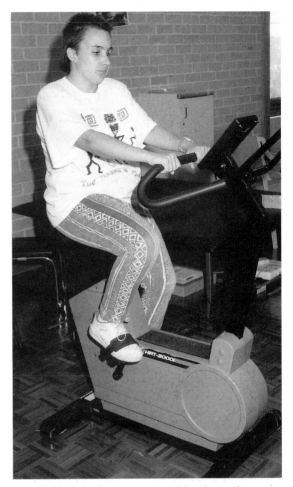

Fig. 12.12 Pedalling a stationary bicycle can improve muscle strength in the lower limbs and endurance, the individual competing against herself to improve performance

muscle strength, cardiorespiratory endurance, agility, power, balance, speed and coordination. Specific items tested included: agility run, standing broad jump, hand grip strength, vertical jump, 50 yard dash, soft ball throw, soccer dribble test and chin-up hang. It has been reported that successful reintegration into sports and physical activities, whether for health, leisure or competition, provides children and adolescents following TBI with a sense of accomplishment (Haley *et al.* 1990). It is probably similar for adults.

Community reintegration

Cognitive disabilities such as problem-solving, memory and organizational skills are the problems most often complained of by the TBI individual and relatives. These disabilities may prevent the individual from re-entering the work force and educational and vocational systems. They also present difficulties for the individual in maintaining an independent lifestyle and often require financial assistance for basic living requirements. Post-traumatic epilepsy can also be an important factor in terms of family and social acceptance and employment opportunities.

Return to work remains the leading indicator of recovery after a TBI and it is often what the individual strives for most (Cook, 1990). The literature is rather confusing on this issue but it appears that a large percentage of people with TBI who enter the workforce lose their jobs within the first 3 months. Unfortunately, it is evident that many of those individuals who are unable to work face years of social isolation and hardship.

Some form of **continuing assistance** is needed for many individuals and their families. Education, support, self-help and sports for the disabled groups assist in fulfilling some of these needs. Ongoing assistance to promote improvement in language and cognitive function and ongoing medical and behavioural assistance to ameliorate mood swings and frustration are some of the issues raised by TBI individuals and their families. Community mobility may be limited for a variety of reasons ranging from physical to the purely cognitive. Lack of adequate recreational facilities whether for health, leisure or competition is viewed as a major obstacle to successful reintegration.

There are relatively few published studies on *sexuality* following TBI. Disturbances in sexual function, either organic or behavioural, may include hypersexuality, hyposexuality, impotence, loss of feeling of attractiveness and an inability to engage in intimate interpersonal relationships (Griffith *et al.* 1990). Individuals with these problems may need specialized assistance.

In conclusion, improved medical and surgical techniques are saving the lives of many TBI victims who, 10–20 years ago, would have succumbed to the metabolic, haemodynamic and other complications that follow brain trauma (Bontke, 1990). As a result, there are an ever-increasing number of survivors of severe injury, mostly children and young adults, who are rapidly familiarizing us with the tragic phenomenon of physically fit young people whose brains have been damaged significantly (Lezak, 1995). The occurrence of some of the once commonly seen physical sequelae, such as contracture and heterotopic ossification, have been lessened, but cognitive and behavioural deficits in many individuals still represent the most significant obstacles to reintegration in the community. There are a variety of financial and medicolegal issues which can also complicate the rehabilitation process, and complex ethical issues related to the treatment of patients in coma or persistent vegetative state. For those who emerge from coma, the goal of successful community reintegration should guide all rehabilitation intervention.

References

Ada, L. and Herbert, R. (1988) Measurement of joint range of motion. *Australian Journal of Physiotherapy*, **34**, 260–262.

Ada, L., Canning, C. and Paratz, J. (1990) Care of the unconscious head-injured patient. In *Key Issues in Neurological Physiotherapy* (eds L. Ada and C. Canning) Butterworth Heinemann, Oxford, pp. 249–286.

Adamovich, B.B. (1990) Treatment of communication and swallowing disorders. In *Rehabilitation of the Adult and Child with Traumatic Brain Injury* (eds M. Rosenthal, M.R. Bond, E.R. Griffith and J.D. Miller), 2nd edn, F.A. Davis, Philadelphia, pp. 374–392.

Akeson, W.H., Amiel, D. and Woo, S.L-Y. (1980) Immobility effects on synovial joints. The pathomechanics of joint contracture. *Biorheology*, **17**, 95–110.

Becker, E., Bar-Or, L. Mendelson, L. *et al.* (1978) Pulmonary responses to exercise of patients following cranio-cerebral injury. *Scandinavian Journal of Rehabilitation Medicine*, **10,** 47–50.

Ben-Yishay, Y., Silver, S., Piasetsky, E. and Rattok, J. (1987) Relationship between employability and vocational outcome after intensive holistic cognitive rehabilitation. *Journal of Head Trauma*, **21**, 35–48.

Blumbergs, P.C., Jones, N.R. and North, J.B. (1989) Diffuse axonal injury in head trauma. *Journal of Neurology, Neurosurgery and Psychiatry*, **52**, 838–841.

Bond, M.R. (1986) Neurobehavioural sequelae of closed head injury. In *Neuropsychological Assessment of Neuropsychiatric Disorders* (eds I. Grant and K.M. Adams) Oxford University Press, New York, pp. 347–373.

Bond, M.R. (1990) Standardized methods of assessing and predicting outcome. In *Rehabilitation of the Adult and Child with Traumatic Brain Injury* (eds M. Rosenthal, M.R. Bond, E.R. Griffith and J.D. Miller) 2nd edn, F.A. Davis, Philadelphia, pp. 59–76.

Bontke, C.F. (1990) Medical advances in the treatment of brain injury. In *Community Integration Following Traumatic Brain Injury* (eds J.S. Kreutzer and P. Wehamn) Paul H. Brookes, Baltimore, MD.

Booth, B.J., Doyle, M. and Montgomery, J. (1983) Serial casting for the management of spasticity in the head-injured adult. *Physical Therapy*, **63**, 1960–1966.

Braakman, R., Jennett, W.B. and Minderhoud, J.M. (1988) Prognosis of the posttraumatic vegetative state. *Acta Neurochirurgica (Wien)*, **95**, 49–52.

Briccolo, A., Turazzi, S. and Feriotti, G. (1980) Prolonged post traumatic unconsciousness. *Journal of Neurosurgery*, **52**, 625–634.

Brooks, D.N. (1990) Cognitive deficits. In *Rehabilitation of the Adult and Child with Traumatic Brain Injury* (eds M. Rosenthal, M.R. Bond, E.R. Griffith and J.D. Miller) 2nd edn, F.A. Davis, Philadelphia, pp. 163–178.

Brooks, D.N. *et al.* (1986) Head injury and the rehabilitation profession in the west of Scotland. *Health Bulletin (Edinburgh)*, **44**, 110.

Carr, J.H. and Shepherd, R.B. (1987) *A Motor Relearning Programming for Stroke*, 2nd edn. Butterworth-Heinemann, Oxford.

Carr, J.H., Shepherd, R.B., Nordholm, L. *et al.* (1985) A motor assessment scale for stroke. *Physical Therapy*, **68**, 1371–1380.

Cook, J.V. (1990) Returning to work after traumatic head injury. In *Rehabilitation of the Adult and Child with Traumatic Brain Injury* (eds M. Rosenthal, M.R. Bond, E.R. Griffith and J.D. Miller) 2nd edn, F.A. Davis, Philadelphia, pp. 493–505.

Dresser, A., Meirowsky, A., Weiss, G., McNeel, M., Simon, G. and Caveness, W. (1973) Gainful employment following head injury. *Archives of Neurology*, **29**, 111–116.

Eames, P. and Wood, R.L. (1985) Rehabilitation after severe brain injury: a follow-up study of a behaviour modification approach. *Journal of Neurology, Neurosurgery and Psychiatry*, **48**, 613.

Eames, P., Haffey, W.J. and Cope, N. (1990) Treatment of behavioural disorders. In *Rehabilitation of the Adult and Child with Traumatic Brain Injury* (eds M. Rosenthal, M.R. Bond, E.R. Griffith and J.D. Miller) 2nd edn, F.A. Davis, Philadelphia, pp. 410–432.

Ellis, D.W. and Rader, M. (1990) Structured sensory stimulation. In *Physical Medicine and Rehabilitation – State of the Art Reviews: The Coma Emerging Patient* (eds M.W. Sandal and D.W. Ellis), **4**.

Ellis, E. (1990) Respiratory function following head injury. In *Key Issues in Neurological Physiotherapy* (eds L. Ada and C. Canning), Butterworth-Heinemann, Oxford, pp.237–248.

Frankowski, R.F. (1985) The demography of head injury in the United States. In *Neurotrauma, Vol 1* (eds M. Miner and K.A. Wagner), Butterworth, Boston, pp. 1–17.

Freeman, E.A. (1987) *Catastrophy of Coma*. David Bateman, Buderim, Australia.

Frost, E.A.M. (1985) Management of head injury. *Canadian Anaesthetic Society Journal*, **32**, S32–S39.

Frost, E.A.M. (1987) Central nervous system trauma. *Practical Neuroanaesthetics Anaesthesiology Clinics of North America*, **5**, 565–585.

Garner, S.H. and Valadka, A.B. (1994) Medical management and principles of head injury rehabilitation. In *Brain Injury Rehabilitation: Clinical Considerations* (eds M.A.J. Finlayson and S.H. Garner) Williams and Wilkins, Baltimore, MD, pp. 83–101.

Giles, G.M. and Clark-Wilson, J. (1988) The use of behavioral techniques in functional skills training after severe brain injury. *American Journal of Occupational Therapy*, **42**, 658–665.

Goldspink, G. and Williams, P. (1990) Muscle fibre and connective tissue changes associated with use and disuse. In *Key Issues in Neurological Physiotherapy* (eds. L. Ada and C. Canning), Butterworth Heinemann, Oxford, pp.197–218.

Gossman, M.R., Sahrmann, S.A. and Rose, S.J. (1982) Review of length-associated changes in muscle. *Physical Therapy*, **62**, 1799–1808.

Griffith, E.R., Cole, S. and Cole, T.M. (1990) Sexuality and sexual dysfunction. In *Rehabilitation of the Adult and Child with Traumatic Brain Injury* (eds M. Rosenthal, M.R. Bond, E.R. Griffith and J.D. Miller) 2nd edn, F.A. Davis, Philadelphia, pp. 206–224.

Gronwall, D. (1989) Behavioural assessment during the acute stages of traumatic brain injury. In *Mild Head Injury* (eds H.S. Levin, H.M. Eisenberg and A.L. Benton) Oxford University Press, New York.

Gronwall, D. and Wrightson, P. (1975) Cumulative effects of concussion. *Lancet*, **ii**, 995–997.

Haley, S.M., Cioffi, M.I., Lewin, J.E. *et al.* (1990) Motor dysfunction in children and adolescents after traumatic brain injury. *Journal of Head Trauma Rehabilitation*, 5, 77–90.

Hans, P., Albert, A., Franssen, C. and Born, J. (1989) Improved outcome prediction based on CSF extrapolated creatine kinase BB isoenzyme activity and other risk factors in severe head injury. *Journal of Neurosurgery*, **71**, 54–58.

Hegel, M.T. (1988) Application of a token economy with a non-compliant closed head injured male. *Brain Injury*, **2**, 333–338.

Hitchcock, E.R. (1971) Summary of emergency care of head and multiple injury. In *Head Injuries. Proceedings of an International Symposium*, Churchill Livingstone, Edinburgh and London, pp. 201–203.

Horn, L.J. and Garland, D.E. (1993) Medical and orthopaedic complications associated with traumatic brain injury. In *Rehabilitation of the Adult and Child with Traumatic Brain Injury* (eds M. Rosenthal, M.R. Bond, E.R. Griffith and J.D. Miller), 2nd edn, F.A. Davis, Philadelphia, pp. 107–126.

Howieson, D.B. and Lezak, M.D. (1995) Separating memory from other cognitive problems. In *Handbook of Memory Disorders* (eds. A.D. Baddeley, B.A. Wilson and F.N. Watts), John Wiley, New York, pp. 411–426.

Hunter, M., Tomberlin, J.A., Kirkikis, C. *et al.* (1990) Progressive exercise testing in closed head-injury subjects: comparison of exercise apparatus in assessment of a physical conditioning program. *Physical Therapy*, **70**, 363–371.

Jankowski, L.W. and Sullivan, S.J. (1990) Aerobic and neuromuscular training: effect on the capacity, efficiency and fatiguability of patients with traumatic brain injuries. *Archives of Physical Medicine and Rehabilitation*, **71**, 500–504.

Jennett, B. (1986) *High Technology Medicine – Costs and Benefits*, Oxford University Press, Oxford.

Jennett, B. (1989) Some international comparisons. In *Mild Head Injury* (eds H.S. Levin, H.M. Eisenberg and A.L. Benton), Oxford University Press, New York.

Jennett, B. (1990) Scale and scope of the problem. In *Rehabilitation of the Adult and Child with Traumatic Brain Injury* (eds M. Rosenthal, M.R. Bond, E.R. Griffith and J.D. Miller), 2nd edn, F.A. Davis, Philadelphia, pp. 3–7.

Jennett, B. and Bond, M. (1975) Assessment of outcome after severe brain damage. *Lancet*, **i**, 480–485.

Jennett, B. and Plum, F. (1972) Persistent vegetative state after brain damage: a syndrome in search of a name. *Lancet*, **i**, 734–747.

Jennett, B. and Teasdale, G. (1981) *Management of Head Injuries*, F.A. Davis, Philadelphia.

Jennett, S. (1985) Pulmonary function in the head-injured patient. In *Head Injury and the Anaesthetist* (eds W. Fitch and J. Barker), Elsevier Science Publishers, Amsterdam, pp. 53–62.

Kelly, J.P. and Dodd, J. (1991) Anatomical organization of the nervous system. In *Principles of Neuroscience* (eds. E.R. Kandel, J.H. Schwartz and T.M. Jessell), 3rd edn, Appleton and Lange, Norwalk, CT, pp. 273–282.

Levin, H.S., Amparo, E., Eisenberg, H.M. *et al.* (1987) Magnetic resonance imaging and computerised tomography in relation to the neurobehavioural sequelae of mild and moderate head injuries. *Journal of Neurosurgery*, **66**, 706.

Levin, H.S., Benton, A.L. and Grossman, R.G. (1982) *Neurobehavioural Consequences of Closed Head Injury*, Oxford University Press, New York.

Lezak, M.D. (1995) *Neurophysiological Assessment*, 3rd edn, Oxford University Press, New York, pp. 87–95.

Lincoln, N.B. (1978) Behaviour modification in physiotherapy. *Physiotherapy*, **64**, 265–267.

Lincoln, N.B. (1981) Clinical psychology. In *Rehabilitation after Severe Head Injury* (ed. C.D. Evans), Churchill Livingstone, Edinburgh, pp. 146–165.

Lincoln, N. and Leadbitter, D. (1979) Assessment of motor function in stroke patients. *Physiotherapy*, **65**, 48–51.

Lindboe, C.F. and Platou, C.S. (1984) Effect of immobilization of short duration on the muscle fibre size. *Clinical Physiology*, **4**, 183–188.

MacFlynn, G., Montgomery, E.A., Fenton, G.W. *et al.* (1984) Measurement of reactive time following minor head injury. *Journal of Neurology, Neurosurgery and Psychiatry*, **47**, 1326–1331.

McKinlay, W.W., Brooks, D.N., Bond, M.R. *et al.* (1981) The short-term outcome of severe blunt head injury as reported by relatives of the injured persons. *Journal of Neurology, Neurosurgery and Psychiatry*, **44**, 527–533.

McLellan, D.L. (1993) Rehabilitation in neurology. In *Brain's Disorders of the Nervous System* (ed. J. Walton), 10th edn, Oxford University Press, Oxford, pp. 768–783.

McMillan, T.M. (1990) *Minor Head Injury: A Booklet for Professionals*, National Head Injuries Association, Nottingham.

MacNiven, E. (1994) Factors affecting head injury rehabilitation outcome: premorbid and clinical parameters. In *Brain Injury Rehabilitation: Clinical Considerations* (eds M.A.J. Finlayson and S.H. Garner), Williams and Wilkins, Baltimore, MD, pp. 57–82.

Mendelow, A. D. (1993a) Head injury. In *Brain's Diseases of the Nervous System* (ed. J. Walton), 10th edn, Oxford University Press, Oxford, pp. 184–196.

Mendelow, A. D. (1993b) Raised intracranial pressure, cerebral oedema, hydrocephalus, and intracranial tumours. In *Brain's Diseases of the Nervous System* (ed. J. Walton) 10th edn, Oxford University Press, Oxford, pp.144–183.

Mendelow, A.D. and Teasdale, G.M. (1983) Pathophysiology of head injuries. *British Journal of Surgery*, **70**, 641–650.

Milton, S.B. and Wertz, R.T. (1986) Management of persistent communication deficits in patients with traumatic brain injury. In *Clinical Neuropsychology of Intervention* (eds B.B. Uzzell and Y. Gross), Martinus Nijhoff Publishing, Boston, pp. 223–256.

Mitchell, S., Bradley, V.A., Welch, J.L. and Britton, P.G. (1990) Coma arousal procedure: a therapeutic intervention in the treatment of head injury. *Brain Injury*, **4**, 273–279.

Moran, A.J. (1972) Problems of a head-injured patient. *Medical Journal of Australia*, 30 September, pp. 782–783.

Moran, A.J. (1976) Six cases of severe head injury treated by exercise in addition to other therapies. *Medical Journal of Australia*, 20 March, pp. 396–397.

Moseley, A.M. (1997) The effect of casting combined with stretching on passive ankle dorsiflexion in adults with traumatic head injury. *Physical Therapy*, **77**, 240–247.

Murray, L.S., Teasdale, G.M., Murray, G.D. *et al.* (1993) Does prediction of outcome alter patient management? *Lancet*, **341**, 1487–1491.

Newcombe, F. (1993) Frontal lobe disorders. In *Neurological Rehabilitation* (eds R. Greenwood, M.P. Barnes, T.M. McMillan *et al.*) Churchill Livingstone, London, pp.377–386.

Oppenheimer, D.R. (1968) Microscopic lesions in the brain following head injury. *Journal of Neurology, Neurosurgery and Psychiatry*, **31**, 299–306.

Pierce, J.P., Lyle, D.M., Quine, S. *et al.* (1990) The effectiveness of coma arousal intervention. *Brain Injury*, **4**, 191–197.

Plum, F. and Posner, J.B. (1980) *The Diagnosis of Stupor and Coma*, 3rd edn, Blackwell, Oxford.

Povlishock, J.T., Becker, D.P., Cheng, C.L.Y. *et al.* (1983) Axonal change in minor head injury. *Journal of Neuropathology and Clinical Neurology*, **42**, 225–242.

Prigatano, G. (1986) *Neuropsychological Rehabilitation After Brain Injury*, Johns Hopkins University Press, Baltimore, MD.

Rappaport, M. (1986) Evoked potential and head injury in a rehabilitation setting. In *Neurotrauma: Treatment, Rehabilitation and Related Issues* (eds M. Miner and K. Wagner), Butterworths, Boston, pp. 189–194.

Rappaport, M., Hall, K.M., Hopkins, K. *et al.* (1982) Disability rating scale for severe head trauma: coma to community. *Archives of Physical Medicine and Rehabilitation*, **63**, 118–123.

Rimel, R.W., Giordini, B., Barth, J.T., Boll, T.J. and Jane, J.A. (1981) Disability caused by minor head injury. *Neurosurgery*, **9**, 221–228.

Rossi, C. and Sullivan, S.J. (1996) Motor fitness in children and adolescents with traumatic brain injury. *Archives of Physical Medicine and Rehabilitation*, **77**, 1062–1065.

Rowland, L.P., Fink, M.E. and Rubin, L. (1991) Cerebrospinal fluid: blood–brain edema and hydrocephalus. In *Principles of Neuroscience* (eds E.R. Kandell, J.H. Schwartz and T.M. Jessell) Appleton and Lange, Norwalk, CT, pp. 1050–1060.

Russell, W.R. (1932) Cerebral involvement in head injury. *Brain*, **35**, 549–603.

Sarno, M.T. (1980) The nature of verbal impairment after closed head injury. *Journal of Nervous and Mental Disease*, **168**, 685–692.

Sarno, M.T. (1984) Verbal impairment after closed head injury: report of a replication study. *Journal of Nervous and Mental Disease*, **172**, 475–479.

Shapiro, H.M. (1975) Intracranial hypertension: therapeutic and anaesthetic considerations. *Anaesthesiology*, **43**, 445.

Shores, E.A. (1989) Comparison of the Westmead PTA Scale and the Glasgow Coma Scale as predictors of neuropsychological outcome following severe blunt head injury. *Journal of Neurology, Neurosurgery, and Psychiatry*, **52**, 126–127.

Shores, E.A., Marosszeky, J.E., Sandanam, J. *et al.* (1986) Preliminary validation of a clinical scale for measuring the duration of post-traumatic amnesia. *Medical Journal of Australia*, **144**, 569–572.

Silver, J.R. (1969) Heterotopic ossification: a clinical study of its possible relationship to trauma. *Paraplegia*, **7**, 220.

Sosin, D.M., Sacks, J.J. and Holmgreen, P. (1990) Head injury-associated deaths from motorcycle crashes. Relationship to helmet use laws. *Journal of the American Medical Association*, **264**, 2395–2399.

Sparedo, F.R. and Gill, D. (1989) Effects of prior alcohol use on head injury recovery. *Journal of Head Trauma Rehabilitation*, **4**, 75–82.

Sullivan, S.J., Richer, E. and Laurents, F. (1990) Programme development. The role of and possibilities for physical conditioning programmes in the rehabilitation of traumatically brain-injured persons. *Brain Injury*, **4**, 407–414.

Sullivan, T., Conine, T.A., Goodman, M. and Mackie, T. (1988) Serial casting to prevent equinis in acute traumatic head injury. *Physiotherapy Canada*, **40**, 346–350.

Tabary, J.C., Tabary, C., Tardieu, C. *et al.* (1972) Physiological and structural changes in the cat's soleus muscle due to immobilization at different lengths by plaster cast. *Journal of Physiology (London)*, **224**, 231–244.

Tabary, J.C., Tardieu, C., Tardieu, G. *et al.* (1976) Functional adaptation of sarcomere number of normal cat muscle. *Journal de Physiologie (Paris)*, **72**, 277.

Tabary, J., Tardieu, C., Tardieu, G. and Tabary, C. (1981) Experimental rapid sarcomere loss with concomitant hypoextensibility. *Muscle and Nerve*, **4**, 198–203.

Teasdale, G. and Jennett, B. (1974) Assessment of coma and impaired consciousness. *Lancet*, **ii**, 81–84.

Tornheim, P.A., Prioleau, G.R. and McLaurin, R.L. (1984) Acute responses to experimental blunt head trauma: topography of cerebral cortical edema. *Journal of Neurosurgery*, **61**, 695–699.

Wade, D.T. and Langton Hewer, R. (1987) Epidemiology of some neurological diseases with special reference to work load on the NHS. *International Rehabilitation Medicine*, **8**, 129–137.

Walsh, K. (1985) *Understanding Brain Damage: A Primer of Neurophysiological Examination*, Churchill Livingstone, Edinburgh.

Wasserman, R.C. and Buccini, R.V. (1990) Helmet protection from head injuries among recreational bicyclists. *American Journal of Sports Medicine*, **18**, 96–97.

White, M.J. and Davies, T.M. (1984) The effects of immobilization after lower leg fractures on the contractile properties of human triceps surae. *Clinical Science*, **66**, 277–282.

Whyte, J. and Rosenthal, M. (1993) Rehabilitation of the patient with traumatic brain injury. In *Rehabilitation Medicine: Principles and Practice* (ed. J.A. DeLisa) 2nd edn, J.B. Lippincott Company, Philadelphia, pp. 825–860.

Williams, P.E. (1990) Use of intermittent stretch in the prevention of serial sarcomere loss in immobilized muscles. *Annals of the Rheumatic Diseases*, **47**, 316–317.

Williams, P.E. and Goldspink, G. (1973) The effect of immobilization on the longitudinal growth of striated muscle fibres. *Journal of Anatomy*, **116**, 45–55.

Wilson, B.A. (1995) Management and remediation of memory problems in brain-injured adults. In *Handbook of Memory Disorders* (eds A.D. Baddeley, B.A. Wilson and F.N. Watts) John Wiley and Sons, New York, pp. 451–479.

Winstein, C.J. (1983) Neurogenic dysphagia, frequency, progression and outcome in adults following head injury. *Physical Therapy*, **63**, 1992–1996.

Wood, R.L. (1987a) *Brain Injury Rehabilitation: A Neurobehavioural Approach*, Croom Helm, London.

Wood, R.L. (1987b) Neurophysiological assessment in brain injury rehabilitation. In *Advances in Rehabilitation* (ed. M.G. Eisenberg) Springer, New York.

Wood, R.L. (1991) Critical analysis of the concept of sensory stimulation for patients in vegetative states. *Brain Injury*, **5**, 401–409.

Yarkony, G.M. and Sahgal, V. (1987) Contracture: a major complication of craniocerebral trauma. *Clinical Orthopaedics*, **219**, 93–96.

Ylvisaker, M. and Urbanczyk, B. (1994) Assessment and treatment of speech, swallowing and communication disorders following traumatic brain injury. In *Brain Injury Rehabilitation: Clinical Considerations* (eds M.A.J. Finlayson and S.H. Garner) Williams and Wilkins, Baltimore, MD, pp. 157–186.

Zencius, A., Wesolowiski, M.D., Burke, W.H. and Hough, S. (1990) Managing hypersexual disorders in brain injured clients. *Brain Injury*, **4**, 175–181.

Further reading

Adams, R. (1990) Attention control training and behaviour management. In *Key Issues in Neurological Physiotherapy* (eds L. Ada and C. Canning), Butterworth-Heinemann, Oxford, pp. 81–97.

Baddeley, A.D., Wilson, B.A. and Watts, F.N. (1995) *Handbook of Memory Disorders*. John Wiley, New York.

Ben-Yishay, Y. and Prigatano, G.P. (1990) Cognitive remediation. In *Rehabilitation of the Adult and Child with Traumatic Brain Injury* (eds M. Rosenthal, M.R. Bond, E.R. Griffith and J.D. Miller), 2nd edn, F.A. Davis, Philadelphia, pp. 393–409.

Diller, L. and Ben-Yishay, Y. (1987) Outcomes and evidence in neuropsychological rehabilitation in closed head injury. In *Neurobehavioural Recovery from Head Injury* (eds H.S. Levin, J. Graffman and H.M. Eisenberg), Oxford University Press, New York, pp. 146–165.

Knight, R.G. and Godfrey, P.D. (1995) Behavioural and self-report methods. In *Handbook of Memory Disorders* (eds. A.D. Baddeley, B.A. Wilson and F.N. Watts) John Wiley, New York, pp. 393–410.

Lezak, M.D. (1995) *Neurophysiological Assessment*, 3rd edn, Oxford University Press, New York.

Sullivan, A.E., Jankowski, L.W., Fleury, J. *et al.* (1995) Screening of health factors prior to exercise or a fitness evaluation of adults with traumatic brain injury: a consenus by rehabilitation professionals. *Brain Injury*, **10**, 367–375.

Wood, R.L. and Burgess, P.W. (1987) The physiological management of disorders of behaviour. In *Rehabilitation of the Severely Brain Injured Adult: A Practical Approach* (eds I. Fussey and G. Giles), Croom Helm, London, pp. 43–68.

13

Parkinson's disease

Introduction

The **basal ganglia** are made up of five large and well connected subcortical nuclei: the caudate nucleus, putamen, globus pallidus, subthalamic nucleus and substantia nigra, which participate in the control of movement. These ganglia do not make direct output to or receive input from the spinal cord. Their primary input is from the cerebral cortex and their output is directed through the thalamus back to the prefrontal, premotor and motor cortices (Fig. 13.1). Diseases which affect the basal ganglia produce characteristic types of motor dysfunction: tremor and other involuntary movements; poverty and slowness of movement without paralysis; and changes in muscle tone and posture. Two nuclei – the caudate nucleus and the putamen – are together called the neostriatum.

Almost all afferent connections to the basal ganglia terminate in the neostriatum, the major input being from the entire cerebral cortex (Côté and Crutcher 1991). The substantia nigra is made up of two zones, a ventral pale zone, the pars reticulata, and a dorsal, darkly pigmented zone, the pars compacta. The globus pallidus together with the pars reticulata comprise the major output nuclei of the basal ganglia, projections going to three nuclei in the thalamus which in turn project to the prefrontal cortex, premotor cortex, the supplementary motor cortex and the motor cortex.

The role of the basal ganglia in movement control remains unclear despite anatomical studies (e.g., Schell and Strick 1984; Parent 1990), cerebral blood flow studies (e.g., Roland et al. 1980, 1982; Seitz and Roland 1992), single cell recordings in conscious animals (e.g., Tanji and Kurata 1985; Brotchie et al. 1991a,b) and clinical studies (e.g., Schwab et al. 1954; Talland and Schwab 1964). It is now clear from anatomical studies that the motor component of the basal ganglia is incorporated in a loop originating in the motor sensory cortex and terminating in the supplementary motor area (SMA) and premotor area. The basal ganglia are considered to be involved in higher-order aspects of motor control; i.e., the planning and execution of complex motor performance. It appears that the SMA and the basal ganglia may work together to run well-learned and predictable movement sequences. Based on the numerous inputs from virtually all areas of the cerebral cortex to the basal ganglia, it has been speculated that the basal ganglia may

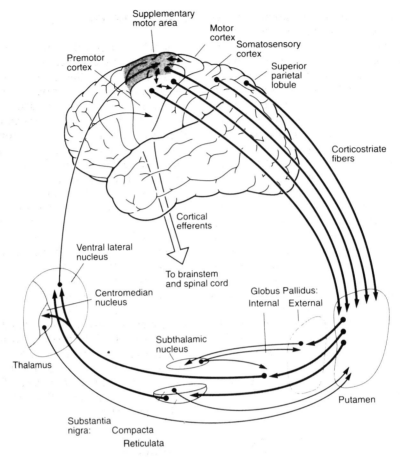

Fig. 13.1 The motor circuit of the basal ganglia is a subcortical feedback loop from the motor and somatosensory areas of the cortex, through restricted portions of the basal ganglia and thalamus, and back to the premotor cortex, supplementary motor area and motor cortex, all of which have direct descending projections to brain stem motor centres and the spinal cortex. (Reprinted from Kandel, E.R., Schwartz, J.H. and Jessell, T.M. (eds.) (1991) *Principles of Neural Science*, 3rd edn, Appleton and Lange, Norwalk, CT, by permission)

also be involved in many functions besides motor control.

Motor disturbances in diseases of the basal ganglia characteristically produce either excessive movements or diminished movement (Wichmann and DeLong 1993). A major breakthrough in understanding how basal ganglia dysfunction may lead to either excessive movements as in Huntington's disease or to reduced movement (akinesia) in Parkinson's disease has come from the finding that there are two pathways that mediate striatal influences over activity of the thalamocortical neurons: a direct pathway that tends to facilitate ongoing motor behaviour and an indirect pathway that dampens motor activity (Goldman-Rakic and Selemon 1990). Excessive involuntary movements

are characterized by: tremor (rhythmic, oscillatory), athetosis (writhing movements), chorea (abrupt movements of the limbs and facial muscles), and ballismus (wild swinging movements of the limbs). Diminished movement is characterized by: dystonia (a persistent posture of the body which can result in distorted alignment of the body) and poverty and slowness of movement without paralysis.

Parkinson's disease (paralysis agitans) is the most common disease affecting the basal ganglia and is the major subject of this chapter. The clinical features of other diseases of the basal ganglia, e.g., Huntington's disease and Wilson's disease, can be found in general neurology texts (e.g., Walton 1993).

Parkinsonism is a clinical syndrome characterized by a disorder of movement consisting of tremor, rigidity, elements of bradykinesia (slowness of movement), hypokinesia (reduced excursion of movement) and akinesia (slowness in initiating movement and loss of spontaneous movement) and postural abnormalities (e.g., Marsden 1994). **Parkinson's disease** (PD) consists of the clinical syndrome of parkinsonism associated with a distinctive pathology. It was James Parkinson (1817) who first described the 'shaking palsy' which now bears his name. Since then the site of neurologic degeneration that results in PD has been identified but the aetiology of the disease is still unknown (idiopathic PD). Over the past two to three decades a change in the understanding of the pathogenesis and treatment of PD has followed new concepts of biochemical and physiological function. There are many other diseases that present with clinical features of parkinsonism and these are commonly referred to as causing a secondary form of PD. These include 'senile' parkinsonism, post-encephalitic parkinsonism and vascular parkinsonism (Jellinger 1987).

PD is the third most common neurologic disease. It is a slowly progressive degenerative disease that affects some 1 in 1000 of the population, both men and women (Marsden 1994) and 1 in 100 people over 75 (Schoenberg 1987). The age of onset is variable with a mean average onset of 58 years when it becomes clinically obvious but younger individuals are not exempt. Incidence in those over the age of 50 rises exponentially. Recent epidemiological community-based data suggest that PD may be more prevalent in Europe and North America compared with some other countries, notably China and Africa (Tanner 1989).

PD was the first disease to be identified as a molecular disease (Côté and Crutcher 1991). In the late 1950s, Carlsson (1959) observed that 80% of the dopamine in the brain is localized in the basal ganglia, an area that contributes to less than 0.5% of the total brain weight. Not long after this, Hornykiewicz (1966), on post mortem examination, found that dopamine was drastically reduced in patients with PD and that a specific defect in transmitter metabolism was shown to have a causal role in the disease. These findings led to the development of replacement therapy. Prior to these advances, PD progressed relentlessly and was a cause of miserable disability (Hoehn and Yahr 1967).

Pathophysiology

Neurochemically, PD is characterized by a disturbance of the central dopaminergic pathway from the substantia nigra to the striatum (Agid *et al.* 1990). In addition to a reduction of dopamine, PD is characterized by neural loss and depigmentation of the substantia nigra at the pars compacta level and the locus coeruleus with consequent changes to neural conduction in the nigrostriatal pathway. Neural degeneration is also evident at the raphe nuclei, and within the motor nucleus of the vagus. Approximately 80% of nigrostriatal dopaminergic neurons are lost before symptoms become noticeable (Korman and James 1993). In 80% of cases, Lewy bodies (intracytoplasmic inclusions) may be observed at both cortical and spinal cord levels but are not specifically indicative of PD. The severity of changes in the substantia nigra parallels the reduction of dopamine in the striatum (Côté and Crutcher 1991). Although the loss of striatal dopamine is considered to account for most of the symptoms in PD, there is also depletion of noradrenergic neurons in the locus coeruleus and serotonergic neurons in the raphe nuclei (Marsden 1990; Côté and Crutcher 1991). Cortical changes are more widespread than previously thought (Marsden 1994).

Aetiology

Although about 15% of individuals with PD have a close relative with the disease (Marsden 1990), inheritance does not appear to be a major factor in its aetiology. Observations of a clinical illness similar to PD produced by a substance containing a highly toxic contaminent to the dopaminergic neurons in the substantia nigra, has suggested that an environmental toxin may play a role in the development of the disease. However, no such toxic agent has been identified (Tanner 1989). Another explanation is that the individual may have been exposed to a toxin early in life, even in utero, that caused subclinical nigral damage. Alternatively, there may be an inherited inability to deal with such a toxin (Marsden 1990). The additional effect of normal nigral ageing may subsequently cause a large enough nigral depletion to result in PD later in life (Calne and Langston 1983).

Diagnosis is primarily clinical and is based on medical history and physical examination. It is now thought that patients with PD may have a long preclinical or asymptomatic period (Korman and James 1993). Although there are no 'markers' for the preclinical phase of PD, positron emission tomography (PET) is being used to determine striatal dopamine concentrations which may indicate an increased likehood of presymptomatic PD. This finding of decreased dopamine concentration, however, is not specific to the disease (Langston and Koller 1991).

Clinical signs

Hughlings Jackson (1932) divided all motor disorders into two classes: positive signs or release phenomena, caused by abnormal patterns of action in neurons when their controlling input is impaired, and negative signs attributed to the loss of function of specific neurons. In PD, rigidity and tremor represent positive signs resulting from release of the brain mechanisms normally inhibited by the basal ganglia, whereas akinesia is the major negative feature representing lack of movement and bradykinesia representing slowness in initiating and carrying out motor acts (Marsden 1982).

Tremor is defined most simply as the rhythmic, mechanical oscillation of a body part. By convention, tremor is classified by the behavioural situation in which it occurs, regardless of the underlying mechanism (Findley 1988). Tremor at rest is a cardinal sign of PD and is often the first sign of the disease (Marsden 1994). Several types of tremor can coexist within the parkinsonian syndrome, including enhanced physiological tremor, essential tremor and writing tremor. EMG recordings of tremor at rest show rhythmic activity alternating in antagonistic muscles at frequencies between 3.5 and 7 Hz (Shahani and Young 1976). EMG recordings can display variations in frequency between upper and lower limbs and between the two upper limbs. In some instances EMG recordings have been shown to change to synchronous discharge (Delwaide and Gonce 1988). Tremor activity is usually suppressed by willed activity, sleep and complete relaxation.

Although the origin of the resting tremor is still disputed, it appears that it results from oscillations in a hyperactive long loop reflex pathway, triggered by an endogenous mechanism at the thalamic level which is influenced by peripheral afferents, chiefly the 1A afferents (Delwaide and Gonce 1988).

Rigidity is characterized by increased stiffness throughout range of passive movement at a joint. This stiffness has the same intensity in both extensor and flexor muscles and may be regularly interrupted at a 5–6 Hz frequency by the cogwheel phenomenon, a result of rigidity superimposed on, or interrupted by tremor. The degree of rigidity is relatively independent of stretch velocity. In some instances, however, the resistance to stretch is inversely proportional to velocity, being greatest when movement is slow.

The degree of rigidity is not necessarily constant, stiffness being reinforced by stress, anxiety and movement of a contralateral limb or in a standing rather than a seated individual. The major cause of rigidity in PD is thought to be excessive and uncontrollable supraspinal drive to the α-motor neurons (Marsden 1982). There are currently two major theoretical explanations: the first suggests that spinal mechanisms are modified by abnormal control of some interneurons; the second proposes hyperactivity in the long loop reflex pathways, probably in the cortex (Delwaide and Gonce 1988).

Mechanical changes in the muscles have also been shown to contribute to resistance to passive movement, particularly in more severe cases (Dietz *et al*. 1981; Watts *et al*. 1986; Dietz *et al*. 1988). Rigidity is taken to indicate the operation of the remaining intact motor systems and offers little insight into the normal function of the basal ganglia (Marsden 1982). It has also been proposed that rigidity may be partly due to adaptive behaviour (Horak *et al*. 1992).

Akinesia is the most disabling manifestation of PD. According to Delwaide and Gonce (1988), akinesia includes a complex variety of motor deficits not all of which can be measured objectively: slow performance of voluntary movement (bradykinesia) which can be measured by the time required to perform a simple stereotyped movement (e.g., Evarts *et al*. 1981); difficulty reaching a target with a single continuous movement (hypokinesia), i.e., reduced excursion of movement, the movement stopping and starting to reach the intended object; delayed initiation of movement possibly reflected in prolonged action time (e.g., Flowers 1976; Evarts *et al*. 1981); rapid fatigue with repetitive movement; and difficulty in both executing simultaneous actions (Talland and Schwab 1964) and sequential movements (Hallett and Khoshbin 1980).

Akinesia affects the performance of all motor actions and their associated postural adjustments (e.g., reaching and manipulation, body transport), and articulation and phonation. Furthermore, the individual with PD demonstrates a loss of spontaneous movements easily recognized by reduced facial expression and reduced arm swing during gait.

Little is known about the mechanisms responsible for the various manifestations of akinesia, which may evolve largely independently and are not necessarily present in a given individual, largely because the role of the basal ganglia in normal movement remains unclear. Furthermore, the effect of therapeutic intervention may vary with the component of akinesia. For example, levodopa has been found to reduce movement time more than reaction time (Delwaide and Gonce 1988).

The *freezing phenomenon*, difficulty in starting or continuing rhythmic repetitive movements such as speech, handwriting and gait, is a well-known and incapacitating problem in PD. Several investigators have suggested that freezing should be considered a distinct clinical sign of PD and independent of akinesia (Narabayashi and Nakamura 1985; Achiron *et al.* 1993). The neural mechanism responsible for freezing remains unclear. It particularly affects gait, patients typically experiencing freezing when walking through an enclosed space or when turning (Giladi *et al.* 1992). The feet appear to get stuck to the floor while momentum carries the centre of body mass forward, with an increasing likelihood of falls as postural adjustments are impaired. Giladi and colleagues (1992) have suggested the use of a broad term 'motor blocks' to characterize all sudden episodes of freezing, breaks in motion and hesitation when switching from one movement to another. The clinical evaluation of motor blocks is difficult because of variability both within and between individuals and the relationship of blocks to time of drug ingestion.

Classification

One of the difficulties in getting a clear and consistent picture of the nature of the movement deficits in PD is that there is no uniform method of classifying the stage of the disease. Furthermore, differences can be observed in the same subject when tested at different times of the day or when subjects are asked to withhold their drugs for a period of time prior to testing (Evarts *et al.* 1981). Despite the variability within and between patients, there have been several attempts to classify the degree and extent of clinical disability in PD. Two commonly utilized scales (Hoehn and Yahr 1967; Webster 1968) are included in Chapter

3. These scales are essential to document clinical disability at the onset of treatment and the rate of progression. Pearce (1992) provides a summary of other scales in clinical use.

Motor control and motor performance deficits

A decline in function may occur even before a diagnosis of PD is established. Early symptoms may be vague and non-specific, such as inexplicable tiredness, unwarranted fatiguability and mild muscular aches and cramps, all potentially contributing to increasing incapacity (Stern and Lees 1991). Depression may compound the situation and may influence the individual's participation in activities. As the disease progresses, clinical signs and symptoms, including tremor, which may result in spills of drinks and food, speech difficulties, diminished facial expression and the possibility of drooling may lead to embarrassing and upsetting incidents causing the individual to feel socially unacceptable and isolated. Difficulty in initiating movement such as in gait and 'freezing' on a social outing may compromise independence and confidence.

Individuals with PD have been studied performing meaningful tasks in an attempt to add insight into the role of the basal ganglia in motor control. Since these studies illustrate the motor control deficits as well as motor performance deficits, the findings should assist the physiotherapy clinician to understand these and to develop and test more scientifically based intervention strategies. Studies typically involve the investigation of reaction time (RT), movement time (MT) and the ability to perform simultaneous or sequential movements.

Reaction time and movement time

Patients with PD undoubtedly have difficulty initiating movement. In 1925, Wilson reported delayed RT in a patient with unilateral parkinsonism when asked to sit up from a supine position by using dynamometers to record contraction of the rectus femoris. More recently, Evarts and colleagues (1981) reported a high degree of variability in RT between patients and within the same individual at different times in a simple pronation/supination arm movement. The authors reported that, although in general RT and MT were prolonged in PD, overall, MT was more severely affected than RT. The degree of slowing in simple movements, however, is often not correlated with the degree of clinical akinesia (Berardelli *et al.* 1986; Benecke *et al.* 1986).

Execution of sequential movements

The generalized movement slowing seen in PD is characterized clinically by slowness of both simple single joint ballistic movements which usually undershoot (Hallett and Khoshbin 1980) and movement sequences (Benecke *et al.* 1987). It has been suggested that slowness of movement may be more marked for movement sequences performed automatically (Schwab *et al.* 1954).

Many of the critical everyday actions that individuals with PD have difficulty in performing, such as sit-to-stand (Fig 13.2) and walking, are made up of sequential movements. In a series of studies,

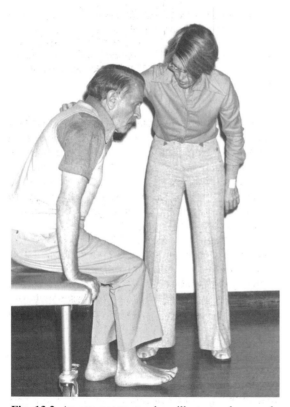

Fig. 13.2 An attempt to stand up illustrates decreased amplitude of trunk flexion at the hips and dorsiflexion at the ankles. He has difficulty initiating horizontal momentum and changing from the horizontal to vertical sequence of the action. Note he has not moved his right foot back

Benecke and colleagues (1987) demonstrated that movement sequences are slower in patients with PD compared with normal subjects. When patients performed sequential movements, not only were the individual movements slower than normal but the interval when switching between the two sequences was also prolonged. Georgiou and colleagues (1993) suggest that the greater severity of deficit with movement sequences compared with individual movements, may arise from the decrease in amplitude and velocity of each component the further down the sequence it is produced. In their study, PD subjects were greatly affected by the length of the individual sub-movements especially in the absence of external cues.

Execution of simultaneous movements

Patients with PD not only have difficulty in executing a motor plan involving sequential motor acts but also in carrying out a plan involving simultaneous motor acts. A striking clinical feature of PD is the difficulty experienced when attempting to perform two motor tasks at the same time. Schwab and colleagues (1954) provided several graphic descriptions of the difficulty PD individuals have in performing simultaneous movements. For example, an individual reported that 'when walking across the hotel lobby in front of the usual number of strangers to pay his bill, he reached into his inside pocket with his left hand to get his wallet. At once he stopped walking, standing immobile before the strangers. Becoming aware of this, he then resumed walking but his left hand remained in his inside pocket, suggesting perhaps a planned holdup.'

Schwab and colleagues (1954) had patients with PD draw lines perpendicular to the midpoint of each side of a triangle with the dominant hand while squeezing the bulb of an ergometer with the other hand. Able-bodied subjects were able to perform these two acts simultaneously with ease whereas this ability was lost or impaired in the PD subjects who tended to make sequential movements by performing first one task then the other.

In an attempt to elucidate further the deficit in performing simultaneous movements, Benecke and colleagues (1986) had PD subjects perform several simple movements as rapidly as possible and then combine these – for example, squeeze an isometric force transducer and flex the elbow. Movement times for each simple movement were slower than able-bodied subjects. This appeared to be due to a failure to deliver a large enough initial burst of agonist EMG activity. When two movements were combined, there was a further slowing of the movement seen in an increase in MT.

The extra slowness found in both sequential and simultaneous movements has been reported to be closely related to the degree of clinically evaluated akinesia and conventional neurological examination (Benecke *et al.* 1986). Akinesia was evaluated on time taken to complete a pegboard task and the number of touches between thumb and finger in a specified time.

The underlying mechanisms responsible for the motor deficits in PD remain unclear. These mechanisms appear to fall into two categories: deficits in the planning of movement, referred to as disorders of the motor plan, motor programme or motor set; problems with muscle activation, which include an inability to produce and time appropriately a certain magnitude of force and inability to produce force consistently for any particular movement (Sheridan and Flowers 1990); and the relationship between these two mechanisms. One function of the basal ganglia may be the provision of internal cues for the performance of well-learned activities or movement sequences (Phillips *et al.* 1993; Morris *et al.* 1995).

The *performance deficits* in PD have been studied in several actions critical to independence – gait, postural adjustments and reach-to-grasp as well as respiratory and oromotor function.

Gait

The most frequently observed gait disorders are slowness of movement and difficulty in initiation. The individual with PD is observed to walk with short, shuffling steps (marche á petit pas), uneven step lengths, a typical flexed posture (Fig. 13.3), reduced movement of the arms and decreased angular displacement of the lower limb joints (Knutsson 1972; Murray *et al.* 1978; Forssberg *et al.* 1984; Blin *et al.* 1990, 1991). These problems tend to become more severe as the disease progresses and are associated with a loss of independence and an increased incidence of falls. Freezing, either in the initiation of or during gait, is also commonly observed and has been found to be particularly evident on turning or in narrow spaces, i.e., context-dependent (Stern *et al.* 1980; Giladi *et al.* 1992). In addition to a shuffling and frozen gait, festination, i.e., an involuntary increase in velocity with a decrease in amplitude of motion, may also be observed in some individuals.

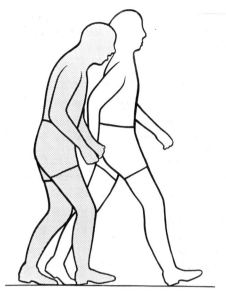

Fig. 13.3 Illustration of a man with Parkinson's disease (shaded) showing relatively flexed posture compared with an able-bodied man at the point of heel contact of the right lower limb. (From Murray, M.P., Sepic, S.B., Gardner, G.M. *et al.* (1978) Walking patterns of men with Parkinsonism. *American Journal of Physical Medicine*, **57**, 278–294, by permission)

Typically, investigations into the gait of individuals with PD have been concerned with describing the deficits in relation to able-bodied subjects, the change in deficits before and after medication, and with and without visual cues. The results of many of these studies have been used in an attempt to determine the role of the basal ganglia in movement organization.

Attempts to quantify gait deficits in PD (Knutsson 1972; Stern *et al.* 1983; Forssberg *et al.* 1984; Blin *et al.* 1990; Wall and Turnbull 1992) have typically found slowness in gait to be associated with decreased stride length, decreased cadence and an increase in the proportion of time spent in double support phase (DS).

In a series of studies with PD subjects and age-matched controls, Morris and colleagues (1994a,b) examined the relationship between walking velocity, cadence and stride length. The authors found that, although PD subjects could vary their gait velocity similar to controls, when speed of walking was controlled, stride length was shorter and cadence higher in these subjects than in control subjects. An increase in stride length could be achieved only in the presence of an external visual cue. The authors suggest that an increase in cadence for any given velocity in PD is a compensation for difficulty in regulating stride length.

Morris and colleagues also found that both PD subjects and age-matched controls showed an increase in the time spent in DS compared with younger subjects. The duration of DS when matched for speed of walking, however, was not significantly different between PD subjects and their age-matched controls. Since DS is considered to be the most stable phase of the gait cycle, this finding may reflect balance deficits and reduced vigour, older subjects spending a longer time in the 'safer' DS phase. Although it could be expected that the semiflexed posture associated with PD would affect gait parameters, there has been as yet no investigation of this.

Reach-to-grasp

Numerous normative studies of the reach-to-grasp movement have shown that the movement consists of two components, the transport or reach component, and the manipulation or grasp component. Both components are activated in parallel. Castiello and colleagues (1993) studied the reach-to-grasp movement in both PD and control subjects. The reach was either 15, 27.5 or 40 cm while the grasp was of a small (0.7 cm) or a large (8 cm) dowel. Analysis of the movement in PD subjects showed a slowed MT but, similar to able-bodied controls, the PD subjects had no difficulty in regulating the spatiotemporal characteristics of the movement related to changes in object distance or size. However, for the PD subjects, it was the coordination of the two components that showed abnormality in that the onset of the grasp component was delayed in relation to the onset of the transport component. In another study (Castiello *et al.* 1994), which involved reaching to grasp a glass filled with water and take it to the lips in order to take a sip, control subjects showed no transition phase between the two movements. On the other hand, PD subjects showed a transition phase in 38% of trials of, on average 337 msec or 7% of movement time. Difficulty in the transition phase has also been reported by Muller and Abbs (1990).

Postural adjustments

Postural instability is considered a major contributor to the disability associated with PD. Clinically, it is evident that people with PD lose their balance more easily and have an increased incidence of falls (Dick *et al.* 1986; Schieppati and Nardone 1991). A disturbance of standing posture has long been considered a characteristic of PD (Martin 1967) and it has been argued that the basal ganglia are primarily responsible for the automatic execution of learned motor plans (Marsden 1982).

The underlying mechanism of the postural instability is not, however, clear. Studies of PD patients' standing balance under different conditions have so far produced variable results, perhaps reflecting differences in the tasks investigated, the timing of testing in relation to ingestion of medication, the changing clinical status and each individual's adaptive behaviour.

Hypotheses regarding reasons for postural instability can be broadly categorized in two groups: (1) alterations in central responsiveness or defective utilization of sensory inputs; (2) defects in central programming, deficits including: the inability to make rapid, accurately coordinated postural responses due to slowed reaction and movement times, i.e., bradykinesia or akinesia (Berardelli *et al.* 1984); reduced amplitude of muscle activation (Hallett and Khoshbin 1980); and defective sensorimotor integration preventing flexible adaptation in various environments (Bronstein *et al.* 1990; Schieppati and Nardone 1991). Impaired reflex function results in difficulty compensating for unexpected perturbations and, therefore, instability, with a greater reliance on vision and other attentional processes as a consequence. However, it is also considered that changes in muscle properties and the person's own adaptive behaviour may play a part in the variations in postural adjustments seen in PD patients when they are compared with able-bodied individuals. Changes in muscle stiffness, for example in gastrocnemius muscle, have been suggested to underlie abnormalities in gait (Dietz *et al.* 1981) and the relatively slow ankle joint displacement and velocity observable in support surface perturbation studies.

What is clear, however, is that the inability to make appropriate postural adjustments (i.e., task- and context-specific muscle activations related to balancing the body mass) is deficient in any individual with a primary motor control problem. Instability is due both to abnormal coordination resulting from the brain impairment and to secondary adaptations (both behavioural and soft tissue).

Postural adjustments are generally considered to occur both in response to external (e.g., support surface) perturbations and before and during a volitional movement as an integral part of the action (see Chapter 7). Much of the research into postural instability in PD has involved studies of PD subjects standing on a movable support surface in order to test postural 'reflex' activity and tests of rapid arm raising in standing individuals. The perturbation studies provide information related to the ability of PD patients, at various clinical stages, to act in responsive ('reactive') mode. The fast arm raising studies provide information particularly related to the presence and timing of preparatory postural adjustments. Recently, the findings of studies of more typical everyday tasks have been reported which provide information about the integration of postural adjustments with volitional movements during complex actions performed at their natural velocities.

The location of the centre of foot pressure (CFP) in relation to the body mass in standing will affect the postural muscle activations occurring during both volitional and responsive movement. Given the *flexed posture* typical of individuals with PD (Fig. 13.4), it is interesting that, in the group of people studied by Schieppati and Nardone (1991), the CFP was found to be shifted backward in less severe cases and forward in the more severe. The

authors suggested that, since maintaining the centre of body mass further back than normal is potentially destabilizing, causing the individual to overbalance backward, the movement of CFP forward (by flexing at the hips and and trunk) may be an adaptive response to maintain balance.

Studies of *postural sway* during quiet standing have generally shown that postural sway oscillations are similar to those of able-bodied subjects whether eyes are open or closed (Bronstein *et al.* 1990; Schieppati and Nardone 1991). However, a recent study of eight individuals with PD (Horak *et al.* 1992) has suggested an abnormally small postural sway area in this group compared with both young and elderly control subjects. This small sway excursion may reflect increased intrinsic musculoskeletal stiffness (Dietz *et al.* 1988). It may also be an adaptation in which the individual stands stiffly, as immobile as possible, in an attempt to avoid overbalancing by limiting movement of the centre of body mass.

One of the possible reasons for poor balance in standing could be an inability to make relevant and appropriately timed *preparatory (or anticipatory) postural adjustments* (muscle activations). Preparatory postural adjustments have been studied in PD patients in relation to several different tasks. A study of rising on tip-toes (Diener *et al.* 1990), which included individuals with PD and age-matched able-bodied subjects, showed that the order of onsets for both groups of subjects was tibialis anterior (to move body mass forward), quadriceps femoris (to stabilize the knee) followed by triceps surae to execute the heel-raising action. Tibialis anterior and quadriceps were active prior to the target movement as preparatory postural adjustments. Although the subjects with PD showed this same basic pattern of muscle activations, the action was performed more slowly and the build-up of muscle tension appeared slower.

Preparatory adjustments have also been investigated by having PD subjects raise one or both arms fast in standing (Bazalgette *et al.* 1986; Dick *et al.* 1986; Rogers *et al.* 1987). Most notably, in one study postural muscle activations in the PD subjects were not specific to the action, i.e., they were the same whether one arm or two was raised (Bazalgette *et al.* 1986). This is in contrast to the pattern of adjustments in the able-bodied subjects, which varied according to task.

Some studies have reported similar muscle latencies to normal. Others have noted delays in agonist onsets of postural muscles (Rogers *et al.* 1987). One

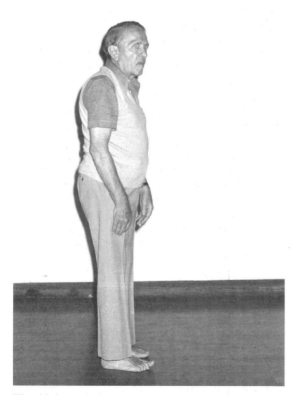

Fig. 13.4 A relatively flexed posture in standing

difficulty in investigating and comparing preparatory postural adjustments is the slowness of movement typical of PD. Such adjustments are known in able-bodied individuals to be particularly evident prior to fast movement (such as arm raising) but not necessarily so when movements are slow. Hence, although preparatory muscle activations have been reported as absent or different from the able-bodied in studies of individuals with PD, this result may have been due to the relative slowness of arm movement compared with able-bodied subjects (Bazalgette *et al*. 1986; Rogers *et al*. 1987).

Evidence that PD individuals have difficulty preparing for an upcoming self-initiated perturbation comes from a study of a bimanual load-lifting task (Viallet *et al*. 1987). Subjects held a 1 kg weight in one hand, with elbow flexed to 90°. When the load was lifted off the hand, either by the investigator or by the subject, the elbow flexed after the unloading and the brachioradialis muscle showed less inhibition than in the group of able-bodied subjects. These findings indicate a relative lack in the regulation of force in response to the changing requirements of the action.

Several studies have investigated the response of subjects with PD to *unexpected externally-induced support surface perturbations* as they stand on a movable platform. The latencies of muscle activations in response to the platform movement have been shown to be similar to those of able-bodied subjects (Dichgans *et al*. 1985; Schieppati and Nardone 1991). Responses tend, however, to be more variable than normal (Schieppati and Nardone 1991).

Several studies have employed rotational platform perturbations which project the individual into a toe-up position as a means of testing postural 'reflexes' (Scholz *et al*. 1987; Beckley *et al*. 1991). Able-bodied subjects, standing on a movable platform tilted to produce a toe-up movement, show short and medium latency electrophysiological responses in the stretched calf muscles (gastrocnemius) and long latency responses in the shortened anterior tibial muscles. The gastrocnemius response would be destabilizing, projecting the subject backward and the anterior tibial activation would be stabilizing/restorative (Nashner 1977). However, in subjects with PD, enhanced amplitudes of medium latency responses have been found (Scholz *et al*. 1987) and the activation sequence of long latency responses reversed (Horak *et al*. 1984). In another study (Beckley *et al*. 1991), whereas able-bodied subjects used a so-called 'ankle strategy' in which tibialis anterior

was active prior to vastus lateralis as a means of regaining the vertical position, PD subjects reversed this order and stiffened the knee. The authors pointed out that, although this stiffening could contribute to postural instability, the initial posture of the subjects would have affected the results by requiring a different motor pattern. The early activation of the more proximal muscles linking thigh and shank (and perhaps other muscles linking trunk and thigh which were not monitored) may also indicate an adaptive stiffening of the limb to counter the perturbation.

More recently, a study of PD individuals (Horak *et al*. 1992) showed similar latencies in both gastrocnemius and tibialis anterior in response to backward and forward platform translations respectively. However, excessive antagonistic activity was noted. These findings illustrate a functionally inappropriate response to this novel task and such abnormalities would be expected to cause instability in real world unexpected situations. Even on levodopa, individuals with PD appear to lack flexible adaptation to changing support surface conditions in standing (Horak *et al*. 1992). These abnormalities would be expected to change over time in a progressive disease and this has been illustrated in a study of 10 PD subjects (5 subjects: Hoehn and Yahr stage III; 5 subjects: Hoehn and Yahr stage IV) (Beckley *et al*. 1991). An enhanced medium latency response was found and a reversed order of activation in only one person in stage III but in 4 subjects in stage IV.

It is not clear, therefore, whether difficulties with balance reflect increased intrinsic stiffness of muscle to dampen body sway (Woollacott *et al*. 1988), or inability to activate muscles with enough force or speed to respond automatically to a perturbation or to anticipate a forthcoming perturbation. It may also be that patients adapt to their inability to generate sufficiently fast muscle activations by self-limiting behaviours such as holding the body stiffly (note the increased activation of antagonists in Horak and colleagues' findings) and by decreasing the excursion of the body mass movement and decreasing destabilization by moving very slowly (e.g., flexing the body at trunk and lower limb joints in standing or taking small shuffling steps when walking).

The view is commonly expressed that PD individuals can generate appropriate postural muscle activation patterns and seem to be able to improve balance control by relying more than usual upon conscious effort, utilizing visual information and other external cues (Waterston *et al*.

1993). It may be that these individuals can use cognitive strategies (e.g., by concentrating attention on preparing for a movement) to override the defective mechanisms.

Respiratory function

Respiratory dysfunction is a common finding in individuals with PD (e.g.,Vincken *et al.* 1984). This dysfunction is thought to result from the motor control deficits associated with PD. The flexed posture and immobility generally associated with PD could also contribute to respiratory impairment and cardiovascular deconditioning. Patients with moderate to severe PD have been found to have both decreased work capacity and exercise efficiency on a similar level of external work compared with age-matched controls performing one-legged exercise (Saltin and Landin 1975). The authors concluded that general muscle weakness secondary to the neurological disorder may have led to these results. Inactivity could also be expected to contribute.

A recent study (Canning *et al.* 1997) examined the exercise capacity of subjects with mild to moderate PD in order to determine whether or not respiratory dysfunction and gait disorders affect exercise capacity. The results suggest that these individuals have the potential to maintain exercise capacity within normal limits for age with regular aerobic exercise.

Oromotor function

Swallowing and speech disorders are among the least studied effects of PD. Speech disorders have been found to be present in as many as 92% of patients (Martin *et al.* 1973) and include abnormal voice modulation (dysphonia), with hoarseness, decreased volume and monotonous tone (Robbins *et al.* 1986). Swallowing disorders have been reported to exist in as many as 50% of patients assessed by barium swallow (Lieberman *et al.* 1980). Radiography (Silbiger *et al.* 1967) and videofluoroscopy (Robbins *et al.* 1986) have demonstrated that abnormal oropharyngeal movement patterns and timing occur in both the initial or volitional stage as well as the pharyngeal stage of swallowing. Problems include tongue tremor, slowness in initiating the swallow, difficulty forming the bolus and propelling it backward to the posterior third of the tongue for stimulating the pharyngeal stage of swallowing, and disturbances in pharyngeal motility. Interestingly, Robbins and

colleagues (1986) found that aspiration was a problem in 33% of their subjects, yet they lacked awareness of aspiration which may explain why bronchopneumonia is a major cause of death in PD (Hoehn and Yahr 1967).

Adaptive motor behaviour

The human system is highly adaptive and the musculoskeletal periphery, being multisegmented, has the potential to produce a variety of alternate movement patterns in order to achieve a specific goal. Indeed, movement patterns appear to emerge from musculoskeletal flexibility, the goal of the task and the environmental context in which it is to be carried out (Shepherd and Carr 1991). Normally, individuals adapt the way they move in response to both internal and external circumstances, for example, favouring an unaffected leg when muscles are sore, avoiding bearing weight through the part of the sole that has a stone underneath, moving more slowly than usual when balance in threatened.

It is possible in individuals with PD that moving slowly (bradykinesia) may reflect in part an adaptation to the difficulty in activating muscles (including postural muscle activations); that freezing and resistance to externally-imposed movement may be adaptations that enable the individual to avoid perturbations for which it is difficult to prepare. Less than optimal motor performance may, therefore, be adaptive in the sense that it is an attempt to avoid failure in task performance. The view that altered motor patterns in PD may be adaptive rather than due to a primary disorder has recently been expressed by Latash and Anson (1996). Phillips and colleagues (1994) argue that PD bradykinesia, rather than being an inability to energize muscles (Hallett and Khoshbin 1980), may reflect a problem in specifying the appropriate rate of force production necessary for accurate movement. In investigations of targeted limb movements, it has been suggested that bradykinesia may enable greater variability and be a means of ensuring an acceptable level of accuracy (Sheriden and Flowers 1990); i.e., an adaptation rather than a primary deficit (Latash and Anson 1996).

The variability between subjects evident in studies of movement in subjects with PD may in part be due to the different adaptations developed by individuals as they attempt to function effectively despite their neural deficits.

Slowness of movement and rigidity of posture may reflect adaptations to the pathological postural reactions rather than primary deficits in themselves (Latash and Anson 1996). Individuals with PD may prefer safer options in order to avoid a total loss of control (see Muller and Abbs 1990, on precision grip tasks.

Future studies of individuals (single case studies) may elucidate this issue by examining and comparing the ability of individuals to perform ordinary functional tasks rather than looking only at group results.

Cognitive deficits

When James Parkinson first described PD, he observed that the senses and intellect were unimpaired. Although this observation has been challenged by more recent research, much remains to be learnt about the nature of cognitive deficits in PD and the influence of motor impairment on cognitive performance both in a test situation and in the individual's daily life. There are many possible reasons for cognitive impairment in PD. For example, the drugs used to control the clinical signs may cause a decline in cognitive abilities. Life expectancy for individuals with PD has approached that of the normal population with the possibility of some individuals developing Alzheimer's disease. Lewy body pathology in the cerebral cortex, which could contribute to cognitive impairment, is more widespread than previously thought (Marsden 1994).

Fisk and Doble (1992), in a review of research into the cognitive deficits, discuss the findings under the headings of generalized behavioural deficits and specific cognitive deficits. Most of the research into cognitive deficits in PD has utilized clinical neuropsychological and experimental methods. For the clinician working with patients with PD, an important factor to understand is the impact of cognitive deficits on the lives of patients and their relatives, and how to cope with them.

Generalized behavioural deficits

Dementia

The central feature of dementia is impairment of memory along with slowed information processing, and mood and personality disturbances. Although the literature varies on the prevalence of dementia in PD, it appears to be more common in patients with PD than with matched controls from the general medical population (Rajput *et al.* 1984).

It also appears to be a more significant issue in older and more functionally impaired individuals (Mayeux et al. 1983; Ebmeir *et al.* 1990). Variations in reported prevalence of dementia reflect a number of factors including the criteria used for detecting its presence and the age of the subjects. The term 'subcortical dementia' is sometimes used in the clinical description of PD in an attempt to distinguish dementia found in PD from cortical dementia associated with Alzheimer's disease (Fisk and Doble 1992). The use of the term subcortical dementia, however, remains controversial.

Mood disturbances

Depression has been reported to be common in PD patients (Mayeux *et al.* 1981) and it is well known that cognitive changes associated with depression, such as slowed performance of motor tasks and slowness of thought can be similar to those of dementia. The possibility that depression in PD arises as a reaction to a disabling neurodegenerative disease and the relation between disability and depression in PD is not clear. Fisk and Doble (1992) comment that depressive symptoms appear to be related to a number of factors including age, physical disability, and rate of progression of disability. They consider that a more important issue than the level of disability or rate of change of disability, is the person's perception of the significance of a change in functional ability for their own life.

It may be difficult for clinicians to recognize the presence of depression in their patients if/when it occurs since many of the symptoms of depression, lack of variation in facial expression, slowness of movement and apparent slowness of thought and lack of variation in speech production, mimic those of PD. Depression, however, may be amenable to either pharmacological or psychotherapeutic intervention whereas there is no known treatment for the cognitive deficits of PD (Fisk and Doble 1992).

Specific cognitive deficits

Memory impairment

Although the presence of dementia implies memory disturbances, the investigation of the pattern of memory impairment in PD compared with that associated with other neurological conditions has functional significance. An issue of considerable importance to clinicians working with individuals with PD is their ability to learn new information. Overall, studies into the ability to learn new information have usually revealed a decreased capacity or slowed rate of early learning in patients with PD, although this group do not differ from control groups in their ability to retain whatever information has been learned (e.g., El-Awar *et al.* 1987). An important finding is that PD patients are able to benefit from cues to aid their memory retrieval. These findings have important implications for rehabilitation. The use of external cues, memory aids and practice of tasks in environments in which they will be typically performed may be all essential in the training of patients.

Conceptual ability

An interesting neuropsychological finding with functional significance from a study of a group of patients with PD was revealed on a deductive reasoning ability test (Lees and Smith 1983). Although subjects with PD did not differ from age-matched control subjects on tests of general intellectual ability or on forced-choice recognition memory tests, significant differences were revealed on a test that required the subjects to use feedback provided by the investigator.

This type of inflexibility or perseverant behaviour on a neuropsychological test may have implications in the performance of everyday actions and affect the person's ability to utilize new or alternative solutions to problems and they may, therefore, require more explicit and overt guidance. It is essential that clinicians and relatives recognize this and do not judge the individual's behaviour to be stubborn or uncooperative.

Spatial abilities

One of the problems in examining spatial ability in PD is that a wide variety of neuropsychological tests have been used and have produced a variety of findings. Many of the discrepancies amongst findings, however, can be explained by differences in the operational definition of spatial behaviour, in the choice of experimental tasks and in patient selection criteria (Fisk and Doble 1992). Another confounding factor is the difficulty in distinguishing between impairments in motor and spatial abilities. In spite of this, there does exist a body of evidence that suggests PD patients do have some visuospatial and visuomotor deficits.

The issues of the *speed of information processing* and *attentional processing* in patients with PD also

remain controversial. In general, performance on both simple and complex RT tasks that have increased information processing demands have failed to reveal differences between PD and control subjects (Evarts *et al.* 1981; Brown and Marsden 1986), although PD subjects may be slower to respond to the onset of the stimulus. Research so far on attentional processing in PD suggests that attentional deficits may work at two levels. When a simple motor response to an unexpected stimulus is required, PD subjects appear to have difficulty in recruiting additional attentional resources that are normally available. In slightly more complex tasks, when these additional resources are not routinely available, the slowed response in PD may reflect a slowing of motor responses as opposed to slowing of information processing. Under more complex situations, when responses are less obviously constrained by motor abilities, the attentional capacity of the PD patients may be exceeded (Fisk and Doble 1992).

It may be implied from these findings that situations that require planning and decision making will be the most difficult for patients with PD. In contrast, structuring and simplifying the environment in a way that provides guidance will assist in focusing the patient's attentional processing and should, therefore, improve the patient's functional performance (Fisk and Doble 1992).

Therapeutic intervention

Medical management

In the late 1960s and early 1970s, it was reasoned that the symptoms associated with PD may be relieved if the amount of dopamine in the brain was restored to normal. Eventually oral levodopa therapy was established as the most effective therapy for PD (Marsden and Parkes 1977; Agid *et al.* 1987) and a significant advance in the treatment of PD was made. In particular, the most disabling symptoms of the disease, akinesia and bradykinesia, which had not shown any marked improvement when previously treated by anticholinergic medication and stereotaxic surgery, responded very well to levodopa (Marsden 1990). Most patients, irrespective of the extent of their disability, responded to the drug and seriously disabled patients, previously chair bound or bedridden by their illness, became mobile. Although the administration of levodopa produced these promising results, many patients suffered from side effects and over time, fluctuations in response, with some patients experiencing end-of-dose deterioration a few hours after each dose of levodopa (the 'on-off' response), with some eventually becoming resistant to the drug (Marsden 1990; Côté and Crutcher 1991). In spite of attempts to counter the 'on-off' response, a symptom of the disease documented before the advent of levodopa (Birkmayer *et al.* 1985), by administering smaller quantities of the drug more frequently, many patients begin to get increasingly severe deterioration in mobility.

Side effects are numerous and include gastrointestinal complaints, such as nausea and vomiting, CNS effects such as confusion and delirium, behavioural changes, neurologic abnormalities (dyskinesia, dystonia) and cardiovascular effects (orthostatic hypotension) (Korman and James 1993). Over the past couple of decades many strategies have been devised in an attempt to prevent or overcome these problems (Quinn *et al.* 1984; Obeso *et al.* 1986; Frankel *et al.* 1990). The medical management of PD, however, continues to be challenging, and despite the development of new forms of medication, including selegiline, which has been shown to delay the need for levodopa therapy (Myllyla *et al.* 1992) and α-tocopherol (an antioxidant agent), there is still no ideal or preventative treatment (for review see Korman and James 1993).

At this stage, no drugs have been found to prevent levodopa-induced dyskinesias without diminishing the drug's benefit to mobility. Similarly, no selective antipsychotic medication has been found to control mental side effects without increasing motor disability (Marsden 1994).

The use of stereotaxic surgery which involves lesioning of different sites in the thalamus to alleviate various kinds of tremor and movement disorders decreased markedly following the introduction of pharmacological treatments. Some patients, however, are resistant to drug therapy and others, after several years of levodopa treatment, develop disabling side effects particularly involuntary movements (Blond *et al.* 1992). This has led to a renewed interest in stereotaxic procedures. High frequency chronic stimulation of the ventral intermediate thalamic nucleus, the globus pallidus internus and subthalamic nucleus for tremor, dyskinesias and dystonia appear to be a safer and more effective procedure than destruction of tissue (Benabid *et al.* 1993,1996).

As a result of the successful restoration of function of the damaged brain in laboratory animals (Lindvall 1989) and the stimulus to overcome fluctuations associated with levodopa therapy, brain grafting techniques are being developed to affect striatal dopaminergic delivery (Madrazo *et al.* 1987; Lindvall *et al.* 1990). Adrenal medullary autografts were attempted initially; however, more recently, human fetal nigral tissue has provided more promising results. Although there is some evidence for the survival of fetal grafts in some circumstances (Lindvall *et al.* 1990), many issues remain controversial. Further work is necessary to both refine the procedures and evaluate their role in treatment (Marsden 1990).

Physiotherapy: an overall view

Before the advent of levodopa therapy, physiotherapy played a role in the management of the movement disorders associated with PD. In general, physiotherapy techniques focused on the musculoskeletal sequelae and were aimed at increasing range of motion, decreasing rigidity, improving coordination and maintaining functional abilities (Rusk 1964; Ball 1967). Massage, relaxation techniques and soft tissue stretching (Doshay 1962) and a gymnasium programme (Bilowit 1956) were amongst the methodologies advocated. Alternative approaches in which therapy was directed more toward the CNS were advocated from the 1960s, in particular proprioceptive neuromuscular facilitation (PNF) (Knott and Voss 1968). Once medication was established as the primary tool in medical therapeutics, the emphasis in physiotherapy changed somewhat. This change reflected the differing needs of individuals with PD who could be broadly divided into two groups: those whose control of movement and postural stability were still deficient despite the reduction in clinical signs brought about by medication; and those who could not tolerate medication or for whom this intervention had little effect.

A common belief expressed in the therapy literature is that methodologies involving relaxation, trunk rotation, bilateral symmetrical and reciprocal PNF patterns, rhythm and auditory cues would improve movement by decreasing rigidity (e.g., Knott and Voss 1968; Goff 1972; Schenkman *et al.* 1989; Melnick 1995). Rigidity is generally considered by physiotherapists to be the major deficit underlying the disability (Schenkman 1992; Melnick 1995) and therapy aimed at decreasing rigidity is thus expected to lead automatically to an improvement in functional ability (Schenkman 1992).

PNF methods are still advocated by some clinicians (Schenkman 1992; Melnick 1995). However, there is no evidence that either PNF or relaxation techniques are effective in reducing rigidity or improving functional performance beyond a sometimes immediate effect. Some clinicians also promote Bobath therapy or conductive education methods (Gibberd, *et al.* 1981; Kinsman 1986; Schenkman *et al.* 1989). Again, there is no objective evidence of effectiveness. One study of PD patients who were in a relatively stable medicated state (Gibberd *et al.* 1981) showed that an individually planned programme of physiotherapy (using a combination of PNF, Bobath and conductive education methods), showed no significant change in post-testing after 4 weeks' treatment (eight sessions). Aims of physiotherapy intervention were: to improve rotation, balance, and walking, reduce festination and increase range of motion where this was decreased due to rigidity. Occupational therapy was given concurrently and was aimed at personal independence and functional activities (feeding, dressing, mobility, cooking). Rigidity and tremor were not affected by the interventions, nor were the functional tasks tested. Another study (Franklyn 1983) has shown deterioration of PD subjects receiving conductive education.

It is probable that the lack of significant results in these studies may have been due to the inappropriate nature of the physiotherapy given, together with some incorrect assumptions about the nature of the motor deficit. It is important that these results should not be taken to infer that physiotherapy as such is ineffective but rather that the methods used were not sufficiently directed toward either the underlying deficits or toward improving functional performance in everyday life. The assumption behind the PNF, Bobath and conductive education methods is that there will be a carry-over from treatment sessions into improved functional performance. As discussed elsewhere (Chapter 2), there is no evidence from the literature on muscle, motor control or motor learning that passive or therapist-controlled movements or active non-specific exercises will carry-over into improved performance of specific actions. Approaches such as Bobath and PNF are based on the belief that rigidity (a positive sign) is the major bar to mobility/function, rather than on findings from recent literature that provide evidence that the slowness of movement and difficulty initiating muscle activation (the negative signs) are the major deficits underlying the poverty of motor performance (Yekutiel *et al.* 1991; Morris *et al.* 1995). In addition, secondary (adaptive) musculoskeletal changes also affect speed and effectiveness of movement. There is in addition the possibility that rigidity may be, at least in part, an adaptive or compensatory phenomenon used to mask the effects of hypokinesia (Horak *et al.* 1992; Morris *et al.* 1995; Latash and Anson 1996).

It is only recently that the effects of physiotherapy methods have been subjected to formalized scrutiny in terms of their effectiveness. A gradually increasing understanding of the basic dyscontrol mechanisms underlying the clinical signs together with biomechanical studies of both able-bodied and deficient motor performance are stimulating the development and testing of new methods of physiotherapy which it is hoped will assist PD individuals to optimize their functional effectiveness and improve their sense of wellbeing. There is sufficient evidence already accumulated of the effectiveness of physical activity and home exercise programmes designed to maintain optimal mobility and fitness and improve wellbeing (e.g., Banks and Caird 1989; Hurwitz 1989; Yekutiel *et al.* 1991) to persuade individuals with PD to seek advice and a training and exercise plan from a physiotherapist.

The need for early physiotherapy remains controversial in the medical literature, possibly because of a lack of understanding of the potential role of physiotherapy. Nevertheless, there is the effect on function, wellbeing and general health caused by the decrease in activity which can occur following the diagnosis as well as due to the increasing deficits in motor control mechanisms and to the ageing process itself. Two obvious reasons for *early referral* of the PD individual to a physiotherapist include the need for advice in preserving musculoskeletal flexibility, including thoracic expansion, and advice in maintaining an active lifestyle and minimizing the deconditioning and mental decline which can result from reduced physical and mental activity. Orofacial function (i.e., eating, drinking) should also be addressed with the patient.

In the later stages of PD, activities may need to be organized in the middle hour between medications, as this may be the only time during which activity is possible (Turnbull 1992). When the patient demonstrates decreasing activity and increasing dependence, the physiotherapist, with the occupational therapist, will need to show a relative or other caregiver methods of assisting changes in position and the general aspects of care needed at the severely dependent stage of any disease. Assistance with oromotor function (i.e., eating and drinking) and methods of optimizing lung function may also be necessary at this stage.

In the following section on movement rehabilitation, physiotherapy methods which are directed at training the PD individual to optimize performance are outlined. Although it is probable that these more scientifically based and specific methodologies will have some degree of effectiveness in improving motor performance, other significant aspects of physiotherapy are critical in addressing the secondary musculoskeletal and cardiovascular deficits which result from the effect of the pathophysiological mechanisms, inactivity and ageing upon general mobility. Similar deficits are common in many older individuals who tend to be less mobile than the young.

New directions in movement rehabilitation

Today it is generally accepted that physiotherapy is necessary as an adjunct to medication and a number of physiotherapy practitioners and others are attempting to redefine the role of physiotherapy (e.g., Yekutiel *et al.* 1991; Turnbull 1992; Morris *et al.* 1995). Developing interest in the ability of the movement sciences to provide the scientific basis of intervention (Carr and Shepherd 1987), developments in the medical sciences regarding the nature of the basal ganglia deficit, together with an increased understanding of the importance of physical fitness and flexibility are driving the development of new methodologies. These are producing more promising results than conventional interventions. A recognition of the need to test effectiveness of interventions in terms of functional performance is also driving the development of a more scientifically rigorous, effective and accountable clinical practice.

The major roles for the physiotherapist seem to lie in promoting physical activities as a means of maintaining an active lifestyle, a flexible neuromusculoskeletal system and physical fitness; establishing with the individual effective means of developing and practising strategies for solving everyday functional problems. It is likely that the physiotherapist would best assist the individual to accomplish an activity programme by working together in his/her own environment and by being available for discussion and advice by telephone and through regular visits.

Task- and context-related practice

Intervention to improve performance of everyday actions should focus on practising tasks in the environments in which they usually take place, with emphasis on improving both motor and spatial abilities and with information and feedback provided by the physiotherapist.

Strategies for improving functional performance by *overcoming slowness and difficulty initiating movement, including methods of improving postural stability* are being developed. A study of 12 PD subjects (Hoehn and Yahr stage III–IV) on stable medication (Yekutiel *et al.* 1991) shows the results of a 3-month, bi-weekly programme given in the person's home. Subjects spent 10 minutes learning and practising throwing and catching; 15 minutes learning and practising whole-body actions in different positions including sitting, standing, and walking; 5 minutes rest; 15 minutes developing and practising strategies for solving problems encountered by each person (e.g., getting up at night, walking out of a small lavatory, turning, negotiating narrow spaces). Simple biomechanical explanations of movement were given with the aim that the person would learn to move more effectively. Environmental restrictions were discussed; for example, walking around the corner of the bed was conceived as a continuous curve rather than as two paths at right-angles.

Subjects were tested before and after the training period on three timed tasks: standing up, walking around another chair and sitting down on first chair; standing up from supine in bed; standing up from supine on the floor. Time taken on a task was taken as an indication of the ease with which subjects performed it. Two subjects who had a history of falling kept a record of where and when each fall occurred. Overall there was a significant decrease in total test time of 40% although there was a great deal of intersubject variability. Although all subjects improved, the most disabled improved more than the least disabled, some of whom had pre-test scores only a little more than normal. One of the 'falling' subjects significantly decreased both the overall number of falls and the number of falls in specific areas of the house. Importantly, the authors report that not all the subjects had maintained their gains when visited several months later, and point out that an effective regime might include a 4–6 week period of training followed by short 'booster' periods every few months.

Motor learning (skill acquisition) is said to involve a change from controlled attention-demanding processes (Fitts' cognitive stage) to more automatic and less attention-demanding processes (Fitts' automatic stage) (Soliveri *et al.* 1992). It seems that PD patients need to practise difficult tasks with an emphasis on 'getting the idea of' the movement (cognitive stage) in order to develop strategies for overcoming the problem. Several studies have shown recently that individuals with PD can learn to adapt their motor performance to the needs of a task or to learn a new task (Frith *et al.* 1986; Worringham and Stelmach 1990; Soliveri *et al.* 1992). What seems certain is that very specific practice in an appropriate context is necessary – as it is in healthy subjects who want to become skilled in a particular action.

For example, turning in bed at night can be a distressing problem for people with PD. In training this action, it is necessary to understand the difference between rolling over and turning in bed. The latter involves turning to the left or right side, raising the body mass sufficiently between the underneath shoulder and feet to move the 'hips' backward. This provides a stable sidelying position. Canning (1996) trained an individual to turn on to either side. Initially the training resulted in a decrease in speed of turning by four secs. However, when a top sheet was added in training, performance deteriorated markedly. This emphasizes the importance of training an action in the context in which it is to be performed, not only in an artificial physiotherapy environment.

By teaching the critical biomechanical features of an action, the physiotherapist helps the individual use cognitive strategies to cue into an effective motor pattern. For example, in standing up, the necessary information for the person to learn is foot placement backward, swinging the upper body forward at the hips and upward into standing. The person who cannot stand up independently may be attempting to extend the legs without doing the preparatory (pre-extension) movements which enable the sit-to-stand action to take place. Stick figure drawings may help the person develop a visual picture of the action required.

One recent study had encouraging results in terms of the ability of people with PD to do two things at once (Soliveri *et al.* 1992), which is critical to effective function. PD subjects (most of them graded III on the Hoehn and Yahr scale) and age-matched controls were tested on the time taken to perform a skilled task, doing up buttons, a task reported to be difficult for PD individuals, and on

their ability to tap their foot at the same time at two different speeds. The PD group were slower than the controls on the buttoning task but both groups improved their time (i.e., performed more quickly) over trials (i.e., as they practised). Performance of both groups on buttoning deteriorated with the addition of foot tapping, although it was more marked in the PD group. However, both the control and the PD group showed a decrease in the effect of interference over successive trials, with PD subjects achieving the same performance level as the controls at the slower tapping speed. The PD group's buttoning speed and tapping speed increased. These findings suggest, according to the authors, that by the end of practice the degree of 'learning' and the level of automaticity was similar in the two groups. The authors suggest that subjects were actually learning a completely new skill (buttoning and tapping as one task), indicating that this process is relatively normal in PD subjects. Although the combination of foot tapping with buttoning is a relatively meaningless task, the study provides a rationale for training more meaningful combinations of actions. The ability to learn a new skill is important to someone who may need to learn to perform a task utilizing different strategies.

The results of other studies suggest that PD individuals can learn to make anticipatory movements in a particular task (Frith *et al.* 1986) and to reduce simple RT (Worringham and Stelmach 1990). Several studies seem to reinforce the view that PD individuals may need to have meaningful explanations of what is essential to the performance of a task as well as accurate feedback, particularly in the early stages of practice. It seems also that the individual with PD may need to practise more than the able-bodied, and with very explicit and specific feedback about critical components of the task.

In training more effective performance of specific tasks, consideration is given to musculoskeletal factors such as soft tissue length. Shortened calf muscles, for example, will affect the ability to stand up (may actually prevent it) and to walk. Environmental manipulation could also be expected to assist the individual to be more effective at home. The environment can be structured to enhance motor performance, by, for example, rearranging furniture to avoid difficult areas. Placing markers on the floor to indicate appropriate step length may help the person negotiate narrow doorways or hallways. The physiotherapist should attempt to identify those aspects of movement that are probably adaptive and those that reflect the primary deficit. Some adaptive behaviours may impair the individual's ability to carry out particular goals. The investigation of adaptive motor behaviour is only in its early stages (see Latash and Anson 1996) but the issue may become clearer with future investigation.

The reader should refer to Chapters 4–7 as a guide to the critical biomechanical features of everyday actions and ways in which more effective performance can be achieved. However, given the particular motor control deficits and adaptive motor behaviours evident in individuals with PD, some ways of using external cueing to improve speed, accuracy and initiation of movement, and of developing exercise and activity programmes, are outlined below.

Visual cueing   Visual cueing with parallel lines on the walking surface was described by Martin in 1967 for use with individuals with freezing episodes. He found that the optimal placement of the lines was in front (full view) of the subject so they could be 'walked over'. Lines were not effective when they were either running parallel to the walking course or off to the side of the subject.

Visual cueing to help individuals overcome episodes of freezing has been described more recently (Dietz *et al.* 1990). However, one method used, which involved having individuals step over the curved portion of an inverted walking stick as a means of aborting the freezing episode (Dunne *et al.* 1987), appears not to be as effective as was hoped. A descriptive study of eight subjects compared the effect of stepping over an inverted stick, walking with a stick in the usual manner and walking over lines (Dietz *et al.* 1990). The results (movement time and number of freezes) indicated overall that only walking over lines, as suggested originally by Martin, had a positive effect; walking with the stick, whether inverted or not, was associated with a decrease in performance. These results fit with the view that PD patients perform better when they pay attention to a visual stimulus directly related to stepping. Use of the stick in both conditions may have required a dividing of attention between the walking and the irrelevant manipulation of the stick, resulting in the decrement in walking performance.

Visual cueing is used to enable PD individuals to overcome the effect of bradykinesia/hypokinesia on stride length during walking, with visual cues placed on the floor at the desired step length (Bagley *et al.* 1991; Morris *et al.* 1994a,b). Bagley and colleagues (1991) showed that visual cues (triangular strips of coloured cardboard placed at a customized distance along a translucent walkway) improved spatial (stride length, step length) and temporal (double support time) parameters of walking and that improvement was maintained for one walk after visual cues were removed. In another more recent study (Morris 1996), PD subjects were found to have relatively normal stride length when they attended to their walking, during presentation of visual cues and after removal of these cues. However, when they were covertly monitored immediately after testing, stride length had deteriorated. The results suggest that PD patients are able to generate an appropriate gait at will when they attend to it. The results of these studies, together with those of Yekutiel and colleagues, indicate the importance of planning training programmes that carry over beyond the training session into real life. Whether or not PD individuals *can* learn to improve their gait pattern (particularly stride length, a critical feature of effective gait) without utilizing cognitive strategies (i.e., at a more automatic level) is not yet known.

Auditory cueing techniques   Auditory cueing techniques such as moving in time to a metronome or musical beat or clapping have also been suggested as strategies for improving walking (Nanton 1986; Quintyn and Cross 1986). One study of eight subjects (Eni 1988) in which knee angular displacement was measured before and after subjects walked along a walkway to a tape recording of JS Bach, suggests that the use of music with a strong beat may benefit some individuals. Similarly, external cueing from a metronome has been shown to improve sequential finger movements (Georgiou et al. 1994) and repetitive tracking movements of the hands (Martin *et al.* 1994). It may be, however, that again it is the attentional factor that is predominant. It appears that some individuals may respond better to auditory cuing (e.g., metronome, entrainment to music) rather than focusing on the movement itself (Morris *et al.* 1995).

Attentional strategies   In one of the studies described above (Morris *et al.* 1995), the authors proposed that, rather than the visual cues as such it was likely that paying attention to stride length, the attentional factor, was critical in improving walking. Once subjects no longer gave the goal of increasing stride length such attention, performance decreased. In support of this proposal, the study by Yekutiel and colleagues also demonstrated the effectiveness of cognitive strategies which utilized attention. Mental practice or mental rehearsal may also be beneficial (Morris *et al.* 1995).

Whereas non-specific exercise therapy has been utilized to increase mobility and decrease rigidity, for example, the effects of specific forms of exercise therapy are now being investigated for a number of other reasons including decreasing depression (Melnick 1995), increasing cardiorespiratory fitness (Bridgewater and Sharpe 1996; Canning *et al.* 1997), improving function (Palmer *et al.* 1986; Banks and Caird 1989; Hurwitz 1989; Formisano *et al.* 1992) and the sense of wellbeing.

Exercise to promote physical activity   Physical activity has been shown in one structured interview study to decline more in PD individuals than in healthy elderly subjects (Fertl *et al.* 1993). It was found that, although people in both groups were similar in their physical activity profiles, once symptoms developed in the PD group, there was a significant reduction in physical activity, although participation in sports such as swimming, hiking and gymnastics continued as it did in the healthy group. The assumption sometimes expressed that sport and exercise may cause a deterioration in physical condition in PD individuals has not been proved (Stern 1982), although there is some suggestion that hard exercise may cause lengthy periods of exhaustion and the possibility of reduced duration of drug effect (Fertl *et al.* 1993). Moderation in physical activity is probably advisable until the issue of the relationship between strenuous exercise and deterioration is better understood, individuals being encouraged to go on with their sporting activity for as long as they can. Interestingly, this study reports that the decrements in the PD group differed from those of the healthy elderly group and included: a feeling of stiffness associated with the fear of drowning while swimming; a shorter 'free and easy' walking distance while hiking; a reduced ability to make quick changes of position while playing tennis.

Anecdotal reports provide examples of the subjective effects of training sessions, illustrating that exercise can help an individual increase the level of confidence, self-esteem and feeling of wellbeing. There is also a suggestion that performing physical exercise in daily life is a factor influencing survival rate in PD by preventing decline from disuse (Kuroda *et al.* 1992).

Exercise to maintain flexibility   The most effective way for an individual to preserve musculoskeletal flexibility is by maintaining an active

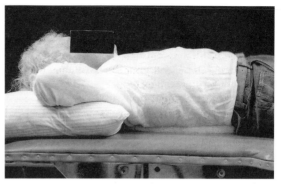

Fig. 13.5 Supine lying on a firm surface with a small towel roll under the thoracic spine. Both arms are abducted and externally rotated to put a further stretch on soft tissues likely to become stiff and short. A small pillow under the knees may be necessary to prevent excessive extension of lumbar spine if spine is very stiff

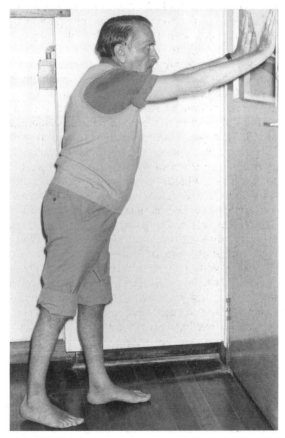

Fig. 13.6 Stretching the R calf muscles. Note he needs to concentrate on keeping his heel on the floor

lifestyle, involving at least three times weekly periods of walking, swimming and general exercise. Such a regime would be expected to optimize cardiorespiratory fitness and general wellbeing as well as musculoskeletal flexibility and strength. There are particular problems associated with PD and the inactivity which commonly ensues, as well as being associated with getting older, and these are considered briefly below.

The tendency to develop an overall flexed posture (the cause of which is uncertain) may be countered by a simple stretching programme including lying in supine on a firm surface and stretching upper limb and upper trunk flexors by active raising and lowering of arms, with the use of a small roll along the thoracic spine to gain further extension (Fig. 13.5). The preservation of thoracic expansion may also be aided by this type of exercise. Since the flexed posture evident in standing in some patients may be an adaptation to avoid a tendency to fall backward, activities performed in standing with the body shifted forward at the ankles may be effective in giving the person an alternative strategy (Figs 13.6, 13.7).

A daily exercise programme designed to enhance flexibility may have effects beyond an increase in range of motion. In one study of a simple exercise programme carried out by nurses, PD subjects (majority graded in the early stage of the disease) reported that they had become more aware of the importance of regular exercise, particularly those who had been experiencing progressive 'stiffness' before the exercise programme (Hurwitz 1989). Although there is no report of significant functional improvement, individuals reported that they felt less 'stiff', indicating that benefits of such a programme may include not only a change in attitude toward exercise but also improved musculoskeletal flexibility.

The authors also report that the regular visit (once a week) by the nurse helped individuals become more disciplined about their exercise

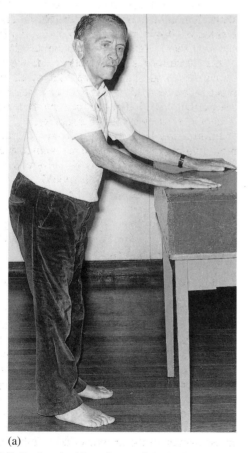 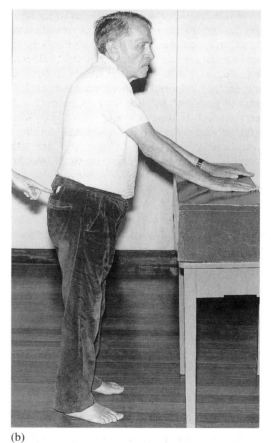

(a)   (b)

Fig. 13.7 Getting the idea of extending the hips and bringing body mass forward in standing. He is also stretching the calf muscles

routine. The findings of the study also reinforce the importance of giving some form of ongoing encouragement to people who are on home exercise programmes.

There is increasing evidence that a programme designed to improve *aerobic fitness* may also be effective. One report of 15 PD subjects who underwent a 12 week, bi-weekly group aerobic exercise programme showed a significant improvement in aerobic fitness as shown by treadmill test duration, estimated VO_2max and heart rate (Bridgewater and Sharpe 1996). Another study (Canning *et al.* 1997) found a significant correlation between exercise habits and maximum exercise capacity in subjects with mild to moderate PD. Individuals who performed regular aerobic exercise produced higher percentage predicted maximum oxygen consumption values than those who were sedentary. The authors concluded that individuals with mild to moderate PD have the potential to maintain normal exercise capacity with regular exercise.

The benefit of *group exercise programmes* designed to improve strength, mobility and fitness is not so clear, although group exercise has been shown in several studies to benefit non-PD elderly subjects (e.g., Grimby 1986). There are anecdotal reports of the benefits of group exercises in PD subjects (e.g., Murray 1956; Szekely *et al.* 1982; Palmer *et al.* 1986), however there is little evidence of improvement in functional abilities. Pedersen and colleagues (1990) reported that PD subjects, mildly to moderately impaired (Hoehn and Yahr I-III), had an overall impression of the beneficial effects of a 12-week training programme, although there was no measurable effect. The programme consisted of exercises to increase coordination, mobility, strength, balance and speed of movement. Subjects were tested before and after the programme and again 4 months later. Measures included gait analysis and muscle strength measurement. Muscle strength did not improve, and gait velocity and stride length were decreased. The authors made the interesting comment that it is possible that benefits to be obtained from a group exercise programme would not be achieved where weakness is not merely the result of disuse, or when there is no weakness but a lack of activation.

Vestibular stimulation To test the proposal that vestibular stimulation might improve gait, Tamlin and colleagues (Tamlin *et al.* 1993) gave PD subjects vestibular stimulation for 6 minutes in a rotating chair with vision occluded. The results showed an increase in velocity of walking and cadence (steps per minute), but there was no significant increase in stride length. Although the authors suggest that vestibular stimulation was effective, the fact that stride length did not increase with the increased velocity suggests otherwise. Subjects showed a mean change in stride length of 0.96 m and 1.01 m, well short of normal values reported for able-bodied subjects of 1.3 to 1.5 m (Morris *et al.* 1994a). Furthermore, subjects with PD typically increase walking speed by increasing cadence *without* having received vestibular stimulation. In this study, the carryover effect was not tested.

Evaluation and measurement

Evaluation by the physiotherapist involves seeking information from the medical notes related to general medical condition and the clinical grading used to establish the level of impairment. Clinical scales in common use include the Hoehn and Yahr Degree of Disability Scale and Webster's Parkinson's Disease Rating Scale (Chapter 3). Wade (1992) describes several tests of disability and impairment and suggests the McDowell Impairment Index be used to assess disease severity and the Barthel ADL Index and the Nine-hole peg test (Chapter 3) as measures of disability.

Information is also sought from the individual regarding motor performance in common everyday actions, particularly details of difficulties being experienced. This evaluation should take place in the environment in which the person is having difficulty. As a guide to the development of an exercise and training programme, the physiotherapist evaluates the individual's performance on the relevant motor actions.

For the physiotherapist and patient to monitor changes occurring during motor training, exercise, fitness or stretching programmes, it is necessary to utilize methods of measurement which provide quantitative information related specifically to what is being trained or exercised. That is to say, methods of measurement need to reflect the goals of intervention which need to be relevant and meaningful. It should be clear whether improvements are short term only (i.e., lasting several minutes to several hours) or more long term (days, weeks or months). Some form of self-monitoring in assessment of therapeutic effects (Yekutiel *et al.* 1991), using, for example, analogue scales provides useful feedback to the therapist about the person's own feelings of change. Pre- and post-testing needs to take into account the stability of medication and the time medication is given.

Tests of functional activities and methods of measuring range of motion and muscle length are outlined in Chapter 3. Simple tests of time on task (e.g., time taken to stand up, walk a given distance) can provide evidence of change in performance. There are available several methods of measuring aspects of gait (e.g., stride length, cadence, speed, time in double support), including simple measurement of distance between powdered footprints and computerized systems such as the Clinical Stride Analyser (B & L Engineering, Sante Fe Springs, California, USA). The Spiral Test (Verkerk *et al.* 1990) (Chapter 3) is a quantitative test designed to evaluate coordination of the hand.

The value to the physiotherapist or patient of tests of isolated clinical signs such as tremor or rigidity is questionable, since it is unlikely that they provide any indication of functional performance. This is particularly so given the present lack of understanding of the primary motor deficits in PD. However, there are tests available for tremor, rigidity and bradykinesia and these are described by several authors (Potvin and Tourtellotte 1984; Sharpe 1992).

Tests of respiratory function may provide useful information at various stages, particularly when a person is undergoing a programme to improve cardiorespiratory fitness. Vital capacity, forced expiratory volume in 1 second (FEV_1), peak inspiratory and expiratory flows are some of the measures in common use. Although inspiratory flow limitation has been documented in individuals with PD (Boggard *et al.* 1989), the relationship between inspiratory flow limitation and exercise limitations is unclear.

In conclusion, physiotherapists have typically utilized a variety of different methodologies as their contribution to the management of individuals with PD. However, there is as yet evidence only that certain methods have short-term positive effects. Encouraging results are emerging of methods which involve ways of providing and teaching the patient strategies (usually cognitive) for dealing with their motor deficits (e.g., Yekutiel *et al.* 1991; Morris *et al.* 1995) and of improving cardiorespiratory fitness.

There are two principal roles of physiotherapy for the individual with PD. The first relates to the preservation of optimal musculoskeletal flexibility, physical activity and fitness. This role involves the provision of advice regarding physical activity and of a regular exercise-stretching-activity programme. The second role is more complex and relates to the provision of strategies, e.g., attentional cues, for dealing with motor deficits during the performance of specific everyday tasks such as sitting down and standing up in different contexts, walking on the street and in the house with kerbs, ramps and steps, and reaching to grasp and manipulate objects. There is evidence that patients respond well to the provision of accurate information about the critical features in the effective performance of everyday tasks. It seems evident also that physiotherapy intervention is most realistically provided by short periods of intervention by the therapist, followed by continuing, regular and monitored practice, with follow-up sessions at intervals.

References

Achiron, A., Ziv, I., Goren, H. *et al.* (1993) Primary progressive freezing gait. *Movement Disorders*, **8**, 293–297.

Agid, Y., Javoy-Agid, F. and Ruberg, M. (1987) Biochemistry of neurotransmitters in Parkinson's disease. In *Movement Disorders 2* (eds. C.D. Marsden and S. Fahn), Butterworth Heinemann, Oxford, pp. 166–230.

Agid, Y., Ruberg, M., Raisman, R. *et al.* (1990) In *Parkinson's Disease* (ed. G. Stern) Chapman and Hall Medical, London, pp. 99–125.

Bagley, S., Kelly, B., Tunnicliffe, N. *et al.* (1991) The effect of visual cues on the gait of independently mobile Parkinson's Disease patients. *Physiotherapy*, **77**, 6, 415–420.

Ball, J.M. (1967) Demonstration of the traditional approach in the treatment of a patient with parkinsonism. *American Journal of Physical Medicine*, **46**, 1034–1036.

Banks, M.A. and Caird, F.I. (1989) Physiotherapy benefits patients with Parkinson's disease. *Clinical Rehabilitation*, **3**, 11–16.

Bazalgette, D., Zattara, M., Bathien, N. *et al.* (1986) Postural adjustments associated with rapid voluntary arm movements in patients with Parkinson's disease. In *Advances in Neurology, 45* (eds M.D. Yahr and K.J. Bergmann), Raven Press, New York, pp. 371–374.

Beckley, D.J., Bloem, B.R., van Dijk, J.G. *et al.* (1991) Electrophysiological correlates of postural instability in Parkinson's disease. *Electroencephalography and Clinical Neurophysiology*, **81**, 263–268.

Benabid, A.L., Pollak, P., Seigneuret, E. *et al.* (1993) Chronic VIM thalamic stimulation in Parkinson's disease, essential tremor and extra-pyramidal dyskinesias. *Acta Neurochirugie*, **58** (Suppl.), 39–44.

Benabid, A.L., Pollak, P., Limousin, P. *et al.* (1996) Why deep brain stimulation should replace ablative neurosurgery as a rehabilitation procedure for Parkinson's disease. *European Journal of Neurology*, **3**, (Suppl. 2), 11.

Benecke, R., Rothwell, J.C., Dick, J.P.R. *et al.* (1986) Performance of simultaneous movements in patients with Parkinson's disease. *Brain*, **109**, 739–757.

Benecke, R., Rothwell, J.C., Dick, J.P.R. *et al.* (1987) Disturbance of sequential movements in patients with Parkinson's disease. *Brain*, **110**, 361–379.

Berardelli, A., Rothwell, J.C., Day, B.L. *et al.* (1984) Movements not involved in posture are abnormal in Parkinson's disease. *Neuroscience Letters.*, **47**, 47–50.

Berardelli, A., Dick, J.P.R., Rothwell, J.C. *et al.* (1986) Scaling of the size of the first agonist EMG burst during rapid wrist movements in patients with Parkinson's disease. *Journal of Neurology, Neurosurgery and Psychiatry*, **49**, 1273–1279.

Bilowit, D.S. (1956) Establishing physical objectives in the rehabilitation of patients with Parkinson's disease. *Physical Therapy Review*, **36**, 176–178.

Birkmayer, W., Danielczk, W. and Riederer, P. (1985) Symptoms and side effects in the course of Parkinson's disease. *Journal of Neural Transmission*, Supplement 9, 185–199.

Blin, O., Ferrandez, A. M. and Serratrice, G. (1990) Quantitive analysis of gait in Parkinson patients: increased variability of stride length. *Journal of Neurological Science*, **98**, 91–97.

Blin, O., Ferrandez, A.M., Pailhous, J. *et al.* (1991) Dopa-sensitive and dopa-resistant gait parameters in Parkinson's disease. *Journal of Neurological Science*, **103**, 51–54.

Blond, S., Caparros-Lefebvre, D., Parker, F. *et al.* (1992) Control of tremor and involuntary movement disorders by chronic stereotactic stimulation of the ventral intermediate thalamic nucleus. *Journal of Neurosurgery*, **77**, 62–68.

Boggard, J.M., Hovestadt, A., Meerwaldt, J.D. *et al.* (1989) Maximum expiratory and inspiratory flow volume curves in Parkinson's disease. *American Review of Respiratory Disease*, **139**, 610–614.

Bridgewater, K.J. and Sharpe, M.H. (1996) Aerobic exercise and early Parkinson's disease. *Journal of Neurological Rehabilitation*, **10,** 233–241.

Bronstein, A.M., Hood, J.D., Gresty, M.A. *et al.* (1990) Visual control of balance in cerebellar and parkinsonian syndrome. *Brain*, **113**, 767–779.

Brotchie, P., Iansek, R. and Horne, M.K. (1991a) Motor function of the globus pallidus: 1. Neuronal discharge and parameters of movement. *Brain*, **114**, 1667–1683.

Brotchie, P., Iansek, R. and Horne, M.K. (1991b) Motor function of the globus pallidus: 2. Cognitive aspects of movement and phasic neuronal activity. *Brain*, **114**, 1685–1702.

Brown, R.G. and Marsden, C.D. (1986) Visuospatial function in Parkinson's disease. *Brain*, **109**, 987–1002.

Calne, D.B. and Langston, J.W. (1983) Aetiology of Parkinson's disease. *Lancet*, **ii**, 1457–1459.

Canning, C. (1996) Personal communication.

Canning, C., Alison, J., Syms, N. *et al.* (1997) Parkinson's disease: an investigation of exercise, respiratory function and gait. *Archives of Physical Medicine and Rehabilitation*, **78**, 199–206.

Carlsson, A. (1959) The occurrence, distribution and physiological role of catecholamines in the nervous system. *Pharmacological Review*, **11**, 490–493.

Carr, J.H. and Shepherd, R.B. (1987) A motor learning model for rehabilitation. In *Movement Science. Foundations for Physical Therapy in Rehabilitation* (eds J.H. Carr and R.B. Shepherd) Aspen, Rockville, MD, pp. 31–91.

Carr, J.H. and Shepherd, R.B. (1996) 'Normal' is not the issue – it is 'effective' goal attainment that counts. *Behavioral Brain Sciences*, **9**, 72–73.

Castiello, U. and Bennett, M.B. (1977) The bilateral reach-to-grasp movement of Parkinson's disease subjects. *Brain*, **120**, 593–604.

Castiello, U., Bennett, K.M.B. and Scarpa, M. (1994) The reach to grasp movement of Parkinson's disease subjects. In *Insights into the Reach to Grasp Movement* (eds K.M.B. Bennett and U. Castiello), Elsevier Science, New York, pp. 215–237.

Castiello, U., Stelmach, G,E. and Lieberman, A.N. (1993) Temporal dissociation of the prehension pattern in Parkinson's disease. *Neuropsychologia*, **31**, 395–402.

Côté, L. and Crutcher, M.D. (1991) The basal ganglia. In *Principles in Neural Science*, (eds E.R. Kandell, J.H. Schwartz and T.M. Jessell), 3rd edn, Elsevier/North Holland, New York, pp. 647–659.

Delwaide, P.J. and Gonce, M. (1988) Pathophysiology of Parkinson's signs. In *Parkinson's Disease and Movement Disorders* (eds J. Jankovic and E. Tolosa), Urban and Schwarzenberg, Baltimore/Munich, pp. 59–73.

Dichgans, J., Diener, H.C. and Muller, A. (1985) Characteristics of increased postural sway and abnormal long loop responses in patients with cerebellar diseases and parkinsonism. In *Electromyography and Evoked Potentials: Theories and Applications* (eds A. Struppler and A. Weindl), Springer, Berlin, pp. 68–74.

Dick, J.P.R., Rothwell, J.C., Berardelli, A. *et al.* (1986) Associated postural adjustments in Parkinson's disease. *Journal of Neurology, Neurosurgery and Psychiatry*, **49**, 1378–1385.

Diener, H-C., Dichgans, B., Guschlbauer, M. *et al.* (1990) Associated postural adjustments with body movement in normal subjects and patients with parkinsonism and cerebellar ataxia. *Revue de Neurologie (Paris)*, **146**, 10, 555–563.

Dietz, V., Berger, W. and Horstmann, G.A. (1988) Posture in Parkinson's disease: impairment of reflexes and programming. *Annals of Neurology*, **24**, 660–669.

Dietz, M., Goetz, C.G. and Stebbins, G.T. (1990) Evaluation of a modified inverted walking stick as a treatment for Parkinsonian freezing episodes. *Movement Disorders*, **5**, 243–247.

Dietz, V., Quintern, J. and Berger, W. (1981) Electrophysiological studies of gait in spasticity and rigidity: evidence that mechanical properties of muscles contribute to hypertonia. *Brain*, **104**, 431–449.

Doshay, L.J. (1962) Method and value of physiotherapy in Parkinson's disease. *New England Journal of Medicine*, April, pp. 878–879.

Dunne, J.W., Hankey, G.J. and Edis, R.H. (1987) Parkinsonism: upturned walking stick as an aid to locomotion. *Archives of Physical Medicine and Rehabilitation*, **68**, 380–381.

Ebmeir, K.P., Calder, S.A. and Crawford, J.R. (1990) Clinical features predicting dementia in idiopathic Parkinson's disease: A follow-up study. *Neurology*, **40**, 1222–1224.

El-Awar, M., Becker, J.T., Hammond, K.M. *et al.* (1987) Learning deficits in Parkinson's disease: Comparison with Alzheimer's disease and normal aging. *Archives of Neurology*, **44**, 180–184.

Eni, G.O. (1988) Gait improvement in Parkinsonism: the use of rhythmic music. *International Journal of Rehabilitation Research*, **11**, 272–274.

Evarts, E.V., Teravainen, H. and Calne, D.B. (1981) Reaction time in Parkinson's disease. *Brain*, **104**, 167–186.

Fertl, E., Doppelbauer, A. and Auff, E. (1993) Physical activity and sports in patients suffering from Parkinson's disease in comparison with healthy seniors. *Journal of Neural Transmission*, **5**, 157–161.

Findley, L.J. (1988) Tremors differential diagnosis and pharmacology. In *Parkinson's Disease and Movement Disorders* (eds J. Jankovic and E. Tolosa), Urban and Schwarzenberg, Baltimore/Munich, pp. 243–261.

Fisk, J.D. and Doble, S.E. (1992) Cognitive deficits. In *Physical Therapy Management of Parkinson's Disease* (ed. G. I. Turnbull), Churchill Livingstone, New York, pp. 69–89.

Flowers, K.A. (1976) Visual 'closed loop' and 'open-loop' characteristics of voluntary movement in patients with Parkinsonism and intention tremor. *Brain*, **99**, 269–310.

Formisano, R., Pratesi, L., Modarelli, F.T. *et al.* (1992) Rehabilitation and Parkinson's disease. *Scandinavian Journal of Rehabilitation Medicine*, **24**, 157–160.

Forssberg, H., Johnels, B and Steg, G. (1984) Is Parkinsonian gait caused by a regression to an immature walking pattern? In *Advances in Neurology*, *40*, (eds R.G. Hassler and J.F. Christ), Raven Press, New York, pp. 375–379.

Frankel, J.P., Lees, A.J., Kempster, P.A. *et al.* (1990) Subcutaneous apomorphine in the treatment of Parkinson's disease. *Journal of Neurology, Neurosurgery and Psychiatry*, **53**, 96–101.

Franklyn, S. (1983) The value of physiotherapy for Parkinson's disease. *International Journal of Rehabilitation Research*, **6**, 271.

Frith, C.D., Bloxham, C.A. and Carpenter, K.N. (1986) Impairments in the learning and performance of a new manual skill in patient with Parkinson's disease. *Journal of Neurology, Neurosurgery and Psychiatry*, **49**, 661–668.

Georgiou, N., Bradshaw, J., Iansek, R. *et al.* (1994) Reduction in external cues and in movement sequencing in Parkinson's disease. *Journal of Neurology, Neurosurgery and Psychiatry*, **57**, 368–370.

Georgiou, N., Iansek, R., Bradshaw, J.L. *et al.* (1993) An evaluation of the role of internal cues in the pathogenesis of parkinsonian hypokinesia. *Brain*, **116**, 1575–1587.

Gibberd, F.B., Page, N.G.R., Spencer, K.M. (1981) Controlled trial of physiotherapy and occupational therapy for Parkinson's disease. *British Medical Journal*, **282**, 1196.

Giladi, N., McMahon, D., Przedborski, S. *et al.* (1992) Motor blocks in Parkinson's disease. *Neurology*, **42**, 333–339.

Goff, B. (1972) The application of recent advances in neurophysiology to Miss M. Rood's concept of neuromuscular facilitation. *Physiotherapy*, **58**, 409–415.

Goldman-Rakin, P.S. and Selemon, L.D. (1990) New frontiers in basal ganglia research. *Trends in Neuroscience*, **13**, 241–244.

Grimby, G. (1986) Physical activity and muscle training in the elderly. *Acta Medica Scandinavica*, **711**, 233–237.

Hallett, M. and Khoshbin, S. (1980) A physiological mechanism of bradykinesia. *Brain*, **103**, 301–314.

Hoehn, M.M. and Yahr, M.D. (1967) Parkinsonism: onset, progression and mortality. *Neurology*, **17**, 427–442.

Horak, F.B., Esselman, P., Anderson, M.E. (1984) The effects of movement velocity, mass displaced, and task uncertainty on associated postural adjustments made by normal and hemiplegic individuals. *Journal of Neurology, Neurosurgery and Psychiatry*, **47**, 1020–1028.

Horak, F.B., Nutt, J.G. and Nashner, L.M. (1992) Postural inflexibility in parkinsonian subjects. *Journal of Neurological Science*, **111**, 46–58.

Hornykiewicz, O. (1966) Metabolism of brain dopamine in human parkinsonism: Neurochemical and clinical aspects. In *Biochemistry and Pharmacology of the Basal Ganglia* (eds E. Costa, L.J. Côté and M.D. Yahr), Raven Press, New York, pp.171–185.

Hurwitz, A. (1989) The benefit of a home exercise regimen for ambulatory Parkinson's disease patients. *Journal of Neuroscience and Nursing*, **21**, (3), 180–184.

Jackson, J.H. (1932) In *Selected Writing of John Hughlings Jackson* (ed. J. Taylor), Hodder and Stoughton, London.

Jellinger, K. (1987) The pathology of parkinsonism. In *Movement Disorders 2* (eds C.D. Marsden and S. Fahn), Butterworth Heinemann, Oxford, pp. 124–165.

Kinsman, A. (1986) Conductive education for the patient with Parkinson's disease. *Physiotherapy*, **72**, 385–388.

Knott, M. and Voss, D.E. (1968) *Proprioceptive Neuromuscular Facilitation*, 2nd edn, Harper and Row, New York.

Knutsson, E. (1972) An analysis of parkinsonian gait. *Brain*, **95**, 475–486.

Korman, L.B. and James, J.A. (1993) Medical management of Parkinson's disease in the elderly. *Topics in Geriatric Rehabilitation*, **8**, 1–13.

Kuroda, K., Tatara, K., Takatorige, T. *et al.* (1992) Effect of physical exercise on mortality in patients with Parkinson's disease. *Acta Neurologica Scandinavia*, **86**, 55–59.

Langston, J.W. and Koller, W.C. (1991) The next frontier in Parkinson's disease: presymptomatic detection. *Neurology*, **41** (Suppl. 2), 5–7.

Latash, M.L. and Anson, J.G. (1996) What are 'normal movements' in atypical populations? *Behavioral Brain Sciences*, **19**, 55–106.

Lees, A.J. and Smith, E. (1983) Cognitive deficits in the early stages of Parkinson's disease. *Brain*, **106**, 257–270.

Lieberman, A.N., Hirowitz, L. and Redmond, P. (1980) Dysphagia in Parkinson's disease. *American Journal of Gastroenterology*, **74**, 157–160.

Lindvall, O. (1989) Transplantation into the human brain: present status and future possibilities. *Journal of Neurology, Neurosurgery and Psychiatry*, **52** (Special Suppl), 68–77.

Lindvall, O., Brundin, P., Widner, H. *et al.* (1990) Grafts of foetal dopamine neurons survive and improve motor function in Parkinson's disease. *Science*, **247**, 574–577.

Madrazo, I., Drucker-Colin, R., Diaz, V. *et al.* (1987) Open microsurgical autograft of adrenal medulla to the right caudate nucleus in two patients with intractable Parkinson's disease. *New England Journal of Medicine*, **316**, 831–834.

Marsden, C.D. (1982) The mysterious motor function of the basal ganglia: the Robert Wartenberg lecture. *Neurology (New York)*, **32**, 514–539.

Marsden, C.D. (1990) Parkinson's disease. *Lancet*, **335**, 948–952.

Marsden, C.D. (1994) Parkinson's disease. *Journal of Neurolology, Neurosurgery, and Psychiatry*, **57**, 672–681.

Marsden, C.D. and Parkes, J.D. (1977) Success and problems of long-term levodopa therapy in Parkinson's disease. *Lancet*, **i**, 345–349.

Martin, J.P. (1967) *The Basal Ganglia and Posture*, Pitman, London.

Martin, K.E., Phillips, J.G., Iansek, R. *et al.* (1994) Inaccuracy, instabilities of sequential movements in Parkinson's disease. *Experimental Brain Research*, **102**, 131–140.

Martin, W.E., Loewenson, R.B., Resch, J.A. *et al.* (1973) Parkinson's disease: clinical analysis of 100 patients. *Neurology (Minneappolis)*, **23**, 783–790.

Mayeux, R., Stern, Y., Rosen, J. (1981) Depression, intellectual impairment, and Parkinson's disease. *Neurology*, **31**, 645–650.

Mayeux, R., Stern, Y., Rosen, J. (1983) Is 'subcortical dementia' a recognizable clinical entity? *Annals of Neurology*, **14**, 278–283.

Melnick, M.E. (1995) Basal ganglia disorders. Metabolic, hereditary and genetic disorders in adults. In *Neurological Rehabilitation* (ed. D. Umphred), 3rd edn, C.V. Mosby, St Louis, pp. 606–640.

Morris, M.E. (1996) Gait hypokinesia in Parkinson's disease. Unpublished doctoral thesis, LaTrobe University, Melbourne.

Morris, M.E., Iansek, R., Matyas, T.A. *et al.* (1994a) Ability to modulate walking cadence remains intact in Parkinson's disease. *Journal of Neurology, Neurosurgery and Psychiatry*, **57**, 1532–1534.

Morris, M.E., Iansek, R., Matyas, T.A. *et al.* (1994b) The pathogenesis of gait hypokinesia in Parkinson's disease. *Brain*, **117**, 1169–1181.

Morris, M.E., Iansek, R., Summers, J.J. *et al.* (1995) Motor control considerations for the rehabilitation of gait in Parkinson's disease. In *Motor Control and Sensory Motor Integration* (eds D. Glencross and J. Piek), Elsevier, Amsterdam, pp. 61–93.

Muller, F. and Abbs, J.A. (1990) Precision grip in Parkinsonian patients. In *Advances in Neurology 53: Parkinson's Disease: Anatomy, Pathology and Therapy* (eds. M.B. Streifler, A.D. Korczyn, E. Melamed *et al.*) Raven Press, New York, pp. 191–195.

Murray, W. (1956) Parkinson's disease: aspects of functional training. *Physical Therapy Review*, **36**, 587–594.

Murray, M.P., Sepic, S.B., Gardiner, G.M. *et al.* (1978) Walking patterns of men with parkinsonism. *American Journal of Physical Medicine*, **57**, 278–294.

Myllyla, V.V., Sotaniemi, K.A., Vuorinem, J.A. *et al.* (1992) Selegiline as initial treatment in de novo parkinsonian patients. *Neurology*, **42**, 339–343.

Nanton V. (1986) Parkinson's disease. In *Conductive Education. A System for Overcoming Motor Disorder* (eds P.J. Cottam and A. Sutton), Croom Helm, London.

Narabayashi, H. and Nakamura, R. (1985) Clinical neurophysiology of freezing in Parkinsonism. In *Clinical Neurophysiology in Parkinsonism* (eds P.J. Delwaide and A. Agnoli), Elsevier, Amsterdam, pp. 49–57.

Nashner, L.M. (1977) Fixed patterns of rapid postural responses among leg muscles during stance. *Experimental Brain Research*, **30**, 13–24.

Obeso, J.A., Luquin, M.R. and Martinez-Lage, J.M. (1986) Lisuride infusion pump: a device for the treatment of motor fluctuations in Parkinson's disease. *Lancet*, **i**, 467–470.

Palmer, S.P., Mortimer, J.A., Webster, D.D. *et al.* (1986) Exercise therapy for Parkinson's Disease. *Archives of Physical Medicine and Rehabilitation*, **67**, 741–745.

Parent, A. (1990) Extrinsic connections of the basal ganglia. *Trends in Neuroscience*, **13**, 254–258.

Parkinson, J. (1817) *An Essay on the Shaking Palsy*, London.

Pearce, J.M.S. (1992) *Parkinson's Disease and its Management*, Oxford University Press, Oxford, pp. 71–89.

Pedersen, S.W., Oberg, B., Insulander, A. and Vretman, M. (1990) Group training in parkinsonism: quantitative measurements of treatment. *Scandinavian Journal of Rehabilitation Medicine*, **22**, 207–211.

Phillips, J.G., Bradshaw, J.L., Iansek, R. *et al.* (1993) Motor functions of the basal ganglia. *Psychological Research*, **55**, 175–181.

Phillips, J.G., Martin, K.E., Bradshaw, J.L. *et al.* (1994) Could bradykinesia in Parkinson's disease simply be compensation? *Journal of Neurology*, **241**, 439–447.

Potvin, P.E. and Tourtellotte, M.D. (1984) *Quantitative Evaluation of Neurological Function*, CRC Press, Boca Raton, FL.

Quinn, N., Parkes, J.D. and Marsden, C.D. (1984) Control of on/off phenomenon by continuous intravenous infusion of levadopa. *Neurology*, **34**, 1131–1136.

Quintyn, M. and Cross, E. (1986) Factors affecting the ability to initiate movement in Parkinson's disease. *Physiotherapy and Occupational Therapy in Geriatrics*, **4**, 51–59.

Rajput, A.H., Offord, K., Beard, C.M. *et al.* (1984) Epidemiological survey of dementia in Parkinsonism and control population. In *Advances in Neurology*, **40** (eds R.G. Hassler and J.F. Christ), Raven Press, New York, p. 229.

Robbins, J.A., Logemann, J.A. and Kirshner, H.S. (1986) Swallowing and speech production in Parkinson's disease. *Annals of Neurology*, **19**, 283–287.

Rogers, M.W., Kukulka, C.G. and Soderberg, G.L. (1987) Postural adjustments preceding rapid arm movements in parkinsonian subjects. *Neuroscience Letters*, **75**, 246–251.

Roland, P.E., Larsen, B., Lassen, N.A. *et al.* (1980) Supplementary motor area and other cortical areas in organization of voluntary movements in man. *Journal of Neurophysiology*, **43**, 118–136.

Roland, P.E., Meyer, E., Shibasaki, T. *et al.* (1982) Regional cerebral blood flow changes in cortex and basal ganglia during voluntary movements in normal human volunteers. *Journal of Neurophysiology*, **48**, 467–480.

Rusk, H.A. (1964) *Rehabilitation Medicine*, 2nd edn, C.V. Mosby, St Louis.

Saltin, B. and Landin, S. (1975) Work capacity, muscle strength and SDH activity in both legs of hemiparetic patients and patients with Parkinson's disease. *Scandinavian Journal of Clinical Laboratory Investigations*, **35**, 531–538.

Schell, G.R. and Strick, P.L. (1984) The origin of thalamic inputs to the arcuate premotor and supplementary motor areas. *Journal of Neuroscience*, **4**, 539–560.

Schenkman, M. (1992) Physical therapy intervention for the ambulatory patient. In *Physical Therapy Management of Parkinson's Disease* (ed. G.I. Turnbull), Churchill Livingstone, New York, pp. 137–192.

Schenkman, M., Donovan, J., Tsubota, J. *et al.* (1989) Management of individuals with Parkinson's disease: rationale and case studies. *Physical Therapy*, **69**, 944–955.

Schieppati, M. and Nardone, A. (1991) Free and supported stance in Parkinson's disease. *Brain*, **114**, 1227–1244.

Schoenberg, B.S. (1987) Epidemiology of movement disorders. In *Movement Disorders 2* (eds C.D. Marsden and S. Fahn), Butterworth Heinemann, Oxford, pp. 17–32.

Scholz, E., Diener, H.C., Noth, J. *et al.* (1987) Medium and long latency EMG responses in leg muscles: Parkinson's disease. *Journal of Neurology, Neurosurgery and Psychiatry*, **50**, 66–70.

Schwab, R.S., Chafetz, M.E. and Walker, S. (1954) Control of two simultaneous voluntary motor acts in normals and parkinsonism. *Archives of Neurology and Psychiatry*, **72**, 591–598.

Seitz, R.J. and Roland, P.E. (1992) Learning of sequential movements in man: a combined kinematic and positron emission tomography (PET) study. *European Journal of Neuroscience*, **4**, 154–165.

Shahani, B.T. and Young, R.R. (1976) Physiological and pharmacological aids in the differential diagnosis of tremor. *Journal of Neurology, Neurosurgery and Psychiatry*, **39**, 772–783.

Sharpe, M.H. (1992) Physical therapy evaluation. In *Physical Therapy Management of Parkinson's Disease* (ed. G.I. Turnbull) Churchill Livingstone, New York, pp. 121–136.

Shepherd, R.B. and Carr, J.H. (1991) An emergent or dynamical systems view of movement dysfunction. *Australian Journal of Physiotherapy*, **37**, 4–5.

Sheridan, M.R. and Flowers, K.A. (1990) Movement variability and bradykinesia in Parkinson's disease. *Brain*, **113**, 1149–1161.

Silbiger, M.C., Pikielney, R. and Donner, M.W. (1967) Neuromuscular disorders affecting the pharynx: cineradiographic analysis. *Investigative Radiology*, **2**, 442–448.

Soliveri, P., Brown, R.G. and Jahanshahi, M. (1992) Effect of practice on performance of a skilled motor task in patients with Parkinson's disease. *Journal of Neurology, Neurosurgery, and Psychiatry*, **55**, 461–465.

Stern, G.L.A. (1982) *Parkinson's Disease*, Oxford University Press, Oxford, pp. 52–57.

Stern, G. and Lees, A. (1991) *Parkinson's Disease: the Facts*, Oxford University Press, Oxford.

Stern, G.M., Franklyn, S.E., Imms, F.J. *et al.* (1983) Quantitative assessments of gait and mobility in Parkinson's disease. *Journal of Neural Transmission*, Suppl, **19**, 201–214.

Stern, G.M., Lander, C.M. and Lees, A.J. (1980) Akinetic freezing and trick movements in Parkinson's disease. *Journal of Neural Transmission*, Suppl, **16**, 137–141.

Szekely, B.C., Kosanovich N.N. and Sheppard, W. (1982) Adjunctive treatment in Parkinson's disease: physical therapy and comprehensive group therapy. *Rehabilitation Literature*, **43**, 3–4, 72–76.

Talland, G.A. and Schwab, R.S. (1964) Performance with multiple sets in Parkinson's disease. *Neuropsychologia*, **2**, 45–53.

Tamlin, B., McDonald, K., Correll, M. *et al.* (1993) The immediate effects of vestibular stimulation on gait in patients with Parkinson's Disease. *Journal of Neurology and Rehabilitation*, **7**, 35–39.

Tanji, J. and Kurata, K. (1985) Contrasting neuronal activity in supplementary and precentral motor cortex of monkeys. 1. Responses to instructions determining motor responses to forthcoming signals of different modalities. *Journal of Neurophysiology*, **53**, 129–141.

Tanner, C.M. (1989) The role of environmental toxins in the etiology of Parkinson's disease. *Trends in Neuroscience*, **12**, 49–54.

Turnbull, G.I. (1992) The role of physical therapy intervention. In *Physical Therapy Management of Parkinson's Disease* (ed. G.I. Turnbull) Churchill Livingstone, New York, pp. 91–120.

Verkerk, P.H., Schouten, J.P. and Oosterhuis, H.J.G.H. (1990) Measurement of the hand coordination. *Clinical Neurology, Neurosurgery*, **92–2**, 105–109.

Viallet, F., Massion, J., Massarino, R. *et al.* (1987) Performance of a bimanual load-lifting task by Parkinsonian patients. *Journal of Neurology, Neurosurgery and Psychiatry*, **50**, 1274–1283.

Vincken, W.G., Gauthier, M.D., Dollfuss, R.E. *et al.* (1984) Involvement of upper-airway muscles in extrapyramidal disorders. A cause of airflow limitation. *New England Journal of Medicine*, **311**, 438–442.

Wade, D.T. (1992) *Measurements in Neurological Rehabilitation*. Oxford University Press, New York.

Wall, J.C. and Turnbull, G.I. (1992) The kinematics of gait. In *Physical Therapy Management of Parkinson's Disease* (ed. G. I. Turnbull), Churchill Livingstone, New York, pp. 49–67.

Walton, J. (1993) *Brain's Diseases of the Nervous System*, 10th edn, Oxford University Press, Oxford.

Waterston, J.A., Hawken, M.B., Tanyeri, S. *et al.* (1993) Influence of sensory manipulation on postural control in Parkinson's disease. *Journal of Neurology, Neurosurgery, and Psychiatry*, **56**, 1276–1281.

Watts, R.L., Wiegner, A.W. and Young, R.R. (1986) Elastic properties of muscles measured at the elbow in man: II patients with parkinsonian rigidity. *Journal of Neurology, Neurosurgery and Psychiatry*, **49**, 1177–1181.

Webster, D.D. (1968) Critical analysis of the disability in Parkinson's disease. *Modern Treatment*, **5**, 257–282.

Wichmann, T. and DeLong, M.R. (1993) Pathophysiology of Parkinsonian motor abnormalities. *Advances in Neurology*, **60**, 53–61.

Wilson, S.A.K. (1925) Disorders of motility and muscle tone, with special reference to the striatum. *Lancet*, **2**, 1–53.

Woollacott, M.H., von Hosten, C. and Rosblad, B. (1988) Relation between muscle response onset and body segmental movements during postural perturbations in humans. *Experimental Brain Research*, **72**, 593–604.

Worringham, C.J. and Stelmach, G.E. (1990). Practice effects on the preprogramming of discrete movements in Parkinson's disease. *Journal of Neurology, Neurosurgery and Psychiatry*, **53**, 702–704.

Yekutiel, M.P., Pinhasov, A., Shahar, G. (1991) A clinical trial of the re-education of movement in patients with Parkinson's disease. *Clinical Rehabilitation*, **5**, 207–214.

Further reading

Allum, J.H.J., Keshner, E.A., Honegger, F. *et al.* (1988) Disturbance of posture in patients with Parkinson's disease. In *Posture and Gait: Development, Adaptation and Modulation* (ed B. Amblard *et al.*), Elsevier, Amsterdam, pp. 245–257.

Dietz, V. (1993) Reflex behavior and programming in Parkinson's disease. In *Advances in Neurology*, **60**, (eds H. Narabayashi, T. Nagatsu, N. Yanagisawa *et al.*), Raven Press, New York, pp. 375–380.

Freeman, J.S., Cody, F.W.J., Schady, W. (1993) The influence of external timing cues upon rhythm of voluntary movements in Parkinson's disease. *Journal of Neurology, Neurosurgery, and Psychiatry*, **56**, 1078–1084.

Kamsma, Y.P.T., Brouwer, W.H. and Lakke, J.P.W.F. (1994) Prevention of early immobility in patients with Parkinson's disease: a cognitive strategy training for turning in bed and rising from a chair. In *Neuropsychology and Cognitive Rehabilitation* (eds M.J. Riddoch and G.W. Humphreys), Lawrence Erlbaum, Hove, UK, pp. 245–270.

Marsden, C.D. (1986) Associated postural adjustments in Parkinson's disease. *Journal of Neurology, Neurosurgery, and Psychiatry*, **49**, 1378–1385.

Robbins, J.A., Logemann, J.A. and Kirshner, H.S. (1986) Swallowing and speech production in Parkinson's disease. *Annals of Neurology*, **19**, 283–287.

Wissel, J. and Poewe, W. (1992) Dystonia – a clinical, neuropathological and therapeutic review. *Journal of Neural Transmission*, Suppl, **38**, 91–104.

14

Multiple sclerosis

Multiple sclerosis (MS) is a demyelinating disease causing a widespread degeneration of the central nervous system (CNS) which gradually results in severe neurological deficits. MS usually presents in early adult life when it has a major impact on family, and on vocational and social life. Since lack of myelin slows down the conduction of the action potentials, MS manifests itself as impaired performance that can have a devastating effect on behaviour. MS usually involves a more or less progressive development of neurological symptoms and behavioural deficits, however, the exact aetiology and pathogenesis is still unclear. The disease is characterized by remissions and relapses, erratic onset and duration of symptoms that flare up acutely. Each relapse may involve a quite different area of the white matter of the CNS. The remissions are rarely complete and may last for either a long or short period. Since the disease remains poorly understood, there is no effective treatment of the disease process itself. New insights into the pathophysiology, however, are suggesting new strategies for intervention. Health professionals working with individuals with MS need to focus on those factors arising from the disease they can prevent or change in order to improve the quality of the individual's life.

Epidemiology and aetiology

MS is thought to involve an interplay between genetic and environmental factors, which result in an immunologically mediated inflammatory response within the CNS. Although immunological abnormalities have been consistently reported, the relative role of each component of the immune response in mediating tissue damage, and the extent to which these changes are the cause or consequence of myelin injury, remain to be established (Compston 1993a). There is compelling evidence for genetic susceptibility to MS while the evidence for environmental initiators or triggers is less convincing (Compston 1990).

Epidemiological studies indicate that MS is a common disorder in young adults in Northern Europe, North America and Australasia but is less prevalent in the Orient, Africa, South America and India (Kurtzke 1975; Compston 1990). It affects white races principally, although it has been known to affect black immigrants living in Europe and North America. In Australia and New Zealand, MS is rarely seen in the Aboriginal or Maori races but occurs in the white population. In South Africa, the disease occurs more commonly in English speaking whites than in Afrikaaners but is not seen in native Africans.

Further evidence for genetic susceptibility is provided by epidemiological studies within and between ethnic groups. The results of a survey of individuals with MS in Israel in 1973 showed that the disease was common among immigrants from Europe, and rare among immigrants from Afro-Asian countries (Leibowitz *et al.* 1973). Approximately 15% of individuals with MS have an affected relative. This risk rises to 1:50 for offspring and 1:20 for siblings of affected persons (Sadovnick *et al.* 1988). The risk of the disease in northern Europeans is said to be approximately 1:800.

There is decreasing incidence of the disease in individuals of northern European ancestry as one approaches the tropics, suggesting that certain environments may be relatively more protective. For example, in Australians of northern European descent and in English-speaking white South Africans, the frequency of MS is only about half that of northern Europe. Age is also a factor in immigrant populations. Dean (1967) showed that the risk of MS is higher for English-speaking South African whites who migrated as adults rather than as children. Dean (1972) suggested that in countries where the disease is relatively rare, early contact with the causative agent, probably a virus, protects the population by making them immune. On the other hand, there is some evidence that exposure to viral illnesses such as measles, mumps, rubella rather late in childhood may be a factor in those who are at risk of developing the disease.

It would appear, therefore, that MS does not have a single cause. New episodes of demyelination are more likely to occur following a viral infection but no single agent has been implicated, suggesting that in the context of genetic susceptibility and immunological priming, demyelination is a physiological response to many pathogens (Compston 1993a). In summary, the epidemiological evidence implicates environmental factors operating against a background of genetic susceptibility or resistance during childhood manifesting as altered immune responsiveness (Compston 1993a).

Pathophysiology

Demyelination is a disintegration of the myelin sheath caused by an inflammatory and destructive process, the axon being partly or completely denuded. Destruction of the myelin sheath disrupts the normal tranmission of nerve impulses resulting in the neurological signs and symptoms. The axons themselves are preserved initially although some loss of axons may occur, particularly in large chronic plaques.

The hallmark features of MS lesions are perivascular inflammation followed by myelin depletion, oligodendrocyte loss and astroglial proliferation, and these processes are accompanied by limited remyelination. There are four stages of evolution of focal inflammation (Compston 1993b). The initial stage is characterized by the accumulation of inflammatory cells, lymphocytes and monocytes around venules within the CNS. Inflammation is sufficient to cause a functional block in conduction through myelinated axons. Next, there is active destruction of the oligodendrocyte and its myelin sheath as a result of contact with macrophages and microglia. This is followed by depletion of oligodendrocytes in which denuded axons are seen within the lesion. Finally, the lesion heals by scar formation dependent upon astrocytic reactivity, producing hardened patches or plaques from which the disease gets its name.

The most common sites of plaques are in the grey–white boundary in the cerebrum, the periventricular regions, cerebellar white matter, optic nerves and cervical portion of the spinal cord and brain stem, but the disease can involve any part of the CNS. Slowed velocities characterize nerve conduction rates in demyelinated areas (Reder and Antel 1983). Partially demyelinated axons cannot transmit fast trains of impulses and this may explain the fatigue complained of by many patients. These partially demyelinated axons may also discharge spontaneously, accounting for unpleasant distortions of sensation reported by a high percentage of patients (Compston 1993a). Increased temperature sensitivity experienced by many patients after exercise or immersion in hot water may also be explained by the partially demyelinated axons (Compston 1993a).

These pathophysiological explanations for the symptoms of MS, however, do not explain many puzzling aspects of the symptomatology of the disease. Magnetic resonance imaging may show more extensive involvement of the nervous system than may be suggested by clinical examination, and physiological principles can neither explain the rate of onset of new symptoms nor offer an explanation for the recovery of symptoms (Compston 1993a). The question of the possibility of functional remyelination in the CNS and the contribution this may make to recovery of function still remains unanswered although there is some evidence that a limited degree of remyelination occurs naturally even in an acute lesion (Heard 1993). The contribution of this limited remyelination to recovery of function, and of adaptive neural processes in general, is, as yet, unknown.

The disease process

Although clinical signs are variable, several patterns can be identified: benign; a relapsing-remitting (RR) course; a relapsing-progressive form; and a chronic-progressive form. Clinical onset in 80% of patients is manifested by episodic neurological symptoms, either multifocal or anatomically discrete, which initially recover fully. A focal lesion may cause a blurring of vision, or a feeling of numbness and tingling in a limb. Typically, further episodes occur at a random frequency and for an unpredictable period involving the same or different CNS regions. Both rate and severity of disease progression may differ considerably among patients, with as many as 20–30% continuing to work 20–25 years after disease onset and with only minimal cognitive impairments (Filley *et al.* 1990). The longer the delay in new symptoms after disease onset the more likely the course will be benign.

With frequent relapses, however, a chronic-progressive form of the disease may evolve. In 10% of patients the disease is progressive from onset and almost always affects the spinal cord. Involvement of optic nerves, cerebrum and brain stem may also be present. The course tends to have a later age of onset and the disease evolves without either exacerbation or remissions with new symptoms appearing on average twice as frequently as that of the RR form (Sibley 1990). Cognitive functions are more likely to be affected and more severely in chronic-progressive MS than in the RR form of the disease.

In population studies, at the one time approximately one-third of individuals are in a quiescent phase of the disease and not significantly disabled, a further third are slowly deteriorating, and the remainder are stable but disabled having had the disease for many years (Swingler and Compston 1992). MS tends to impact on the quality of life rather than on its duration, life expectancy only decreasing slightly in individuals with MS. However, in very disabled individuals, the probability of death is more than four-fold that of the general population.

Clinical symptomatology

The pattern of symptoms is complex, variable and unpredictable.

Cognitive and affective symptoms

There has been considerable development in the understanding of cognitive impairments over recent years. Attentional deficits, both visual and auditory, appear to be major contributors to impaired cognitive ability, including memory disorders. These deficits are more severe and prevalent in patients with the progressive form of the disease than in the relapsing disease. Surveys of patients with advanced MS have documented a high incidence of global intellectual deterioration (Beatty *et al.* 1989). Cognitive deficits are said to occur usually without psychiatric symptoms.

Lezak's clinical observations (1995) suggest that slowed mental processing makes it difficult for individuals with attention deficits to grasp all aspects of a verbal message, particularly when long, complicated and delivered rapidly in a complex environment. When patients have no recollection of what has been said or what is happening around them, they and their families interpret this as a problem of memory rather than slowed processing of information. Once patients, families and health professionals understand the nature of the problem, careful attention to how, when and where information and messages are given and activities organized may greatly improve the patient's 'memory'.

Personality and psychosocial behaviour

Changes in personality, preferences and attitudes tend to accompany impairments in focusing attention and distractability (Lezak 1995). Individuals with MS describe feelings of being mentally blocked, of dissatisfaction with themselves and of diminished spontaneity of action (Lezak 1995).

Depression is said to be more commonly observed in patients with MS than in those with comparable medical disorders (Minden and

Schiffer 1990). Although this is not surprising, given depression is an appropriate reaction to what can be a devastating disease, the appearance of depression does not seem to be related to the severity of the disease. It is not clear whether depression arises as a manifestation of the disease or from physical and social disability.

Individuals with MS have also been described as being prone to 'euphoria'. The term euphoria, however, is inappropriate when applied to individuals with MS who attempt to face the future with courage (Compston 1993a). True euphoria is a relatively rare phenomenon, typically associated with advanced disease involving frontal lobes. Emotional lability may however be associated with frontal lobe dysfunction.

Stress may exacerbate symptoms and precipitate onset. *Emotional distress* increases with flare-ups of symptoms and in patients experiencing increasing severity of symptoms.

Special senses

The involvement of the visual pathways is very common. The episodic visual blurring so often described by patients early in the disease may later deteriorate further, with some patients losing sight in one eye or suffering double vision. Deafness is more often seen in individuals with established disease. Acute vestibular symptoms with severe positional vertigo (an illusion of movement in the person's relationship with the environment), vomiting, ataxia and headache are typically seen in acute brain stem demyelination. Other senses such as taste and smell may be involved.

Sensorimotor impairments

Weakness may develop gradually in one or more limbs, increasing with use and often described as a feeling of heaviness and clumsiness. Depending on the site of the lesion, signs of an upper motor neuron lesion (Chapter 8) may be present while involvement of the cerebellum and its connections produces ataxic symptoms (Chapter 9), which usually occur in combination with corticospinal damage. Spinal demyelination causes progressive weakness in both legs. In individuals where there is extensive demyelination adjacent to the dorsal root entry zones, lower motor neuron signs may be present.

Spasticity is typically listed as a common impairment in MS. The influence of spasticity in MS is, however, hard to assess. The term is seldom defined and no distinction may be made between resistance to passive movement due to reflex hyperactivity, and increased mechanical stiffness. Added to this, the Ashworth Scale (1964) is typically used to measure spasticity although this scale measures muscle length and stiffness. As discussed in Chapter 8, increased resistance to passive movement can be caused by an increase in passive stiffness of soft tissue or joints, an increase in stiffness mediated by the stretch reflex, or an increase in intrinsic stiffness which reflects the stiffness of the contractile properties of the engaged cross-bridges.

Sinkjaer and colleagues (1993) measured the passive, the intrinsic and the reflex-mediated response to stretch in the ankle extensors and flexors in MS subjects and able-bodied subjects. The major findings suggest that spastic muscles in individuals with MS have an increased non-reflexive stiffness (passive and intrinsic) and that reflex-mediated stiffness in the ankle extensors during a sustained voluntary contraction does not differ significantly from able-bodied subjects.

Altered *sensation* occurs at some stage in almost every individual with MS. Sensory symptoms, such as paraesthesia of a limb or of the face, with numbness, tingling or burning, may be the first clinical signs. Involvement of the posterior columns of the spinal cord results in impairments in position and movement sense, vibration sense and touch. Pain and temperature sense may also be affected. Due to the unpredictable nature of the disease, sensory deficits may affect one limb, one side of the body or all four limbs.

Fatigue

Fatigue, a poorly understood manifestation of MS, is experienced by most patients and may be more disabling than any of the milder symptoms, compromising the person's efficiency and sense of well-being (Lezak 1995). Individuals with MS report that fatigue generally occurs daily, interferes with physical and social function, and worsens with heat. Individuals with MS, their families and friends can misjudge the impact of fatigue by misinterpreting it as laziness. Individuals who are working complain that they have no energy for recreational activities because of needing to rest at the weekend. Furthermore, fatigue is one of the two major reasons for unemployment among MS individuals (Edgley *et al.* 1991). Many patients are unable to be actively engaged for more than a few hours without fatigue and tend to limit activity to avoid fatigue and overheating. A vicious cycle occurs, with decreased physical and social activity tending to have a further deleterious effect.

Schapiro and colleagues (1987) have described four types of fatigue: fatigue following *physical exertion*, experienced by the general population and which recovers after a period of rest; *nerve impulse* fatigue following extreme activity which, again, recovers with rest; fatigue related to *depression*, and associated with sleep disturbances, low self-esteem and mood fluctuations; and *lassitude*, or an abnormal sense of tiredness of unknown aetiology. All four types described may contribute to fatigue in MS. However, the sense of tiredness or lassitude is little understood and people with MS appear to be particularly vulnerable to this. However, an additional cause of fatigue is the underlying slowing of nerve impulses along partially demyelinated axons.

A nine-item Fatigue Severity Scale (Krupp *et al.* 1989) has demonstrated sensitivity to fatigue in MS patients. This scale has been shown to have acceptable internal consistency, stability over time and reflects the effect of fatigue on daily functioning. Interestingly, Krupp and colleagues found that the severity of fatigue did not correlate significantly with depression in individuals with MS, suggesting that fatigue and depression are separate, although overlapping, entities.

Heat in the form of hot weather, overheated rooms and immersion in hot water, increases fatigue as well as other symptoms of MS, tending to weaken the individual (Lezak 1995). Increased temperature sensitivity, with a reduction in the safety factor for conduction in partially demyelinated axons, may explain the temporary increase in the severity of symptoms experienced by patients after exercise or hot baths (Honan *et al.* 1987). On the other hand, cold may help to improve performance.

Autonomic involvement

Autonomic involvement occurs in most patients with MS. Bladder symptoms are more common in women than men. Impotence may be prevalent in males. Sphincter control may be lost or impaired. Disinhibition causes urgency and frequency which leads to incontinence. Bowel incontinence may also be present.

Other manifestations of brain stem involvement

Compston (1993a) reports several manifestations of brain stem demyelination. Abnormalities of eye movement are common in MS. Facial palsy is reported to be present in individuals with established MS. Extensive brain stem demyelination may produce disturbances of consciousness or central respiratory failure. Paroxysmal episodes (tonic spasms), in which painful tetanic posturing of the limbs occurs for up to 1 or 2 minutes, may also be present.

Medical management

There is at present no accurate laboratory-supported diagnostic test for MS. Investigations such as magnetic resonance imaging (MRI), transcranial magnetic stimulation and cerebrospinal fluid analysis in individuals with MS are used to document the site and extent of lesions, to confirm the presence of intrathecal inflammation and to exclude conditions that may mimic demyelinating disease. MRI is thought to have increased the accuracy in diagnosing MS from 60% to 90% (Ebers 1994) and appears to be a more sensitive indicator of disease activity than the clinical history or neurological examination (Polman and Hartung 1995).

A large body of experimental evidence implicating immune-mediated processes in activation and progression of MS has led to a search for immunotherapies that not only abrogate acute relapses, but also modify the progression of the disease. Clinical trials using immuno-suppressant drugs are still progressing (Polman and Hartung 1995). A promising new approach is the use of interferon beta to suppress exacerbations (Panitch *et al.* 1993).

Drugs such as baclofen and diazepam may be useful in the reduction of hyperactive reflexes. When given to individuals experiencing severe flexor and adductor spasms associated with spinal cord lesions, these agents may reduce hyperactivity sufficiently to enable the individual to sit and stand more comfortably or to be nursed more easily. Orally administered drugs such as these, however, can cause severe side-effects. More recent studies using botulinum toxin to relieve adductor spasms (e.g., Snow *et al.* 1990) have reported easier nursing care and no significant side-effects.

While aetiology remains unclear and because of the possibility of spontaneous remission, treatment and evaluation of effectiveness is difficult and must rely on empirical evidence. The use of steroids has been widely practised, but there is still no evidence to indicate that they influence the eventual outcome of the disease, although they may accelerate the onset of a remission when given during an acute relapse. High-dose intravenous methylprednisolone is now thought to be more effective and less complicated than steroids given orally or by intramuscular injection (Milligan *et al.* 1987).

Documenting the course, assessing the prognosis, and validating the effects of intervention in MS requires standardized measures of disability. The most extensively used scale appears to be the Expanded Disability Status Scale (Kurtzke 1983). However, this scale is widely criticized on theoretical grounds, on its insensitivity to change, its emphasis on ambulation with neglect of other relevant functions, and on its lack of objectivity and reliability (Goodkin *et al.* 1988; Willoughby and Paty 1988; Polman and Hartung 1995). Wade (1992) suggests that one should only consider using the Kurtzke scale in order to be able to compare results with other studies. He further suggests that it is preferable otherwise to measure change in specific impairments and disabilities using measures which are valid and reliable.

Physiotherapy: an overall view

Many of the challenges associated with progressive neurological disease are well exemplified in MS. Progressive disease presents a series of difficulties and burdens that impact on the quality of life of the individual, their families and health professionals. Coping with functional limitations, explicit uncertainty about the future and possibility of loss of function and family role has a negative impact on quality of life, social interaction, vocational and leisure activities and is extemely stressful.

Almost any manifestation of neurological impairment can be observed in individuals with MS and the reader is referred to Chapters 8–10 for details of specific impairments. The nature of the impairments which arise from one individual to another, but also in the same individual at different times, are wide-ranging, variable and unpredictable. Physiotherapists, as part of a team working with individuals with MS, need to be sensitive to the individual's wishes in working out strategies to enable that individual to preserve dignity and lifestyle. The physiotherapist needs to have sufficient knowledge and expertise to address wide-ranging problems, and the flexibility to cope with the unpredictable nature of the disease. If physiotherapy is to be effective, it needs to be focused and expert, and demonstrate clearly to the patient the benefits of interventions.

The overall aims of physiotherapy as part of a multidisciplinary team are to:

- Optimize performance in everyday activities and skills.
- Maximize functional ability.
- Prevent unnecessary disability and handicap.
- Improve the individual's quality of life.

The reader should refer to Chapters 2, 4–7 for task-related training.

More specific aims for an individual may be to:

- Preserve musculoskeletal integrity.
- Preserve aerobic capacity.
- Manage fatigue.
- Collaborate with the individual to ensure that interventions are relevant to the person's needs and desires.
- Collaborate with the individual in setting goals and defining expectations.
- Provide necessary aids to living.

Preserving musculoskeletal integrity

The need to prevent secondary adaptation to disuse is critical for the maintenance of performance of everyday actions as well as for continued participation in social and vocational activities. Individuals need advice and instruction about what muscles and soft tissues are at risk of shortening and becoming stiffer, what stretches to do and how often. In the very disabled person, this may require equipment.

It is interesting to note that subjects participating in a baclofen drug trial reported that muscle stretching provided them with a subjective sense of control over stiffness (Brar *et al.* 1991), although the stretches were performed for only a short period which would not be considered to be of sufficient duration to prevent contracture in inactive individuals (Williams 1990). People who are wheelchair-bound should spend at least 30 minutes a day stretching hip and knee flexors and ankle plantarflexors. A tilt-table is probably essential for some individuals in order to prevent severe contractures.

The role of muscle strengthening to prevent unnecessary disability and improve functional motor performance in MS is unclear. It is interesting to note at the conclusion of a study designed to increase aerobic fitness (e.g., Petajan *et al.* 1996) that there were also increases in muscle strength, indicating that individuals with a demyelinating disease can improve muscle performance. The effects of more *specific* muscle training for these individuals requires further investigation. There is some evidence that cooling methods (e.g., ingestion of ice slurry or wearing of wet clothing) result in a trend toward improvement in work capacity in individuals with MS (Woyciechowska *et al.* 1995) and some patients may benefit from some form of cooling prior to and during exercise.

Aerobic exercise

The benefits of regular exercise in the able-bodied and disabled population are well documented and include: increased wellbeing and improved mental state; increased cardiorespiratory fitness; reduction in depression and anxiety; decreased excess body fat. A particularly interesting paper on this topic published recently (Petajan *et al.* 1996) demonstrated a positive impact on cardiovascular responses and facets of wellbeing in individuals with MS. Subjects were randomly assigned to either an exercise group or non-exercise group. The exercise group participated in three supervised training sessions per week for 15 weeks. Subjects adhered to the training programme, which involved use of a combined arm and leg ergometer. Subjects wore light clothing, exercised in a well-ventilated room, were encouraged to socialize with one another and to drink adequate liquid.

The results indicated significant improvement in cardiovascular fitness, with increases in VO_2max comparable with those reported in studies involving healthy sedentary subjects. The improvement did not seem to be related to the degree of neurological impairment. Although training did not involve *specific* strengthening exercises, increases in strength of most upper limb muscles and knee extensors were reported, indicating that muscle strength can be increased in a demyelinating disease.

The exercise group also experienced improvement on factors related to the quality of life: on physical function assessed on the Sickness Impact Profile (Gilson *et al.* 1979); depression, anger and fatigue on the Profile of Mood States (McNair *et al.* 1992); and improvement on the bladder and bowel score on the Expanded Disability Status Scale (Kurtzke 1983). They did not improve on the Fatigue Severity Scale (FSS) (Krupp *et al.* 1989). Petajan and colleagues suggest that this may be because subjects interpreted the FSS item 'fatigue interferes with my physical functioning' in a way which was insensitive to change. Non-exercise subjects retained their pre-trial sedentary habits and scores.

We agree with Petajan and colleagues that individuals with MS should both be encouraged and assisted to engage in regular aerobic exercise. The arm and leg ergometer used in their study has the advantage of enabling the individual to compensate for deficits due to weakness in the upper and lower extremities. For more disabled individuals, an arm ergometer may be more appropriate, however, Canning (1992) describes the use of a leg ergometer placed in front of a patient with Friedreich's ataxia who was unable to balance on the bicycle ergometer but was able to pedal it while sitting in her wheelchair.

Managing fatigue

Management of fatigue involves discussion with the individual and gathering of information about the nature, extent and precipitating factors in fatigue. Strategies to implement may include relaxation breaks, simplification of, for example, work, dressing or food preparation, and time management. It is interesting to note that subjects reported less difficulty performing leisure activities of their choice and increased energy levels while participating in an aerobic training programme (Petajan *et al.* 1996).

Coping with disability and handicap

Reduction of handicap in MS is to some extent dependent on national health policy, structures for rehabilitation and disability services. Health professionals have an important role in being familiar with and referring patients to the appropriate agency which may include: a multiple sclerosis society; an independent living centre; technical aids to the disabled; accessible leisure centres; respite care provision; sporting groups for the disabled; self-help groups; carer support groups; vocational rehabilitation services. These agencies can be valuable sources of information.

Health professionals also need to keep up-to-date with technological advances designed to increase environmental interaction to improve the quality of life for individuals with MS and their families. Some recent publications are helpful, for example, The Multiple Sclerosis Society of Australia has published a booklet (1990) for the newly diagnosed person.

The stress on families assisting an individual with MS can be high. A survey in the United Kingdom, for example, found that 15% of carers were depressed and 24% suffered from clinical anxiety (University of Southampton 1989). Information regarding availability of services, practical help at home and access to respite facilities appear to be some of the more important factors to address in order to relieve family stress. A hoist (Fig. 14.1) enables the person to be moved, thus diminishing some of the physical stress on family members.

A wheelchair is necessary for individuals who may be coping with walking about the house but who otherwise are confined to the house. Wheelchair training should be instituted to train the individual to negotiate a more complex environment than the home. An electric wheelchair and/or a three wheel scooter will give more freedom to a person who is unable to walk effectively and efficiently or is having difficulty operating a hand-driven chair. In some instances the energy required to walk may be better put to more beneficial activities, and the use of a wheelchair or scooter may be critical to remaining employed and maintaining social contact outside the house.

Measurement

Specific measures used need to be reliable and valid and be clinically relevant to the intervention (Chapter 3).

Coping with chronic illness and uncertainty can be very stressful. Schwartz and colleagues (1996) have developed and tested a *self-efficacy scale* specifically for MS. Self-efficacy is a term used to describe the degree of confidence an individual has in his/her ability to cope with a specific situation or condition. The test was found to have high internal consistency and test-retest reliability. This scale should be valuable in measuring the outcome of intervention in terms of enhancing the patient's wellbeing and confidence. High self-efficacy in

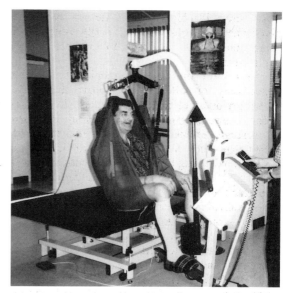

Fig. 14.1 A hoist decreases the physical burden for carers and ensures greater comfort for the individual when being moved from one place to another

individuals with MS has previously been found to be associated with better adjustment and less psychological dysfunction (e.g., Schnek *et al.* 1995).

The use of *integrated care pathways* (ICPs) appears to be useful in identifying key factors influencing outcome of intervention. An ICP is a document that details the interventions expected to occur during a specific period of clinical intervention (Rossiter and Thompson 1995). Several recent audits have shown that the introduction of ICPs in an inpatient setting resulted in decreased length of stay, a framework for identifying not just how many goals were achieved but also for identifying why goals were not met, and improved record keeping (Rossiter and Thompson 1996).

In summary, as Compston (1990) has pointed out a clearer understanding of the epidemiological and biological factors that determine the geographical and anatomical dissemination of multiple sclerosis may provide a solution to this disease. The most exciting development in neurological rehabilitation for persons with multiple sclerosis is the impact of aerobic training, with adequate temperature control, on fitness, together with factors related to quality of life. Therapists are encouraged to become familiar with the literature on aerobic training in patients with MS in order to prescribe effective exercise programmes. Other critical interventions include prevention of unnecessary disability and advice on reducing unnecessary fatigue in everyday, social and vocational activities.

References

Ashworth, B. (1964) Preliminary trial of carisoprodol in multiple sclerosis. *Practitioner*, **192**, 540–542.

Beatty, W.B., Goodkin, D.E. and Monson, N. (1989) Cognitive disturbances in patients with relapsing remitting multiple sclerosis. *Archives of Neurology*, **46**, 1113–1119.

Brar, A.P., Smith, M.B., Nelson, L.M. *et al.* (1991) Evaluation of treatment protocols on minimal to moderate spasticity in multiple sclerosis. *Archives of Physical Medicine and Rehabilitation*, **72**, 186–189.

Canning, C. (1992) Friedreich's ataxia – improve your fitness. *Friedreich's Ataxia Association Quarterly Newsletter*, July, pp. 4–6.

Compston, D.A.S. (1990) The dissemination of multiple sclerosis. The Langdon-Brown Lecture 1989. *Journal of the Royal College of Physicians of London*, **24**, 207–218.

Compston, A. (1993a) Multiple Sclerosis. In *Brain's Diseases of the Nervous System* (ed. J. Walton), Oxford University Press, Oxford, pp. 366–382.

Compston, A. (1993b) Limiting and repairing the damage in multiple sclerosis. *Schweizerische Medizinische Wochenschrift*, **123**, 1145–1152.

Dean, G. (1967) Anual incidence, prevalence and mortality of multiple sclerosis in white south African born and in white immigrants to South Africa. *British Medical Journal*, **2,** 724.

Dean, G. (1972) On the risk of multiple sclerosis according to age at immigration. In *Multiple Sclerosis Progress in Research* (eds E.J. Field, T.M. Bell and P.R. Carnegie), North-Holland, Amsterdam and London, pp.197–207.

Ebers, G.C. (1994) Treatment of multiple sclerosis. *Lancet*, **343**, 275–279.

Edgley, K., Sullivan, M. and Dehoux, E. (1991) A survey of multiple sclerosis: 11. Determinants of employment status. *Canadian Journal of Rehabilitation*, **4**, 127–132.

Filley, C.M., Heaton, R.K., Thompson, L.L. *et al.* (1990) Effects of disease course on neuropsychological functioning. In *Neurobehavioural Aspects of Multiple Sclerosis* (ed. S.M. Rao) Oxford University Press, New York, pp. 136–148.

Gilson, B.S., Bergner, M., Bobbit, R.A. *et al.* (1979) *The Sickness Impact Profile: Final Development and Testing, 1975–1978*, Department of Health Services, School of Public Health and Community Medicine, University of Washington, Seattle.

Goodkin, D.E., Hertsgaard, D. and Seminary, J. (1988) Upper extremity function in multiple sclerosis: improving assessment sensitivity with box-and-block and nine-hole peg tests. *Archives of Physical Medicine and Rehabilitaiton*, **69**, 850–854.

Heard, R.N.S. (1993) New horizons in the treatment of multiple sclerosis. *Medical Journal of Australia*, **158**, 714–716.

Honan, W. P., Heron, J. R., Foster, D.H. *et al.* (1987) Paradoxical effects of temperature in multiple sclerosis. *Journal of Neurology, Neurosurgery, and Psychiatry*, **50**, 1160–1164.

Krupp, L.B., LaRocca, N.G., Muir-Nash, J. *et al.* (1989) The fatigue severity scale. Application to patients with multiple sclerosis and systemic lupus erythematosus. *Archives of Neurology*, **46**, 1121–1123.

Kurtzke, J.F. (1975) A re-assessment of the distribution of multiple sclerosis, parts 1 and 2. *Acta Neurologica Scandinavia*, **51**, 110–136.

Kurtzke, J.F. (1983) Rating neurologic impairment in multiple sclerosis: an expanded disability status scale (EDSS). *Neurology*, **33**, 1444–1452.

Lezak, M.D. (1995) *Neuropsychological Assessment*, 3rd edn, Oxford University Press, New York, pp. 241–248.

Liebowitz, S., Kahana, E. and Alter, M. (1973) The changing frequency of multiple sclerosis in Israel. *Archives of Neurology*, **29**, 107.

McNair, D.M., Lorr, M. and Droppleman, L.F. (1992) *Profile of Mood States (POMS)*. Educational and Industrial Testing Service, San Diego, CA.

Milligan, N.M., Newcombe, R. and Compston, D.A.S. (1987) A double blind controlled trial of high dose methylprednisolone in patients with multiple sclerosis. 1. Clinical effects. *Journal of Neurology, Neurosurgery and Psychiatry*, **50**, 511–516.

Minden, S.L. and Schiffer, R.B. (1990) Affective disorders in multiple sclerosis. *Archives of Neurology*, **47**, 98–104.

Multiple Sclerosis Society of Australia (1990) *Living with Multiple Sclerosis – a Book for the Newly Diagnosed*. Sydney, Australia.

Panitch, H.S. and Bever, C.T. (1993) Clinical trials of interferons in multiple sclerosis. *Journal of Neuroimmunology*, **46**, 155–164.

Petajan, J.H., Gappmaier, E., White, A.T. *et al.* (1996) Impact of aerobic training on fitness and quality of life in multiple sclerosis. *Annals of Neurology*, **39** (4), 432–441.

Polman, C.H. and Hartung, H. (1995) The treatment of multiple sclerosis: current and future. *Current Opinion in Neurology*, **8**, 200–209.

Reder, A.T. and Antel, J.P. (1983) Clinical spectrum of multiple sclerosis. In *Neurologic Clinics: Symposium on Multiple Sclerosis* (ed. J.P. Antel), W.B. Saunders, Philadelphia.

Rossiter, D. and Thompson, A.J. (1995) Introduction of integrated care pathways for patients with multiple sclerosis in an inpatient neurorehabilitation setting. *Disability and Rehabilitation*, 17, 443–448.

Rossiter, D. and Thompson, A.J. (1996) Integrated care pathways (ICPs) in multiple sclerosis management: a three series audit review. *European Journal of Neurology*, **3**, 49.

Sadovnick, A.D., Baird, P.A. and Ward, R.H. (1988) Multiple sclerosis: updated risks for relatives. *American Journal of Medical Genetics*, **29**, 533–541.

Schapiro, R.T., Harris, L., Lenling, M. *et al.* (1987) Fatigue. In *Symptom Management in Multiple Sclerosis* (ed. R.T. Schapiro), Demos Publications, New York, pp. 23–28.

Schnek, Z.M., Foley, F.W., LaRocca, N.G. *et al.* (1995) Psychological predictors of depression in multiple sclerosis. *Journal of Neurological Rehabilitation*, **9**, 15–23.

Schwartz, C.E., Coulthard-Morris, L. and Zeng, Q. (1996) Psychosocial correlates of fatigue in multiple sclerosis. *Archives of Physical Medicine and Rehabilitation*, **77**, 165–170.

Sibley, W.A. (1990) The diagnosis and course of multiple sclerosis. In *Neurobehavioural Aspects of Multiple Sclerosis* (ed. S.M. Rao), Oxford University Press, New York, pp. 5–14.

Sinkjaer, T., Toft, E., Larsen, K. *et al.* (1993) Non-reflex and reflex mediated ankle joint stiffness in multiple sclerosis patients with spasticity. *Muscle and Nerve*, **16**, 69–756.

Snow, B.J., Tsui, J.K.C., Bhatt, M.H. *et al.* (1990) Treatment of spasticity with botulinum toxin: a double blind study. *Annals of Neurology*, **28**, 512–515.

Swingler, R.J. and Compston, D.A.S. (1992) The morbidity of multiple sclerosis in south east Wales. *Quarterly Journal of Medicine*, **83**, 325–337.

University of Southampton (1989) *Multiple Sclerosis in the Southampton District*. Rehabilitation Unit and Department of Sociology and Social Policy, University of Southampton.

Wade, D.T. (1992) *Measurement in Neurological Rehabilitation*, Oxford University Press, New York.

Williams, P.E. (1990) Use of intermittent stretch in the prevention of serial sarcomere loss in immobilised muscles. *Annals of the Rheumatic Diseases*, **47**, 316–317.

Willoughby, E.W. and Paty, D.W. (1988) Scales for rating impairment in multiple sclerosis: a critique. *Neurology*, **38**, 1793–1798.

Woyciechowska, J., Israel, D.J., Hoffman, R.G. *et al.* (1995) Application of cooling techniques during exercise in MS patients. *MS Management*, **2**, 25–29.

Further reading

Fuhrer, M.J. (1994) Subjective well-being: implications for medical rehabilitation outcomes and models of disablement. *American Journal of Physical Medicine and Rehabilitation*, **73**, 358–364.

Kidd, D., Howard, R.S., Losseff, N.A. and Thompson, A.J. (1995) The benefit of inpatient neurorehabilitation in multiple sclerosis. *Clinical Rehabilitation*, **9**, 198–203.

Kosich, D., Molk, B., Feeney, J. *et al.* (1987) Cardiovascular testing and exercise prescription in multiple sclerosis. *Journal of Neurological Rehabilitation*, **4**, 167–170.

Rose, F.D., Attree, E.A. and Johnson, D.A. (1996) Virtual reality: an assistive technology in neurological rehabilitation. *Current Opinion in Neurology*, **9**, 461–467.

Schapiro, R.T., Petajan, J.H., Kosich, D. *et al.* (1988) Role of cardiovascular fitness in multiple sclerosis: a pilot study. *Journal of Neurological Rehabilitation*, **2**, 43–49.

Index